Total patient care

FOUNDATIONS AND PRACTICE

Total patient care

FOUNDATIONS AND PRACTICE

DOROTHY F. JOHNSTON, R.N., B.S., M.Ed.

Formerly Director, Athens School of Practical Nursing, Athens, Ga.;
Director, Department of Nursing, Georgia Southwestern College,
Americus, Ga.; Assistant Professor of Nursing, Duke University,
Durham, N. C.; Educational Director, Grady Memorial Hospital School
of Nursing, Atlanta, Ga.; Assistant Professor of Nursing, University of
Georgia, Athens, Ga.; Assistant Nurse Officer (R), United States
Public Health Service

GAIL H. HOOD, R.N., B.S., M.S.

Instructor, Medical-Surgical Nursing, Northern Illinois
University, DeKalb, Ill.; formerly Administrative Assistant in
Curriculum and Research, The Reading Hospital School of
Nursing, Reading, Pa.

with 311 illustrations

FOURTH EDITION

The C. V. Mosby Company

Saint Louis   1976

FOURTH EDITION

Copyright © 1976 by The C. V. Mosby Company

All rights reserved. No part of this book may be reproduced
in any manner without written permission of the publisher.

Previous editions copyrighted 1964, 1968, 1972
Printed in the United States of America
Distributed in Great Britain by Henry Kimpton, London

Library of Congress Cataloging in Publication Data

Johnston, Dorothy F
    Total patient care: foundations and practice.

    Includes bibliographies and index.
    1. Nurses and nursing.   I.   Hood, Gail H., joint
author.   II.   Title.   [DNLM: 1.   Nursing, Practical.
WY195 J72t]
RT41.J6   1976   610.73   75-15563
ISBN 0-8016-2573-4

CB/CB/B   9   8   7   6   5   4   3   2

Preface

The delivery of health care is shared by many persons with different kinds of preparation. Each individual is recognized for his unique contribution to health care. The quality of care depends heavily on the quality of preparation and on continuing education through inservice programs, refresher courses, and independent study. *Total Patient Care* is a textbook of medical-surgical nursing designed for students in one-year programs of nursing education. It may also serve as a reference for those students who have graduated. Nurses are now helping to provide care in every clinical unit of the hospital. They serve the needs of persons employed in industry, as public health nursing assistants, in health care centers, and in institutions caring for the aged, disabled, and emotionally disturbed.

Total Patient Care has been thoroughly revised to provide greater depth and understanding of illness and nursing care. The latest available knowledge has been incorporated, and the sociologic and psychologic factors have been expanded.

The format for the fourth edition of *Total Patient Care* is the same as that for previous editions; however, it reflects considerable new material. The textbook now contains twenty-four chapters rather than twenty-three as in the previous editions. A new chapter on death and dying has been written to help students develop a personal philosophy and to familiarize themselves with some of the present concepts about terminal illness and death.

Several chapters have been completely rewritten or extensively revised. Some of the major inclusions are elementary material on microbiology and pathology, intravenous solutions, hematogenic shock, cardiac arrhythmias, cardiac monitoring, mechanical ventilation, blood, blood fractions, electrolytes, drug dependency, and expanded material on hospital-acquired infections.

The lists of key words have been expanded, defined, and placed in the glossary. Answers to the review questions following each chapter have been transferred from the textbook to the teaching guide. Annotated films are correlated with each chapter; however, few new films are available on loan. When the rental charge is known, it has been listed with the film. A few illustrations have been eliminated and twenty-six new illustrations added.

Consideration should be given to Dr. Annette Lefkowitz, Department Head, and Dr. Ann Hart, Assistant Department Head, Northern Illinois University School of Nursing, for their invaluable assistance and encouragement. A particular acknowledgment goes to family members, friends, colleagues, and students for their fresh ideas and continued support. Special thanks belong to S. Roger Hood and Michael and Karen Merrill for their patience, understanding, and, above all, sense of humor.

Dorothy F. Johnston

Gail H. Hood

Contents

Part one

CHAPTER 1

Introduction to medical-surgical nursing

KEY WORDS

aerobic

Ascaris

coccidioidomycosis

congenital

dermatomycosis

disease

droplet nuclei

embryonic

frostbite

histoplasmosis

malformation

malaria

mental retardation

Metazoa

mycotic infection

Nematoda

phenylketonuria

pinworm

Platyhelminthes

Protozoa

rickettsiae

sunstroke

trichinosis

trichomoniasis

virology

viruses

DEVELOPMENT OF MEDICINE AND SURGERY

The background of modern medicine and surgery is rich in the achievements of men whose lives were dedicated to the search for truth and knowledge. Much of their early work was ridiculed, and some lost their lives in the pursuit of knowledge. However, without their contributions medicine could not have achieved its present status. Today medical science builds on its past heritage but looks to the future. The achievements of modern medicine and surgery are intricately linked to the insatiable desire of mankind to prevent and cure disease and to prolong a healthy life.

History shows that all kinds of operations were performed long before present civilization. The early history of India indicates that a concise classification of operations was in existence. As early as 400 B.C. Hippocrates, called the "father of medicine," was familiar with various surgical procedures for disorders of the skeletal system, and many kinds of prostheses were in use. However, aseptic surgery had its beginning about 1867 with the work of Joseph Lister, an English surgeon. Wound infection complicated most surgical operations, and puerperal infection was common in the obstetric wards. After observing the process of wound infection Lister concluded that it was caused by microbes. Based on his belief, he began using a solution of carbolic acid in the operating room, as well as saturating dressings over wounds. These measures resulted in a remarkable decrease in the incidence of wound infection. Although Lister was severely criticized by others and his work was not accepted for a number of years, he had laid the foundation for modern aseptic surgery.[2]

A further major achievement was the discovery of ether as an anesthetizing agent. In 1842 Crawford W. Long was the first to use ether when he performed surgery on a man's neck.

Dr. William Halsted, Professor of Surgery at Johns Hopkins School of Medicine, introduced the use of rubber gloves in the operating room during the 1880s.

Although hardly more than a hundred years old, modern surgery has made rapid advances. Surgical teams are performing some of the most complicated surgical procedures. Along with the surgical techniques, advances in anesthesia, equipment, and drugs have contributed to the progress of surgery. Today wound infection is rare, and mortality from surgery is minimal.

In the beginning, surgery progressed much more rapidly than did medicine. One of the earliest and most significant contributions occurred in the sixteenth century with the discovery of the circulation of blood by William Harvey, an English physician.

Although many physicians believed that disease was caused by microbes, the evidence was lacking until the seventeenth century when the Dutch scientist Anton van Leeuwenhoek invented a crude type of microscope with which he examined many different substances. In 1674 he observed what are now known as bacteria and protozoa, which he called *animalcules*. The microscope was gradually improved until the nineteenth century, when the modern microscope came into use.

With the discovery of bacteria and the invention of the microscope a new era of investigation into the causes of disease began. Louis Pasteur, a French chemist, conducted many studies that finally led to the discovery of the cause of rabies and a vaccine against the disease. From his work came the "Pasteur treatment" used to prevent rabies. In 1798 Edward Jenner, an English physician, discovered how to prevent smallpox by vaccination with the virus of cowpox. The work of these men was the forerunner of the modern program of immunization against infectious disease.[2]

The contributions of scientists to the prevention and cure of disease are many. In 1884 Charles Chamberlain devised the filter that led to the discovery of viruses, and in 1909-1910 Howard Ricketts discovered rickettsiae, which causes Rocky Mountain spotted fever and endemic typhus fever. In more recent years tribute has been paid to Alexander Fleming, who discovered penicillin. Other discoveries are those of insulin in 1922 and cortisone in 1935. New drugs and new forms of old drugs to treat and cure disease are constantly being discovered, but of equal or more importance is the technologic development without which many medical and surgical procedures could not be done—the heart-lung machine, respirators, artificial heart valves, pacemaker, hemodialysis machine, and intricate monitoring equipment, to mention only a few.

The scientific progress made in medicine has brought about many changes in nursing, as well as social changes, which in turn have had an impact on nursing. More patients are entering hospitals for complicated examinations and radical surgical procedures. The nurse, as always, is the right arm of the physician, but in a new role.

CAUSES OF DISEASE

Disease is any condition in which either the physiologic or psychologic functions of the body deviate from what is regarded as normal. Most diseases are characterized by specific symptoms related to a specific disease. Since in a state of health the body functions as a whole, with each part interdependent, the malfunctioning or abnormal condition of any part of the body may affect the entire body. Often more than one specific disease, each resulting from a different cause, may be present in the same person at the same time.

Many superstitions and fallacies exist concerning the cause, prevention, and cure of disease. Millions of dollars are spent annually on patent medicines for self-diagnosed and self-treated conditions. Often medical care is delayed until treatment is difficult and prolonged or until care is improbable. The nurse will often be asked questions concerning disease and some advertised remedy and should remember that reputable physicians do not advertise and that the physician is the only person qualified to diagnose and treat disease.

The causes of many diseases still remain unknown to medical science, but a partial grouping of the known causes of disease includes (1) microorganisms, (2) metazoa, (3) malnutrition, (4) physical agents, (5) chemical agents, and (6) congenital and hereditary disorders.

Microorganisms

Some of the most serious diseases are caused by pathogenic (disease-producing) forms of microorganisms called *bacteria*. Many of these bacterial infections are transmitted from person to person by direct contact, by inhaling droplet nuclei, and by articles contaminated with the pathogen (indirect contact); some are transmitted through the ingestion of contaminated food and drink. Microscopic bacteria have been divided into three major groups: (1) cocci, (2) bacilli, and (3) spirilla (Fig. 1-1). The nurse will more frequently encounter diseases caused by the cocci and the bacilli.

Streptococci, staphylococci, and diplococci. The streptococcus bacterium is responsible for more diseases than is any other organism. Some strains produce serious or even fatal diseases, others will produce disease only under special conditions, and other strains are nonpathogenic.

Disease-producing strains include betahemolytic streptococci and the viridans group, also called *alpha-hemolytic streptococci*.

The beta-hemolytic group of streptococci is responsible for about 90% of streptococcal infections.[2] Some of the diseases caused by this group are extremely serious and may be fatal. They include osteomyelitis, septicemia, scarlet fever, rheumatic fever, pneumonia, tonsillitis, and impetigo. The organisms may also invade surgical wounds or malignant lesions. Wound infection may occur as the result of improper handwashing prior to changing dressings. The organisms live in the upper respiratory tract and may be spread from one person to another by direct or indirect contract.

Viridans streptococci may cause subacute bacterial endocarditis, in which the valves of the heart may be affected. Viridans streptococci may also be found in the nose and throat of well persons (p. 63).

There are two species of staphylococcus bacteria: *Staphylococcus aureus* and *Staphylococcus epidermidis*. *Staphylococcus aureus* belongs to the pyogenic (pus-producing) group. Staphylococci may be found on the skin at all times and cause boils, abscesses, and carbuncles. Sometimes they get into the bloodstream and cause serious complications. A more intensive review of this organism and the nursing responsibilities related to it will be found in Chapter 4.

Staphylococcus epidermidis is a nonpathogenic species of the staphylococcus organism that inhabits the human skin. Al-

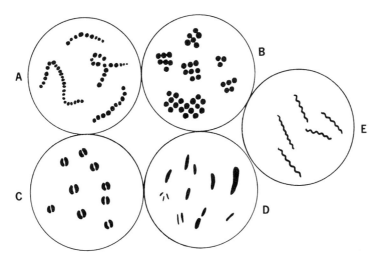

Fig. 1-1. Common disease-producing bacteria. **A,** Streptococci. **B,** Staphylococci. **C,** Diplococci. **D,** Bacilli. **E,** Spirilla.

though this species may cause minor infections, the incidence of such infections is low, and they are not serious.

There are several kinds of diplococcus bacteria. One type is the cause of pneumonia and is called the *pneumococcus*, of which thirty different types have been found to exist. One characteristic of the pneumococcus is that it is encased in a capsule, or gelatinous envelope. Two other forms of the diplococci cause gonorrhea (gonococcus) and meningitis (meningococcus).

Bacilli. The name *bacilli* means "little rod" (Fig. 1-1); however, its rodlike shape is extremely variable. Certain forms of the bacillus produce spores. These forms are present in the intestinal tract of humans and animals and are discharged onto the soil. These spore-forming bacilli produce tetanus (p. 550), gas gangrene (p. 550), and anthrax. Numerous other diseases are caused by these organisms, including tuberculosis, diphtheria, pertussis, typhoid fever, and bacillary dysentery.

Spirilla. Spirilla organisms are spiral shaped, or like a corkscrew. Some forms of spirilla are rigid, whereas others are flexible. One form, which resembles a comma, is the cause of Asiatic cholera. Most of the diseases caused by the spirilla bacteria are fairly uncommon. At one time the spirochetes that cause syphilis were considered in the same classification as spirilla. Now they have been separated and classed in a separate order of bacteria.

Viruses. Viruses are the smallest known agents that cause disease. Before 1900 scientists discovered that certain agents, unlike bacteria, would pass through a laboratory filter. In addition, they were unable to observe these tiny bodies with the ordinary microscope. In 1898 Martinus W. Beijerinck called these small bodies viruses, and they became known as filterable viruses.

For years scientists knew little about viruses, even though they were able to observe their effect on humans and animals. In 1941 the electron microscope became available, and a whole new era in the study of human disease was opened. With this advancement the science of virology was born. In addition to the electron microscope the use of certain dyes that become luminous when exposed to ultraviolet light (fluorescent microscopy), tissue culture methods, ultracentrifuge, cytochemistry, and the development of other technical laboratory aids have resulted in rapid advances in the science of virology (the study of viruses).[2]

The virus may gain entrance to the body through the respiratory tract, the gastrointestinal tract, or the broken skin resulting from an animal bite, or it may be injected by a mosquito or hypodermic needle. Viruses are selective in the type of body cells they attack, but once they have found cells showing affinity, they enter the cell and reproduce rapidly. As they multiply, they interrupt the cell activities and use the cell material to produce new virus material.

Virus infections are usually self-limiting. They run a given course, and recovery occurs. One exception is rabies, which is almost always fatal (p. 555). Other virus diseases may be fatal if complications occur or if they attack extremely weak, elderly, or debilitated persons. The common cold is caused by a virus, and the aching feeling, fever, and chilly sensations may be relieved by staying in bed and taking certain medicines. No medicine will cure the cold, only relieve the discomfort that it causes. A person who gets a cold often goes to a physician and asks for an antibiotic. In nearly all viral diseases antibiotics and sulfonamide agents do not alter the course of the disease.

Viruses are classified in various ways. They can be classified according to the human diseases they cause. A specific group of viruses may be divided into subgroups, and each subgroup may have many types or strains. Following is an example of such a division:

I. Picornavirus
  A. Enterovirus
    1. Poliovirus—poliomyelitis
    2. Coxsackie virus—encephalitis, hepatitis
    3. Echovirus—gastroenteritis, aseptic meningitis
    4. Other subgroups

A partial list of the major groups of viruses and some of the diseases they cause follows:

Papovavirus—papilloma (wart)
Adenovirus—bronchitis, pneumonitis, pharyngitis

Herpesvirus—herpes simplex (cold sore), herpes zoster (shingles)
Poxvirus—rubella, rabies, smallpox
Picornavirus—poliomyelitis, common cold
Reovirus—believed to cause acute respiratory diseases

Fungi. The fungus (mycotic) infections are among the most common diseases found in man. Fungi belong to the plant kingdom, and although many of them are harmless, some are responsible for infections. Types of fungi that almost everyone is familiar with include mildew, mold, mushrooms, and toadstools. Mycotic infections may be superficial, involving the skin and mucous membrane. The most frequently involved areas include the external layers of the skin, hair, and nails. These infections are commonly referred to as *ringworm* (dermatomycosis). The most frequent site in children is the scalp. The condition is considered infectious, and the child may not be permitted to attend school until the infection has been cured. Other sites include the beard (barber's itch) in adolescent and adult males, and the feet (athlete's feet). The latter may occur in any person but appears more often in males. The infection may also occur on other parts of the body, frequently about the nails. Domestic pets may also have ringworm infection and are frequently the source of infection for humans.

Fungi also invade the deeper tissues of the body. Most of these infections produce no symptoms; however, some become serious and may be fatal. Those most common in the United States are coccidioidomycosis (valley fever) and histoplasmosis.

Coccidioidomycosis was discovered in southern California, although the disease is found in other areas of the Southwest where the climate is hot and dry. The disease affects the lungs and is believed to be contracted by inhaling the spores present in the soil, which is blown about by the wind. Histoplasmosis also affects the lungs. This disease is widespread throughout the world; in some areas 80% of the population may be infected with it. The disease occurs as the result of inhaling spores present in the soil, and there is some possibility that ingestion of the spores may cause the disease. Histoplasmosis has often been associated with various kinds of birds; however, it is now believed that the only rela-

tionship is that bird droppings enrich the soil, providing fertile media in which the fungi may proliferate.[4]

Protozoa. The protozoa are single-celled animals existing everywhere in nature in some form. Some of the parasitic forms are often found in the intestinal tract of human beings and animals. The disease-producing protozoa are responsible for malaria, amebic dysentery, and African sleeping sickness. Another form of protozoa causes vaginal trichomoniasis in women, often as a complication of pregnancy. It may also live in the male urethra and may be acquired or transmitted through coitus (p. 372). Of the diseases caused by protozoa, the two of importance in the United States are malaria and amebic dysentery. The latter is more prevalent where sanitation is poor and personal hygiene is neglected. The source of infection is the excreta of convalescent patients or carriers, and the disease is transmitted by food handlers, contaminated food, or contaminated water supplies. The common housefly may be an intermediary vector by transmitting the organism to food.

The malaria protozoan is transmitted to humans through the bite of the *Anopheles* mosquito. Malaria is a worldwide health problem and is one of the most serious handicaps to the development of many countries. Between 1964 and 1968 less than 600 cases of malaria occurred annually in the United States. Servicemen returning from Vietnam with malaria produced a dramatic increase in the incidence of malaria. In 1970, 3051 cases were reported to the Center for Disease Control. After termination of the Vietnam conflict and the return of servicemen the incidence has declined. For the first 22 weeks of 1975, 116 cases were reported. During this period a total of 90 cases have been reported among refugees from Vietnam. Malaria causes morbidity, and some forms of the disease may be extremely serious, resulting in death[6] (p. 560).

Rickettsiae. Rickettsiae appear as tiny microorganisms, but some of their characteristics have led researchers to believe that they may hold an intermediate position between bacteria and viruses. The most serious diseases caused by rickettsiae are typhus fever and Rocky Mountain spotted fever. There are two types of typhus fever, the epidemic typhus and the murine typhus. The latter has been of special importance in the United States. The United States Public Health Service has set up control centers in areas where the disease has been prevalent, and through preventive and control measures the incidence of the disease has decreased. The disease is an infection of rats and is carried from rat to rat by rat fleas. Humans become infected when they are bitten by the flea and feces from the flea are rubbed into the skin about the bite. In epidemic typhus the disease is carried from person to person by the body louse. This type of typhus is common in European countries and has been responsible for the death of millions of persons over the past centuries.

Rocky Mountain spotted fever has been found in almost every area of the United States, and its prevalence seems to be increasing. It is transmitted to humans through the bite of an infected tick. Several varieties of ticks have been found to be carriers of the disease. The ticks live on many different kinds of animals found in rural and wooded areas. They may also live on common house pets such as cats and dogs. Persons working in areas where ticks are known to be abundant are more likely to become infected. The tick attaches itself to the skin, and the longer it remains attached to the skin the more likely the person is to become infected. In removing the tick from the skin, great care should be taken not to crush or squeeze it.

Symptoms of Rocky Mountain spotted fever and typhus fever are similar; in both diseases patients are usually extremely ill. Preventive vaccines are available for both diseases, and persons going into areas where the diseases are known to exist should avail themselves of the preventive vaccines (p. 360).

Metazoa

Metazoa are parasites that belong to the animal kingdom. When they invade the human body, this is referred to as a helminth infection. The Metazoa of concern here are divided into two groups: (1) Platyhelminthes, which includes tapeworms and (2) Nematoda, or roundworms. This group includes *Ascaris* parasites, hookworms, pinworms, and *Trichinella* parasites. (See Fig. 1-2.)

Some of the reasons nurses are interested in these parasites are as follows:

1. They may feed on the host's blood, causing severe anemia.
2. Some utilize nutrient materials, depriving the host of essential nutritive elements.
3. They may cause irritation and damage to the host's tissue.
4. Some may undergo abnormal growth or increase in number so as to block vital ducts and passageways.
5. It appears that some may produce poisons and toxins that injure the host.
6. Some cause severe allergic tissue reactions.*

Platyhelminthes (flatworms)

Tapeworms (Cestoda). The tapeworm is a flatworm, and nearly all flatworms are segmented. At one end there is a head and a neck called the *scolex;* in relation to the size of the worm the head is tiny. The scolex contains a mechanism enabling the worm to attach itself to the mucous membrane of the intestinal tract. (See Fig. 1-2.) Three forms of the worm are known to infect humans in the United States: (1) dwarf tapeworm, (2) beef tapeworm, and (3) fish tapeworm.

The dwarf tapeworm is the smallest of the tapeworms. It is most prevalent in areas where the sanitation is extremely poor. Infection occurs as the result of ingestion of the eggs of the worm, which hatch in the human intestinal tract. The cycle begins when the worms produce eggs that are discharged in the feces. Lack of proper handwashing after using the toilet is the medium by which the eggs are conveyed to the mouth and thus to the intestinal tract.

The beef tapeworm reaches the human intestinal tract through the ingestion of insufficiently cooked or raw beef containing the larvae of the worm. The cycle begins when the larvae produce worms. The eggs produced by the worms are present in human feces and are deposited onto the soil where cattle graze. A cow ingests the eggs, which hatch in the small intestine. The larvae (an intermediate stage

*From McInnes, Mary Elizabeth: Essentials of communicable disease, ed. 2, St. Louis, 1975, The C. V. Mosby Co., p. 349.

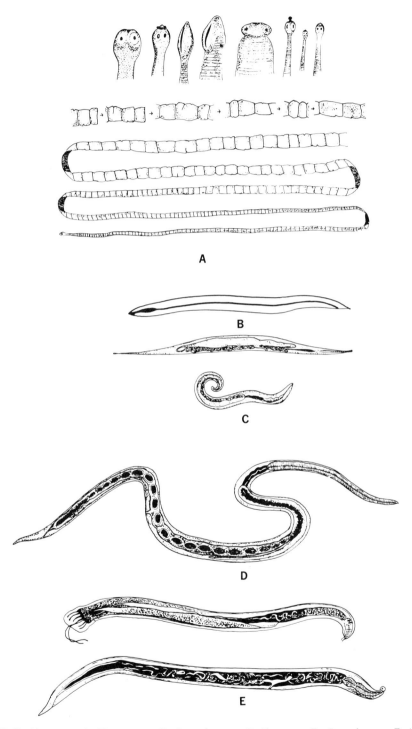

Fig. 1-2. Metazoa. **A,** Tapeworm. **B,** Roundworm. **C,** Pinworm. **D,** Roundworm. **E,** Hookworm.

in the development of the worm) lodge in the animal's tissues. A person who eats beef containing the larvae may become infected. The beef tapeworm is known to grow to a length of 25 feet, and as long as the head remains attached to the mucous membrane of the intestinal wall it will continue to grow and produce eggs. The beef tapeworm is the one most commonly found in the United States.

The fish tapeworm, like the beef tapeworm, requires an intermediary host, and human infection occurs in a similar way. Human feces containing the eggs are deposited into fresh water where the eggs mature into tiny embryos. The embryos are usually eaten by small shellfish, which are ultimately eaten by larger fish. The embryo then matures in the tissues of the fish. In areas where fish is eaten raw or is insufficiently cooked, infection may occur. The fish tapeworm may grow to 30 feet in length and may live for many years in the human intestine. Fish tapeworm infection is believed to be more prevalent than previously thought. Infection is known to result in severe anemia, and it is reported that the worm absorbs large amounts of vitamin B_{12} from the intestinal tract.[4]

Nematoda (roundworms)

Ascaris. Ascaris is a large roundworm resembling the common earthworm (fishworm). It varies in length from 4 to 12 inches, and the female worm may produce as many as 27 million eggs. When human feces are deposited on the ground, they become mixed with the soil, where the eggs may live for indefinite periods. Infection results from ingestion of the eggs containing the larvae, which reach the small intestine where the worms mature. Infection with *Ascaris* may be serious and cause complications such as intestinal obstruction, perforation of ulcers, appendicitis, and similar conditions.

Hookworm. There are two species of hookworm, and both may cause human infection. One species is most common in the southern United States, whereas the other species is most prevalent in Europe and Asia. As with many other kinds of worms, the source of infection is soil that has been contaminated with human feces

containing the eggs. The larva of the hookworm will penetrate the unbroken skin of the feet and legs and enter the body by way of the hair follicles and sweat glands. It penetrates lymph and blood vessels and may reach the lungs, where it is often coughed up and expectorated. If swallowed,. the larva will reach the small intestine, where the worms mature. The worm attaches itself to the intestinal mucosa by a pinching kind of hook. A mature worm will produce from 5000 to 10,000 eggs daily. The hookworm is reported to ingest as much as 50 ml. of the host's blood daily, which results in a severe iron-deficiency anemia. It also damages and ingests bits of tissue from the intestinal mucosa and frequently causes allergic reactions.

Pinworm (threadworm, seatworm). The pinworm is a tiny worm, and infection is self-induced by the anal-oral route. The ingested eggs pass into the stomach, and the worm matures in the large intestine. When the mature worm is ready to lay its eggs, it crawls to the outside and deposits its eggs in folds about the rectum and anus, after which it dies. Severe itching occurs about the area and through scratching the hands become infected with the eggs, which are then carried to the mouth and the entire cycle begins again.

Trichina. Trichina is a parasitic organism responsible for trichinosis. The primary source of trichinosis is insufficiently cooked pork and pork products that are infected with the worm. The larva that is present in the meat passes into the intestinal tract, and the worm matures in the intestine, where it becomes embedded in the mucosa. The larva is then released and eventually reaches the bloodstream. After entering the general circulation the larva is carried to skeletal muscle tissue and becomes encased into a cyst. There are several stages of the infection during the development of the worm and its passage through the body. During the various stages, symptoms of the infection may be acute, with fever, increased leukocyte count, allergic manifestations, and psychic symptoms. After encasement the primary symptom is rheumatic-like pain. The disease is serious in that 5% to 10% of persons infected will die. During 1974, 120 human cases were reported in the United States.

Malnutrition

Malnutrition may be due to insufficient diet, unbalanced diet, or failure of the body to utilize nutrients. There has never been greater emphasis on diet than at the present time. For many years it has been known that a deficiency of certain vitamins can cause scurvy, beriberi, and pellagra. Present research is concerned not only with the kinds of food necessary for health but also with how the body utilizes the nutrients. The diet may be entirely adequate from a nutritional standpoint, but because of the malfunctioning of some organ or part of the body, the diet is not properly utilized and the person is ill. In diabetes the body cannot utilize carbohydrates, and the person becomes ill with a specific set of symptoms (p. 404).

In some countries the lack of food is so serious that people are predisposed to develop various diseases or die from starvation. The United States has made millions of dollars worth of surplus food and grains available to many of these countries to help combat malnutrition.

More recently the United States government has been concerned with the problem of hunger and malnutrition in this country. In an affluent society such as exists in the United States it has been taken for granted that everyone has had enough to eat. Investigation and examination have shown that this is not true. In spite of opposition in some areas, Congress has moved to increase purchasing power through a program of food stamps for many low-income families.

Physical agents

Physical agents that result in injury to the body include changes in external temperature, electric current, exposure to radiation, and changes in atmospheric pressure. Exposure to extremes of heat may cause heat exhaustion or sunstroke. Overexposure to the sun's rays may result in severe burns. For example, Mrs. Y., wearing a sunback dress, went to the golf course on a very hot sunny day and played nine holes of golf. The following morning she reported to the emergency clinic with second-degree burns over her shoulders and upper back. Exposure to extremes of cold may cause frostbite or actual freezing of the body and possible death. Electric current may cause slight tingling such as may be experienced in the home due to faulty wiring, or it may result in severe shock, burns, or death when a person is exposed to high voltage. Severe and harmful radiation injury may occur from exposure to atomic radiation, and unless proper precautions are taken, injury may result when x-ray or radium therapy is used. Deviation from normal atmospheric pressure to increased or decreased pressure may cause illness or death. Persons traveling by air may experience extreme pain in the ears because of the rapid increase in atmospheric pressure. A condition known as the *bends,* in which severe abdominal and leg pain is suffered by divers or persons working below the land surface, is due to the rapid decrease in the atmospheric pressure.[8]

Chemical agents

Studies indicate that poisoning by various chemicals constitutes a major health problem. Substances known to be poisonous or nonpoisonous substances, such as medicines in large enough doses to be toxic, may be taken accidentally or intentionally. There are many new drugs on the market for which no satisfactory antidote may be available. Overdoses of some drugs cause respiratory and cardiovascular depression. Some chemical agents are inhaled in the form of gas such as carbon monoxide; others, like lye, may be ingested. Various industrial processes use chemicals that are injurious if inhaled or if they come into contact with the skin. There are certain high-risk occupations such as mining in which exposure to gases or dust may cause acute or chronic illness. The problem of drug and chemical poisoning has become so serious that programs have been instituted to assist the persons involved and help save lives. Some hospitals, clinics, and other institutions have established poison control centers where information concerning a drug is available, usually on a 24-hour basis. Special educational displays, posters, and printed material have been placed in public buildings to inform the public about the harmful effects from poisons. The United States government has curtailed the use of the artificial sweetener cyclamate and some drugs because of the possible harmful effects resulting from their use. State and local governments are becoming increasingly aware of the necessity for more public information and legislation for the control of hazardous drugs, chemicals, insecticides, and sprays.

Congenital and hereditary disorders

Congenital means "existing at birth." The causes of many congenital defects are unknown. Some are known to be hereditary, or caused by a defect in the genes that carry the traits of inheritance. Others are caused by malformation in the developmental stage of intrauterine life. Many are believed to occur during the first few weeks of embryonic life, even before the mother realizes she is pregnant. If a mother has German measles during the first trimester of pregnancy, there is a possibility that the baby will have a congenital defect. There is increasing evidence that other infectious diseases, including mumps, infectious hepatitis, and influenza, may play some part in abortion, premature birth, stillbirth, and birth defects. Some defects believed to be the result of birth injury may actually be the result of developmental abnormalities.

Congenital birth defects may affect any organ or system of the body, and frequently several defects involving different organs or systems may occur in the same child. The largest number of defects occur in the skeletal system. Many defects are believed to be the result of prematurity, whereas others are the result of the birth process and are classified as birth injuries. In recent years certain drugs, including the hallucinogenic agents (e.g., LSD) and antimetabolites, have come under investigation. Some researchers are of the opinion that such agents cause chromosome patterns that result in certain defects. The traits for specific diseases are known to be carried in the genes and are passed on from parents to offspring. These are known as hereditary diseases and include sickle cell anemia and hemophilia.

Because of medical science, many children with congenital disorders survive and reach adulthood. Some survive without medical care if the defect is minor. One of the problems concerning birth defects is that the parents may believe that the defect is a stigma or that they are in some way to blame. Superstition also plays a part, since many parents still believe that a child may be marked because of some abnormal craving or accident of the mother during pregnancy.

PREDISPOSING FACTORS TO DISEASE

In addition to specific pathogenic agents and known causes of diseases, there are factors associated with predisposition to disease. These include the aging process, tumor growth, emotional disturbances, various types of sensitivity reactions, and inadequate self-care.

Normal aging process

The normal aging process brings about changes in the human organism. These changes are contributing factors in many diseases affecting elderly persons. With advancing years the blood vessels lose some of their elasticity (hardening of the arteries). As they become narrowed, there is a decreased blood supply to vital parts of the body, with the result that degenerative changes occur in some of the organs. Some organs will become affected and wear out sooner than others. The loss of fluid and thinning of the intervertebral disks cause the person to bow forward. This bowing causes changes in the contour of the thoracic cage and predisposes the individual to diseases of the lower respiratory system. The branch of medicine that deals with the problems of the aging process is called geriatrics, and it will be reviewed in detail in Chapter 8.

Tumor growth

Tumor growth, both benign and malignant, is a cause of increasing incidence of illness among persons between 45 and 65 years of age. The presence of tumors anywhere in the body will result in impaired functioning of the affected part. Scientists now feel certain that viruses cause certain kinds of malignant tumors. It has been predicted that soon it may be possible to have a vaccine to prevent certain kinds of cancer.

3/ Emotional disturbances

Many diseases are the result of more than one cause. There is a close relationship between bodily disease and emotion. In some persons the disease may be entirely the result of emotional factors, whereas in others a severe disease condition may precipitate emotional problems. However, it may be said that physical illness always results in some emotional problems. When emotional problems are so severe as to result in total personality disintegration, a true psychosis develops.

4/ Sensitivity reactions

Some persons are hypersensitive to certain substances that ordinarily do not affect most people. The hypersensitive person may have a mild to severe or even fatal reaction if he comes into contact with these substances or takes them into his body. These hypersensitive responses are called *allergic reactions*. (See Chapter 22.)

5/ Inadequate self-care

Persons may be predisposed to disease because of improper living. Extended loss of sleep and rest, improper diet, alcoholism, excessive cigarette smoking, and poor habits of personal hygiene leave the body susceptible to disease. Poverty, unemployment, lack of education, and severe crippling conditions are contributing factors. Even when frank disease cannot be demonstrated, the functioning of the body may be impaired to the extent that symptoms of disease do appear. Conditions of this type are called functional disorders.

CLASSIFICATION OF DISEASES

Diseases are sometimes classified according to their cause, such as diseases caused by fungi, or they may be classified by the body system affected, as in diseases of the respiratory system. The physician is able to identify a particular disease by the symptoms peculiar to it, often utilizing laboratory tests, microscopic examinations, and special kinds of examinations before making a diagnosis. Some diseases have symptoms so similar that the physician must compare and contrast the symptoms before making a diagnosis. This process is called *differential diagnosis*. In these situations the physician may rely heavily on the nurse to make and record careful, accurate observations of the patient.

made by comparing & contrasting similar symptoms of different diseases

NURSE-PATIENT RELATIONSHIPS

The patient is an individual member of a family, and the family is the unit of society. The illness of any member of the family will indirectly affect other members of the family. How the patient reacts to his illness may be conditioned by the way his family feels about it or by the way he thinks society feels about it. The patient's reaction to his illness is affected by what happens to him when he enters the hospital, his age, his position in the family, his standing in the community, his economic status, and the nature of his illness. The family may be under emotional tension and anxiety or economic stress that consciously or unconsciously is transmitted to the patient.

When the patient enters the hospital, he is stripped of his clothing and loses his identity in the world. He becomes subject to unfamiliar time schedules, and his patterns of activity are not his own. He is expected to play a passive role and to conform to the role of a hospital patient. The patient may become submissive and regress to a childlike dependency, or he may rebel and be labeled uncooperative. Nurses often stereotype and place the patient in the category of being a good patient or a poor patient without trying to understand how he feels about the new role he is expected to play.

The way in which nurses react to patients and their illnesses will depend to a great extent on their feelings about people in general. Patients may have different illnesses and different problems, but they are all human beings in need of acceptance and understanding.

It is important for nurses to have confidence in their technical competence. However, of equal or even more importance is an ability to see the patient as an individual with certain physical, psychologic, social, and spiritual needs. Skills and procedures can be memorized, but the ability to understand human behavior must be gained through experience and living. The kind of physical care that nurses give and the comforting measures that contribute to the patient's well-being will convey their attitudes toward the patient and his illness. When the nurse takes time to listen to the patient's feelings in relation to his problems, the patient may feel accepted. When the patient feels accepted and understood, he also has a feeling of trust and confidence.

The nurse should be aware that the patient's family also need to feel accepted. In many instances the family can supply information about the patient that will give the nurse insight into his particular needs. This is especially important when the patient is a child. Members of the family should be given the opportunity to do things for the patient and should be given an explanation concerning his care. For example, a nurse comes on duty with Mrs. X, who has had major surgery this morning. Mrs. X is lying on her back and seems comfortable. The physician's orders state that the patient is to be turned from side to side every 2 hours, so the nurse turns the patient to her side. Mrs. X's husband is in the room and feels that she is comfortable and asks why it is necessary to turn her. When Mr. X is given an explanation of the importance of turning, he accepts it with understanding and assists with the care. Satisfying nurse-patient relationships must include the patient's family and will be fostered only in an atmosphere of mutual confidence, understanding, and trust.

NURSE-CHILD RELATIONSHIPS

The nurse should remember that children are not miniature adults but individuals with special problems and needs. The child may need physical and psychologic care, but above all his sense of security and trust must be preserved. Much has been written about the traumatic experiences to which the hospitalized child is exposed, and physicians, nurses, and others have a long way to go in relieving these situations. The child is thrust into a totally strange environment, where parents are excluded in many instances and where strange people do strange and painful things to him. Is it any wonder that the child screams and must be held, re-

strained, or sedated? Often children are threatened by parents so that the physician, nurse, and hospital come to be feared and avoided. In no field of nursing is tender loving care more important than in working with children.

Pediatric practice usually includes children through 12 years of age. However, children under 4 years of age are particularly susceptible to environmental change. The separation and deprivation engendered by hospitalization cause a loss of mothering and the stimulation of the home environment that is essential to the child's growth and development and feeling of security. Studies have indicated that the child's future intellectual, social, and emotional growth and development may be seriously compromised because of the loss.[1]

Every year thousands of children are brought into hospitals who have been abandoned by parents or otherwise mistreated. Often these children have been so severely denied the mother's love and care that their personalities are already affected.

Studies made by the World Health Organization and reported by Blake and associates[1] indicate that many factors are involved in the child's loss of mothering. Some hospitals permit the mother to remain with the hospitalized child. When this is not possible, it becomes the responsibility of the nursing staff to supply substitute mothering to help relieve anxiety and fear related to the child's separation. (Students should consult a pediatric textbook for more information.)

MENTAL RETARDATION

Mental retardation is a condition in which there is an absence of normal mental growth and development. In some cases physical growth may also be affected. There are a great many causes of mental retardation, and some are not completely understood. A general grouping places the causes into various periods: (1) prenatal, (2) natal, and (3) postnatal. During the prenatal period, mental retardation may be the result of traits carried by the genes, as in phenylketonuria. Others may be caused by infections of the mother during the prenatal period, for example, syphilis and rubella. Injury during the birth process may cause damage to the infant's brain. Birth accidents, poisoning, and some infectious diseases such as encephalitis may retard mental growth and development.[1]

The extent of mental retardation varies. Some children are so severely affected that institutional care is required. Others are able to attend school and through special education and vocational training are able to take care of themselves. Some mentally retarded individuals die during infancy or childhood, whereas others reach adulthood. It may not be possible to distinguish between the mildly retarded and a normal person.

In the past, mental retardation was looked on as a stigma, and families sought to conceal the existence of a retarded child. Today public education and programs to help retarded persons to achieve the maximum of their potential have eliminated much of the secrecy previously associated with the condition.

Mental retardation affects all races and all segments of society, regardless of economic status. The nurse should remember that mental retardation is not the fault of the individual involved. The nurse will care for persons of all ages who are mentally retarded; all will need the same care as normal individuals.[1]

The mentally retarded child has the same needs as the normal child, but in addition has special needs that must be met in special ways. The ways in which the child's needs will be met will depend on the degree of retardation and the presence of physical limitations. Each child must be treated as an individual and his care planned on an individual basis. In general it may be expected that the child will be unable to remember things told to him and that he will be able to remember only one thing at a time. He may not be toilet trained, and frequent bed changes may be necessary. He may be unable to feed himself or may play with his food and be messy with it. In working with and providing care for these children it should be remembered that patience and lavish praise will be necessary to achieve results.[3]

The mentally retarded adult may have been rejected or overprotected throughout life. In either case he may not have the feeling of security and belonging afforded the normal person. The nurse may expect speech problems to be present. If moderately or severely retarded, the person may be unable to bathe himself or perform other personal care. He may be unable to read or write, will have a short memory span, and will have difficulty following directions. An important nursing function is to help the patient have a feeling of security and trust. If coordination is poor, the patient must be protected from injury.

The family of the retarded person need special consideration. They may have feelings of guilt and shame. They may have had ambitions for the child that have had to be abandoned. The nurse can do much to make them feel accepted and to maintain their self-respect and dignity. When the patient is dismissed from the hospital, any orders for medications, treatments, or other care should be explained to a responsible member of the family.

THE ADOLESCENT PATIENT

Adolescents are frequently admitted to the hospital for care. Admission may follow an accidental injury such as an automobile accident. Under emergency conditions it may be expected that the individual will be anxious, fearful, and insecure. Unlike younger patients or more mature persons, adolescents may be impatient and want their questions answered at once. Adolescents view themselves as adults, and in many respects they are, although lacking in experience. In caring for the patient, involvement and communication are the key words. The patient should be accepted as an individual and given the right to be included in decisions concerning his treatment and prognosis and should be consulted in matters concerning his care. He should be allowed to participate in his own care and whenever possible should be placed in a room with other persons. The adolescent has his own vocabulary, and the nurse should try to understand it. He needs constant reassurance concerning his progress and will be happier if he has something to do and his family and friends are encouraged to visit him.[5]

THE MEDICAL-SURGICAL PATIENT

The medical service usually includes those patients with the most serious conditions such as myocardial infarction, terminal cancer, congestive heart failure, leu-

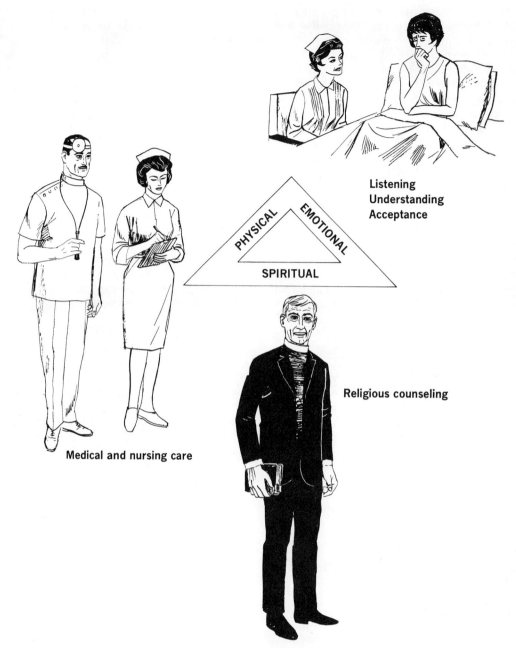

Listening
Understanding
Acceptance

Religious counseling

Medical and nursing care

Fig. 1-3. The triangle of life.

kemia, and similar serious conditions. The medical patient may have entered the hospital for a series of diagnostic tests and examinations because there is some question as to what is wrong with him. On completion of the examinations and when a diagnosis is established, the patient may be transferred to the surgical service or

dismissed. In some hospitals the medical and surgical services are not segregated so that the nurse may be caring for both medical and surgical patients on the same clinical unit. Other patients have both medical and surgical conditions at the same time.

The care of the medical patient who is

acutely ill offers the greatest challenge to the nurse's skill and understanding. Although every patient may anticipate danger, the seriously ill medical patient may be acutely aware of an impending crisis. A critically ill medical patient was extremely restless and anxious. He said to the nurse, "I am worried; something is going to happen tonight, and I don't know what." He died 2 hours later! Such experiences make it easy to understand why the critically ill patient is fearful of the unknown and is afraid of the loneliness and weakness, the suffering and the pain that await him. (See Chapter 7.)

Many medical patients are not seriously ill and show improvement day by day. Some are wholly or in part ambulatory and provide a large portion of their own care. As the patient improves, he should be encouraged in self-help and a return to normal routines, within the limits of his ability and environment. This period will provide the nurse's greatest opportunity for teaching on the medical service. The diabetic patient needs to be taught to administer his own insulin and to understand his diet and the importance of personal hygiene. The patient with a cardiovascular condition may need help with the sodium-restricted diet and with planning rest periods, suitable recreational activities, and exercise within the limits of his disease. The nurse should be a messenger of good health, constantly alert to the opportunities for helping people to maintain good health, as well as taking care of them in illness. Many times it is easier to help a person stay well than to try to cure him if he becomes sick.

Most surgical patients are plagued by fear, although they may not verbalize their fear. When faced with surgery, the person often puts up a "front." He may appear calm and cheerful, but behind the outward manifestation of bravery he is probably scared to death. Almost all patients dread and fear anesthesia. They fear they will die during surgery; they fear mutilation, cancer, and pain. Perhaps the most traumatic experience for the surgical patient is the loss of a limb. The patient who is confronted with removal of the female reproductive organs may have mixed feelings. The patient may welcome the relief from fear of pregnancy and at the same time may be depressed in realizing that surgery marks the end of the ability to reproduce. American women have placed great emphasis on the size and contour of the human breast. Patients undergoing mastectomy have many anxieties concerning disfigurement. Also, a mother may worry about the care of her children; a father may worry over loss of income, loss of employment, and costs of surgery and hospitalization. The patient fears prolonged dependency and worries that he might never be well again.

The nurse as a member of the team can do much to assist the surgical patient through this difficult period. The surgical patient should be informed of everything he should know. This is a joint responsibility of the surgeon and the nurse. It should not be assumed that the intelligent patient is free from fears or that the less intelligent patient is without fear. It is not unusual for the nurse to think that a patient is uncooperative when he does the opposite thing from what he is asked to do. The nurse should understand that a worried patient may unconsciously respond in this manner. The nurse must be able to discriminate carefully between patients regarding what they need to be told. When fear is not relieved, it may seriously interfere with heart action and the induction of anesthesia.

The patient should be told what to expect after surgery. If there are to be tubes, machines, side rails, and dressings, a careful explanation of these articles and the reasons for their use should be given. The nurse will find it much easier to care for the patient postoperatively if he knows that he will have a Levin tube or retention catheter and why. The patient should be told that he will be turned, that he may have intravenous fluids, or that he may be given nothing by mouth. The patient should be assured that his pain will be relieved. When preoperative medication is administered, the nurse should reassure the patient, encouraging him to trust those responsible for his care. He should be told that he will become sleepy and that he might not realize when he is taken to surgery, but nevertheless the nurse will be waiting for him to return.

The nurse must never allow an anxious, fearful patient to go to surgery and find out things for himself.

The nurse should remember that a surgical patient's family may be anxious. The family should be told approximately how long the patient will be in surgery. They should know that after surgery he will be taken to the recovery room. In some cases the patient may be transferred to the intensive care unit. One way to reassure the family is to make periodic checks on the condition of the patient while he is in surgery and the recovery room.

When possible, a close relative should be permitted to see the patient before he goes to surgery, and in some cases it may be desirable for the relative to remain with the patient after surgery.

No matter how serious the surgery may be, the nurse must seek to inspire confidence, relieve anxiety, and reassure the patient and his family and must not allow the patient to give up hope. The will to live must be strengthened, since without it the patient may have less chance for recovery.

Psychosocial, family, and adjustive situations

Many of the situations and/or problems of the medical-surgical patient and his family may be classified as psychosocial, family, and adjustive or any combination of these factors. The goal of most persons is health oriented, and few can be completely objective when illness occurs. Each person is an individual, and each individual will differ from every other individual in any illness situation. As a person faces illness or surgery, the way in which he reacts to it will depend on his lifetime patterns of growth and emotional development, the culture to which he belongs, and to society in general.

Psychosocial situations. Society establishes expectations for its individual members. When serious illness occurs, the social values of society and those of the individual may be affected. Most illness creates a crisis situation for the individual. The patient looks to the physician and the nurse for understanding and amelioration of the situation. Illness, if prolonged, may create

to make better, improve

a poverty situation and force the family to seek public assistance. It may mean loss of employment and/or inability to secure employment. Society may be affected by the loss of irreplaceable services. It may mean retraining of a person for another type of employment. In some cases the person may remain an invalid for the rest of his life.

In any serious illness it may be expected that normal patterns of behavior will be affected. There may be anxiety, frustration, feelings of guilt, uncertainty, and at times regression to earlier forms of behavior. As indicated earlier in this chapter, the patient who is going to have surgery is anxious. He is concerned about what the surgeon will find, whether he will live, the financial cost, his job, and his family. The patient having a gastrectomy may have feelings of guilt because he failed to follow the dietary regimen advised by his physician. The patient who recovers from an acute myocardial infarction will thereafter live in a world of apprehension, fearing that he may have another heart attack and that it may be fatal. There is increasing evidence that the excardiac patient is being rejected for employment. The patient with cancer may not be told of his diagnosis and lives with uncertainty and worry about what will happen to him.

Family. The way in which the family reacts to a serious illness depends on several factors—age of the patient, his position and social role in the family, and his physiologic and psychologic state as well as his ability to recover and assume family functions. It should not be assumed that babies, small children, sick people, and the elderly are able to care for themselves and direct their activities toward recovery and wellness. The family members must be the motivating force and accept the responsibility for care if the member is to survive and recover. The best medical and hospital care available should be provided. When financial resources are not available, community social agencies may assist the family. When elderly persons require care, the government program of Medicare provides assistance.

Adjustment. Medical and/or surgical illness always means adjustment for the family as well as for the patient. The patient may try to adjust by employing defense mechanisms. If he is emotionally mature, he may seek to adjust by analyzing the situation, developing a plan of action, and utilizing previous experiences to guide him in the immediate crisis.

When the breadwinner is the victim of prolonged illness, problems of adjustment may be developed by calling the family together. Through communication and understanding each family member decides how he or she can contribute to the present situation. The same procedure may be employed if the mother is ill. The sharing of responsibility by all members of the family develops togetherness and provides stability of the home.

Adjustment may be made by placing an elderly person in a nursing home or convalescent facility. A severely mentally retarded child may have to be placed in an institution for the welfare of other children in the family. A mother may have to seek temporary employment outside the home, and a father may need to secure extra work to meet the financial responsibility of illness. Reorganization of the home routine may be necessary to care for a severely handicapped member or one with chronic illness.

In everyday life most well persons are confronted with problems that require adjustment. Every person should be taught and learn early in life how to cope with problem situations and to make emotionally mature decisions.

TOTAL PATIENT CARE

The concept of total patient care implies that all the patient's needs will be met. Total is defined as "entire" or "whole," and to give this kind of care the whole patient must be considered. It is well beyond the nurse's scope to give total care, but the nurse is a very important participant in the entire care of the patient.

Each patient is an individual, and when he enters the hospital, he brings with him a lifetime of behavior patterns, hopes, ambitions, frustrations, and problems. He enters the hospital because of a diseased physical body or a deranged mind. He does not want to be sick, and he does not want to be in the hospital; because of his illness, he is beset by a whole new range of fears, apprehensions, and anxieties. His problems are physical, emotional, social, and economic. In addition, depending on the individual, his religious beliefs may be involved.

No one person can give total care that meets all the patient's needs. Each patient has individual needs, and it may require many persons within and without the hospital to provide total care. For example, the business office may have to assist the patient in the financial arrangements for his hospitalization. The social worker may have to plan with a community agency regarding economic assistance for the family. The psychiatrist may see the patient to determine his emotional and mental state, and the court may be brought in to arrange commitment to a mental hospital.

The internist and the surgeon request certain examinations, and the laboratory and x-ray personnel carry out the requests. The dietitian visits the patient to explain his diet or how to select his food from menus. The nurse on the clinical unit plans for the care of the patient and assigns certain aspects of care to other personnel on the unit.

The physical therapist, occupational therapist, religious counselor, visiting teacher, and vocational rehabilitation counselor may become members of the team necessary to give total patient care.

The patient wants to feel accepted, secure, and in good hands. The nurse may help the patient by accepting him as an individual; by having a warm, friendly, understanding attitude; by providing skillful, thorough, unhurried nursing care; and by listening to his problems, fears, or complaints and reporting them. The nurse should remember that every patient needs comfort and understanding in time of illness and a feeling that everything possible is being done to hasten his recovery.

NURSING HISTORY AND NURSING CARE PLAN
Nursing history

The objective of the *nursing history* is so that the nurse will know the patient. Becoming familiar with his lifetime patterns, interests, and health problems will enable the nurse to plan care for the patient in a more enlightened manner. The nurse will be able to make better use of

Table 1-1. Nursing history

1. Name _____
2. Age _____ Sex _____
3. Occupation _____
4. Religion _____
5. Date admitted _____
6. Diagnosis _____
7. Family members _____
8. Food: Breakfast
Lunch
Dinner
Likes
Dislikes
9. Sleep habits _____
10. Physical or recreational activities _____
11. Hobbies _____
12. Previous hospitalizations _____
Patient's reaction to them _____
13. Other information _____
14. Nurse's observations _____
15. Problems that may be anticipated _____

time, and the patient will be better satisfied, believing that the nurse is interested in him as an individual.

Most well persons have developed a daily routine designed to meet their own needs. The patterns for the day become fixed: eating, sleeping, bathing, eliminating, work, play, and religious meditation. When the patient becomes ill, these fixed patterns are disrupted, possibly causing acute discomfort to the patient. When the patient enters the hospital, he has consciously or unconsciously set goals for himself. These goals may include recovery and a return to health with the least discomfort and in the shortest time possible. He expects that his physicians and his nurses will provide the care and understanding to expedite his recovery and accomplish his objectives.

To work with the patient in accomplishing his objectives the nurse must know something about the patient as an individual. This information is provided in the nursing history which may include biologic information such as age, sex, race, nationality, family, etc. It may also include religion, occupation, date of admission, and diagnosis or reason for admission. It should include information concerning activities

of daily living, food likes and dislikes or special diets, sleeping habits, recreational activities, previous hospital experiences and the patient's reaction to them, and what he hopes to accomplish from this hospitalization. It should include the nurse's observations and notes about any special problems that may be encountered in his care. The nursing history may be extensive or it may be modified, but it should always present a written picture of the patient that will enable the nurse to prepare a plan of action for meeting his needs (Table 1-1).

Nursing care plan

A careful examination and study of the nursing history will aid the nurse in establishing objectives and the kinds of actions necessary to realize these objectives and will improve the quality of patient care. This is called a *nursing care plan.* The plan is made for the individual patient and should provide for modification and change as the patient's needs change. When nursing care is given by a team, the professional nurse is the team leader. Each member of the team should assist in preparing the nursing care plan, establishing objectives, and carrying out the actions necessary to im-

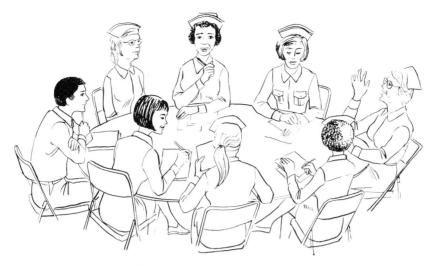

Fig. 1-4. Many different persons contribute to the nursing care plan.

Table 1-2. Simple nursing care plan for Mr. Hill, age 60

Name_____ Age_____ Sex_____ Race_____Nationality_____
Religion_____Occupation_____ Economic status_____
Family_____Diagnosis_____Date admitted_____

Record hours	Items of care	Needs, actions, problems, etc.
6:00 A.M.		Patient likes coffee early; has cup and coffee in room; get hot water for him
7:00	Personal hygiene	Patient likes to take shower and shave before breakfast; check items that he may need
8:00	TPR and B/P	Check blood pressure in both arms
	Breakfast	Wants his eggs scrambled and no orange juice
	Up in chair	Always wants morning paper
11:00		Patient says he always rests before lunch
12:00	Lunch	Will make coffee in room; says hospital coffee not very good
1:00 P.M.	Exercise	Patient wants to walk in hall for exercise; says he walks a lot and is not used to being so confined
2:00 to 4:00	Recreation	Watching television
4:00	TPR and B/P	Check blood pressure in both arms
5:00	Supper	Wants very light supper
6:00		Patient visits with nurse; says his wife has been dead 5 years; patient seems to be lonely
8:00	Recreation	Enjoys sports and always listens to ball game
Bedtime		Does not want to go to sleep until after game is over
	ECG in A.M.	Explain procedure to patient and reassure him
		Be sure high-low bed is down and night light is on
	Observation	Patient might be told about clubs for older citizens so that he could meet other persons who would keep him from being so lonely

plement the desired goals. The team should consist of all levels of nursing personnel, including the orderly. Persons other than nurses such as the physical therapist or the social worker may provide helpful suggestions for specific patients. In the case of a terminally ill patient the hospital chaplain may contribute by interpreting specific needs of the dying patient and his family.

Nurses employed in nursing homes should be familiar with the new federal law that requires nursing care plans for each patient, including long-range plans. This law applies to all homes receiving government money through Medicare and Medicaid (p. 127).

Medications, treatments, special tests, and examinations are usually placed on a cardex and do not have to be carried on a nursing care plan. However, procedures may vary. Table 1-2 is an example of a simple nursing care plan that might be prepared, based on information secured from the nursing history.

Summary outline

1. Development of medicine and surgery
2. Causes of disease
   A. Microorganisms
   B. Metazoa
   C. Malnutrition
   D. Physical agents
   E. Chemical agents
   F. Congenital and hereditary disorders
3. Infections caused by microorganisms
   A. Streptococci, staphylococci, and diplococci
      1. Beta-hemolytic streptococci and viridans (alpha-hemolytic) streptococci may be cause of rheumatic fever or bacterial endocarditis
      2. *Staphylococcus aureus* (pyogenic, or pus-producing group) may cause boils, abscesses, and carbuncles: *Staphylococcus epidermidis* (nonpathogenic group) rarely causes infections
      3. Diplococcus—several kinds:
         a. Pneumococcus—thirty different types
         b. Gonococcus—causes gonorrhea
         c. Meningococcus—causes meningitis
   B. Bacilli
      Cause many infectious diseases, including tuberculosis, pertussis, typhoid fever, and diphtheria
      1. Some forms produce spores, including those that cause tetanus, gas gangrene, and anthrax
   C. Spirilla (corkscrew in shape)
      Several kinds
      1. Spirochete now classified separately from spirilla

   D. Viruses
      1. Virology is the study of viruses
      2. May gain entrance to the body through
         a. Mucous membranes of the gastrointestinal tract or respiratory tract
         b. Broken skin from animal bites
         c. Injected by mosquito or hypodermic needle
      3. Viruses selective in type of tissue attacked; infections self-limited
   E. Fungi (mycotic infections)
      Many harmless; common fungi include mildew, mold, mushrooms, and toadstools
      1. Superficial infections involve nails, skin, and hair
      2. Deep infections cause coccidioidomycosis and histoplasmosis
   F. Protozoa
      Single-celled animals; some parasitic forms cause disease
      1. Malaria protozoan transmitted by *Anopheles* mosquito
      2. Amebic dysentery
      3. African sleeping sickness
      4. Trichomoniasis
   G. Rickettsiae
      Microorganisms causing
      1. Rocky Mountain spotted fever through bite of tick
      2. Murine typhus transmitted by rat flea from rat to rat; bite of flea transmits disease to humans
      3. Epidemic typhus transmitted by body louse; most common in European countries
4. Metazoa (helminths)
   Parasites that belong to the animal kingdom
   A. Platyhelminthes (flatworms)
      1. Tapeworms (Cestoda)
         a. Dwarf tapeworm
         b. Beef tapeworm
         c. Fish tapeworm
   B. Nematoda (roundworms)
      1. *Ascaris*
      2. Hookworm
      3. Pinworm
      4. Trichina
5. Malnutrition
   May result from
   A. Insufficient food
   B. Unbalanced diet
   C. Failure of body to utilize nutrients
6. Physical agents
   A. Changes in external temperature
   B. Electric current
   C. Exposure to radiation
   D. Changes in atmospheric pressure
7. Chemical agents
   Poisoning a major health problem
   A. The ingestion of poisonous substances or nonpoisonous substances in toxic doses
   B. Drugs taken in overdoses
   C. Inhalation of gases such as carbon monoxide
   D. High-risk occupations such as coal mining in which inhalation of dust may cause acute or chronic illness

E. Establishment of poison control centers
F. United States government control of food additives (cyclamate), some drugs, pesticides, and sprays
8. Congenital and hereditary disorders
Some conditions hereditary, other caused by developmental errors or birth injuries
   A. German measles in pregnant mother during first trimester may result in birth defects
   B. Some evidence that mumps, infectious hepatitis, and influenza in pregnancy may cause abortion, stillbirth, premature birth, and birth defects
   C. Largest number of defects affect skeletal system
   D. Many defects believed to be due to prematurity
   E. Some defects due to birth injury
   F. Hallucinogenic agents (e.g., LSD) may change chromosome patterns and cause defects
   G. Hereditary defects due to traits carried in genes and transmitted by parents to offspring
      1. Sickle cell anemia
      2. Hemophilia
9. Predisposing factors to disease
   A. Normal aging process
   B. Tumor growth
   C. Emotional disturbances
   D. Sensitivity reactions
   E. Inadequate self-care
10. Classification of disease
    A. According to cause
    B. According to part or system of body affected
    C. Differential diagnosis necessary when same symptoms are common to more than one disease
11. Nurse-patient relationships
Patient's reaction to illness affected by what happens to him when he enters hospital, age, position in family, standing in community, economic status, nature of illness
    A. Illness disrupts patient's patterns and normal routines
    B. Each patient has individual set of behavior patterns
    C. Patient expected to conform to role of hospital patient
    D. Patient may regress to childlike dependency
    E. How nurse reacts to patient's illness dependent on how nurse feels about people in general
    F. Acceptance and understanding of patient's feelings results in his trust and confidence in nurse
    G. Nurse must see patient with physical, psychologic, social, and spiritual needs
    H. Nurse needs confidence in technical competence
    I. Patient's family needs to feel accepted
    J. Satisfying nurse-patient relationships fostered by mutual understanding and trust
12. Nurse-child relationships
    A. Child must be treated as individual with his own needs
    B. Child must have sense of security and trust
    C. Pediatric practice includes children through 12 years of age
       1. Children under 4 years susceptible to environmental change
       2. Separation and deprivation causes loss of mothering and stimulation of home
       3. Social, intellectual, and emotional growth and development may be seriously compromised
       4. Nursing staff should supply substitute mothering
13. Mental retardation
Absence of normal growth and development
    A. Many causes
    B. Extent will vary
    C. Some will die in infancy or childhood, others will reach adulthood
    D. Mentally retarded child has special needs
    E. Mentally retarded adult may not have feeling of security and belonging
    F. Family of retarded need special consideration
    G. In adolescent care, involvement and communication are key words
14. Medical-surgical patient
    A. Medical patients expect to feel better each day; surgical patients expect to feel worse before they feel better
    B. Medical patients may be most critically ill patients in hospital
    C. Some of the greatest teaching opportunties present themselves on medical service
    D. Nurse is messenger of good health
    E. Surgical patient should be informed of everything that he needs to know; a joint responsibility of surgeon and nurse
    F. Surgical patient often scared to death; fears anesthesia, death, mutilation, cancer, and pain
    G. Nurse must seek to inspire confidence, reassure, and relieve anxiety in surgical patient
15. Psychosocial, family, and adjustive situations
    A. Psychosocial factors
       1. Most illness creates crisis situation
       2. Normal patterns of behavior will be affected
    B. Family
       1. Numerous factors may affect how family reacts to serious illness
       2. Family must be motivating force if member is to survive
    C. Adjustment
       1. Illness always means that family and patient must make adjustments
       2. Communication and understanding among family members may help situation
       3. All members should share responsibility
16. Total patient care
    A. Total means entire or whole
    B. No one person can give total patient care
    C. Total care may require a team that includes many persons
    D. Nurse may assist by giving skillful nurs-

ing care, listening to patient, and reporting problems, fears, or complaints
E. Every ill person needs comfort and understanding
17. Nursing history and nursing care plan
A. Objective is to individualize patient care
B. Effectiveness of plan depends on communication and cooperation between all shifts
and personnel
C. Nursing history is written picture of patient
D. Patient sets goals for himself to speed his
recovery; nurse must assist patient in
realizing his goals
E. Nursing care plan provides for
1. Nursing objectives in caring for patient
2. Plan of action to accomplish objectives

Review questions

1. List two diseases that may be caused by the
herpesvirus.
a. *cold sore – herpes simplex*
b. *shingles " zoster*
2. Where would Rocky Mountain spotted fever
be found?
a. *anywhere there is infected ticks!*
3. List two foods in which tapeworm may be
found.
a. *beef*
b. *raw fish*
4. List four conditions that the nurse may encounter in caring for a mentally retarded
adult.
a. *speech problems*
b. *short memory span*
c. *incontinence*
d. *illiterate*
5. Discuss how serious illness may affect society
and the family.
6. List four persons who may help in preparing
and maintaining a nursing care plan.
a. *dietary worker*
b. *chaplain*
c. *nurse*
d. *orderly*
7. Discuss how the nursing care of an adolescent
may differ from that of an adult.
8. What three bacterial diseases may form spores?
a. *tetanus*
b. *gas gangrene*
c. *anthrax*
9. What is a microorganism that grows only in
the presence of air called?
a. *aerobic*
10. What person has been credited with the discovery of ether as an anesthetic?
a. *1842 - Crawford Long*

Films

1. Early clinical aspects of mental retardation—
M-664 (37 min., sound, black and white, 16
mm.), Media Resources Branch, National
Medical audiovisual Center (Annex), Station
K, Atlanta, Ga. 30324. Prenatal and perinatal
etiologic factors in mental retardation. Types
responding to specific therapy.
2. Mental retardation: the long childhood of
Timmy, Part 1—M-2077-X, (21 min., sound,
black and white, 16 mm.), Media Resources
Branch, National Medical Audiovisual Center
(Annex), Station K, Atlanta, Ga. 30324. Part
2—M-2078-X (32 min., sound, black and
white, 16 mm.). Shows a mongoloid child
making the transition from a family setting
to a residential training school.
3. The nurse combats disease—M-543 (12 min.,
sound, color, 16 mm.), Media Resources
Branch, National Medical Audiovisual Center
(Annex), Station K, Atlanta, Ga. 30324. Shows
how nurses help prevent disease and promote
recovery from illness.
4. The problem of hookworm infection—M-157
(8 min., sound, color, 16 mm.), Media Resources Branch, National Medical Audiovisual
Center (Annex), Station K, Atlanta, Ga. 30324.
Emphasizes dangers of hookworm infection,
life cycle of worm, and conditions conducive
to infection.

References

1. Blake, Florence G., Wright, F. Howard, and
Waechter, Eugenia H.: Nursing care of children, ed. 8, Philadelphia, 1970, J. B. Lippincott Co.
2. Burdon, Kenneth L., and Williams, Robert F.:
Microbiology, ed. 6, New York, 1968, The
Macmillan Co.
3. Durand, Barbara A.: Helping retarded children, Bedside Nurse 2:19-22, July-Aug., 1969.
4. Johnston, Dorothy F.: Essentials of communicable disease, St. Louis, 1968, The C. V.
Mosby Co.
5. Meyer, Herbert L.: Predictable problems of
hospitalized adolescents, American Journal of
Nursing 69:525-528, March, 1969.
6. Morbidity and mortality weekly report 53,
year ending Dec. 28, 1974, Atlanta, 1975,
Center for Disease Control.
7. Palisin, Helen E.: Nursing care plans are a
snare and a delusion, American Journal of
Nursing 71:63-66, Jan., 1971.
8. Young, Clara G., and Barger, James D.:
Introduction to medical science, ed. 2, St.
Louis, 1973, The C. V. Mosby Co.

CHAPTER 2

How the body reacts to and combats disease

KEY WORDS

aerosol *atomized into a fine spray*
anaerobic *absence of O₂*
anaphylactic shock *immediate sensitivity to a foreign substance*
antibody *immune substance*
antigen *the body mfgs. antibodies against*
antitoxin *serum used to combat toxin*
attenuated *weaken*
capsule
carrier *carries the disease organism + doesn't get sick*
chemotherapy *Rx of disease w/drug*
cilia *hairlike projections*
endogenous *from in*
endotoxin *toxin released when cell disintegrates*
exogenous *from outside the body*
exotoxin *produced by bacteria*
exudate *pus + tissue fluids*
flagella *hairlike projections from a bacterial cell*

gangrene *necrosis of tissue*
gram-negative *color being removed*
gram-positive *or retained*
host *an organism from which another gains its nourishment*
immunity *resistance to a specific disease*
immunization *process of becoming immune*
leukocytosis *increased WBC*
live attenuated vaccine
macrophage *class of*
microphage *phagocyte*
noninfective vaccine
Pasteur treatment
phagocytosis *pathogens ingested + destroyed*
septicemia *bacteria + toxins in the bloodstream*
serum sickness
toxemia *presence of toxins in the blood*
urticaria
virulence *strength of an organism to produce disease*

MICROBIOLOGY AND PATHOLOGY

In Chapter 1 you were introduced to microorganisms that cause disease. Microbiology is the study of microbes. The microbiologist studies, identifies, and classifies microbes, good and bad, that exist in the environment. Pathology is the study of the changes that occur in humans and animals caused by microbes. When microbes invade the human body, they cause changes in the physiologic functioning of the body. The physician studies these changes and the symptoms they cause and is then able to establish a diagnosis and prescribe treatment. Thus the physician depends on both the microbiologist and the pathologist for information needed in the practice of medicine.

The study of bacteria has shown that they have many different characteristics. In addition to the three basic shapes, round, oblong, and spiral (Fig. 1-1), there are many variations of these shapes. Some may be elongated or have pointed ends, or they may be flattened on one side. Some are shaped like a comma, and others may appear square. Spirilla may be tightly coiled like a corkscrew. During cell division some remain together to form pairs, whereas others may form long chains. All of these modifications are important in identifying specific kinds of bacteria.

Bacteria may also have different chemical compositions, require different nutrients, and form different waste products. Some bacteria grow only in the presence of oxygen (aerobic), whereas others grow only in the absence of oxygen (anaerobic). Some bacteria are capable of movement. Their motility is possible because of fine

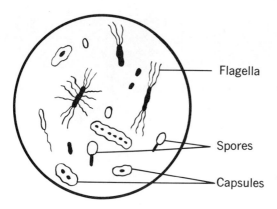

Fig. 2-1. Flagella, spores, and capsules.

hairlike projections (flagella) that arise from the bacterial cell (Fig. 2-1). These projections cause a wavelike motion that moves the cell along. A bacterium may have only one flagellum attached to one end of the cell, or there may be many flagella surrounding the cell. Locomotion of the spirochete is achieved by a wiggling motion involving the entire cell body.

Some bacteria form spores (Fig. 2-1). Certain conditions must be present for sporulation to take place. Spores may form in the presence or absence of oxygen. Depending on conditions, they may form in as short a time as 5 hours or as long as 13 hours. Only one spore forms in a single bacterium, and their formation appears to occur when conditions are unfavorable for growth of the bacterium. The spore is a round body that is formed by the bacterial cell. The body enlarges until it is as large as the bacterial cell and is surrounded by a capsule. Eventually the portion of the cell surrounding the spore distintegrates. Characteristically, spores have a high degree of resistance to heat and disinfectants (p. 48). They cannot be stained by the usual laboratory methods but require special staining techniques.

Some bacteria have the ability to form capsules about the cell wall. These mucilaginous envelopes seem to form when the bacterial environment is unfavorable; it is also believed that the formation may be defensive to protect the bacteria. Capsules may also occur when the invading organism is highly virulent. The composition of the capsule varies with the species of bacteria. However, they may be composed of protein substances, wax, or fat, and some contain nitrogen and phosphorus. As with spores, staining in the laboratory may require special procedures. When capsules are present, antibiotic therapy may be difficult because the capsule prevents the drug from reaching the bacteria within the capsule.

Many diseases cannot be diagnosed and properly treated until the specific microorganism causing the illness has been identified. Identification of microorganisms is made by specially trained laboratory personnel. Most bacteria cannot be seen until a special staining process has been done. In some instances examination may be done prior to staining, but usually this is less satisfactory. Staining is accomplished by the use of a dye, usually gentian violet and crystal ·violet applied to a specially prepared glass slide containing a small amount of the material to be examined. Most bacteria can be identified by this simple process; however, other bacteria require additional staining. Depending on whether a color can be removed by a solvent or if the color is retained after the use of the solvent, the organism is identified as being gram positive or gram negative. This identification is important in the treatment of the patient. The gram-positive bacteria are more sensitive to sulfonamides and penicillin than are the gram-negative bacteria. However, gram-positive and gram-negative bacteria may require different antibiotics for their destruction.[3, 11] Some bacteria are known as acid-fast bacteria, depending on the staining process. Special staining is required for bacteria having flagella, spores, or capsules.

As a member of the health team, the nurse is an extremely important person. The nurse is responsible for collecting many specimens for laboratory examination. Careful collection and prompt routing to the laboratory may avoid delay in the diagnosis and treatment of the patient.

BACTERIAL INVASION

Microorganisms enter the body by several routes, called *portals of entry,* and leave the body by *portals of exit.* Pathogenic organisms may enter the body by way of the (1) respiratory system, (2) digestive system, (3) urinary system, and (4) skin.

They may leave the body through discharges from the nose and throat, vomitus, feces, urine, and draining wounds. In addition, certain pathogenic organisms may be transferred from a donor's blood to that of a recipient through a blood transfusion, as in malaria and hepatitis B. Placental transfer of microorganisms to the fetus from the mother may occur such as in syphilis.

Endogenous infection may occur when microorganisms already present in the body produce disease because the normal defense mechanisms of the body break down or become weakened.

Exogenous infection results when pathogenic microorganisms gain entrance to the body from the outside.

Another way in which bacteria may harm the body is by the production of powerful poisons, or toxins. These toxins are classified as _endotoxins or exotoxins._ Endotoxins are present in the cells of the bacteria and cause damage to the body only when the cells disintegrate. Most endotoxins are contained in organisms that cause enteric diseases such as typhoid fever and bacillary dysentery. Exotoxins are produced by the bacteria outside the cell and are the most poisonous substances known to injure humans. Examples of diseases in which exotoxins are produced are diphtheria, tetanus, and botulism.

FACTORS INFLUENCING PATHOGENICITY

There are five factors that influence the ability of invading pathogens to survive and cause disease, that is, pathogenicity:
1. Whether the pathogens gain entrance by their characteristic route
2. Whether they have an affinity for only certain types of tissue
3. The degree of virulence
4. The number of pathogens that enter the body at a given time
5. The degree and character of resistance offered the invading pathogens by the host

Most bacteria enter the body by a specific route, and unless they are successful in gaining entrance by their characteristic route, they may not cause disease. Bacteria whose characteristic route is the respiratory system may be rendered harmless if they are swallowed.

Some pathogens have a particular affinity for certain types of tissue. Once they gain entrance to the body, they go directly to that tissue, leaving other tissues unaffected. The virus causing poliomyelitis attacks only nerve tissue; other pathogens attack only the respiratory system.

Pathogens vary in their power to invade the body and produce toxins. This factor is called _virulence_. Pathogens may be highly virulent, possessing great power of invasion, with the ability to produce deadly exotoxins. Others may be of low virulence and, although able to invade the body, are too weak to produce disease.

The occurrence of disease may depend on the number of pathogens that enter the body at a given time. If a large number of pathogens enter the body, disease is more likely to occur than if only a few invade the host. However, the presence of a few highly virulent pathogens may result in disease, whereas a large number of pathogens of low virulence may be destroyed without causing disease.

A final factor is the degree and character of resistance offered invading pathogens by the host. The human body has certain natural barriers against invasion of bacteria. The individual may also have an artificially acquired resistance to specific pathogens, which is called immunity.[6]

DEFENSES AGAINST BACTERIAL INVASION

Nature has provided the body with various defense mechanisms that limit microorganisms in their ability to invade the body and cause disease. There are certain external body defenses, which play a major role, and internal body defenses, about which there still is much to be learned. Immunity is another way in which the body may be prepared to ward off disease (p. 36).

External defenses. The first line of defense is the unbroken skin and the mucous membranes, which serve as mechanical barriers against invading pathogens. The intact skin protects the deeper tissues from injury and infection caused by bacteria. Many bacteria do not survive in an acid medium. Perspiration, the excretion of the sudoriferous (sweat) glands, has an average acid content on the skin of 5.65%; thus many bacteria die on the unbroken skin without invading the body. Lysozyme, an antibacterial enzyme present on the skin, dissolves some bacteria. This enzyme is also present in saliva and in tears.

The mucous membranes lining the respiratory tract, gastrointestinal tract, and urinary tract secrete substances that are bacteriostatic. The lacrimal fluid (tears) has the ability to destroy some microorganisms, and the secretions continuously bathe and wash foreign materials, including pathogens, from the eye. The high acid content of the stomach acts as a formidable barrier for pathogens that are swallowed. Any pathogens entering the intestines may be destroyed by certain enzymes secreted by the cells along the intestinal route. Vaginal secretions are normally acid, and pathogens entering the vagina are usually destroyed. Frequent vaginal irrigations will reduce the pH (acid) concentration of the vagina and thereby reduce the effectiveness of the natural barrier.

The nasal cavities, trachea, and bronchi contain fine hairlike projections called *cilia*, which are in constant wavelike motion. The cilia sweep pathogens toward the pharynx, where they may be swallowed or expectorated. If swallowed, they are destroyed by the stomach acids. The fine hairs about the external nares help prevent pathogens from entering, and if they do enter, they are trapped by the sticky mucus secreted by the cells lining the nasal cavities. The mouth has a high concentration of microorganisms. Many are swallowed and destroyed. Pathogens in the mouth usually do no harm as long as the mucous membrane remains intact. Involuntary acts also assist the body to rid itself of pathogens. Through these acts or reflexes, such as sneezing and coughing, pathogens may be eliminated from the respiratory tract. Vomiting and diarrhea eliminate bacteria and their toxins from the gastrointestinal system.[6]

Internal defenses (nonspecific). Internal body defenses against pathogens are less understood than are the external defenses. It is believed that the blood and body fluids such as the peritoneal fluid provide limited defense against bacteria. An important internal defense is called *phagocytosis.* In this process pathogens are ingested and destroyed by specific cells. (See following section.) Scientists believe that a serum protein called *properdin* in combination with other substances (properdin system) defends the body against certain bacteria and viruses.

Inflammation

The most common defense against bacteria is an inflammation reaction. Inflammation occurs when any agent, including a chemical substance, foreign body, severe blow, or bacteria, injures the tissue. The process of inflammation is characterized by five classic signs: redness, heat, pain, swelling, and limitation of movement. When pathogenic bacteria invade the tissue, a defensive process begins in which the body tries to localize or eliminate the injurious agent, to neutralize or destroy its poisons, and finally to repair the injured tissue[10] (Fig. 2-2). The inflammatory process begins with an increased flow of blood to the area. The tiny capillary blood vessels become dilated, allowing a larger amount of blood to pass through them. The leukocytes (white blood cells) have the power to move about, and they begin to migrate out of the capillaries to the area where the pathogen has invaded the tissue. Certain leukocytes, called phagocytes, begin to engulf and ingest the bacteria or foreign material. This process is called phagocytosis, meaning cell eating. There are two classes of phagocytes, the microphages, which ingest and carry away the bacteria, and the macrophages, which are large cells capable of ingesting dead tissue and cells. As the microphages ingest the bacteria, they carry it away by the blood and lymph streams. In the process some phagocytes are killed, some pathogens are destroyed, and some tissue is destroyed. The dead phagocytes, the pathogens and cells that have been destroyed, and some tissue fluid accumulate at the site. This is called the *exudate,* or pus. The characteristic heat and redness at the site are caused by the increased flow of blood to the area. The swelling results from the accumulation of exudate, and its pressure on the nerves in the area causes the pain. Depending on the location, any effort to move the part may be painful, causing the individual to limit

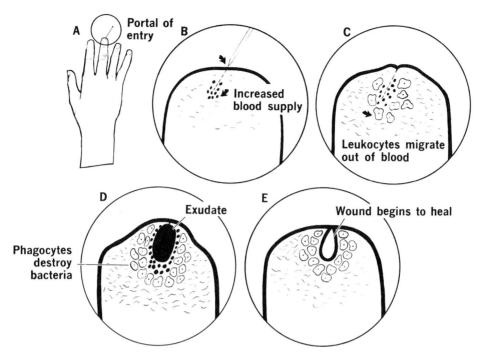

Fig. 2-2. Inflammatory process. **A,** Pathogenic bacteria are introduced into the tissue through a portal of entry such as a pinprick. **B,** Blood supply to the area begins to increase. **C,** Leukocytes begin to move out of the blood capillaries. **D,** Phagocytes begin to engulf and digest the bacteria, and dead phagocytes, cells, and tissue fluid escape as exudate. **E,** When phagocytosis is complete, the wound begins to heal.

movement to a minimum. When phagocytosis is complete, the inflammatory condition subsides and healing begins. (See Fig. 2-2.)

During the healing process new cells begin to fill in the injured area. When large numbers of body cells have been destroyed, they may be replaced in part by normal cells and in part by a fibrous type of tissue called scar tissue.

Sometimes the bacteria are picked up by the lymphatic vessels and carried to one or more of the lymph nodes. The lymph nodes are located at various places along the lymphatic channels and act as filters. If this occurs, leukocytes are brought into the lymph node to ingest and destroy the bacteria. The lymph node may then become swollen and tender because of the accumulation of destroyed tissue, phagocytes, and pathogens. If pathogens get into the bloodstream, the macrophages that are located in various organs throughout the body will ingest and destroy them, along with dead cells or other foreign material.[10] When macrophages enter the bloodstream, they are called monocytes.

The system by which this defensive process occurs, the destruction and removal of pathogens, is called the reticuloendothelial system. The system also plays a part in the development of immunity.

Infection

Some bacteria are powerful enough to resist the leukocytes and will destroy many of them, or the bacteria may produce powerful toxins that kill the leukocytes. If this occurs, the bacteria will cause disease, and their toxins will be carried by the bloodstream and lymphatic vessels to various parts of the body. The individual is then said to have an infection. The time factor is extremely important in an infection, since the longer the bacteria have to multiply the more severe the infection will be. The physician may order drugs that are bacteriostatic in action to be administered to the patient to prevent the rapid multiplication of the bacteria.

Infection is classified in a number of different ways, according to location, extent, and severity.

acute infection A severe infection that often runs a rapid course and may terminate quickly and fatally.

chronic infection An infection that develops slowly and extends over a period of weeks or months.

primary infection Original infection.

secondary infection Usually a complication of the primary infection. Bacteria causing a secondary infection may not always be the same as those causing the primary infection.

local infection An infection confined to a single area.

generalized infection An infection that spreads and involves the entire body.

focal infection An infection in which bacteria spread from the original site of the infection to other parts of the body.

latent infection A condition in which bacteria are still present in the body but are not active and do not cause any symptoms.

specific infection An infection caused by one kind of microorganism.

mixed infection An infection caused by more than one kind of microorganism.

When pathogenic microorganisms invade the body and cause inflammation or infection, they may give rise to certain symptoms or conditions. Following are some of the conditions with which the nurse should be familiar:

abscess A collection of pus in a cavity or a walled-off area surrounded by inflamed tissue.

bacteremia The presence of bacteria in the bloodstream.

gangrene Healing does not occur, and tissue dies.

necrosis The death of tissue or small groups of cells.

purulent discharge A discharge containing pus.

pyemia Pus in the bloodstream, causing multiple abscesses in various parts of the body.

sanguineous discharge Discharge containing blood.

septicemia The presence of bacteria and their toxins in the bloodstream.

serous discharge A clear thin discharge.

toxemia The absorption of bacterial toxins into the bloodstream.

Nursing care

Patients with infections and inflammatory conditions may have only minor discomfort from a local inflammation, or they may be seriously ill, and some infections may cause death. The treatment and nursing care depends on the kind of microorganism, the extent of involvement, and the effectiveness of the defense mechanisms of the body. The infection may be local, as in the case of a boil, it may involve an entire body system such as the respiratory system, or if there is a bloodstream infection, it may affect the entire body.

Local inflammatory conditions may be painful and may cause the patient considerable discomfort. The treatment and care of the patient is directed toward relieving the discomfort and terminating the inflammatory condition before it can affect other parts of the body. Treatment includes rest, elevation of the part affected, application of heat or cold, use of mild counterirritants, and occasionally incision and drainage.

It may be necessary for the patient to remain in bed to keep the affected part at rest. By elevating the part, the pain and throbbing will be relieved, bringing comfort to the patient. Elevation may be accomplished by the use of pillows, which for this purpose should have plastic covers. Elevation usually means raising the affected part above the level of the heart.

Moist or dry heat or cold may be used. Moist heat is in the form of warm moist compresses or hot wet dressings. The treatment may be continuous, or compresses may be applied at intervals for specified periods of time. An electric heating pad should not be used with wet dressings unless it is well insulated. Rubber covers are frequently used, since rubber is a poor conductor of electricity. The Aquamatic K pad described on p. 442 is one way to maintain a safe, constant temperature. Moist heat may also be applied by warm irrigations, soaks, or baths such as the sitz bath. If moist heat is applied to an extensive area of the body, a bathtub or whirlpool bath may be used. Solutions commonly used include physiologic saline solution, boric acid solution, and magnesium sulfate (Epsom salt) solution, or the physician may order an antiseptic solution. Dry heat is applied by a hot-water bottle, an electric pad, or a heat lamp. A hot-water bottle should always have a cover, and when it is applied to an extremity, it is better to place it alongside the extremity, since weight over a sensitive area may be uncomfortable. The nurse should be careful when applying any form of heat because of the danger of burning the patient.

Moist cold is applied in the form of cold compresses usually for short intervals at specified periods. Dry cold is provided by an ice bag. An uncovered ice bag should never be applied directly to the skin and should not be used to cover wet dressings because of danger of injury to the tissues.

In some conditions such as sprains or arthritis a liniment with counterirritant action may be ordered and is gently rubbed on the skin over the inflamed area.

When local inflammation does not respond to the methods of treatment just discussed, surgical incision may be required to provide for escape of the accumulated exudate.

Patients with generalized infection may be very ill. The temperature may be extremely high, with corresponding increase in the pulse and respiratory rates. The white blood cell count is increased (leukocytosis), and chills may occur, as well as loss of appetite, sweating, and delirium. The patient is usually confined to bed. The nurse must understand the physician's instructions concerning bed rest because in some cases the physician may allow bathroom privileges.

Acetylsalicylic acid (aspirin) and alcohol sponge baths may be given to lower the temperature. In some infections antibiotic or sulfonamide drugs may be given to assist the body in overcoming the infection. The skin should be kept clean by warm sponge baths. Because of the increased perspiration, an increased elimination of body wastes occurs through the skin. Special mouth care should be given several times a day or as indicated. A water-soluble jelly such as petroleum jelly may be used to lubricate the lips and nose to prevent dryness and crust formation. Fluid intake should be maintained to permit a daily urinary output of 1000 ml. for an adult, 500 ml. for a child, and 300 ml. for an infant. Careful records should be maintained, and if the output falls below the amount just indicated, the physician should be notified. Approximately 3000 ml. of fluid should be taken daily, with a corresponding decrease in the amount for children and infants.[10] If sufficient oral fluids are not taken, the physician may order fluids to be

administered intravenously. During the febrile period the diet should be liquid, followed by soft, easily digested foods and a gradual return to general diet.

Providing back rubs, a quiet well-ventilated room, and freedom from annoying disturbances will add to the patient's comfort. The nurse should be careful to see that young children and delirious patients are protected from injury. Since most patients generally feel ill, the number of visitors should be kept to a minimum.

Most patients with superficial or generalized infections caused by bacteria will be isolated. The nurse should be careful to maintain medical asepsis, with special attention to handwashing. (See Chapter 3.)

CHEMOTHERAPY

Chemotherapy means the treatment of disease with chemical drugs. Among these agents are the sulfonamide drugs. In the past the term *chemotherapy* did not apply to the antibiotic agents. Antibiotics consisted of substances produced in nature by certain microorganisms that had the capacity to destroy or retard growth of other microorganisms. Recently some of the antibiotics have been produced synthetically from chemicals. Therefore chemotherapy has been broadened to include some of the antibiotics. Some chemotherapeutic drugs are bacteriostatic and arrest the multiplication of pathogenic bacteria, whereas others are bactericidal in action and kill bacteria.

Sulfonamides. The sulfonamide drugs were the first chemotherapeutic agents to be discovered and came into use after 1935. Since that time, more than 6000 sulfonamides have been developed, but only about thirty are in use today. Those in use are generally effective in treating the diseases for which they are administered. All are highly toxic and may produce severe reactions. For this reason the antibiotics are often used rather than the sulfonamides, or they may be used in combination. With the development of new and improved antibiotics some sulfonamide agents are used to a limited extent. However, there are conditions in which the sulfonamides are the preferred treatment.[5]

Some sulfonamide drugs are especially effective against infections of the urinary tract and as a preventive against infection when long-term therapy is required. They may cause severe damage to the urinary tract by the formation of drug crystals in the kidneys, ureters, and bladder. When a patient is receiving a sulfonamide drug, he should be observed for evidence of hematuria or any decrease in urinary output. Fluid intake should be encouraged to provide from 1200 to 2000 ml. of urinary output in 24 hours.

Other sulfonamide drugs that are poorly absorbed are used to treat diseases of the intestinal tract. Some surgeons prescribe a sulfonamide agent or an antibiotic prior to intestinal surgery to limit the number of microorganisms present in the bowel and provide a form of sterilization. However, other surgeons doubt the value of the procedure and place emphasis on good aseptic surgical technique.[9]

In the treatment of some diseases sulfonamide drugs are useful because they diffuse easily into body fluids. Some diseases in which they are effective include meningitis, empyema, and rheumatic fever.

Some bacteria are known to become resistant to the sulfonamide agents. Therefore it is important to identify the specific

Table 2-1. Partial list of sulfonamide agents

Generic name	Trade name	Route of administration	Average dose	Toxic and/or side effects
Systemic use				
Sulfacetamide	Sulamyd	Oral and topical	Initial dose 4 Gm.; maintenance dose 1 Gm. q. 4 h.	Almost all sulfonamide drugs will cause toxic reactions such
Sulfadiazine	Pyrimal	Oral	2 to 4 Gm. daily	as the following if
Sulfadi- methoxine	Madribon Madriqid	Oral	Initial dose 1 Gm.; maintenance dose 0.5 Gm. daily	continued for long periods:
				1. Damage to urinary system and
Sulfamethizole	Thiosulfil	Oral	250 mg. daily	ultimately fatal
Sulfamethoxa- zole	Gantanol Azo Gantanol	Oral	Initial dose 2 Gm.; maintenance dose 1 Gm. t.i.d.	uremia 2. Nausea, vomiting, and headache in sensitive individ-
Sulfisomidine	Elkosin	Oral	Initial dose 3 Gm.; maintenance dose 1 to 1.5 Gm. q. 6 h.	uals 3. Urticaria and various skin erup-
Sulfisoxazole	Gantrisin Azo Gantrisin	Oral	Initial dose 4 Gm.; maintenance dose 1 Gm. q. 4 h.	tions 4. Central nervous system distur-
Acetyl sul- fisoxazole	Gantrisin acetyl	Oral	Initial dose 4 Gm. maintenance dose 1 to 2 Gm. q. 4 to 6 h.	bances, dizziness, vertigo 5. Blood dyscrasias
Intestinal use				6. Topical prepara- tions for eye, ear,
Phthalyl- sulfathiazole	Sulfathalidine	Oral	10 to 20 Gm. daily	skin may cause systemic reactions
Salicylazo- sulfapyridine	Azulfidine	Oral	4 to 8 Gm. daily adjusted to individual	
Succinyl- sulfathiazole	Sulfasuxidine	Oral	1 Gm. q. 4 h.	
Sulfamethoxy- pyridazine	Kynex Midicel	Oral	Initial dose 1 Gm.; maintenance dose 0.5 Gm. daily	

bacteria causing the disease so that the drug that will be most effective may be administered.

The nurse administering any of these drugs should adhere to the principles of promptness and accuracy. Patients should be observed carefully for signs of nausea, vomiting, dizziness, headache, cyanosis, or any signs of sensitivity such as sneezing, itching of the skin, or skin rash. Careful attention should be given to urinary output, since any decrease may indicate the formation of sulfonamide crystals in the kidney tubules. (See Table 2-1.)

Antibiotics. The development of antibiotic drugs began in 1928 when Alexander Fleming, a British bacteriologist, discovered a substance that he called *penicillin.* His findings were not immediately accepted, and it was not until about 1941 that the United States began intensive work in the development of penicillin. In the early days only penicillin and streptomycin were available, but today there are a large number of antibiotic agents. Some antibiotic drugs are effective against only gram-positive or gram-negative bacteria, whereas others are called broad-spectrum antibiotics because they are effective against both gram-positive and gram-negative bacteria. Although antibiotics have saved many lives, there still are many diseases for which they are not effective.

Penicillin is available in different forms and under a variety of trade names. The most common method of administering it is through intramuscular injection, but it may be given intravenously, orally, subcutaneously, or sublingually. It is also given as an aerosol inhalant and is used in ointments, lotions, and troches. Under usual conditions penicillin is nontoxic; however, in some patients allergic reactions may occur. These reactions vary from mild skin rashes to fatal anaphylactic shock. The nurse administering penicillin in any form should first be sure that the patient has had no previous reaction to it, and, second, should observe the patient carefully for several hours after administration of the drug. Reactions do not always develop immediately, and fatal reactions have occurred several hours after the drug has been given.

During the past few years a large number of semisynthetic penicillins have been developed. When bacteria are found to be resistant to penicillin, as in staphylococcus infections, the semisynthetic agents are often useful. Since a specific antibiotic may be ineffective against a particular organism, sensitivity tests are usually done, if possible, before any antibiotic is administered. By identifying the microorganism causing the illness, the physician can prescribe the most suitable antibiotic to cure the disease. (See Table 2-2.)

Corticosteroids. The corticosteroids are hormones produced by the adrenal cortex and include cortisone and hydrocortisone, commonly referred to as adrenal steroids. One adrenal gland is located above each kidney and is composed of two parts. The inner part is the medulla, and its primary secretion is epinephrine. The outer part is the cortex, which produces several substances, some of which are necessary for life. It also produces cortisone and hydrocortisone. When the adrenal glands are surgically removed because of disease or when they fail to function, hydrocortisone is administered to replace the normal secretion.

Cortisone is produced naturally from the bile of oxen and sheep, but scientists have developed synthetic corticosteroids. It was hoped that the synthetic products would eliminate some of the undesirable side effects and reduce the toxic reactions; however, most of the side effects remain.

The beneficial effects derived from corticosteroids are the relief of inflammation, reduction of fever, and production of a feeling of well-being. The latter is probably due to the relief of symptoms. For example, when cortisone is administered for an inflammatory condition, the classic signs of inflammation described on p. 28 may be absent. Patients receiving cortisone feel encouraged because of the absence of symptoms; however, cortisone used therapeutically does not cure disease or alter its course, and it does not reverse any preexisting damage such as crippling in arthritis.

The corticosteroids are powerful and dangerous drugs and have the potential of causing serious side effects. Most physicians prescribe these drugs extremely cautiously because of the toxic effects. The

Table 2-2. Partial list of antibiotic drugs

Generic name	Trade name	Route of administration	Average dose	Toxic and/or side effects
Natural penicillins				Urticaria, dermatitis, erythema, nausea, vomiting, diarrhea, and anaphylactic shock possible in persons hypersensitive to penicillin
Benzathine penicillin	Bicillin	IM	1.2 million units single dose	
	Permapen	IM		
Hydrabamine phenoxymethyl penicillin	Compocillin-V	Oral	200,000 to 600,000 q. 6 to 8 h.	
Potassium phenoxymethyl penicillin	Compocillin-VK	Oral	200,000 to 400,000 units 4 to 6 doses daily	
Potassium penicillin G	Pentids	Oral	Varies with sensitivity of organism	
		IM, IV	400,000 units daily	
	Pfizerpen G	Oral	200,000 to 250,000 units	
	Kesso-Pen	Oral	q. 6 to 8 h.	
Procaine penicillin G	Duracillin	IM	600,000 to 1 million units daily	
	Crysticillin	IM	600,000 to 1 million units daily	
Sodium penicillin G		IM	400,000 units daily	
		IV	10 million units daily	
Semisynthetic penicillins				In many instances dose varies with severity of disorder and sensitivity of invading organism
Ampicillin	Amcill-S	IM, IV	500 mg. q. 8 to 12 h.	
	Amcill	Oral	500 mg. t.i.d., dose varies	
	Penbritin	IM, IV	4 to 12 Gm. daily, varies with sensitivity of organism	
	Polycillin	Oral		
Methicillin	Staphcillin	IM, IV	1 to 2 Gm. q. 4 to 6 h.	
Nafcillin sodium	Unipen	Oral	250 to 500 mg. q. 4 to 6 h.	
		IV	500 mg. q. 4 h.	
		IM	500 mg. q. 6 h.	
Phenethicillin	Chemipen	Oral	125 to 250 mg. t.i.d.	
	Maxipen	Oral	250 to 500 mg. q. 4 to 6 h.	
	Syncillin	Oral	125 to 250 mg. t.i.d.	
Cloxacillin monohydrate sodium	Tegopen	Oral	500 mg. q. 6 h.	
		IV	500 mg. q. 4 h.	
Oxacillin sodium	Prostaphlin	Oral	250 to 500 mg. q. 4 to 6 h.	
Alternate to penicillin				Mild urticaria, jaundice, diarrhea, nausea, vomiting, overgrowth of bacteria or fungi
Erythromycin	Erythrocin	Oral	250 mg. q. 6 h.	
	Ilotycin	IV	1 to 2 Gm. daily	

Table 2-2. Partial list of antibiotic drugs—cont'd

Generic name	Trade name	Route of administration	Average dose	Toxic and/or side effects
Erythromycin estolate	Ilosone	Oral	1 to 2 Gm. daily	
Erythromycin ethylsuccinate	Pediamycin	Oral	400 mg. q. 6 h.	
Tetracycline and chloramphenicol agents				Broad-spectrum antibiotics; nausea, vomiting, and diarrhea may occur;
Chlortetracycline	Aureomycin	Oral	1 to 2 Gm. in divided doses	prolonged or overuse may cause damage to kidneys or liver
		Ophthalmic ointment		
Oxytetracycline	Terramycin	Oral	1 to 2 Gm. q.i.d.	
		IM	250 mg. daily	
		IV	250 to 500 mg. q. 12 h.	
Tetracycline	Achromycin	Oral	250 to 500 mg. q. 6 h.	
		IM	250 mg. daily	
		IV	500 mg. q. 6 to 12 h.	
Chloramphenicol	Chloromycetin	Oral	50 mg./kg. of body weight q.i.d.	Patient must be under close medical supervision because of toxic side effects; frequent blood studies required; nausea, vomiting, diarrhea, blood dyscrasias
		IV	50 mg./kg. of body weight at 6 h. intervals	
		Otic drops topical	2 to 3 drops in ear b.i.d. or t.i.d.	

drug is usually started with minute doses gradually increasing to the desired amount. Abrupt withdrawal is avoided by a gradual decrease in the dose.

When hospitalized patients are receiving any of the corticosteroid preparations, nurses have a grave responsibility. The dose must be accurate, and the patient must be carefully observed for undesirable or toxic effects. When a patient is admitted to the hospital, the nurse must know if he has been receiving cortisone because any abrupt withdrawal of the drug may be serious. When a patient is transferred from one clinical unit to another, care must be exercised to see that the medication order is clearly understood. A patient may be discharged home while receiving cortisone, and the nurse must be sure that the patient understands the physician's orders. If the drug is to be decreased, the patient should be told and should understand why and exactly how it is to be done. Any patient receiving cortisone must remain under his physician's care.[10] All patients are not suitable candidates for corticosteroid therapy. Some of the conditions in which steroids are contraindicated follow as well as some of the toxic and side effects. (See Table 2-3.)

Toxic and side effects
1. Headache and dizziness
2. Increase in blood pressure
3. Moon face, increased sweating, and growth of hair on the face
4. Gain in weight
5. Purpura, thrombophlebitis, and embolism
6. Depression, psychic disturbances, and convulsions

Table 2-3. Partial list of corticosteroid preparations

Generic name	Trade name	Route of administration	Average dose	Toxic and/or side effects
Natural steroids				Side effects from oral or parenteral administration are essentially the same:
Cortisone acetate	Cortogen acetate	Oral	All doses of steroids must be planned and carefully supervised for the individual patient	1. Hypertension
	Cortone	Parenterally Ophthalmic ointment		2. Potassium and calcium retention
Hydrocortisone	Cortef	Oral, IM, IV		3. Fluid and sodium retention
	Cortril Hydrocortone	Topical		4. Hyperacidity and peptic ulcer
Hydrocortisone acetate	Cortef acetate	Ophthalmic		5. Masking infection
	Cortril acetate	Intra-articular		6. Weakness of involuntary muscles
Hydrocortisone sodium succinate	Solu-Cortef	IV		7. Adrenocortical insufficiency
Synthetic steroids				Side effects are essentially the same as for natural steroids; toxic effects from prolonged administration of steroids:
Prednisone	Meticorten Deltasone	Oral		1. Cushing's syndrome
Prednisolone	Delta-Cortef	Oral		2. Moon face
	Meticortelone	Topical		3. Acne
Triamcinolone	Aristocort Kenacort	Oral		4. Electrolyte imbalance
Triamcinolone acetonide	Aristocort Kenalog	Oral		5. Hyperglycemia
				6. Osteoporosis
				7. Spontaneous fractures
				8. Purpura
				9. Hypertension
				10. Convulsions

7. Muscle weakness and loss of sleep
8. Increase in blood sugar and worsening of diabetes
9. Sodium retention and potassium excretion
10. Increase in leukocytes
11. Disturbance of menstruation

Contraindications
1. A history of tuberculosis, diabetes, and hypertension
2. Severe coronary disease
3. Nephritis or any condition in which the kidneys fail to function adequately

4. Some fungus diseases and most diseases characterized by skin eruptions
5. Myasthenia gravis *muscle weakness*
6. Peptic ulcer
7. Thrombophlebitis
8. Pregnancy
9. Severe emotional disturbance or psychoses
10. Osteoporosis *porous bone*

IMMUNITY

"The word 'immunity' refers to the presence of specific antibodies in the blood and tissues of an individual and to their activity in the prevention or modification of an infectious disease."* There is no such thing as absolute immunity to any specific disease to which humans are susceptible. It is a relative term and indicates degree. The degree of resistance to a certain disease may vary from person to person and may vary within the same person at different times. Immunity is the result of several chemical processes that take place within the body.

Previous reference was made to the cells of the reticuloendothelial system and their function in destruction of pathogens (p. 29). Every microorganism has within itself a substance called an _antigen_. When a microorganism invades the body, its antigen stimulates the body cells to produce certain chemical compounds called _antibodies._ Exactly how the cells of the reticuloendothelial system function in antibody production is not clearly understood. However, it is believed that the antigen of the microorganism stimulates the cells to produce antibodies. The introduction of the antigen by having a disease or by the inoculation of either live or dead antigenic substances is necessary to stimulate the cells to activity. The antibodies are formed in the liver, spleen, bone marrow, and other organs and are carried by the blood and lymph. The antibodies destroy the toxins of the microorganism and render them incapable of harm. Antigens differ from each other in their chemical structure, and antibodies are highly selective. A specific antigen stimulates the body to produce a specific antibody that has little if any effect in protecting a person from disease caused by another microorganism. There are several means by which immunity may be produced. In general, it may be natural or acquired.

Natural immunity

Most newborn infants have a natural immunity. Antibodies from the mother cross the placental barrier and enter the fetal circulation. The immunity will be for those diseases to which the mother is immune, one exception being the pertussis

(whooping cough) antibody, which does not appear to cross the placental barrier. Immunity passed from the mother to the newborn infant is transitory and protects the infant during the first few months of life, the period when mortality from infectious disease is greatest. The period of time that the protection lasts is variable, usually ranging from 3 to 6 months, and the number of diseases resisted by natural immunity is limited.

Species immunity protects against many diseases to which humans are susceptible but are not transmitted to animals, even though contact may be close. A child with measles or pertussis may have close contact with household pets such as cats and dogs, but the animals do not contract the disease. Likewise, most diseases of animals are not transmitted to humans.

Racial and group immunity has been observed in the same species. From studies, it appears that certain races of people are more immune to certain diseases than others are. For example, the black race seems to be more immune to malaria, yellow fever, and poliomyelitis than the white race is. Persons of Jewish ancestry are considered to be more immune to tuberculosis.

Acquired immunity

Immunity acquired during a person's lifetime is called acquired immunity. It may be acquired in several ways: by having an attack of the disease, by carrying the microorganism without becoming ill, and through artificial means.

Active immunity acquired by having the disease is the most durable kind of immunity and usually lasts the person's lifetime. However, by having the disease, the person runs the risk of severe or even fatal complications. Once the microorganism enters the body, its antigen stimulates the production of antibodies. If the person recovers and subsequent exposure to the same disease occurs, the cells will immediately manufacture additional antibodies. In most cases the resistance is great enough to protect the person from a recurrence of the specific disease.

A person may recover from a disease, thereby being immune to it, but continue to harbor the microorganisms. Or the indi-

---

*From Ager, Ernest A.: Immunization as practiced today, American Journal of Nursing 62:74-79, May, 1962.

vidual may never actually have symptoms of the disease, and apparently be immune to it but may harbor the pathogenic organisms and be capable of transmitting the disease to other persons. Such persons are called "carriers." Carriers are dangerous persons in any community because they are unaware of the condition, and their detection by public health personnel may be extremely difficult.

Artificially acquired immunity results from the injection into the body of a vaccine or serum containing the antigen of the microorganism. This type of acquired immunity may be either active or passive. All vaccines are antigens, but not all antigens are vaccines. There are a great many antigenic substances; vaccines are only one small group. Active immunity is acquired by the administration of a vaccine or toxoid. Vaccines may contain live organisms and are referred to as *live attenuated vaccines*, but the organisms have been weakened in such a way that they do not cause disease. Other vaccines contain organisms that have been killed by heat or chemicals. These are called *noninfective vaccines*.

Toxoids may be administered to produce active immunity. The toxoid contains the toxin produced by the organism, but the toxin has been rendered harmless. There are two kinds of toxoid, one in which formalin has been used to detoxify the toxin. The other preparation is absorbed toxoid, a toxoid that has been precipitated by adding potassium alum. This preparation is known as *alum-precipitated toxoid*.

Vaccines are administered before the person has the disease or before exposure to the disease has occurred. Immunity acquired by the injection of a vaccine is less durable than immunity acquired by having the disease; however, it usually lasts several years. Booster doses must be given at intervals to maintain immunity acquired in this manner.

Until 1957 the nervous tissue Semple type of vaccine was the only rabies vaccine available. It was administered after exposure because during the long incubation period for rabies a passive immunity may be established to prevent the disease from developing. This postexposure treatment is known as the *Pasteur treatment* (p. 4).

In 1957 a new kind of vaccine known as *duck embryo vaccine* became available. It is prepared from duck eggs that have been infected with the rabies virus, which is then inactivated. Preexposure vaccine consists of two 1 ml. injections of duck embryo vaccine subcutaneously in the deltoid muscle 1 month apart. A third dose is given 6 to 7 months after the second dose.[7, 8] Preexposure immunization is recommended for all high-risk groups such as veterinarians, dog wardens, forest rangers, and some laboratory workers. Duck embryo vaccine is also used for postexposure immunization to produce a passive immunity.

The administration of vaccines for active immunity should be started early in life. Many young children die every year from infectious diseases or their complications. Many who do not die are left with defects handicapping them throughout their lives. Primary immunization with a triple vaccine, consisting of diphtheria and tetanus toxoids and pertussis vaccine (DTP), should be started at 1½ to 2 months of age. Three doses are given 4 to 6 weeks apart. A fourth dose is given 1 year after the third injection. Children 3 through 6 years of age or entering school should be given one booster dose of DTP. After 6 years of age TD adult vaccine is administered.[7]

The trivalent oral polio vaccine (TOPV) should be started with the first DTP injection. The second dose should be given 6 to 8 weeks later, and the third dose 8 to 12 months after the second dose. One booster dose should be given when the child enters school.[7]

There are two strains of live attenuated measles virus vaccine: the Edmonston B strain and the Schwarz strain. Both require a single injection, and it is believed that this injection will produce immunity for several years and possibly for life. Approximately 30% of children receiving the Edmonston strain have a febrile reaction with elevated temperature and skin rash. The incidence of reaction is reduced by about one half when immunoglobulin is given at the same time as the vaccine. Edmonston B further attenuated vaccine may be given without immunoglobulin. When the Schwarz strain is administered without the immunoglobulin, only about 15% may suffer any reaction. It is recommended that measles vaccine be given at 1 year of age and that, if necessary, immunoglobulin be given to infants under 1 year to prevent or reduce the severity of measles. Early in 1971 two new vaccines were licensed: one "double vaccine" to protect against rubeola and German measles and a "triple vaccine" to protect against mumps as well as the two measles strains. Measles vaccine should not be administered to children who are sensitive to eggs. Contraindications for administration of measles virus vaccine include leukemia or other malignant disorders. Children whose resistance is low because of receiving steroid therapy, radiation, alkylating drugs, and antimetabolites should not be given the measles vaccine. Administration of the vaccine during pregnancy should be avoided.[7] The nurse may reassure parents that if mild symptoms occur, they are not serious and will subside without incident.

Administration of live mumps virus vaccine provides an active immunity against mumps. The vaccine is given in a single dose or as a triple vaccine after 1 year of age. The vaccine is prepared in chick embryo cell culture and therefore should not be given to persons sensitive to the proteins of eggs. Contraindications for its use are the same as for measles vaccine.

Live rubella virus vaccine provides active immunity against rubella (German measles). The vaccine is given in a single dose or as a double or triple vaccine after 1 year of age up to puberty. The vaccine should not be given to pregnant women or adolescent girls. It may be given to women of childbearing age only if pregnancy will be avoided for at least 2 months. It is recommended that priority be given to children of elementary school age and that adolescent and adult males be assigned a lower priority. It should not be given during febrile illnesses but postponed until recovery occurs. Other contraindications are the same as for measles and mumps. The label on the bottle should be read before administering the vaccine to determine the kind of cells from which the vaccine has been prepared. This is important to prevent sensitivity reactions in persons who may be hypersensitive to the particular type of cell used (p. 40).

No person is born immune to smallpox, and during severe epidemics young infants may contract the disease (p. 555).

Schedules for immunization of infants and young children may vary among physicians. The schedules presented in this book are those recommended by The Public Health Service Advisory Committee on Immunization Practices and the American Academy of Pediatrics, Report of the Committee on Infectious Disease.[7, 8] (See Chapter 23 for more information.)

Administration of vaccine. Disposable syringes and needles should be used, or the jet and hypospray may be used. The latter is most often used in mass immunization programs. Syringes and needles that are not disposable should be autoclaved, and multiple dose syringes should not be used. If the preparation being used contains alum or aluminum hydroxide, as in alum-precipitated toxoid, it should be given intramuscularly. In children under 3 years of age it should be placed in the gluteal muscle, and in children over 3 years of age it may be given in the deltoid muscle. Fluid toxoid or vaccines in a saline suspension may be given subcutaneously. When the skin is disinfected with alcohol, it should be allowed to dry before the puncture is made.[2] The nurse should refer to textbooks on basic nursing for the technique of intramuscular and subcutaneous injection.

The liquid Sabin oral poliovirus vaccine may be administered to infants by placing it on the tongue with a dropper. In older children it may be placed on a lump of sugar prior to ingestion.

Passive immunity. Passive immunity is acquired by injecting into the body a serum that produces an immediate but temporary immunity. It is useful in emergency prophylaxis and often in the treatment of specific diseases. In the case of a serum the antibodies are borrowed or are ready-made. Serums do not contain live or dead organisms or their toxins but consist of blood plasma with antibodies added. The immunity acquired is temporary and usually does not last longer than 3 weeks. Most serums are derived from animals, primarily horses. Because of the size of the horse, a larger number of antibodies can be produced.

Antitoxins. Antitoxins are serums that are anti, or against, the toxin that is produced by the particular microorganism infecting the body. Thus the administration of an antitoxin is for the purpose of neutralizing the poisons produced by pathogens and does not have any effect on the organism itself. Chemotherapeutic drugs may be given to the individual to destroy the organism. Examples of antitoxin serums include diphtheria antitoxin, tetanus antitoxin, antiplaque serum, and antisnake (antivenin) serum. Serums are sometimes derived from sources other than animals.

Immunoglobulin (Ig or gamma globulin). Immunoglobulin is a fraction of the plasma of human blood containing antibodies against certain diseases. It is occasionally used in treating or modifying measles in a nonimmune person. It may also be used to prevent infectious hepatitis in exposed persons. Other diseases for which it has been used include rubella, mumps, and poliomyelitis. It has been recommended that it be given at the same time that the Edmonston B strain of live attenuated measles virus vaccine is given to reduce the febrile reaction that may occur from the vaccine. Immunoglobulin is prepared in a sterile solution for subcutaneous or intramuscular injection.[4] It is never given intravenously. When it is administered to prevent disease, it produces only a passive immunity. Emphasis should be placed on active immunization to prevent those diseases for which vaccines are available.

Tests of immunity

Skin tests to determine the presence of circulating antibodies in an individual may be done by injecting a minute amount of the antigen into the skin of the forearm. If some degree of immunity is present, a localized skin reaction will occur within 24 to 48 hours. A large number of tests have been developed, but only a few are in use. Skin tests are also used to test the individual for sensitivity to foods, pollens, and various other substances believed to cause allergic reactions. (See Chapter 22.)

ALLERGY

Serum sickness. Serum sickness is an allergic manifestation due to foreign proteins. Allergy involves antigens and antibodies and is caused by a hypersensitivity in some persons, causing them to react unfavorably to certain substances that are harmless to most people. These substances include many items such as food, drugs, pollens, and horse dander (scales found on horsehair). Repeated exposure to these substances causes the individual to produce antibodies against them or to become sensitized. Serum sickness occurs when a person receives an injection of animal serum, usually horse serum. In some instances the individual may have had no previous experience with the serum, or he may have been sensitized from a previous injection of animal serum. About 10 to 14 days after the injection a delayed response occurs, which is characterized by some uncomfortable symptoms; it is generally uncomplicated and rarely serious, although intermittent recurrence of symptoms may continue in some persons for several weeks. Symptoms include headache, nausea, vomiting, fever, swollen painful joints, enlargement of lymph nodes and spleen, decrease in leukocytes, and a tendency toward bleeding. Serum sickness may occur in any person regardless of age, sex, state of health, or route of administration. Some evidence indicates that certain races (blacks and American Indians) may have less tendency to develop serum sickness.[12]

Serum sickness is usually self-limited, and little or no treatment is required. However, if urticaria is severe, several small injections of epinephrine may be given or one of the available antihistaminic drugs may be administered orally. Before administering any animal serum, intracutaneous skin tests should be done. It should also be realized that there may be a delayed reaction to the skin test, thus it may be desirable to wait 2 or 3 hours after the test to be certain of the results.

Anaphylaxis. The word *anaphylaxis* came into use in 1902 when it was used to describe a shock state that resulted after the injection of a foreign substance into dogs. However, anaphylaxis occurred and was known before the time of Christ. Anaphylaxis usually occurs in persons who have a high degree of sensitivity. Any substance foreign to the body is capable of causing anaphylactic shock in the hypersensitive individual. With the increasing number of new drugs, vaccines, booster doses, and food products containing various insecticides, the potential for severe reactions cannot be overlooked. The route of administration or the amount of antigen alone is not a factor in producing a reaction. Although the intravenous route is more likely to prove fatal, the subcutaneous route could be fatal to certain hypersensitive persons. It has been estimated that 20% of persons who receive penicillin therapy become sensitive to the drug.[12] Most reactions to penicillin are in the form of serum sickness or skin manifestations; however, fatal anaphylactic shock has occurred in some.

The symptoms of anaphylaxis usually begin rather quickly with a local skin reaction about the site of the injection, followed by itching of the scalp, severe respiratory symptoms, hypotension, weak rapid pulse, loss of consciousness, and death. Prompt treatment is necessary. Treatment includes administration of 0.5 to 1 ml. of epinephrine in a 1:1000 solution. Respiratory stimulants such as caffeine sodium benzoate or nikethamide (Coramine) should be given to elevate the blood pressure. The patient should be placed in the Trendelenburg position. A blood pressure cuff may be placed on the arm above the site of the injection and inflated to slow the absorption of the allergen. A mouth gag should be available.

The nurse should remember that hypersensitivity in individuals may create a serious emergency unless extreme care is taken. Persons should always be questioned concerning allergic reactions, and as a precautionary measure it is generally best to test the person before administering a serum. An intradermal skin test may be done on the forearm, or a drop of diluted serum may be placed in the conjunctival sac of the eye. Formation of a wheal on the forearm or redness and lacrimation of the eye indicates that the serum should not be given.[10]

Summary outline

1. Microbiology and pathology
   A. Bacteria—basic shapes
      1. Round
      2. Oblong
      3. Spiral
   B. Many variations of basic shapes
   C. Different chemical composition and different waste products
   D. Aerobic bacteria grow only in presence of oxygen; anaerobic bacteria grow only in absence of oxygen
   E. Motility accomplished by
      1. Flagella
      2. Wiggling motion of entire cell body
   F. Spores have high degree of resistance to heat and disinfectants
   G. Capsules prevent antibiotics from reaching bacteria
      1. Composition variable
   H. Staining bacteria for laboratory examination
      1. Gram-positive bacteria
      2. Gram-negative bacteria
      3. Special staining for presence of flagella, spores, or capsules
   I. Careful collection and prompt routing to laboratory important
2. Bacterial invasion
   A. Portals of entry
      1. Respiratory system
      2. Digestive system
      3. Urinary system
      4. Skin
   B. Portals of exit
      1. Discharges from nose and throat
      2. Vomitus
      3. Feces
      4. Urine
      5. Draining wounds
   C. Blood transfusion
   D. Placental transfer
   E. Endogenous infection—when microorganisms are already in body
   F. Exogenous infection—when microorganisms gain entrance to body from outside
   G. Endotoxins—toxins present in cell of organism released when cell distintegrates
   H. Exotoxins—toxins produced by bacteria outside cell
3. Factors influencing pathogenicity
   A. Whether pathogens gain entrance by their characteristic routes
   B. Whether they have affinity for only certain types of tissue
   C. Degree of virulence
   D. Number of pathogens that enter body at given time
   E. Degree and character of resistance, natural or acquired, offered invading pathogens by host
4. Defenses against bacterial invasion
   A. External defenses
      1. Unbroken skin mucous membranes
      2. Acid medium of skin and antibacterial enzymes
      3. Bacteriostatic substances secreted by mucous membranes lining respiratory tract, gastrointestinal tract, and urinary tract
      4. Lacrimal fluid, which destroys some pathogens and washes foreign material from eye
      5. High acid content of stomach, which acts as barrier to pathogens that are swallowed
      6. Certain enzymes may destroy pathogens that are swallowed and enter intestines
      7. Vaginal secretions, which are normally

acid and usually destroy pathogens that enter vagina

8. Fine hairlike projections (cilia) in nasal cavities, trachea, and bronchi that sweep pathogens toward pharynx, where they may be swallowed or expectorated
9. Fine hairs about external nares that help prevent pathogens from entering and sticky mucus secreted by cells, which traps those that do enter
10. Involuntary or reflex acts that help rid body of pathogens
   a. Sneezing and coughing
   b. Vomiting and diarrhea

B. Internal defenses
1. Less understood
2. Blood and some body fluids provide limited defense
3. Phagocytosis
4. Properdin (serum protein) with other substances defends against certain pathogens

C. Inflammation, most common defense against bacteria
1. Signs
   a. Redness and heat due to increased supply of blood to area
   b. Swelling due to accumulation of exudate
   c. Pain due to pressure on nerves
   d. Limitation of movement due to pain
2. Phagocytes engulf and destroy bacteria; phagocytosis means cell eating
3. Classes of phagocytes
   a. Microphages, which ingest and carry away bacteria
   b. Macrophages, large cells that ingest dead tissue and cells
4. Exudate, or pus, which is accumulation of dead phagocytes, pathogens, tissue cells, and some tissue fluid
5. After phagocytosis is completed, healing begins
   a. Growth of new cells fills in injured area
   b. Replacement by fibrous tissue called scar tissue occurs when large number of cells are destroyed
6. Bacteria sometimes picked up by lymphatic vessels and carried to one or more lymph nodes
   a. Leukocytes brought in to ingest and destroy bacteria
   b. Lymph node may be swollen and tender
7. Pathogens may get into bloodstream, where macrophages ingest and destroy pathogens; macrophages in bloodstream called monocytes

D. Infection
Occurs when bacteria powerful enough to resist leukocytes or their powerful toxins kill leukocytes
1. The longer bacteria have to multiply the more severe infection will be
2. Bacteriostatic drugs sometimes admin-

istered to prevent rapid multiplication of pathogens
3. Classification
   a. Acute infection
   b. Chronic infection
   c. Primary infection
   d. Secondary infection
   e. Local infection
   f. Generalized infection
   g. Focal infection
   h. Latent infection
   i. Specific infection
   j. Mixed infection
4. Conditions that may occur when microorganisms invade body
   a. Abscess formation
   b. Bacteremia—bacteria in bloodstream
   c. Gangrene—follows death of tissue
   d. Necrosis—death of tissue
   e. Purulent discharge—discharge containing pus
   f. Pyemia—pus in bloodstream
   g. Sanguineous discharge—discharge containing blood
   h. Septicemia—bacteria and their toxins in bloodstream
   i. Serous discharge—clear thin discharge
   j. Toxemia—bacterial toxins in bloodstream

E. Nursing care
1. Patient may have minor discomfort, be seriously ill, or fatally ill
2. Treatment and nursing care depend on microorganism, extent of involvement, and body defenses
3. Treatment and care directed toward relieving discomfort and terminating inflammatory condition
4. Treatment and care of local inflammatory conditions
   a. Rest
   b. Elevation of part affected
   c. Dry or moist heat
   d. Dry or moist cold
   e. Use of mild counterirritants
   f. Surgical incision and drainage
5. Generalized infection
   a. Symptoms—fever, increased pulse and respiratory rates, leukocytosis, chills, loss of appetite, sweating, and delirium
   b. Nursing care
      (1) Bed rest
      (2) Aspirin, alcohol baths for fever
      (3) Warm cleansing baths
      (4) Special mouth care, lubricant for lips
      (5) Urinary output should be 1000 ml. for adult, 500 ml. for child, and 300 ml. for infant
      (6) Intake of 3000 ml. in 24 hours for adult
      (7) Liquid diet
      (8) Back rubs, quiet, well-ventilated room
      (9) Protect from injury in delirium

(10) Infections caused by some bacteria are isolated

(11) Special attention to handwashing

5. Chemotherapy
   A. Treatment of disease with chemical drugs
   B. Chemotherapy applies to sulfonamide drugs and some antibiotics
   C. Sulfonamides
      1. Sulfonamide drugs came into use after 1935; all are highly toxic and may produce severe reactions
      2. Antibiotics often used in place of sulfonamide drugs
      3. Some effective against urinary tract infections and as preventive when long-term therapy required
      4. May cause drug crystals in kidneys, ureters, and bladder
         a. Observe for hematuria and decrease in urinary output
         b. Fluid intake 1200 to 2000 ml. in 24 hours
      5. Poorly absorbed sulfonamides used to treat diseases of gastrointestinal tract may be prescribed preoperatively for surgery on the intestines
      6. Sulfonamide drugs that dissolve readily in body fluids are used to treat meningitis, empyema, and rheumatic fever
      7. Specific bacteria should be identified so that most effective sulfonamide drug can be administered
   D. Antibiotics—development began in 1928
      1. Some effective only against certain kinds of bacteria: some are broad spectrum—effective against several kinds of bacteria
      2. Administered by many routes—intravenously, intramuscularly, subcutaneously, orally, sublingually, as aerosol inhalants, and in ointments, lotions, and troches
      3. May produce severe and fatal reactions in some individuals
      4. Many semisynthetic penicillins have been developed
      5. Semisynthetic penicillin useful in staphylococcal infections
      6. Sensitivity tests should be done to identify specific microorganism
   E. Corticosteroids—hormones produced by adrenal cortex (adrenal steroids); include cortisone and hydrocortisone
      1. Produced naturally and synthetically
      2. Beneficial effects
         a. Relieve inflammation
         b. Reduce fever
         c. Produce feeling of well-being
      3. Do not cure or alter course of disease
      4. Have serious toxic and side effects
      5. Nursing responsibilities
         a. Accuracy of dose
         b. Careful observation for side effects or toxic reactions
         c. Instruction of patient
      6. Contraindications

6. Immunity
   Refers to specific antibodies in blood and tissues and to their activity in prevention or modification of infectious disease
   A. Immunity—is relative; no such thing as absolute immunity, only indicates degree
   B. Immunity is result of several chemical processes that take place in body
   C. Microorganisms contain substance called *antigen;* when pathogen invades body, antigen stimulates body cells to produce chemical compounds called *antibodies*
   D. Antibodies destroy toxins of microorganism
   E. Specific antigens stimulate body cells to produce specific antibodies
   F. Ways in which immunity may be produced
      1. Natural immunity
         a. Passed from mother to fetus in utero, with exception of pertussis; this type of immunity temporary, lasting only 3 to 6 months
         b. Species immunity—diseases to which humans are susceptible are not transmitted to animals; most diseases of animals not transmitted to humans
         c. Racial and group immunity observed in same species; blacks more immune to malaria, yellow fever, and poliomyelitis; those of Jewish ancestry appear more immune to tuberculosis
      2. Acquired immunity
         a. Produced by having an attack of disease
         b. Produced by carrying organism, but having no symptoms
         c. Produced artificially by injections of vaccines, toxoids, or serums
            (1) Injection of vaccine, toxoid, or serum can produce active or passive immunity
            (2) Live attenuated vaccines
            (3) Noninfective vaccines
            (4) Toxoid contains toxins that develop in disease, with the poisonous properties eliminated
            (5) Vaccines usually administered prior to exposure
            (6) Rabies vaccine
               (a) Semple type *Pasteur treatment* postexposure
               (b) Duck embryo vaccine preexposure and postexposure; recommended for high-risk groups
            (7) Vaccines for active immunity should be administered early in life
            (8) Triple vaccine consists of diphtheria and tetanus toxoids and pertussis vaccine (DTP)
            (9) Sabin live oral attenuated poliovirus vaccine (TOPV) administered at same time as (DTP)
            (10) Live attenuated measles virus vaccine
               (a) Edmonston B strain
               (b) Schwarz strain

(c) Administer at 1 year of age
(d) Administer immunoglobulin with Edmonston B strain
(e) Double vaccine
(f) Triple vaccine
(g) Contraindications
(11) Live mumps virus vaccine
  (a) Give after 1 year of age
  (b) Contraindications same as in measles
(12) Live rubella virus vaccine
  (a) Administer from 1 year to puberty
  (b) Not to be given to pregnant women or adolescent girls
  (c) If given to childbearing women, pregnancy must be avoided for 2 months
  (d) Recommended for elementary school-age children
  (e) Should not be given during febrile illness
  (f) Contraindicated as in measles
  (g) Label on bottle should be read for contents to avoid sensitivity reactions
(13) No person immune to smallpox
d. Administration of vaccine
(1) Use disposable syringes and needles
(2) If needles and syringes are not disposable, they should be autoclaved
(3) Preparations containing alum or aluminum hydroxide should be given intramuscularly
  (a) In children under 3 years give in gluteal muscle
  (b) In children over 3 years in deltoid muscle
(4) Give fluid toxoids or vaccines subcutaneously
(5) TOPV dropped on infant's tongue or placed on lump of sugar for older children
e. Passive immunity—acquired by injecting a serum into body
(1) Serum—blood plasma with antibodies
(2) Immunity temporary, lasting about 3 weeks
(3) Serums derived from animals, usually horses
f. Antitoxins are serums
(1) Neutralize toxin that is produced by pathogen; do not affect pathogen
(2) Chemotherapeutic drugs may be given to destroy pathogen
(3) Antitoxin serums include diphtheria antitoxin, tetanus antitoxin, antiplague serum, and antivenin serum

g. Immunoglobulin—fraction of plasma of human blood
(1) Contains antibodies against some diseases
(2) May be used to prevent or modify some diseases
(3) Given with Edmonston B type measles vaccine
(4) Given intramuscularly or subcutaneously, never intravenously
(5) Produces passive immunity
3. Tests of immunity
Performed to determine presence of circulating antibodies
a. Many tests developed, few in use
b. Skin tests to determine sensitivity to foods, pollens, and other substances
7. Allergy
A. Serum sickness—allergic response to foreign proteins
1. Delayed response occurs in 10 to 14 days after last injection
2. Symptoms self-limiting, rarely serious
3. May occur in any person—age, sex, state of health, or route of administration not factors
4. Blacks and American Indians have less tendency to serum sickness
5. Treatment may include epinephrine or antihistaminic drugs
6. Skin test should precede administration of serum
B. Anaphylaxis
1. May occur in person with high degree of sensitivity
2. Any substance foreign to body capable of causing anaphylaxis
3. Intravenous injection more likely to be fatal
4. Sensitivity to penicillin may cause
a. Serum sickness
b. Skin rash
c. Death
5. Symptoms begin quickly
6. Prompt treatment necessary
a. Give epinephrine, 0.5 to 1 ml. in 1:1000 solution, immediately; place patient in Trendelenburg position; give caffeine sodium benzoate or nikethamide (Coramine) to elevate blood pressure; blood pressure cuff may be applied above site of injection and inflated enough to occlude arterial pressure; mouth gag should be available
b. Reactions may be prevented by questioning patients concerning allergic reactions
7. Tests for sensitivity
a. Place minute amount of diluted serum just under skin on forearm; sensitivity indicated by formation of wheal
b. Place drop of diluted serum in conjunctival sac; within 10 to 20 minutes eye will become red and watery if individual is sensitive

Review questions

1. Name two methods of identifying bacteria based on their retention or removal of a stain.
   a. *gram negative*
   b. *" positive*

2. What attachment(s) to bacteria enable them to be capable of movement?
   a. *cilia flagella*

3. Name two diseases that may be caused by endotoxins.
   a. *typhoid fever*
   b. *bacillary dysentery* } *enteric diseases (intestinal tract)*

4. List three ways by which active immunity may be acquired.
   a. *natural - to fetus from mother*
   b. *by having the disease - (active)*
   c. *vaccine or serum (passive)*

5. List four diseases for which immunization may be started at 1½ to 2 months of age.
   a. *diphtheria   smallpox*
   b. *tetanus*
   c. *pertussis*
   d. *polio*

6. List three additional diseases for which a child should be immunized.
   a. *measles - rubeola*
   b. *German measles - rubella*
   c. *mumps*

7. What are three beneficial effects of corticosteroids?
   a. *relief of inflammation*
   b. *reduction of fever*
   c. *feeling of well being*

8. How do immunoglobulins (Ig) differ from vaccines?

9. What toxic effects should the nurse watch for after administering penicillin?
   a. *skin rash*
   b. *hives - (urticaria)*
   c. *nausea*
   d. *anaphylactic shock*

10. By what route would you administer a sulfonamide drug?
    a. *orally*

Films

1. Defense against invasion—Mis-038 (10 min., sound, color, 16 mm.), Media Resources Branch, National Medical Audiovisual Center (Annex), Station K, Atlanta, Ga. 30324. Describes principles of immunization by representing the human body as the theater of mechanized warfare.

2. Right from the start—Mis-752 (23 min., sound, color, 16 mm.), Media Resources Branch, National Medical Audiovisual Center (Annex), Station K, Atlanta, Ga. 30324. Dramatizes two of the most common deterrents to immunization of children: ignorance and procrastination.

3. Reprieve from lethal infection (18 min., sound, color, 16 mm.), Ayerst Laboratories, 685 3rd Ave., New York, N. Y. 10017. Deals with the rising mortality rate from bacterial infection and shows how the trend can be reversed.

4. Staining blood films for detection of malaria parasites—M-1432 (7 min., sound, color, 16 mm.), Media Resources Branch, National Medical Audiovisual Center (Annex), Station K, Atlanta, Ga. 30324. Shows steps in staining blood films with Giemsa stain to demonstrate maximum details of blood parasites.

5. Antibiotics: curative drugs—T-1316X (60 min., sound, black and white, 16 mm.), Media Resources Branch, National Medical Audiovisual Center (Annex), Station K, Atlanta, Ga. 30324. Describes history and development of antibiotic drugs, penicillin and streptomycin. Reviews the effectiveness in reducing severity, recovery time, and complications associated with specific diseases. Reviews misconceptions and abuse of antibiotics.

References

1. Ager, Ernest A.: Immunization as practiced today, American Journal of Nursing 62:74-79, May, 1962.
2. Arena, Jay M., editor: The complete pediatrician, ed. 9, Philadelphia, 1969, Lea & Febiger.
3. Baker, Brian H.: Medical bacteriology—an introduction to bacteria, Bedside Nurse 5: 24-27, Feb., 1972.
4. Bergersen, Betty S.: Pharmacology in nursing, ed. 13, St. Louis, 1976, The C. V. Mosby Co.
5. Burdon, Kenneth L., and Williams, Robert F.: Microbiology, ed. 6, New York, 1968, The Macmillan Co.
6. Memmler, Ruth L.: The human body in health and disease, ed. 3, Philadelphia, 1970, The Macmillan Co.
7. Morbidity and mortality weekly report 25, week ending June 24, 1972, ACIP Recommendations 1972, Atlanta, 1972, Center for Disease Control.
8. New immunization schedule issued by AAP, American Journal of Nursing 73:1252, July, 1973.
9. Rodman, Morton J., and Smith, Dorothy W.: Pharmacology and drug therapy in nursing, Philadelphia, 1968, J. B. Lippincott Co.
10. Shafer, Kathleen N., Sawyer, Janet R., McCluskey, Audrey M., Beck, Edna L., and Phipps, Wilma J.: Medical-surgical nursing, ed. 6, St. Louis, 1975, The C. V. Mosby Co.
11. Smith, Alice L.: Microbiology and pathology, ed. 11, St. Louis, 1976, The C. V. Mosby Co.
12. Weiser, Russell S., Myrvik, Quentin N., and Pearsall, Nancy N.: Fundamentals of immunology, Philadelphia, 1969, Lea & Febiger.

CHAPTER 3

Asepsis and disinfection

KEY WORDS

antiseptic
asepsis
autoclave
bactericidal
bacteriostat
contamination
cross infection
disinfectant
ethylene oxide
germicide
iodophors
ophthalmia
  neonatorum
permeable
sterilization
surgical scrub
toxicity
vegetative bacteria

(handwritten annotations: antiseptic — agent that retards the growth of bacteria; asepsis — freedom from pathogenic organisms; autoclave — steam pressure sterilizer; bactericidal — an agent that kills bacteria; bacteriostat — prevents multiplication of bacteria; germicide — an agent that destroys bacteria; iodophors — iodine combined c̄ another agent — antiseptic or disinfectant; ophthalmia neonatorum — newborn eye infection c̄ gonococcus; permeable — able to penetrate; sterilization — destruction of pathogenic organisms; surgical scrub — pre op scrub; toxicity — being poisonous; vegetative bacteria — bacteria that do not form spores; ethylene oxide — a gas used to sterilize surgical supplies & equipment)

ASEPSIS

The work of Louis Pasteur and Joseph Lister ushered in a new era of surgery; in fact, Joseph Lister has been considered the "father of antiseptic surgery." (See Chapter 1.) Although modern science has progressed far since Lister, the basic principle of asepsis is unchanged. Asepsis is a condition in which there is complete absence of germs. Asepsis is absolute; there is no compromise or modification. The nurse will encounter many situations on the clinical unit that require aseptic technique such as catheterization or changing surgical dressings. The slightest error may mean prolonged illness or hospitalization for the patient. Repeatedly throughout this book the nurse will be referred to conditions and procedures in patient care in which asepsis must be employed. This chapter is designed to familiarize the nurse with the methods used to achieve asepsis and the variables that determine the effectiveness or ineffectiveness of the method employed. In general, asepsis is divided into two categories: (1) medical asepsis and (2) surgical asepsis. The basic principles are the same, that is, to prevent the spread and cause the destruction of pathogenic microorganisms.

Medical asepsis. Medical asepsis is employed when a patient is isolated (p. 542). The objective is (1) to confine all pathogens to a given area, thus preventing their spread to other persons and (2) to prevent pathogens from the outside from being carried to the patient in the isolated unit. In other words, the environment both inside and outside the isolated unit must be protected. To accomplish this all infectious material must be destroyed as soon as it leaves the patient. It means that all nurses who enter a contaminated area understand how to protect themselves and the environment outside the unit and how to avoid carrying pathogens into the unit. Medical asepsis does not require that equipment coming in contact with the patient be sterile, but it does require that it be clean and as free from pathogenic organisms as possible. Medical asepsis involves the use of various methods of disinfection, and in conditions in which spores are present, sterilization by autoclaving is necessary (p. 48). The hospital should have a written policy for carrying out medical asepsis, and the nurse should be familiar with the policy. Patients entering the hospital have a right to be protected from infection, and protection of patients rests largely with nurses. When medical asepsis is not properly adhered to and other patients become infected, the result is called cross infection. (See Chapter 23.)

Surgical asepsis. In surgical asepsis any object that comes in contact with a wound must be absolutely free of pathogenic organisms to prevent all contaminants from entering the area of operation or any wound. In surgical asepsis the patient is protected from the environment, whereas in medical asepsis the environment is protected from the patient. Surgical asepsis may be accomplished through various methods of sterilization. Procedures in operating rooms are carried out under strict surgical asepsis. This involves preparation of the patient's skin and sterilization of all instruments, linens, dressings, or other materials coming in contact with the wound. It includes special attire for the surgeon and assistants. Surgical asepsis also includes proper cleaning and disinfecting of all inanimate objects in the room and maintaining proper temperature and humidity and may include sterilization of the air.

The nurse will encounter many situations on the clinical units or in the home that require surgical aseptic technique. Sterile technique is the same as aseptic technique. The nurse will use surgical aseptic technique when administering a hypodermic injection to a patient. This technique includes washing hands, using a sterile syringe and needle, and disinfecting the patient's skin before inserting the needle. In medical asepsis and surgical asepsis various antiseptics and disinfectants may

be used for the purpose of sterilization. Several factors determine the type of disinfectant to be used and the method of use. The nurse should know the factors that determine the usefulness of the various substances used.

ANTISEPTICS AND DISINFECTANTS

antiseptic An agent that inhibits, retards, or kills pathogenic microorganisms.
disinfectant Any process that, when applied to inanimate objects, will destroy microorganisms; usually a chemical, may also be an antiseptic.
germicide Any agent that will destroy microorganisms.

Because of mass means of advertising, the public is constantly being confronted with many different disinfectants for personal and household use, with claims that each product is superior to all the others. Such preparations are often left within the reach of small children who are poisoned by them. Because of the advertising claims made for these products, the public often overrates their germ-killing power. Basically, most disinfectants are the same, with limited modifications. The hospital nurse may be confused when constantly confronted with new and different disinfectants. Two points should be kept in mind. First, there is no disinfectant effective for all purposes. Second, disinfectants effective in a laboratory situation may be completely ineffective in actual use.[3] It should also be remembered that the perfect disinfectant has not been found. When using any disinfectant the nurse should be aware of several factors, including the strength of the solution, time allowed for disinfecting, temperature of the solution, character of the material to be disinfected, and proper disinfectant to be used.

Strength of solution. The greater the strength the greater will be the germicidal power of the disinfectant. However, it must be remembered that bacteria respond differently to disinfectants, depending on their strain and stage of development. A weak solution might have value as an antiseptic. Most throat gargles and mouthwashes are considered antiseptics. Weak solutions having antiseptic value may be completely ineffective for disinfecting highly contaminated instruments. Some microorganisms are so resistive that extremely strong solutions of disinfectants are required to kill them.

Time. Most disinfectants do not act quickly. Usually the greater the strength of the solution the shorter will be the time required to kill bacteria. A weak solution may result in disinfection over a long period of time. Disinfecting time is shortened when the material is clean, that is, free from blood, feces, and pus. The presence of such organic material may render the disinfecting solution completely ineffective. Application of this principle is demonstrated when the nurse is taught to wipe the mucus from a clinical thermometer before placing it in a disinfecting solution.

Temperature. Bacteria are often killed more quickly when the disinfecting solution is heated. However, it may not be possible or even desirable to heat some disinfecting solutions.

Character of the material. As stated earlier, there is no disinfectant suitable for all purposes. Disinfectants are widely used for many purposes such as disinfecting swimming pools, drinking water, floors, dishes, furniture, linens, surgical instruments, and the human skin.

Proper disinfectant for the material to be disinfected. Most disinfectants on the market state the purpose for which they are intended. The nurse should read labels carefully to ensure using the correct disinfectant. All disinfectants should be used for the purpose for which they are intended and for no other purpose.

The hospital is a contaminated environment. It is contaminated by patients, visitors, and hospital personnel. Some areas such as the nurse's station and utility rooms, dressing rooms, and examining rooms are considered to be at risk. To reduce the degree of contamination in these areas, frequent cleaning, mopping, and dusting and using the proper disinfectant are necessary. Much of the equipment used by the nurse in giving patient care becomes highly contaminated, for example, suction equipment, respirators, airways, Isolettes in the nursery, laundry hampers, ice tongs, ice chests, water pitchers used by patients, bedpans, and urinals. All these items should be kept clean and disinfected. Some will require sterilization

by autoclaving, whereas others may require chemical disinfection. The appropriate disinfectant will kill most vegetative bacteria (bacteria that do not form spores), fungi, animal parasites, and some viruses in 10 minutes. Spore-forming bacteria and the virus-causing infectious hepatitis require sterilization. Sterilization differs from disinfection in that sterilization must guarantee the destruction of all forms of microorganisms, whereas disinfection does not destroy all pathogenic organisms.

On p. 47 it was stated that a disinfectant may also be an antiseptic. Most disinfectants are chemical substances and when in solution are used for disinfecting inanimate objects such as those listed in the previous paragraph. However, chemicals may also be used to disinfect the human skin, for example, alcohol prior to a hypodermic injection, iodine in preparation of the skin for surgery, and an aqueous benzalkonium chloride (Zephiran) solution for irrigating a body cavity. When chemicals are used for these purposes they are antiseptics.

Chemical disinfection

Both liquids and gases are used to destroy microorganisms. Following are some of the chemical compounds, their derivatives, and the purposes for which they are used.

Chlorine compounds. Chlorine is a poisonous gas, and its inhalation for even a short time may cause damage to the lungs. Almost no chlorine occurs free in nature; it is prepared by chemical methods. Chlorine dissolves in water, and large amounts are used for purification of drinking water and disinfection of water in swimming pools. Chlorine also combines with other elements to form compounds. Some of these compounds include chlorinated lime, which is used to disinfect urine and feces in certain infectious diseases such as typhoid fever when municipal sewage systems are not available. Chlorine compounds are used in commercial and home laundries for bleaching clothes; Clorox is one such preparation. All chlorine compounds used in the home should be kept out of the reach of small children.

Phenol compounds. Carbolic acid was the first germicide used (p. 3). It is irritating and toxic to the skin and its use has been declining since less toxic germicides have become available. By irritating sensory nerve endings in the skin it acts as a local anesthetic and therefore is used in lotions such as calamine lotion to relieve pruritus. A mixture of phenols (cresol), generally in a 5% solution, is used to disinfect feces in certain infectious diseases such as typhoid fever. A solution of cresol (Lysol) in a 1% to 2% solution is often used to disinfect bedpans, sinks, and toilets.

Ammonium compounds. Ammonium compounds ("quats") are used both as disinfectants and as antiseptics. One preparation that is widely used is Zephiran. It is a colorless, odorless substance available in a tincture and a water solution. It is used as an antiseptic on the skin and mucous membranes as well as for disinfecting instruments. It does not kill spores, viruses, or tubercle bacilli. One of its limitations is that soap inactivates its germicidal activity. Therefore all soap must be removed before using Zephiran as a skin antiseptic. Many hospitals prepare a 1:1000 solution to be kept as a standard stock solution. Since the solution is used for many different purposes, the physician may order a weaker solution for the irrigation of a body cavity. The nurse should know how to prepare a weaker solution from the stock solution of 1:1000. Following is one method for doing this, and the formula can be applied for any strength needed.

    1:5000 strength of weaker solution needed
    1:1000 strength of stock solution
    2000 ml. needed for irrigation
    X ml. amount of 1:1000 solution needed
    1:1 : 1:5 :: X ml. : 2000 ml.
    5X = 2000 ml.
    X = 400 ml. of the 1:1000 solution; add 1600
      ml. of water for 2000 ml. of a 1:5000 solution

Alcohol. Alcohol is available in several preparations, primarily as an antiseptic. Ethyl alcohol is used in a 50% to 70% concentration. Isopropyl alcohol has greater antiseptic values than ethyl alcohol. It may be used in concentrations of 99% (full strength) or as isopropyl rubbing alcohol, which is 70% concentration in a water solution. Isopropyl rubbing alcohol is generally used in the hospital for giving alcohol rubs and sponges and as a skin antiseptic prior to parenteral injections and venipunctures. Some hospitals use it for disinfecting thermometers. Alcohol evaporates, and unless care is taken its germicidal qualities will become ineffective. Alcohol will not kill spores, and its use in disinfecting instruments is limited because it corrodes.[1]

Iodine. Iodine has been in use for many years as an antiseptic and disinfectant. It is often used in preparation of the skin for surgery. Although it is one of the most effective chemical disinfectants, it has certain disadvantages. It may burn the skin and cause tissue damage, it corrodes instruments, and it stains. Iodine is prepared in an aqueous solution and in an alcohol solution. A 2% solution of tincture of iodine contains 2% of iodine, 2.4% potassium iodide, and 46% ethyl alcohol. If tincture of iodine is used in the home, it should be in a dark bottle, kept tightly closed, labeled *poison,* and placed out of reach of children. Iodine is used in the prevention, diagnosis, and treatment of simple goiter and is placed in common table salt. It may also be used for emergency disinfection of drinking water.

Iodophors are available both as disinfectants and as antiseptics. They combine iodine with another agent such as a detergent, and in combination the iodine is gradually released. Iodophors are free from the objectionable properties of iodine and are safe to use as antiseptics on the skin and mucous membranes. They may be employed as disinfecting agents in medical asepsis, and some are used as sanitizers for floors. Iodophors are marketed under a number of trade names that include Wescodyne. Povidone-iodine (Betadine) has been used in the operating room for surgical scrubbing. Another new iodophor is ACU-dyne.

Other common disinfectants that the nurse will encounter include silver nitrate and boric acid. Silver nitrate in a 1% solution is used to treat the eyes of most newborn babies to prevent ophthalmia neonatorum caused by the gonococcus organism. It is also used to cauterize certain types of lesions. Boric acid is a mild antiseptic. A 2% solution may be used for irrigating the eyes and a 3% solution for wet dressings. It is also used in ointments (boric acid ointment) and in dusting powders. It is poisonous if inhaled or ingested, and deaths have been reported as the result of inhaling it.

Hydrogen peroxide solution consists of hydrogen peroxide and water and is used to clean wounds and to treat Vincent's infection (trench mouth). It is generally used in a 3% to 6% solution, and its germ-killing ability is due to its oxygen-releasing ability. The solution should be kept in a tightly closed bottle in a cool dark place because it decomposes rapidly. It should not be used in any closed body cavity where oxygen cannot escape.[1]

The appearance of new chemical disinfectants and the wide divergence in practice between hospitals make it increasingly important for the nurse to be familiar with a disinfectant and its use. Information can usually be secured from a pharmacist, chemist, or bacteriologist.

STERILIZATION

sterilization A process by which all forms of living microorganisms are completely destroyed, including spores and viruses.

Sterilization is accomplished in a number of different ways. Modern methods of sterilization include the use of disinfectants or gases that destroy bacteria by chemical action, the use of dry or moist heat, and the use of ultraviolet radiation. Regardless of the method used, the responsibility rests on the nurse. The method of sterilization should be determined by the purpose for which the supplies are to be used. In surgical asepsis, all supplies and equipment are sterilized before use and are handled only with sterile equipment. In medical asepsis, equipment and supplies should be freed of pathogenic organisms by daily disinfection and terminal sterilization. Three factors are important in determining the type of sterilization to be used:

1. The type of microorganism to be destroyed must be considered, since some pathogens are easily destroyed by ordinary methods of disinfection, whereas others are extremely resistant. When the type of organism is unknown, as is often the case, every nurse should select the method of sterilization that will assure safety.

2. The greater the amount of contamination the longer it will take to ensure complete destruction of pathogenic organisms.

3. Clean articles can be sterilized more quickly than those contaminated with blood, pus, or other cellular debris.

Gas. Ethylene oxide is a chemical found in both liquid and vapor form. If the liquid form comes into contact with the skin, it causes blistering, and inhaling the gas causes nausea, vomiting, dizziness, and irritation of the mucous membranes. Research has demonstrated that exposure to ethylene oxide gas will kill all forms of vegetative bacteria, including spore-forming types, and viruses. During the past decade its use has increased in sterilizing equipment that cannot be subjected to other methods of sterilizing, for example, medical and surgical equipment such as instruments with lenses (the cytoscope, cystoscope, and bronchoscope), also plastic equipment such as infant incubators and the artificial kidney machine. It is also useful for sterilizing polyethylene tubing and some rubber goods.

The use of ethylene oxide gas requires special types of sterilizers. The gas is prepared commercially as a mixture of ethylene gas and other gases and is dispensed in steel cylinders. The process by which sterilization is accomplished is complex and involves several factors, including temperature, time, concentration of the gas, moisture, and proper packaging of materials.

All materials prepared for sterilizing must be clean and dry. The actual sterilizing time varies from 1 to 4 hours, followed by about 24 hours to permit dissipation of all residual gas before materials or equipment can be used.[2]

Boiling. Boiling is a form of moist heat and is one of the oldest methods of sterilization. It is commonly used in the home and under most conditions is satisfactory. Equipment to be sterilized by boiling must be completely immersed in the water, and timing begins when the water begins to boil. Most vegetative forms of bacteria will be killed if boiled for 10 to 20 minutes. Distilled water is generally used when boiling syringes or glassware, or a water softener may be added. This prevents deposits from forming on the items as a result of the minerals in the water.

Many hospitals have automatic bedpan sterilizers that rinse and sterilize bedpans and urinals. If rubber gloves, rubber tubing, or other rubber items are boiled, they should be wrapped in gauze before sterilization.

Many hospitals are eliminating the use of sterilizers on the clinical units. Through the development of prepackaged sterilized equipment that is completely disposable after use, many hours of cleaning, packaging, and sterilizing equipment have been saved. The nurse and the patient can feel confident and safe in having readily available safe equipment. Hospitals are making greater use of central service departments for care of all types of equipment, including disinfecting and sterilizing (Fig. 3-1).

② *Hot air.* Dry heat sterilization utilizes circulating hot air provided by an electric oven sterilizer. It may be compared to an ordinary baking oven. This type of sterilizer is used extensively in the laboratory for sterilizing glassware and for sharp cutting instruments and delicate instruments that would be damaged by moist heat. The use of hot air for sterilizing syringes and needles has the advantage of prolonging the life of the syringe and keeping needles dry. When needles are kept dry, the stylets may be left in place. Hot air is not suitable for textile materials.

The kind of materials, the way they are prepared, and the loading of the oven will determine the length of time necessary for sterilization to be accomplished. In general, the time required for hot air sterilization will vary between 1 and 6 hours, and in some cases may be longer.

③ *Steam under pressure.* Steam under pressure is the most dependable method of sterilizing, since it will destroy all forms of microorganisms. This method of sterilizing is called *autoclaving.*

The principle on which the autoclave operates is that of heat and moisture. The moisture is from the steam; it is the heat that sterilizes and not the moisture. The steam enters the autoclave under pressure, which increases the temperature of the steam. The air is forced out through an outlet at the bottom by the pressure of the steam above. It is important that all air be withdrawn, since the presence of air reduces the temperature of the steam. During the sterilizing process the temperature is maintained at about 250° F. and at 15 to 17 pounds of pressure for a specified period of time. At completion of the process the pressure is reduced to zero, and the load is allowed to dry.

The nurse assigned the responsibility of operating the autoclave will need to become thoroughly familiar with its operation, exposure time for various equipment and supplies, and the pressure required at various altitudes.

For proper sterilization it is important to wrap articles correctly and load the autoclave in such a way that the sterilizing

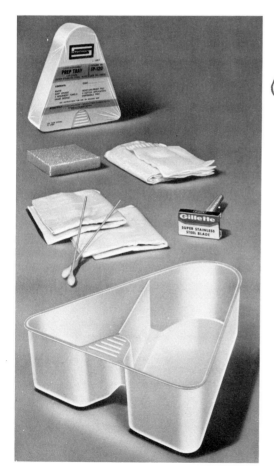

Fig. 3-1. Disposable prep tray, which is newly designed and contoured to the human body for convenient placement. (Courtesy Sterilon Corporation, Braintree, Mass.)

temperature reaches all parts and is maintained at the proper level and pressure.

Ultraviolet light. Sunlight has long been used as a disinfectant. It is the ultraviolet rays of the sun that exert the powerful germicidal effect. The ultraviolet rays cannot be seen and do not penetrate ordinary window glass. Any object to be disinfected must be placed where the direct rays of the sun will fall on it. Exposure to the direct rays of the sun for 6 to 8 hours is often employed as a method of sterilization for bedding such as pillows and mattresses. This method is more commonly used in the home after infectious diseases such as tuberculosis.

Packaging supplies for sterilization

All articles to be sterilized are wrapped and securely fastened before being placed in the sterilizer. Cotton fabrics are commonly used for this purpose. Materials used must be tightly woven, durable, and of double thickness. Various colors are often used to designate supplies for specific clinical areas or certain types of equipment. This speeds the process of sorting supplies and enables a person to secure more quickly an article needed. Before packaging, all wrappers must be inspected for holes or tears and must be clean.

Bundles are fastened in various ways, for example, by tying with string or bandage, adhesive tape, and autoclave tape. The latter offers certain advantages in that it sticks securely and leaves no marks on wrappers. When exposed to the heat of the sterilizer, brown stripes appear on the tape. Although appearance of the stripes attests to the autoclaving process, it may not always assure the sterility of a package.

Metal drums with hinged tops and perforations in the sides are sometimes used. They are lined with a heavy cotton wrapper that is permeable to steam. The perforations are left open during sterilization and closed when the drum is taken from the autoclave. When the drums are packed, areas about the walls should be left free of supplies to allow for effective sterilization. Although some hospitals continue to use drums, the practice is discouraged. Adequate passage of steam to all parts is questionable, and contamination is possible.

All packages must be plainly marked with the contents before they are placed in

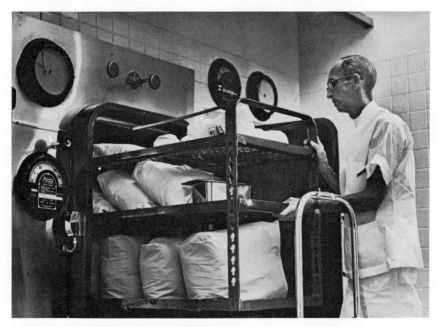

Fig. 3-2. A constant supply of sterile equipment is provided by mammoth autoclaves located in the central service department. (Courtesy Memorial Hospital of Chatham County, Savannah, Ga.)

the sterilizer. This may be done with waterproof ink or pencil. When removed from the autoclave, they should be marked *sterile*. A rubber stamp can be used for this purpose. Most hospitals have an expiration date after which the package is considered to be unsterile.

Hospitals vary in their practice for packaging supplies. However, certain basic principles are applicable in most situations.

1. All linens must be clean and free of holes, and all threads or ravelings must be removed.
2. Sheets, covers, towels, and drapes are fanfolded or folded to avoid undue handling when opened. Towels and covers are folded in such a way that only edges will be handled when opened.
3. Gowns are folded with the wrong side out and rolled from the bottom into a tight, compact roll.
4. The contents of a pack are arranged so that articles appear in the order in which they are used.
5. Basins and instruments should be wrapped separately.

Most hospitals use some type of indicator to ascertain that a package has been autoclaved. The autoclave tape (pressure-sensitive tape) previously referred to is one type of indicator. A sealed glass tube containing a small pellet that melts when sterilizing temperature has been reached is placed in the pack before it is wrapped. There are limitations in the use of most indicators. When properly installed and properly used, the temperature recording gauge is the most valuable means of checking the sterilizing temperature and sterility of supplies. Hospitals generally run special tests at intervals to check the functioning of the autoclave.

Two factors are important in autoclaving medical and surgical supplies: (1) the size of the packages and (2) loading the sterilizer. The time required to sterilize large packages is doubled, and if a package is larger than 12 pounds, the time may be tripled. It is suggested that packages should not be larger than 12 by 12 by 20 inches to assure proper sterilization. The sterilizer should be loaded loosely, with small packages placed on end so that steam may reach every part of them. A basic principle to remember is to avoid crowding and overloading.[2] We have previously said that aseptic technique is absolute. There is no shortcut for sterilizing supplies, regardless of what type of sterilization is used. The nurse should have access to a central clock for timing and should not rely on a wristwatch.

CENTRAL SERVICE DEPARTMENT

A central service department may be simple or elaborate, depending on the particular institution. As the service was originally conceived, it was to relieve ward personnel of certain duties and to allow them more time for patient care. Although this remains true, the unit may actually become an administrative part of the institution. Beside the mechanical operations of the department, it provides uniformity of supplies, contributes to cost analysis for various clinical units, and provides for wider and more practical use of expensive equipment. It can contribute to more economical use of supplies by study of the needs of the various units. It is an essential and integral factor in controlling the spread of infections.

The operations of the central service department will depend to a large extent on the size of the hospital. The autoclaves are usually placed in or near the service. Activities such as cleaning, repairing, packaging, sterilizing, and dispensing supplies are functions of the service. There is a system through which the service secures supplies from stores and through which clinical units secure needed equipment for patient care. Some hospitals maintain a pickup and delivery service to the units. The advantages of such a service are that personnel concerned with patient care are kept on the clinical units and more economical use of time can be made by the central service department personnel.

Regardless of its size, the unit should be divided into clean and contaminated areas. All used and contaminated equipment is received in the contaminated area, and only clean and sterile equipment is kept in the clean area. Ideally, autoclaves should be available in the contaminated unit for sterilizing highly contaminated equipment, such as linen that has come in contact with patients who have infectious diseases, and such autoclaves should be used for no other purpose. Personnel should wear short-sleeved clothing, and hands and arms to the elbows should be thoroughly washed before clean and sterile supplies are handled and packaged. Personnel should wear rubber gloves while handling highly contaminated equipment. Sterile and clean supplies should be placed in plainly marked, closed cabinets where they are not exposed to dust. Large equipment may be stored in specially designed closets or covered to protect it from dust. Only personnel assigned to the service should be allowed in the central service area.

The location of the central service department within the hospital should be carefully planned. In the past the process of autoclaving, packaging, and sterilizing was primarily a function of the operating room staff, and these activities were performed in or near the operating rooms. As a result, in many instances the central service department became simply an expansion of these services, occupying the same areas. With the widespread incidence of hospital infection, the greater centralization of supply service, and the increased amount of contaminated equipment coming into the area, it seems desirable to locate the central service department at some point remote from the operating rooms. However, the location should allow for economical and convenient dispersal of supplies and equipment with a minimum of traffic.

HANDWASHING

Every person has a relatively stable resident bacteria population on the skin. New bacteria may be added and, unless removed, may become part of the resident population and be spread to other persons. Nurses are constantly coming into contact with contaminated equipment and material. They are also going from patient to patient in providing nursing care and may unconsciously transfer pathogenic organisms from one patient to another, or even endanger their own health. The safest way for nurses to protect themselves and their patients is by thorough and careful handwashing. Handwashing in surgery is a precise technique called the *surgical scrub;* however, such extensive washing is not considered necessary in the care of patients on the

clinical units. Nurses are advised to wash their hands after every bed change, every dressing change, and every other exposure to contamination. The hands should be washed before preparing and administering any medication and before as well as after every treatment. Hands should be washed from 30 seconds to 2 minutes with soap and warm water. Bar soap may be used if it is in a drainable dish. Hands should be thoroughly rinsed, carefully keeping them in a downward position to prevent water from running up the arm from which it might drain back and contaminate the hands. Nails and areas between the fingers should receive special attention. Hands should be thoroughly dried; paper towels are available in most hospitals. When caring for patients involves massive exposure of the hands to pathogens, as in changing dressings on draining wounds or caring for seriously ill incontinent patients, gloves should be worn. The gloves should be rinsed under running water, using soap, then placed in a bag to be autoclaved. No jewelry should be worn except a wedding band. The application of hand lotion will help keep the hands in good condition.

Most persons were taught in early childhood to wash their hands after using the toilet and before meals. Many patients in the hospital are ambulatory and need no assistance with this procedure. Others are confined to bed, and the nurse should provide the equipment for and assist when necessary with handwashing for these patients. It should be remembered that patients with certain diseases such as typhoid fever, infectious hepatitis, and pinworms may reinfect themselves because of failure to wash their hands after using the toilet.

Nurses must constantly be alert to situations and practices that provide opportunity for the transmission of infection. They need to understand the importance of their own personal hygiene, including daily bathing and clean clothing, as a factor in preventing the transmission of pathogenic organisms. (See Chapter 4 for more information.)

Summary outline
1. Asepsis
   A. Joseph Lister—father of antiseptic surgery
   B. Condition in which there is complete absence of germs

C. Medical asepsis
D. Surgical asepsis
2. Medical asepsis
Employed when patient is isolated
   A. Objectives
      1. To confine all pathogens to given area and prevent their spread to other persons
      2. To prevent pathogens from outside from being carried to patient
   B. Destruction of all infectious material as soon as it leaves patient
   C. Involves use of various disinfectants
   D. Cross infection occurs when other patients become infected
3. Surgical asepsis
Preventing all contamination from entering area of operation or any wound
   A. Accomplished by methods of disinfection or sterilization
   B. Required in many clinical situations on clinical units
4. Antiseptics
   A. Antiseptic—an agent that inhibits, retards, or kills pathogenic microorganisms
   B. Disinfectant—any process that, when applied to inanimate objects, will destroy microorganisms; usually a chemical and may also be used as antiseptic
   C. Germicide—any agent that will destroy microorganisms
5. Disinfectants
   A. There is no disinfectant effective for all purposes
   B. Disinfectants effective in laboratory may not be effective in work situation
   C. Factors affecting use of disinfectants
      1. Strength of solution—the greater the strength the greater will be germicidal power of disinfectant
      2. Time—most disinfectants do not act quickly; the greater the concentration the shorter will be time required to kill bacteria
         a. Time is shortened when material is clean and free of organic debris
      3. Temperature—heating increases germicidal power
      4. Character of material to be disinfected determines kind of disinfectant to be used
      5. Proper disinfectant for material to be disinfected; read labels on disinfectants carefully
   D. Hospital environment contaminated
      1. Areas of risk need frequent cleaning
      2. Most vegetative bacteria, fungi, animal parasites, and some viruses destroyed in 10 minutes by appropriate disinfectant
      3. Sterilization destroys all forms of microorganisms; disinfection does not destroy all pathogenic organisms
   E. Chemical disinfection
      1. Chlorine compounds—used to disinfect swimming pools and municipal water supplies; used in laundry bleaches
         a. Chlorinated lime used for disinfecting feces and urine in typhoid fever
      2. Phenol compounds—carbolic acid used in calamine lotion
         a. Cresol in 5% solution used to disinfect feces
         b. Lysol—solution of cresol used to disinfect sinks, toilets, bedpans, etc.
      3. Ammonium compounds—used as disinfectants and antiseptics
         a. Benzalkonium chloride (Zephiran) used as antiseptic on skin and as disinfectant for instruments
            1. Soap inactivates germicidal activity of Zephiran
      4. Alcohol
         a. Ethyl alcohol—50% to 70% concentration
         b. Isopropyl alcohol—99% or full strength
            1. Isopropyl rubbing alcohol, 70% in water solution
         c. Alcohol evaporates and germicidal qualities become ineffective
         d. Corrodes instruments
      5. Iodine—one of most dependable disinfectants
         a. Used for disinfecting skin prior to surgery
         b. Repeated use of strong solutions may cause blistering of skin and tissue damage
         c. Used in prevention and treatment of simple goiter
         d. Placed in common table salt
         e. Used for emergency disinfection of drinking water
         f. Iodophors
            (1) Combine iodine with another agent such as detergent; releases iodine slowly
            (2) Used on skin as an antiseptic
            (3) Used as disinfectant in medical asepsis
            (4) Povidone-iodine (Betadine) used in operating room for surgical scrubbing
            (5) Other preparations marketed as Wescodyne and ACU-dyne
      6. Silver nitrate in 1% solution used in eyes of most newborn infants to prevent gonorrheal ophthalmia and is also used to cauterize certain types of lesions
      7. A 2% boric acid solution used for eye irrigation and a 3% solution for wet dressings; also used in ointments and dusting powders; poisonous if inhaled
      8. Hydrogen peroxide in a 3% to 6% solution used to clean wounds
         a. Germicidal action due to oxygen-releasing ability
         b. Cannot be used in closed wounds
6. Sterilization
Process by which all forms of living microorganisms are completely destroyed, including spores and viruses
   A. Factors of importance in determining type of sterilization to be used

1. Type of organism to be destroyed
2. Amount of contamination; the greater the amount of contamination the longer it will take to destroy organisms
3. Degree of contamination (clean articles sterilized more quickly)
4. Purpose for which sterilized material is to be used; whether medical or surgical asepsis

B. Gas sterilization with ethylene oxide
1. Blisters skin in liquid form
2. Vapor may cause nausea, vomiting, and dizziness
3. Kills spores, viruses, and vegetative bacteria
4. Used to sterilize equipment that cannot be subjected to other sterilizing methods
5. Prepared commercially as a mixture of ethylene oxide and other gases
6. Sterilization process is a complex procedure involving factors of time, temperature, moisture, concentration of gas, and proper packaging of materials

C. Boiling—form of sterilization by moist heat; one of oldest methods of sterilization
1. Equipment must be completely immersed in water, timed when water begins to boil, with boiling continuous for required period of sterilization
2. Clean equipment may be sterilized in 10 to 20 minutes
3. Rubber items should be wrapped in gauze before boiling

D. Hot air sterilization accomplished by use of hot air oven similar to ordinary baking oven
1. Used in laboratory for sterilizing glassware
2. Used for sterilizing sharp cutting instruments
3. Used in sterilizing syringes and needles; prolongs life of syringes and needles and keeps needles dry
4. Not suitable for textile materials
5. Time required for sterilizing dependent on kind of materials, their preparation, and loading of the oven; the higher the temperature the shorter will be sterilizing period

E. Steam under pressure—most dependable method of sterilizing; called *autoclaving*
1. Principle of autoclaving based on heat and moisture; heat, not moisture, is sterilizing agent
2. Autoclave should be loaded so that sterilizing temperature reaches all parts; small packages sterilize more evenly than large ones

F. Ultraviolet light exerts powerful germicidal effect; rays do not penetrate ordinary window glass
1. Ultraviolet rays of sun frequently used for sterilization in home after infectious diseases

G. Packaging supplies—supplies must be wrapped, securely fastened, and labeled before being placed in autoclave

1. Wrappers should be tightly woven, durable cotton fabrics of double thickness
2. Autoclave tape (pressure-sensitive tape) has advantage of sticking securely, leaving no marks on bundles; brown stripes appear on tape when exposed to heat; string or bandages may be used
3. Metal drums sometimes used; must be lined and packed so that area about walls is free; use of drums is being discouraged
4. Packages removed from sterilizer should be marked *sterile* and dated with expiration date
5. Some type of indicator to check sterility of package used by most hospitals, and special tests done at intervals to check proper functioning of autoclave
6. Crowding and overloading of packages must be avoided

7. Central service department
May become administrative unit of hospital
A. Advantages of service
1. Uniformity of supplies
2. Contributes to cost analysis of various clinical units
3. Provides for more efficient and economical use of expensive equipment
4. May study needs of various units
5. Assists with control of infection

B. Unit should be divided into clean and contaminated areas
1. Ideal situation—separate autoclaves for contaminated as well as for clean supplies
2. Personnel should wear short-sleeved clothing; if handling contaminated equipment, should scrub hands and arms before handling clean and sterile supplies
3. Personnel should wear rubber gloves when cleaning highly contaminated equipment
4. Clean and sterile supplies should be placed in plainly marked closed cabinets away from dust
5. Only personnel assigned to service should be allowed in area; personnel assigned to service should not work on clinical units

8. Handwashing
A. After every bed change
B. After every dressing change
C. After every exposure to contamination
D. Before preparing and administering any medication
E. Wash hands 30 seconds to 2 minutes with soap and warm water and rinse, holding hands down
F. Nails and areas between fingers need special care
G. Wear gloves when there is exposure to massive infection
1. Rinse gloves under running water using soap; place in paper bag to be autoclaved
H. Assist nonambulatory patients to wash hands before meals and after using bedpan or urinal
I. No jewelry except wedding band should be worn

Review questions

1. What is the name for a process that completely destroys all pathogenic organisms?
   a. *sterilization*
2. Aseptic technique means the same as:
   a. *sterile*
3. For what purposes are chlorine compounds generally used?
   a. *disinfect swimming pools*
   b. *purify drinking H₂O*
   c. *disinfect urine & feces*
4. What percent alcohol would you use to disinfect the skin before giving an injection?
   a. *70%*
5. Which disinfectants may also be antiseptics?
   a. *zephiran*
   b. *alcohol*
   c. *iodine*
6. What preparation is used to treat the eyes of most newborn babies? What is its strength?
   a. *silver nitrate*
   b. *1%*
7. List three methods by which sterilization may be accomplished.
   a. *boiling*
   b. *steam under pressure — autoclave*
   c. *dry heat*
8. When preparing supplies to be autoclaved, what two factors must be kept in mind?
   a. *size of package*
   b. *proper loading of autoclave*
9. Discuss the importance of handwashing in giving patient care.
10. Discuss the difference between medical asepsis and surgical asepsis.

Films

1. Chemical disinfection—M-816 (30 min., color, sound, 16 mm.), Media Resources Branch, National Medical Audiovisual Center (Annex), Station K, Atlanta, Ga. 30324. Chemical disinfection in hospital practice: definitions, factors involved in disinfection, and recommendations.
2. Handwashing in patient care—M-462 (English), M-1045 (Spanish) (15 min., color, sound, 16 mm.), Media Resources Branch, National Medical Audiovisual Center (Annex), Station K, Atlanta, Ga. 30324. Demonstrates the importance of the conscientious practice of handwashing to avoid transmission of pathogens.
3. Medical asepsis—Mis-961 (42 min., black and white, sound, 16 mm.), Media Resources Branch, National Medical Audiovisual Center (Annex), State K, Atlanta, Ga. 30324. Describes basic principles of medical aseptic techniques used during care of patients with communicable disease. Discusses factors related to spread, agents, portals of entry, transmission, isolation, and handwashing.
4. Sterilization problems and techniques—Mis-736 (30 min., color, sound, 16 mm.), Media Resources Branch, National Medical Audiovisual Center (Annex), Station K, Atlanta, Ga. 30324. Describes sterilization in hospital practice: definitions, dry and moist heat (steam), and chemical and radiologic sterilization.

References

1. Bergersen, Betty S.: Pharmacology in nursing, ed. 13, St. Louis, 1976, The C. V. Mosby Co.
2. Perkins, John J.: Principles and methods of sterilization in health sciences, ed. 2, Springfield, 1969, Charles C Thomas, Publisher.
3. Shafer, Kathleen N., Sawyer, Janet R., McCluskey, Audrey M., Beck, Edna L., and Phipps, Wilma J.: Medical-surgical nursing, ed. 6, St. Louis, 1975, The C. V. Mosby Co.

Part two

CHAPTER 4

Nursing the patient with nosocomial infection

KEY WORDS

abscess
aerobic
autogenous
bacteremia
bacteriophage typing
boil
carbuncle
empyema
enterotoxin
Escherichia coli
etiologic
fungi
high-risk patient
impetigo
Klebsiella aerogenes
mononucleosis

necrotic tissue
nosocomial *hospital acquired*
osteomyelitis
pathogen
penicillinase
Proteus morganii
Proteus vulgaris
Pseudomonas aeruginosa
pyogenic *pus forming*
reticuloendothelial system
spores
Staphylococcus aureus
surveillance

HOSPITAL INFECTION

1 in 20 pt. "acquires" it

Nosocomial infection means that the patient develops an infection after he is admitted to the hospital. It may also mean readmission of the patient with an infection acquired on a previous hospital admission. In contrast to nosocomial infection a *community-acquired* infection is one that the patient may have been exposed to and be in an incubation stage at the time of his admission to the hospital. In this case the symptoms of infection may appear during his hospitalization. Any infection, whether hospital acquired or community acquired, may be serious if it spreads to other patients.

We have indicated previously that the patient brings with him to the hospital fixed patterns of behavior (p. 20). In addition he brings with him pathogenic microorganisms in his nose, throat, intestinal tract, and on his skin. Although some of these pathogens are harmless and some may be beneficial, others have the potential for precipitating hospital infection if given the opportunity.

The hospital is a contaminated environment. It is contaminated by patients, visitors, and hospital personnel. Often medical-surgical supplies and equipment become highly contaminated. Evidence indicates that prepackaged sterile supplies designed to protect the patient are not always a guarantee of safety.[14] Between 1970 and 1973 incidents of contaminated intravenous fluids were reported. The use of these fluids caused serious infection and some mortality among patients who received them.[10, 11]

In 1970 an international conference on nosocomial infection was held in Atlanta.

The conference demonstrated that hospital-acquired infection is not a problem confined to the United States. Hospitals in other countries have similar problems. Certain significant factors concerning infection seemed to emerge from the conference. The incidence and kinds of microorganisms vary with the size and type of hospital. One of the most important factors in preventing infection is surveillance by trained persons. There is a need for strong controls over manufacturing concerns that distribute prepackaged sterile supplies. The surveillance of hospital personnel becomes a primary factor in control. What may seem as an innocuous-appearing pimple on the hand of the nurse, maid, or even the patient may become the source of a serious staphylococcal infection. The conference noted that much more research is needed, but it also indicated that if the present knowledge about hospital infection was seriously implemented, the incidence of infection could be reduced.[14]

High-risk patients

Although any patient in the hospital may acquire an infection, certain groups of patients are more susceptible and at a greater risk. These include all surgical patients with any kind of wound, newborn infants, obstetric patients, elderly persons, patients with chronic disease, burned patients, and patients with decreased leukocytes in the blood, as in leukemia. The greatest incidence of nosocomial infection reported during the first 3 months of 1970 occurred among chronic disease patients. *Staphylococcus aureus* bacteria was responsible for most of the infections, with *Escherichia coli* a close second.[14]

Host resistance

There must be some condition in the patient that reduces his normal resistance before an infection can develop. There may be a breakdown of the body's normal defense mechanisms that were outlined in Chapter 2. There may be defects in the internal defenses of the body, including the *immunoglobulins* or the reticuloendothelial system (p. 29). The extensive use of antibiotics may be responsible for decreasing host resistance. Some of these factors are not clearly understood at this time. However, age and the disease process are known to be underlying factors in determining whether the patient will or will not develop an infection.

Surgery increases the risk of infection. Because of medical and technologic advance, more patients who are elderly and who may have chronic disease are undergoing surgical procedures. Before surgery and anesthesia reached its present state, many of these patients would have been rejected as poor surgical risks. The length and extent of the surgical procedure, emergency surgery in contrast to elective surgery, and prolonged hospitalization decrease host resistance and increase host susceptibility.[14]

MICROORGANISMS AND DISEASE

The microorganisms most frequently responsible for nosocomial infection are *Staphylococcus aureus, Escherichia coli, Proteus, Pseudomonas aeruginosa,* and *Klebsiella aerogenes.* These organisms are responsible for wound infection, infections of the urinary tract, abscesses of internal organs, enteric infections, infections of burned patients, respiratory infections, and infections occurring in patients with blood dyscrasias. There are other microorganisms that cause infection but to a lesser degree. It should not be assumed that bacteria are the only pathogens causing infection. Increasing attention is being focused on viruses and their role in nosocomial infection, for example, viral hepatitis B (SH), resulting from blood transfusion, with a large number of cases reported in hemodialysis units. Viral pneumonia, herpes infections, and mononucleosis are other viral diseases that may cause infections in the hospital. Various kinds of fungi infections may be superimposed on other disease conditions. With host resistance compromised the presence of any pathologic microorganism in the hospital environment may pose a serious threat to the patient.

STAPHYLOCOCCI
Characteristics

In Chapter 1 it was stated that the staphylococci belong to the coccus family of bacteria. There are several species of staphylococcus, but the species concerned with nosocomial infection is *Staphylococcus aureus*. It is sometimes called *pyogenic micrococcus*—pyogenic meaning "pus producing," and micrococcus meaning "small berry." As a rule, the organism is arranged in clusters similar to a bunch of grapes. Under some conditions it may occur in other arrangements.

The staphylococcus is one of several cocci that are gram positive (p. 26). They do not form spores and usually are aerobic. This organism has two important characteristics: (1) it is highly resistant to chemical disinfection and to heat, and (2) it has the ability to become resistant to many chemotherapeutic agents.[17] The virulence of *Staphylococcus aureus* depends on its ability to produce substances that are injurious and that help the organism to spread through the tissues. These substances destroy tissues, break down and destroy red blood cells, and destroy leukocytes, which are one of the body's defenses against infection.

Origin

The normal habitat of staphylococcus bacteria is the skin, nose, and throat of all persons. In general, the staphylococcus organism is present on the skin from soon after the day a person is born until the day that he dies. The bacteria on the skin are both transient and resident. The transient population may be removed by proper washing, but ordinary handwashing does not remove the resident population of bacteria on the hands.

Source of infection

In the past the source of hospital-acquired staphylococcal infection has been attributed to carriers, transmission of the organism by air currents, and contaminated fomites such as blankets, pillows, and mattresses. Absolute proof to discredit these as sources is not forthcoming, but proof that they are sources is also lacking. At the present time it is believed that the most likely source is the person with an infection. It may be a patient, or it may be one of the hospital personnel. Exactly how staphylococcus bacteria are transmitted is not clearly known. Some studies have shown that staphylococci are dispersed from the skin into the environment and subsequently find their way into the nose. It has also been indicated that the person with a high concentration of *Staphylococcus aureus* in the nose is more likely to contaminate his skin.[14]

Clinical manifestations

The typical superficial staphylococcal infection is the boil, abscess, or carbuncle. These superficial pustular infections are usually not serious, but they may be potentially hazardous. What may be a simple boil on the face may result in a bloodstream infection if it is squeezed. A common form of staphylococcus infection is impetigo, usually seen in children. The condition generally appears on the face and exposed parts of the body in small pustules. It is quickly spread by contact and will spread rapidly through a nursery of newborn infants. Cutaneous skin infections may become a familial condition, with every member of the family acquiring some type of infection at some time. Studies have been made showing that the same family over a period of years has had repeated infections resulting from person-to-person familial contact. From investigation it has been found that the rate of infection among family members is four times greater than among the general population.[15] One of the characteristics of the staphylococcus organism is its reappearance after cure is believed to have been effected. The development of cutaneous infections attests to the fact that the body's first line of defense (the intact skin) has been invaded. (See Fig. 4-1.)

When staphylococcus bacteria gain entrance to the bloodstream, abscess formation may occur in any organ of the body, but the kidneys are most frequently involved. If the heart has been damaged by rheumatic fever or congenital heart disease, the staphylococcus may cause bacterial endocarditis, and the result may be fatal (p. 272).

Staphylococcal bacteremia occurs when large numbers of the organisms gain entrance to the bloodstream. In this situation the patient is acutely ill and the outlook is grave.

Osteomyelitis may be caused by staphylococcus bacteria. It usually affects young persons and infants under 1 month of age. In infants it is frequently fatal.

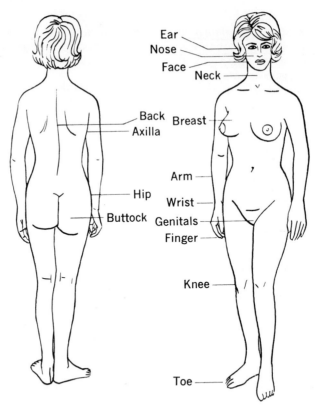

Fig. 4-1. Common sites of staphylococcal infections.

Staphylococcal pneumonia frequently occurs as a complication after viral influenza, or in children it may complicate measles or whooping cough. However, staphylococcal pneumonia may occur as a primary infection, and lung abscess or empyema (pus in the chest cavity) may follow the pneumonia (p. 217).

Staphylococcus is a common cause of meningitis in infants and may occur either from a cutaneous skin lesion such as impetigo or as the result of infection of the cord stump. Meningitis may also be a complication of osteomyelitis in the infant.

Certain strains of the organism produce an enterotoxin that causes a type of food poisoning. A few hours after eating food contaminated by the organism, a person's symptoms begin rather abruptly with nausea, vomiting, diarrhea, abdominal cramping, and prostration. In infants and elderly persons the disorder may be particularly severe and may even result in death.

Development of resistant strains

As many other organisms have been destroyed by antibiotic therapy, pathogenic strains of *Staphylococcus aureus* have become more resistant to treatment. It has been shown that the widespread use of antibiotics, both as prophylactic agents and as therapy, will contaminate the hospital environment. This has contributed to the development of resistant strains of staphylococcus bacteria.[14] Certain strains of the organism become resistant to antibiotics because the bacteria produce enzymes, one of which is penicillinase, which destroys penicillin. Some organisms develop a tolerance for the drug and in spite of large doses will continue to grow, multiply, and survive. Antibiotic resistance has become a serious problem, and many believe that a partial solution is a more rational use of antibiotics, that is, discontinuing their use for minor ailments, for viral infections, and as prophylactic measures.[3]

Diagnosis

Diagnosis of *Staphylococcus aureus* is made by laboratory procedures. Specimens of pus or exudate are collected from a suppurating lesion. The material is placed on a glass slide, stained, and examined under the microscope. A culture may also be made. A slide can be examined rather quickly, whereas a culture has to be incubated and examined at a later time. The slide and culture methods will identify the staphylococcus but will not identify the particular strain of the organism. Identification of specific strains is made by a laboratory process called *bacteriophage typing*. A bacteriophage is a virus that attacks bacteria, and it means "bacteria eating." There are about thirty different bacteriophages, and each is specific for a particular strain of bacteria. Phage typing, as it is called, enables determination of the strain of staphylococcus causing an infection. When this procedure is followed by sensitivity tests, it may be learned which antibiotic will be effective against the particular strain of the organism.[17]

Treatment

Treatment of staphylococcal infection varies with the location and extent of the infection. Most local infections are treated with hot soaks and warm compresses. Occasionally incision and drainage may be required (p. 30). The skin about the lesion should be kept clean by using a germicidal agent to prevent infection of the surrounding area. Alcohol, 70%, or pHisoHex may be used for this purpose. All superficial skin infections should be treated by the physician, since they may involve the underlying tissues such as bones and lymph nodes. Most patients with superficial cutaneous lesions are treated in the physician's office or the outpatient clinic. It is usually unnecessary to administer antistaphylococcal drugs for superficial infections.

When the patient has a general infection or an infection such as staphylococcal pneumonia, the situation is considered an emergency. In severe infections the physician will generally request phage typing and sensitivity tests to determine which antibiotic will be most effective against the particular strain of the organism responsible for the infection. In many types of infections penicillin is considered the most effective agent, but its use will be determined by the sensitivity tests. Several semisynthetic penicillins may be employed including methicillin, oxacillin, nafcillin, ampicillin, and cloxacillin. Their use has saved many lives, and so far they have not been affected by penicillinase. According to some reports, methicillin may be inactivated by the enzyme.[6] Methicillin is administered in staphylococcal pneumonia, 1 to 2 Gm. every 4 to 6 hours by the intramuscular route. Oxacillin may be given orally, 1 Gm. every 4 hours. Nafcillin may be given orally, 250 to 500 mg. every 4 hours, 500 mg. every 6 hours intramuscularly, or 500 mg. intravenously. Ampicillin dosage depends on the purpose for which it is given; it can be given orally 2 to 6 Gm. daily in divided doses, or 250 mg. may be given every 6 hours intramuscularly, or 125 to 500 mg. may be given intravenously. Cloxacillin may be given orally in 500 mg. doses every 4 to 6 hours. Preparations are also available for parenteral injection. In many serious staphylococcal infections physicians will select the antibiotic that they believe will give the best results. The primary objective of therapy is to reduce the number of organisms and their effectiveness as quickly as possible.

In addition to the problem of drug resistance, the physician is often confronted with the problem of patient sensitivity to penicillin. When this is the case, vancomycin may be given intravenously. Vancomycin is also used for patients with staphylococcal resistance to penicillin. When the patient suffers a severe allergic reaction to penicillin, he may be given penicillinase (Neutrapen), an enzyme that lowers the blood level of penicillin. Penicillinase is given intramuscularly in 800,000 units. If allergic symptoms continue, the dosage may be repeated 3 days later.

Nursing care and prevention

The prevention of staphylococcal infection and nursing care of patients with such infection are so intimately related that it is difficult to separate them. Thus they will be considered together. In spite of the voluminous literature on the subject, much is still unknown. Many authorities agree that the best way of controlling staphylococcal infection is through strict aseptic technique and a return to precautions that were followed more carefully before antibiotics became available.[16] Many also believe that there should be restriction of careless or unwarranted use of antibiotics.

A sampling of nurses' uniforms and physicians' coats conducted in two British hospitals revealed the presence of *Staphylococcus aureus*. When samples were taken at the beginning of the day, few organisms were found, but after several hours considerable contamination was found. It was pointed out that the chief danger may be when a nurse is near a patient's bedside changing a dressing over an open wound; the slight friction of the uniform against the bed may release the organism into the air and contaminate the wound. Wearing a plastic apron or disposable paper garment when dressing open wounds might be a solution.[18] Attention has also been called to the stethoscope. Physicians and nurses go from patient to patient using the same stethoscope. A study made in London showed that 21% of the instruments were contaminated with staphylococcus and that many of the strains found were antibiotic resistant. Wiping the instrument with 70% alcohol after each use could reduce the number of organisms.[7] Although similar studies of the sphygmomanometer cuffs are not available, it is probable that they also are contaminated.

It has been said that man is frequently the cause of his own illness and death. In the past the public have often demanded that their physicians administer penicillin even when its beneficial effects might be questioned. In addition, they have purchased over-the-counter remedies such as lozenges, troches, and other preparations containing antibiotics. In some situations these practices may have contributed to drug resistance, and in a life-threatening situation it may be found that penicillin is ineffective. In 1966 the Food and Drug Administration gave orders prohibiting over-the-counter sale of preparations containing antibiotics. Such remedies may now be purchased only with a physician's prescription.

We have previously indicated some of the areas where measures are needed for preventing nosocomial infection (p. 62). Nurses play an extremely important role in preventing infection. In addition to providing nursing care, nurses must have accurate and explicit knowledge and understanding of the high-risk patients under their care, and be certain that these patients are protected from infection. Nurses must constantly be alert to any condition that might lead to infection. The physican depends on the nurse to observe patients for any clinical signs of infection, to record observations, and to report to the physician. The nurse is frequently responsible for the collection of specimens. This procedure should be done carefully, and they should be sent to the laboratory promptly. The nurse should realize that delay may jeopardize the value of the specimen and that the treatment of the patient may be delayed.[2]

Isolation. The strict isolation of all patients with draining wounds is essential in preventing the spread of staphylococcal infection to other patients and personnel. Diagnosis of the etiologic agent should be confirmed by laboratory examination. It is equally important that the patient be isolated in a private room. Research has shown that close environmental contact such as in a ward or cubicle results in dissemination of the organism to other patients in the immediate environment, who in turn were found to become infected and to carry the particular strain in their nose and throat.[5] All personnel should be encouraged to report any skin lesions and should be restricted from contact with patients until lesions have healed.

When a person is isolated, no one except authorized personnel should enter the unit; all cross traffic should be reduced to a minimum, visitors from the outside should be allowed infrequent, limited, and carefully supervised visits, and visiting between patients should be prohibited. The patient with a staphylococcal infection should remain isolated until cultures taken from the lesion or from body fluids are reported negative by the laboratory.

Medical and surgical asepsis. When caring for a patient with staphylococcal infection, the nurse should wear a gown and an effective mask (see below). Gloves should be worn when dressing draining wounds.

Discarded dressings should be securely wrapped and burned immediately. In staphylococcal pneumonia, sputum should be collected in tissues, deposited in a paper bag at the bedside, and burned immediately. Disposable equipment from the unit should be burned, not placed in trash receptacles in utility rooms. Nondisposable items should be thoroughly disinfected with the appropriate disinfectant or autoclaved. Bed linens should be placed in a tightly closed laundry bag, marked *contaminated,* and sent immediately to the laundry. In some situations it may be desirable to autoclave bed linens before sending them to the laundry.[8] An individual clinical thermometer should be available and should be disinfected after its use.

When the patient is released from isolation, the unit should be thoroughly cleaned, using the appropriate disinfectant. All linens, blankets, etc. should be laundered, and pillows and mattresses should be sterilized. The room should be aired and not occupied immediately.

Infection hazards exist on hospital wards in the form of procedures performed by nurses. Many times results do not appear until years later. During recent years bladder catheterization has been considered a potentially dangerous procedure. Studies have confirmed that the prolonged use of indwelling catheters results in urinary tract infection by organisms other than staphylococci.

Handwashing. A most important factor in preventing staphylococcus infection is handwashing. All nurses and physicians should understand the importance of this procedure and should be conscientious in its performance. Hands should be thoroughly washed before leaving an isolated unit. On the regular services hands should be washed after giving care to each patient. Hands should be washed under warm running water. Studies have indicated that bar soap does not transmit infection but should be in a container that provides for drainage. Recent studies on handwashing found that, when povidone-iodine (Betadine) was used for washing the hands, it removed more *Staphylococcus aureus* in 20 seconds than other cleansing agents. The study concluded that the agent was useful in high-risk areas.[19]

A medical expert speaking at a conference of nurses and reported by United Press International stated that "failure of hospital personnel to wash their hands is a frequent cause of infection."

Newborn nursery. The newborn nursery is a vulnerable place for staphylococcal infections, and many of the most serious and publicized epidemics have been in nurseries. The question of how babies become infected has many possible answers, none of which is specific. It has been believed that nurses who are carriers play a major role in the transfer of infection in the nursery.

Nurses assigned to the nursery should not care for patients on other wards. All personnel entering the nursery should wear protective clothing, and their hands and arms should be thoroughly scrubbed. Nurses should wear short-sleeved gowns, and long-sleeved gowns should be worn by other personnel entering the unit. The use of caps is optional, and the use of masks is not recommended. The American Academy of Pediatrics sets standards for the care of newborn infants in the nursery. Infants in isolation should be cared for by one person, and strict medical asepsis should be observed. Gowns worn in the isolation unit should be discarded inside the unit. The nurse needs to observe all infants carefully for evidence of vesicles or pustules with a reddened base, boils, pimples, whiteheads, blisters, or severe diaper rash.

In December, 1971, the Food and Drug Administration issued a warning about the use of hexachlorophene-containing preparations for bathing babies in the newborn nursery.[9] Subsequently reports indicated that outbreaks of staphylococcal infection had occurred after the use of hexachlorophene bathing had been discontinued. After careful investigation the Food and Drug Administration and the Center for Disease Control[12] issued the following recommendations:

1. Adequate numbers and placement of handwashing facilities
2. Ability to isolate and treat neonatal disease promptly
3. Reliability of systems for surveillance of neonatal disease
4. Adequate number and type of personnel involved in patient care

5. Avoiding relative crowding of facilities, and
6. Ability to practice infant cohorting routinely

ESCHERICHIA COLI (COLON BACILLUS)

Escherichia coli belongs to a group of microorganisms known as coliform bacteria. This organism is a gram-negative bacillus and is nonsporulating (p. 26). It may or may not be motile[17] (capable of movement). Nosocomial infections reported by a group of hospitals previously referred to indicated that one fifth of the infections were caused by *Escherichia coli*.[14]

The normal habitat of this organism is the lower intestinal tract. Under normal conditions it does not cause any harm; however, it is known as an "opportunist" and if given a chance will cause infection elsewhere in the body. Colon bacilli as a group may contaminate water supplies. If found during routine examination of water, the source must be carefully investigated and corrected.

Escherichia coli is often the cause of urinary tract infections. One of the most significant problems caused by the organism is gastroenteritis in hospital nurseries. During the latter part of 1972 and early 1973 an epidemic occurred in a hospital nursery. During this outbreak thirty-seven premature infants were affected. Four deaths occurred, and nine infants had prolonged illness.[12] The primary source of this and similar outbreaks in nurseries is from the hands of nursing personnel. Prevention is based on handwashing, isolation of infected infants, and discharge of well babies.

Treatment caused by *Escherichia coli* is based on sensitivity tests and administration of the appropriate antibiotic.

PROTEUS BACILLI

The *Proteus* bacillus is a gram-negative microorganism that does not form spores (p. 26). It is extremely motile. As with *Escherichia coli*, this organism caused nosocomial infection in all of the reporting hospitals, ranking fourth in the percentage of infections.[14]

The organism lives in the intestinal tract and is usually harmless. Two strains of the organism are important. *Proteus morganii* has been implicated as the cause of infectious diarrhea in infants and children.

The most common strain of the organism is *Proteus vulgaris*, which is often the cause of cystitis and other urinary tract infections. It is also found in a variety of suppurating conditions.

A major problem encountered in treating infections caused by this organism is its resistance to most antibiotics. Two antibiotics that have been used with some success are neomycin and kanamycin (Kantrex).[3]

PSEUDOMONAS AERUGINOSA

Pseudomonas aeruginosa is a gram-negative microorganism that does not form spores but will develop flagella (p. 26). A characteristic of the organism is its ability to produce a blue-green color during laboratory procedures and in pus from suppurating wounds.

Pseudomonas inhabits the intestinal tract and may also be found on the skin, as in the soil and water. It is usually harmless and rarely causes a primary infection. High-risk patients (p. 62), especially the very young and elderly, are frequently susceptible to infection caused by this organism. It will cause secondary infections in burned patients or in other areas where there is necrotic tissue. It causes urinary tract infections, pneumonia, and wound infection.

Treatment is difficult because of antibiotic resistance and resistance to destruction by heat and most chemicals. The antibiotic found to be most effective is polymyxin B (Aerosporin), which is administered parenterally to hospitalized patients. It is also available for intrathecal and ophthalmic use.

The source that is believed to be responsible for nosocomial infection caused by *Pseudomonas* is hospital equipment when cleaning has failed to destroy the organism.[4, 17]

KLEBSIELLA AEROGENES

Klebsiella aerogenes is a gram-negative microorganism (p. 26). It will form capsules and is aerobic. The organism resembles the coliform bacterium and may be found in the intestinal tract. It also inhabits the respiratory system.[17] Many serotypes of the organism have been identified.

Infection by *Klebsiella* is frequently hospital acquired. A characteristic of the organism is its high resistance to antibiotics. Studies have indicated that some persons may be carriers of the organism in the intestinal tract, and many develop autogenous infection. Outbreaks caused by this organism have occurred in intensive care units and in pediatric units, and in some situations the mortality has been high.[14] One serotype, Friedländer's bacillus, causes pneumonia. Other types cause urinary tract infection, septicemia, and otitis media.

Although the source of nosocomial infection caused by the *Klebsiella* organism is not always known, it is believed that hospital equipment and nurses' hands are possible sources. Urologic instruments and suction and inhalation equipment have been cited as possible sources of infection.[14] The semisynthetic antibiotic found to be most effective in treating infection caused by this organism is cephalexin (Keflex). The drug is administered orally in doses of 250 mg. every 6 hours.

EMOTIONAL SUPPORT

The nurse should appreciate what hospital-acquired infection means to the patient. The patient may enter the hospital for clean surgery and through no fault of his own acquires an infection in the wound. A newborn infant develops impetigo, or an aged patient develops a urinary tract infection from an indwelling catheter. These situations cause anxiety, apprehension, frustration, and feelings of hostility in the patient and/or his family. It may mean additional hospital days that increase hospital costs, loss of work, or a mother being kept away from her family. An added danger is that the patient returning home may infect other members of the family. The patient may feel depressed and rejected as a result of the restrictions placed on his liberty and freedom of movement. It is important that careful emotional preparation of the patient be done before isolation takes place. The patient's physician can be helpful in interpreting the necessity for the precautions. Much can be done to relieve the patient's anxiety by a sympathetic, understanding nurse. If the patient is made to feel accepted, although isolated, and believes that everything is being done to hasten his recovery, the emotional impact will be lessened.

PUBLIC HEALTH CONTROL

Individual cases of nosocomial infection are not reported to the health department. If epidemics such as impetigo occur among children in summer camps or in any other community group, only the epidemic should be reported to the health department, and efforts should be made to locate the source of the infection. Outbreaks of infectious diarrhea in nurseries should be reported and fully investigated. Examination of public water supplies for coliform bacteria is a function of public health departments. Water carried on trains and airplanes is approved by public health authorities; water carried on ships is not subject to such approval. Because of a recent outbreak of enteric infection occurring on a pleasure cruise ship, an investigation is being conducted toward controls to prevent similar outbreaks.

In 1972 persons interested and responsible for the prevention of nosocomial infection formed an organization with the following objectives: (1) to share information, (2) to improve communication, (3) to establish educational programs, and (4) to develop techniques for control of nosocomial infection. The responsibility for the prevention and control of hospital-acquired infection is the responsibility of all hospital personnel.[1]

Summary outline

1. Hospital infection
   A. Nosocomial means hospital-acquired infection
   B. Community-acquired infection means patient was exposed prior to admission to hospital
   C. Hospital is a contaminated environment
      1. Contaminated by patients, visitors, and hospital personnel
      2. Prepackaged sterile supplies may be contaminated
      3. Contamination of intravenous fluids
   D. Factors related to incidence and prevention of infection
      1. Size and type of hospital
      2. Surveillance by trained persons
      3. Controls over manufacturing and distribution of prepackaged sterile supplies
      4. Surveillance of hospital personnel
   E. More research is needed
2. High-risk patients
   A. All surgical patients
   B. Newborn infants
   C. Obstetric patients
   D. Elderly persons

E. Patients with chronic disease
F. Burned patients
G. Patients with decreased leukocytes in blood
3. Host resistance
   A. Normal resistance must be reduced before infection can develop
      1. Breakdown of normal defense mechanisms
      2. Defects in internal defenses
         a. Immunoglobulins
         b. Reticuloendothelial system
      3. Extensive use of antibiotics
   B. Surgery decreases resistance
      1. Length and extent of surgical procedure
      2. Emergency as opposed to elective surgery
   C. Prolonged hospitalization
4. Microorganisms and disease
   A. *Staphylococcus aureus*
   B. *Escherichia coli*
   C. *Proteus*
   D. *Pseudomonas aeruginosa*
   E. *Klebsiella aerogenes*
   F. Infections caused by organisms
      1. Infections of wounds, urinary tract, internal organs, burned patients, respiratory tract, and in blood dyscrasias
   G. Viruses in nosocomial infections
      1. Viral hepatitis B (SH)
         a. In blood transfusions
         b. In hemodialysis units
      2. Viral pneumonia
      3. Herpes infections
      4. Mononucleosis
   H. Fungi infections
      1. Superimposed on other disease conditions
5. Staphylococci (*Staphylococcus aureus*, pyogenic micrococcus) is species frequently involved in nosocomial infection
   A. Characteristics
      1. Gram-positive organism
      2. Does not form spores
      3. Highly resistant to chemicals and heat
      4. Resistant to many antibiotics
      5. Produces injurious substances
         a. Destroys tissue
         b. Destroys red blood cells
         c. Destroys leukocytes
   B. Origin
      1. Normal habitat in nose, throat, and on skin
      2. Organisms both transient and resident
   C. Source of infection
      1. Method of transmission is unclear
   D. Clinical manifestations
      1. Superficial infections—boils, abscesses, carbuncles
      2. Impetigo, usually seen in children
      3. Superficial infections occur four times more often in same family than among general population
      4. Organism may reach bloodstream, causing abscess formation in any organ; kidneys most often involved
      5. May cause bacterial endocarditis, especially if heart has been damaged from rheumatic fever or congenital heart disease
      6. Large numbers in bloodstream may cause bacteremia
      7. Osteomyelitis in young persons and infants under 1 month of age
      8. Staphylococcal pneumonia may be primary or may complicate viral influenza, measles, or whooping cough
      9. Staphylococcal meningitis may occur in infants from cutaneous skin lesions
      10. Certain strains of staphylococcus produce enterotoxin causing food poisoning
   E. Development of resistant strains
      1. Increasing resistance to treatment
      2. Hospital environment contaminated by widespread use of antibiotics
      3. Certain strains have become resistant to antibiotics
      4. Some strains produce enzyme penicillinase, which destroys penicillin
      5. Some strains may develop tolerance for penicillin
   F. Diagnosis
      1. Slide and culture method to identify staphylococcus—will not identify specific strain
      2. Bacteriophage typing is used to identify strain of organism
      3. Sensitivity tests to determine most effective antibiotic
   G. Treatment
      1. Local cutaneous infections
         a. Hot soaks or warm compresses
         b. Incision and drainage
      2. Severe infections such as staphylococcal pneumonia
         a. Sensitivity tests to determine most effective antibiotic
         b. Several semisynthetic penicillins available—methicillin, oxacillin, nafcillin, ampicillin, cloxacillin
         c. Primary objective of treatment to reduce number of organisms and their effectiveness as quickly as possible
         d. Patient may be sensitive to penicillin
         e. Enzyme penicillinase (Neutrapen) given to treat severe reaction to penicillin
   H. Nursing care and prevention
      1. Strict aseptic technique
      2. Return to precautions that were followed before antibiotics
      3. Restriction of careless and unwarranted use of antibiotics
      4. Nurses' uniforms and physicians' coats found to be contaminated
      5. Stethoscope found to be contaminated with staphylococcus
         a. Wipe with 70% alcohol after each use to reduce number of organisms
      6. Over-the-counter sale of lozenges and troches containing antibiotics restricted by Food and Drug Administration, effective in 1966

7. Nursing factors important in preventing spread of staphylococcal infection
   a. Provide nursing care
   b. Accurate knowledge and understanding of high-risk patients under nurse's care essential
   c. Alert to any condition that might lead to infection
   d. Observe and report to physician any clinical sign of infection
   e. Prompt and careful collection of specimens
I. Isolation
   1. Isolate in private room
   2. Only authorized personnel to enter unit
   3. Reduce cross traffic
   4. Limit visitors
   5. Isolate until negative cultures are obtained
J. Medical and surgical asepsis
   1. Gown and mask
   2. Gloves when changing draining wounds
   3. Disinfection or burning all contaminated supplies and equipment
   4. Autoclave contaminated linens and non-disposable equipment
   5. Terminal airing and cleaning of room
K. Handwashing
   1. Before leaving contaminated unit
   2. Between caring for every patient on all services
L. Newborn nursery
   1. Vulnerability of newborn infant
      a. Protective clothing for all personnel—short-sleeved gowns for nurses; long-sleeved gowns for all other personnel
      b. Masks not recommended in nursery; caps optional
      c. Hands and arms scrubbed before entering
      d. Follow standards of care as set by American Academy of Pediatrics
      e. Strict medical asepsis for infants in isolation
      f. Careful observation for evidence of vesicles, pimples, whiteheads, blisters, or severe diaper rash
      g. Food and Drug Administration issued warning against use of hexachlorophene preparations for bathing babies

6. *Escherichia coli* (colon bacillus)
   A. Coliform bacteria
   B. Gram-negative, nonsporulating organism
   C. Normal habitat
      1. Lower intestinal tract
   D. May contaminate water supplies
   E. Diseases caused by organism
      1. Urinary tract infection
      2. Gastroenteritis in hospital nurseries
   F. Prevention
      1. Handwashing
      2. Isolation of infected babies
      3. Discharge of well babies
   G. Treatment

1. Sensitivity tests and administration of the appropriate antibiotic
7. *Proteus* bacilli
   A. Gram-negative, nonsporulating, extremely motile organism
   B. Normal habitat
      1. Intestinal tract
   C. Important strains
      1. *Proteus morganii*
         a. Causes diarrhea in infants and children
      2. *Proteus vulgaris* most common
         a. Causes cystitis
         b. May be found in suppurating wounds
         c. Resistant to most antibiotics
8. *Pseudomonas aeruginosa*
   A. Gram-negative, nonsporulating organism; will develop flagella
   B. Produces blue-green color
   C. Normal habitat
      1. Intestinal tract and on skin
      2. In soil and water
   D. Young and elderly may become infected with this organism
   E. Secondary infections in burns and other necrotic tissue
   F. Causes urinary infections, pneumonia, and wound infection
   G. Resistance to antibiotics, chemicals, and heat
   H. Source of infection may be improper cleaning of hospital equipment
9. *Klebsiella aerogenes*
   A. Gram-negative, aerobic organisms; will form capsules
   B. Normal habitat
      1. Intestinal tract and respiratory system
   C. Organism highly resistant to antibiotics
   D. Carriers of organism in intestinal tract may be responsible for self-infection
   E. May cause outbreaks in intensive care units and in pediatric units
   F. One serotype is cause of Friedländer's pneumonia
   G. May cause urinary infection, septicemia, and otitis media
   H. Possible sources of infection
      1. Nurses' hands
      2. Hospital equipment
         a. Urologic instruments
         b. Inhalation equipment
         c. Suction equipment
10. Emotional support
    A. Careful preparation of patient for isolation
    B. Make patient feel accepted and that everything is being done to hasten recovery
11. Public health control
    A. Individual cases of nosocomial infection not reported
    B. Outbreaks that should be reported
       1. Impetigo among groups of children
       2. Infectious diarrhea in hospital nurseries
    C. Examination of water supplies for coliform bacteria
    D. Formation of organization to aid in preventing nosocomial infections in hospitals

Review questions

1. List five bacterial organisms that may cause nosocomial infection.
   a. *Staph*
   b. *E Coli*
   c. *Proteus*
   d. *Pseudomonas aeruginosa*
   e. *klebsiella aerogenes*
2. What specific groups of patients are considered to be high risk?
   a. *infants*
   b. *OB pts.*
   c. *chronically ill*
   d. *post op patients*
   e. *burn pts*
   f. *elderly*
   g. *pts. c̄ decreased leukocytes*
3. What three factors increase the risk of infection in the surgical patient?
   a. *the surgical procedure - length + extent*
   b. *emergency surgery*
   c. *prolonged hospitalization*
4. In an apparently well person, where would you expect to find the *Staphylococcus* bacterium?
   a. *nose*
   b. *throat*
   c. *skin*
5. What three kinds of superficial infections may be caused by the *Staphylococcus* bacterium?
   a. *boil*
   b. *abscess*
   c. *carbuncle*
6. How may the laboratory identify specific strains of the *Staphylococcus* bacterium?
   a. *Bacteriophage typing*
7. What four kinds of hospital equipment may be the source of a hospital-acquired infection?
   a. *pillows*
   b. *blankets*
   c. *mattresses*
   d. *instruments*
8. In addition to providing nursing care, what are three responsibilities of the nurse in helping to prevent infection?
   a. *isolation*
   b. *asepsis*
   c. *handwashing*
9. In the prevention of hospital-acquired infection, what one thing may be the most important?
   a. *frequent hand washing*
10. What hospital procedure should be implemented for all patients with draining wounds?
    a. *isolation*

Films

1. Epidemiology of staphylococcal infection—M-335 (13 min., color, sound, 16 mm.), Media Resources Branch, National Medical Audiovisual Center (Annex), Station K, Atlanta, Ga. 30324. Traces staphylococcal infection from reservoir to environment and to host in hospital. Shows how hospital personnel may be carriers of antibiotic-resistant epidemic strains of staphylococcus and how they may infect patients. Supplement with current data.
2. Prevention and control of staphylococcal infection—M-356 (20 min., sound, black and white, 16 mm.), Media Resources Branch, National Medical Audiovisual Center (Annex), Station K, Atlanta, Ga. 30324. Emphasizes techniques and improved housekeeping in hospitals to prevent staphylococcus infections. Supplement with current data.
3. Hospital sepsis—Mis-551 (28 min., sound, color, 16 mm.), Media Resources Branch, National Medical Audiovisual Center (Annex), Station K, Atlanta, Ga. 30324. Film demonstrates ways infection can be spread in a hospital. Uses staphylococcal-infected patient as a prime example.

References

1. Association for Practitioners in Infection Control, Health Services Reports 88:218, March, 1973.
2. Baker, Brian H.: Medical bacteriology—an introduction to bacteria, Bedside Nurse 5: 24-27, Feb., 1972.
3. Bergersen, Betty S.: Pharmacology in nursing, ed. 13, St. Louis, 1976, The C. V. Mosby Co.
4. Burdon, Kenneth L., and Williams, Robert P.: Microbiology, ed. 6, New York, 1968, The Macmillan Co.
5. Burke, John F., and Corrigan, E. A.: Staphylococcal epidemiology on a surgical ward,

New England Journal of Medicine **264**:321-326, Feb. 16, 1961.

6. Dyke, K. G., Jerons, M. P., and Parker, M. T.: Penicillinase production and intrinsic resistance to penicillin in *Staphylococcus aureus*, Lancet **1**:835-838, April 16, 1966.

7. Gerken, A., et al.: Staphylococcus on the stethoscope, Lancet **1**:1214-1215, June 3, 1972.

8. Knudsin, Ruth B., Walter, Carl W., Ipsen, Johannes, and Brubaker, Mary D.: Ecology of staphylococcus disease, Journal of the American Medical Association **185**:159-162, July 20, 1963.

9. Morbidity and mortality weekly report, week ending Feb. 5, Atlanta, 1972, Center for Disease Control.

10. Morbidity and mortality weekly report, week ending March 6, Atlanta, 1971, Center for Disease Control.

11. Morbidity and mortality weekly report, week ending March 17, Atlanta, 1973, Center for Disease Control.

12. Morbidity and mortality weekly report, week ending July 7, Atlanta, 1973, Center for Disease Control.

13. Morbidity and mortality weekly report, week ending July 29, Atlanta, 1972, Center for Disease Control.

14. Proceedings of the International Conference on Nosocomial Infections, Chicago, 1971, American Hospital Association.

15. Roodyn, Leonard: Recurrent staphylococcal infection and duration of the carrier state, Journal of Hygiene **58**:11-19, March, 1960.

16. Shafer, Kathleen N., Sawyer, Janet R., McCluskey, Audrey, Beck, Edna L., and Phipps, Wilma J.: Medical-surgical nursing, ed. 6, St. Louis, 1975, The C. V. Mosby Co.

17. Smith, Alice L.: Microbiology and pathology, ed. 11, St. Louis, 1976, The C. V. Mosby Co. Co.

18. Speers, R., Jr., Shooter, R. A., et al.: Contamination of nurses' uniforms with *Staphylococcus aureus*, Lancet **2**:233-235, August 2, 1969.

19. Studies on handwashing preparations reported, American Journal of Nursing **72**:1976, Nov., 1972.

CHAPTER 5

Nursing the patient with cancer

KEY WORDS

benign
carcinogenic
carcinoma
exfoliative cytology
genetic
immunologist
isotopes

malignant
metastasis
neoplasm
palliative
pulsing therapy
radioactive
sarcoma

The annual number of deaths from cancer in the United States is exceeded only by those resulting from heart disease. In 1974 it was estimated that approximately 355,000 Americans would die of cancer. It is estimated that one out of four people and one out of two families will be affected by cancer at some time. Cancer is no respecter of persons; it attacks rich and poor, young and old with the same devastating effect. The largest number of malignant tumors occur in three areas of the body: the lungs, the colon-rectum, and the breast in order of incidence.

Cancer of the lung in men has been increasing at an alarming rate. The mortality (death) rate from lung cancer has increased in men more than fourteen times in 40 years—a 1400% increase. Women also are increasingly becoming victims of the disease, and the lungs rank as the third most common site of cancer development in females. In 1974 it was estimated that 59,900 men and 15,500 women in the United States would die of lung cancer. The survival rate for cancer of the lung is extremely low, with only about 7% living as long as 5 years after the disease is diagnosed. These statistics are unfortunate because the disease is largely preventable. Most lung cancer is directly related to cigarette smoking.[3]

Cancer of the large intestine and rectum kills approximately 48,000 persons each year and ranks second as a cause of cancer deaths. There has been some small increase in survival rates during the past two decades. Early diagnosis and treatment is the key to survival. It has been estimated that 75% of cancer of the colon and rectum could be discovered by the sigmoidoscopic examination and that 50% could be detected by digital examination.

Cancer of the breast is common in women between 40 and 45 years of age. In 1974 it was expected that 90,000 new cases of breast cancer would be diagnosed, of which 33,000 women would die. When cancer of the breast is diagnosed early, it may be expected that 85% of those affected will survive 5 years or longer, but when diagnosis and treatment is delayed, less than half will survive 5 years. Despite new methods of detection and treatment, the death rate from cancer of the breast has not been substantially reduced. If present trends continue, one of every fifteen women in the United States will develop breast cancer.[3] This fact has effectively been brought to the attention of the American public by the mastectomies performed on two prominent women. As a result, more women are performing breast self-examinations and seeking medical attention when necessary.

CANCER RESEARCH

For the 1973-1974 fiscal year the United States Congress appropriated $500 million to the National Cancer Institute for research and training.[4] In addition to the work done by the National Cancer Institute, Congress provides grants and contracts to other organizations whose research activities may be applied to prevention, detection, diagnosis, and treatment of malignant disease. The ultimate objective of all cancer research is the control of cancer in humans. Progress toward realizing this objective is measured by (1) increased knowledge about malignant disease, (2) identification and control of factors related to cause and prevention, and (3) improvement in detection, diagnosis, and treatment.

Cancer has been defined as comprising a large group of diseases that are characterized by abnormal and unrestricted cell division. It is one of the oldest diseases known to humans, and its cause has been a puzzle for centuries and remains so. Many causative theories have been developed. In some instances an error in a developing embryo may be responsible for uncontrolled cell growth. Wilms' tumor, a cancer involving kidney tissue, occurs primarily in children, and embryonic tissues have been found within the tumor. Certain precancerous conditions have been identified. These are abnormal tissues of the body that tend to become malignant. Polyps of the rectum, solitary lumps in the breast, and black-pigmented moles are a few examples. Chronic irritation of parts of the body can be a contributing cause of cancer. Bladder stones, chronic infections, parasitic infestations, excessive exposure to the sun's rays, smoking, and even continuous exposure to atmospheric pollution can all predispose a person to cancer.[1, 5]

The most emphasis in research, however, has been on viruses as a cause of the various forms of malignant disease. Viruses have been proved to cause cancer in some animals and appear to be related to leukemia in humans. If causative viruses can be isolated, it is possible that protective vaccines can be developed. However, it is probable that many viruses can cause cancer and that human cancer is due to a combination of many factors. For instance, an inherited tendency to acquire cancer has been demonstrated. Some researchers believe that cancer is a result of a chance mutation. This is supported by the fact that many carcinogens, substances that are known to cause cancer, can cause mutations in simple organisms. Also, some investigators believe that every cell contains a gene capable of uncontrolled cell division and that cancerous cells are being produced in the human body constantly. This concept has stimulated research involving the immune system of the body. Some immunologists suggest that cancer may be caused by a failure of this system and that strengthening the body's natural immune defenses may help to destroy malignant tissue. It appears that cancer may eventually be defined as a disease of the genetic material that controls the entire life processes of human body cells.[1, 12, 16]

In 1974 a number of researchers discovered a possible relationship between chlorinated water and cancer. Most water used for human consumption in the United States comes from rivers, lakes, or streams. To ensure the safety of water, chlorine is added. Research appears to indicate that the chlorine reacts with other minerals in the water to form carcinogenic agents. Research in this field is continuing, with the United States Government participating.

Progress has been made in the treatment of some forms of malignant disease. The survival rate for acute lymphocytic leukemia in children has been increased from 40% to 50%. Significant advances have been made in the use of chemotherapy, surgery, irradiation, or a combination of these techniques to increase the survival rates for many cancer patients. Cancer research during the next few years will be exciting, and the nurse should seek to keep informed concerning the most authoritative information available.

PREVENTION AND CONTROL

Cancer usually begins as an alteration in one microscopic cell of the body. At this time the individual is asymptomatic and considered to be an active healthy person. As the cancer cell begins to divide without restraint, eventually symptoms will occur. The first symptoms are insidious and not readily apparent to the victim. A small, painless lump, a vague change in bowel habits, or a chronic cough may be the only prodromal sign of a devastating illness, and often these poorly defined symptoms are not considered valid reasons for seeking medical attention. If left untreated, cancer cells will continue to invade adjacent healthy tissue and eventually will spread to other parts of the body where new cancer growths will be established. Because of this characteristic pattern of development, cancer is difficult to detect in its earliest stages. If the disease is not readily diagnosed, the chances for cure are greatly reduced, since spread of the disease has usually occurred. Early diagnosis and prompt treatment could save 50% of all cancer patients; currently the survival rate is one in three patients. The importance of preventing and controlling cancer through the use of all available resources is obvious.

Most states have enacted legislation dealing with some phase of cancer. Laboratories have been established in which tissue examinations and diagnoses can be made. Cancer clinics provide examination, diagnosis, and treatment services. Many of these clinics are supported by federal, state, and local funds and provide free services for persons financially unable to obtain proper care. Cancer-detection centers provide examination for apparently well persons; a small percentage of those examined in such centers are found to have cancer. Physicians are increasingly alert for signs and symptoms indicative of cancer. Health examinations now include special diagnostic measures for the leading sites of cancer, such as Pap smears for cervical cancer and proctoscopic examinations for rectal cancer. All commercial advertising of cigarettes on television and radio has been banned, and all cigarette packages carry a warning. Educational programs in schools and spot filmstrips on television are designed to acquaint the public with the hazards of smoking and to encourage persons who smoke to discontinue the habit.

Large amounts of money and many services are provided by voluntary agencies such as the American Cancer Society, Inc., which is one of the oldest and has branches in all states and large cities. Its activities include contributions to research, distribution of information through printed material, and improvement in the care of cancer patients through institutes for nurses. Public education programs also are sponsored to encourage people to adopt preventive habits, have physical examinations annually, and learn the warning signs of cancer. Many of the local branches of the American Cancer Society, Inc., provide dressings, drugs, and transportation for patients. Free pamphlets are available from the Metropolitan Life Insurance Company and the John Hancock Life Insurance Company, as well as from the American Cancer Society, Inc. The American National Red Cross and many church groups render volunteer service by making dressings and assisting in centers and clinics.

Nurses are important people in the prevention and control of cancer, as well as in the nursing care of patients with cancer. Almost daily, nurses are asked by friends, neighbors, or family about cancer, and simple correct answers should be given to these questions. Nurses can help to educate people regarding the seven danger signals of cancer, stressing that the individual should seek medical advice at once should one occur. Many persons would have been cured of cancer if ignorance and fear had not kept them from their physician's office. Everyone should be encouraged to have regular health examinations, especially persons over 40 years, since they are in the age group in which 90% of all cancers occur. Nurses must understand the basic pathophysiology of cancer and methods of diagnosis and treatment. It must be realized that although all cancer patients cannot be cured, all can be helped. Cancer is not contagious, there is no stigma attached to having cancer, and there are no home remedies, patent medicines, salves, or ointments that will cure it. Unfortunately widespread quackery often offers false hopes to the patient with cancer and his family.

CHARACTERISTICS OF TUMORS

The reason why a single body cell suddenly goes on a wild rampage of uncontrolled growth is not known, but tumors are found in all kinds of tissue and in all parts of the body. Carcinoma, a malignant tumor, is the most common form of cancer. Carcinomas arise from epithelial cells. These cells form coverings such as the skin, and they line cavities such as the mouth, stomach, and lungs. Other kinds of epithelial cells are found in glandular organs such as the breast. Another form of cancer is the sarcoma, which occurs less frequently than do carcinomas. Sarcomas arise from connective tissue and from bone, muscle, and cartilage. The carcinomas and the sarcomas are called *solid tumors.* They are considered systemic diseases because they spread and start new growths in other parts of the body. Other forms of cancer are considered to be generalized, including those affecting the blood-forming and lymphoid organs. Among these generalized forms are the leukemias, in which there is an abnormal, uncontrolled multiplication of white blood cells. Another kind is the lymphoma, found in organs such as the lymph nodes, which is characterized by overproduction of cells in the organ. Multiple myeloma (cancer of the bone) is due to an overproduction of plasma cells.

New growths of abnormal tissue, whether benign or malignant, are referred to as *neoplasms,* or tumors. Benign tumors do not tend to progress, whereas malignant tumors tend to become progressively worse, often resulting in the death of the individual. Although benign tumors are usually harmless, occasionally they will involve vital organs such as the brain with fatal results. Normally they do not spread and are easily removed.[15] The word ending-*oma* means tumor, and the site of the tumor is indicated by the stem to which the ending is added, as in the general grouping of benign tumors that follows:

adenoma (*ade-* means gland) Thus a tumor in a gland.
angioma (*angi-* means vessel) A tumor composed of a network of blood vessels.
chondroma (*chondr-* means cartilage) A tumor growth of cartilage tissue.
fibroma A tumor composed of fibrous connective tissue.
lipoma (*lip-* means fat) A tumor of fatty tissue.
myoma (*my-* means muscle) A tumor in muscle tissue.
nevus Skin tumors such as moles; there are many different kinds of nevi.
osteoma (*ost-* means bone) A tumor of bone.
papilloma A tumor in epithelial tissue; example of this type is a wart.

Malignant tumors differ from benign tumors in several important aspects (Table 5-1). They are capable of continued

Table 5-1. General characteristics of neoplasms

Benign tumor	Malignant tumor
1. Slow growth	1. Rapid growth
2. Remains localized	2. Metastasizes
3. Usually contained within a capsule	3. Rarely contained within a capsule
4. Smooth, well defined, movable when felt	4. Irregular, more immobile when felt
5. Resembles parent tissue	5. Little resemblance to parent tissue
6. Crowds normal tissue	6. Invades normal tissue
7. Rarely fatal	7. Fatal without treatment

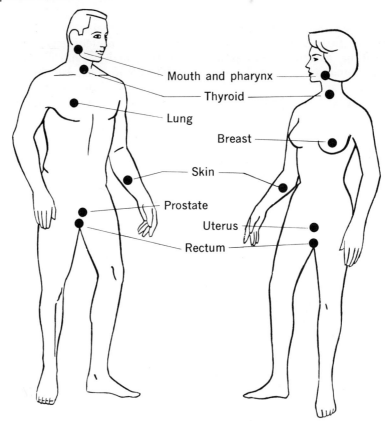

Fig. 5-1. Most frequent sites of malignant neoplasms.

growth, which will compress, invade, and destroy normal tissue. Malignant cells break away from their original sites and are transported by the blood or lymph to new sites where they begin to grow. (See Fig. 5-1.) This is called *metastasis*. During this process of spread, malignant cells are temporarily stopped by the lymph nodes, but they may grow and multiply there. The white blood cells are constantly attempting to rid the body of these metastasizing cells and are generally successful, only a fraction of 1% surviving. However, this 1% is sufficient to establish tumors in other portions of the body.[1] Cancer spreads by direct extension into adjacent tissue, permeation along lymphatic vessels, embolism through lymphatic or blood vessels, and diffusion or seeding within a body cavity.[2]

SYMPTOMS

Cancer is insidious in onset and may often be far advanced before the individual experiences any symptoms. This is especially true of cancers originating in body cavities such as the abdomen. However, there are certain danger signals of which every person should be aware. Any one of these symptoms that exists longer than 2 weeks should receive immediate attention from the physician. The American Cancer Society, Inc., lists seven danger signals.

1. Any unusual bleeding or discharge
2. A lump or thickening in the breast or elsewhere
3. A sore that does not heal
4. A change in bowel or bladder habits
5. Hoarseness or cough
6. Indigestion or difficulty in swallowing
7. Any change in a wart or mole

DIAGNOSTIC TESTS AND PROCEDURES

Exfoliative cytology (Papanicolaou smear test). The Pap test is a means of studying cells that the body has shed during the normal sequence of growth and replacement of body tissues. If cancer is present, cancer cells are also shed. By studying these cells under the microscope, malignant conditions can be diagnosed before symptoms are noticed by the patient. The test was originally developed to diagnose early cancer of the cervix and now can be effectively used to study cells shed from the stomach, esophagus, lung, colon, bladder, and discharge from the breasts.[9] If cancer cells are found, a biopsy is always done.

Secretions from the cervix are secured during a pelvic examination. It is a simple, painless procedure that should be performed annually for all women past 35 years of age. Kits are now available for women to use at home. The specimens are sent to a laboratory, and results are sent to the physician and often to the patient.[6]

The nurse should understand that the test is primarily a screening test and that further examination may be necessary to confirm a diagnosis. The nurse can assist the patient by telling her how to prepare for the examination. The test is not done during a menstrual period. A douche should not be taken for several hours prior to the test, and often the physician may wish the patient to avoid coitus or taking a tub bath for 24 hours prior to reporting for the test.[6] This simple test has resulted in a decrease in the death rate from uterine cancer.

Phosphatase acid test. Acid phosphatase is an enzyme found in the blood. The phosphatase acid test is performed on a sample of blood; it is useful in diagnosing metastasizing carcinoma of the prostate gland. The prostate gland and the carcinoma are abundantly supplied with the enzyme; however, it is not released into the blood serum in large amounts unless the carcinoma has metastasized.

Mammography. Mammography is a safe, simple, nontraumatic technique for detecting the presence of breast tumors. X-ray films of the soft breast tissue are taken without the use of a radiopaque medium. In many instances it is possible to differentiate between a benign and a malignant tumor. The x-ray procedure is recommended for women who have the following:
1. Symptoms of any disease of the breast
2. A history of breast biopsy
3. A history of breast cancer in the family
4. A mastectomy of one breast
5. Large, pendulous breasts, which make palpation difficult
6. A persistent, morbid fear of cancer
7. When adenocarcinoma is suspected, but the exact site is undetermined[8]

Thermography. Thermography is a new technique under investigation designed to locate breast tumors before they are palpable. Its purpose is to locate hot and cold areas of the skin over the breast. The temperature over the breast where a tumor is located is portrayed photographically when an infrared scanner is passed over the skin. In the presence of a tumor, abnormal changes in the infrared heat emissions coming from the area may be detected.[10, 15]

Xerography. A more recent diagnostic technique is xerography. A selenium-coated plate is used and exposed to x rays, then developed. The xerogram provides improved visualization of the breast and its structures including the skin. The xerogram has several advantages over the mammogram. The patient is exposed to less radiation, the procedure is simple, and it provides for improved interpretation. It is believed that xerography will eventually replace mammography when extensive study is required.[7]

Breast self-examination. Every woman should become familiar with the procedure for breast palpation, and self-examination should be made once a month several days after the menstrual period. Women who have had benign tumors removed or have had a mastectomy should be particularly conscientious in the inspection of the breasts. If a lump is felt, palpation should be stopped, and the physician should be consulted immediately.

Biopsy. A biopsy is the surgical removal of a small amount of tissue from a suspicious lesion for microscopic examination. The biopsy may be performed in the physician's office, in the clinic, or in the hospital. If the biopsy is made from an external lesion, preparation will include the use of an antiseptic and injection of a local anesthetic such as 2% procaine solution. Using a special biopsy instrument, the physician removes a small amount of tissue for examination, after which a sterile dressing is applied. The physician advises any woman who has a positive Papanicolaou smear for cancer to follow it with a biopsy of the cervix. Although the biopsy is a simple procedure, the nurse should remember that it may not seem simple to a frightened, nervous patient. The nurse needs to be understanding and sympathetic regarding the patient's feelings.

Proctoscopic and sigmoidoscopic examinations. One of the most frequent sites of terminal cancer is the rectum and the large intestine. Procedures using the proctoscope and sigmoidoscope enable the physician to visualize approximately the lower 10 inches of the gastrointestinal tract so that tumors, polyps, or ulcerations may be studied by observation, examination, and biopsy. In preparing the patient for the examination, it is extremely important that all fecal matter be removed prior to the examination, and this is usually accomplished by cleansing enemas. Laxatives and cathartics are seldom given before the procedure, however, and the nurse should be familiar with the exact preparation desired by the physician. The patient is placed in the knee-chest position and draped to expose only the anal area. In some situations, however, it may be desirable to place the patient in a side-lying position. The patient should be given information about the examination and should know what to expect. He should know that there may be some discomfort but that the procedure is usually not painful. Since the examination is often fatiguing, especially for the elderly person, the nurse should arrange for the patient to rest after the procedure and should provide some light nourishment.

Barium enema. When the physician wishes to visualize the colon above the sigmoid, a more careful preparation of the patient is required. Procedures vary in hospitals and clinics; however, all fecal matter must be removed from the colon. This is extremely important because any residue left in the colon may interfere with a correct diagnosis. Solid food may or may not be withheld prior to the examination. A cathartic such as castor oil or emulsified castor oil (Neoloid) may be given the evening before, and in the morning, at least 2 hours before the examination, enemas are given until the solution returns free of fecal material. Enemas may be of tap water, saline solution, or soapsuds, and there should be a specific understanding as to how many enemas are to be given. Some physicians believe that one enema of disodium phosphate or monosodium phosphate will provide adequate preparation of the bowel. The triple-step enema reduces the number of enemas to one and has been found to provide better preparation of the patient than does giving several enemas by the usual method. Proper positioning of the patient is important in securing the desired results. The steps of the procedure are as follows:

1. Place the patient in the right Sims' position and administer 1000 ml. of warm soap solution under low pressure, with periodic rest periods to avoid cramping and to assist in breaking up pockets of gas. As the colon becomes distended with the solution, gas in the ascending colon is displaced and moves into the transverse colon.
2. The patient is rolled over onto the bedpan with the hips elevated, and as the position is changed, the displaced gas moves into the descending colon.
3. The patient remains in the dorsal recumbent position with the head, shoulders, and chest lower than the hips, and the enema is expelled in this position (Fig. 5-2).

The patient should be protected from chilling, and a small pillow may be placed under the lower back. The nurse should be careful in the preparation of the patient because a poorly prepared patient may delay the examination, resulting in inconvenience to the x-ray department and additional expense to the patient.

The patient reports to the x-ray department at the scheduled hour, at which time he is given an enema of barium, a radiopaque substance, which he is asked to retain. The radiologist observes the filling of the colon, using the fluoroscope, after which x-ray films are taken. The patient is then allowed to evacuate the barium. Sometimes the radiologist has the patient return after evacuation of the barium. The colon is distended with air, and additional x-ray films are taken. The patient may feel exhausted after the examination, and a

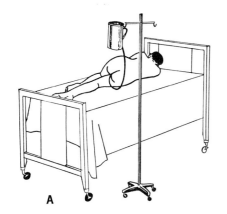

A

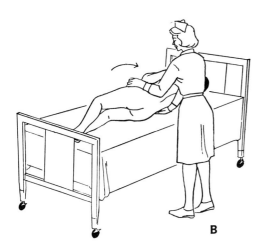

B

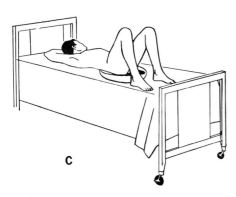

C

Fig. 5-2. Triple-step enema provides for more adequate emptying of the colon and eliminates the necessity for several enemas. **A,** With the patient in the right Sims' position, 1000 ml. of solution is administered. **B,** The patient is rolled onto the pan, keeping the head and shoulders low. **C,** The solution is expelled with the patient in the supine position and the hips slightly elevated on the pan; the head and shoulders remain flat.

period of rest is desirable. A warm oil retention enema may be given to relieve irritation in the rectum caused by the barium and the enemas.

Gastrointestinal series (GI series). The gastrointestinal series is a study of the upper gastrointestinal tract.

The patient is given nothing by mouth, after midnight, and breakfast is withheld prior to the examination. The patient reports to the x-ray department at the scheduled hour, at which time he is given a mixture of barium to drink. The fluoroscope is used to observe the barium as it passes through the esophagus into the stomach. X-ray films are then taken at specific intervals over a period of several hours to study the movement of the barium from the stomach into the small intestine. The patient should not be given any food until the x-ray department notifies the nurse that they are finished with the tests. Many patients find the examination fatiguing, especially elderly persons. The patient is usually hungry and should be served a warm, appetizing meal, made comfortable, and allowed to rest undisturbed.

Radioisotope studies. Radioisotopes are elements that emit rays of energy. They occur naturally as radium or uranium or can be artificially produced from other elements. The most widely used radioisotopes in medicine are altered forms of iodine, phosphorus, cobalt, iron, and gold.[9] The patient needs no specific preparation other than explanation of the procedure. At a specified time he will be given an intravenous injection of an isotope, which has a tendency to accumulate in the organ to be studied. In the radioisotope laboratory a sensing device charts or maps the areas of the organ that have picked up the radioactive material. Variations from normal are seen as lighter or darker areas and indicate pathology of the organ, often a malignancy. For example, radioactive iodine is readily assimilated by the thyroid gland, and pathology can be detected during a thyroid scan. It is now possible to scan most major organs, such as the brain, kidneys, liver, pericardium, and bone. Such minute amounts of radioactive material are used, and it is eliminated so quickly, that the patient is not considered radioactive.[15]

TREATMENT

Cancer may be treated in three ways: surgery, radiation, and chemotherapy. Early diagnosis and treatment may result in cure, whereas delayed diagnosis and treatment may be palliative only, with death the inevitable outcome.

Surgery

Surgery for cancer is performed for varying purposes. It may be preventive, diagnostic, curative, or palliative. The surgical removal of a potentially dangerous mole on the skin may be considered preventive surgery. Sometimes cancer of an internal organ is suspected, but diagnosis cannot be made without surgical biopsy. In many instances the removal of a malignant tumor before metastasis has occurred results in a permanent cure. For example, in cancer of the cervix the surgeon will remove the entire uterus, the cervix being its distal end. When metastasis has become extensive, surgery may be only palliative, such as relieving an intestinal obstruction or controlling pain. Sometimes surgery is extensive, with removal of the regional lymphatics and adjacent tissue. When surgery is performed early before metastasis has occurred, it offers the patient the best chance for cure.

Research is in progress to increase chances of cure by surgery. It is believed that at the time of surgery, cancer cells may be released to metastasize throughout the body. Anticoagulants have been successfully used on laboratory animals to reduce this spread of tumor cells. The effects of cancer drugs and radiation treatment administered before, during, or after surgery are being investigated. Some inoperable tumors have been reduced in size by drugs or radiation so that surgery can be performed. New surgical techniques and tools have been developed. Cryosurgery is being used in many areas of the United States to treat cancer of the skin and mouth. This technique destroys tumors by freezing them with liquid nitrogen.[17]

Nursing patients with operative cancer. The preoperative and postoperative nursing care of patients having surgical procedures involving cancer is essentially the same as for any other kind of surgery and will be reviewed in the appropriate sections.

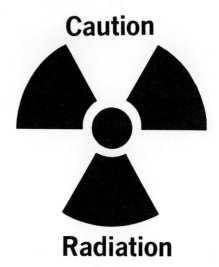

Caution

Radiation

Fig. 5-3. Radiation symbol.

Radiotherapy

Radioactive materials used in diagnostic and therapeutic procedures are x rays, radium or radon, and radioactive isotopes. The symbol indicating the presence of radiation is pictured in Fig. 5-3.

X rays

X rays are electromagnetic waves similar to light and heat waves and are produced in a vacuum tube. They have the ability to penetrate most substances and alter a photographic plate, which takes a picture of those substances through which the rays pass.[17] In this way they allow for visualization of body cavities, organs, and bones, thereby assisting the physician in diagnosis and treatment.

Fluoroscopy is a method by which the radiologist is able to visualize internal structures by means of x rays. The patient is placed in front of a fluorescent screen in a darkened room. The radiologist is protected by an apron and gloves containing lead while operating the fluoroscope and also wears goggles to protect the eyes and to assist in visual adjustment to the dark.

X rays are the form of radiation that has been used the longest in treating cancer. The principle in using various forms of radiation to cure cancer is to give doses large enough to destroy cancer cells but not enough to damage normal tissue surrounding the tumor. X-ray therapy can be used alone or in combination with other methods of treatment. It can be used for external application of radiation or to penetrate into deeper tissues and organs. Improved high-intensity x-ray machines now permit rays to be focused on internal tumors with minimal effect on intervening tissues.[17]

Nursing care. The nurse may be requested to assist in positioning patients or to hold a difficult child or ill older person while diagnostic x-ray films are being taken. Nurses may be employed in operating rooms in which x-ray films are being made during certain surgical procedures, as in orthopedic conditions. When it is impossible to move a patient, x-ray films may be taken in the patient's room with a portable unit. In all these situations the nurse may be exposed to radiation unless precautions are taken. Only the minimum number of persons required to care for the patient should be allowed in the room when x-ray films are being made. In all diagnostic procedures with which the nurse is required to assist, protection by a lead apron and gloves should be used. The nurse should avoid coming into contact with the beam of radiation. Nurses who spend considerable time in areas in which x-ray therapy is being used should wear a badge with a small dental film inside, which is developed at intervals and observed for fogging that might indicate overexposure.

The nurse does not need to have any fear in caring for a patient receiving deep x-ray therapy, since neither he nor his surroundings are radioactive, and it may be helpful to assure the patient that he is no danger to other persons. X-ray therapy may be given on an outpatient or an inpatient basis. Since the preparation of the patient is important, the public health nurse can be helpful by visiting the patient in the home for instruction, observation, and supervision. New patients are usually extremely apprehensive and need much reassurance and support. The nurse should listen to the patient's fears and attempt to explain simply what will happen.[11] Every patient should understand that the treatment is administered while he is lying on a table in a room by himself, but he should know that the radiologist is outside the room observing him.

X-ray therapy is more effective when the patient's nutritional status is good, and a high-calorie, high-protein diet is generally recommended. The patient may be given a glass of fruit juice before and after the treatment. The nurse should see that the bowels are evacuated and that the bladder is emptied before the patient reports for the treatment. This is particularly important if the patient is receiving therapy to the back, abdomen, or pelvis. The patient should be assured of adequate sleep and rest, using mild sedation if necessary. Any ointment or dressings should be removed and the skin thoroughly cleansed before the patient reports to the x-ray department, and unless otherwise directed, the nurse should not apply anything to the skin after x-ray treatments. The nurse should see that the patient is ready and reports to the x-ray department promptly at the scheduled hour. Elderly, debilitated, and seriously ill patients should be accompanied and should not be left alone.

Patients receiving deep x-ray therapy may experience nausea, vomiting, and diarrhea, and several small feedings a day may be tolerated better than regular meals. The food should be attractive and served in such a manner that it stimulates the appetite. If vomiting is severe, food intake may be reduced to liquids only, which should be increased to 3000 ml. a day to compensate for fluid loss. Several drugs, including dimenhydrinate (Dramamine), hydroxyzine hydrochloride (Vistaril), vitamin B, and folic acid, have been helpful in controlling nausea and vomiting, and if diarrhea occurs, it can usually be controlled with paregoric. Indelible ink is used to outline the area that will receive radiation. The patient should be instructed not to remove the markings while he is undergoing treatment. Whether the patient may shower or bathe depends on the policies of the radiation department where he is being treated. Usually bathing of the area outlined for therapy is avoided, but if it is permitted, only mild soaps should be used and scrubbing of the area should be avoided.[11] If radiation is being applied to the trunk, no constricting clothing should be worn. The patient should avoid exposure to the sun and extremes of hot and cold such as the use of hot-water bottles, ice caps, and electric pads. The patient should know that there may be some reddening of the skin, which may turn dark in color, become dry, and slough. The nurse should avoid referring to the reddening as a burn or as a reaction to the treatment. Ointments, deodorants, powders, and other products should not be used unless approved by the radiation department.[11] In the event a break occurs in the continuity of the skin, great care should be taken to avoid infection. The nurse should avoid discussing the course of therapy with the patient but may emphasize that therapy is planned individually for each patient.

Radium and radon

Radium and radon are radioactive materials that produce deeply penetrating rays. Radium is used to provide both internal and external radiation. The supply of radium is limited, and thus it is costly. However, it remains almost unchanged over many years and therefore can be used over and over. Radium is prepared in a number of ways such as in needles, tubes, capsules, applicators, and molds. Molds have limited use at present. The specific form used is determined by the area to which radiation is to be applied; for example, radium needles may be used to treat cancer of the mouth, whereas radium tubes or capsules are generally used for internal radiation of the uterus. When radium is used, the radiologist determines the exact length of time that it should remain in place, and it must always be removed at exactly the specified time. It is removed by the physician using long-handled forceps, washed, and placed in a lead-lined container.

Radon is a gas given off from radium as it slowly disintegrates. It is usually enclosed in gold seeds or in glass tubes. When radon seeds are implanted in a malignant lesion, they are generally left as foreign bodies because they contain only the gas from radium and become harmless in a few weeks. Radon has limited use at the present time.[15]

Nursing care. The patient who is to have radium therapy is prepared in the same way that most surgical patients are prepared. A cleansing enema is given the night before treatment, and if radium is to be inserted into the cervix, the perineum is prepared. The patient is given a bed-time sedative to ensure sleep and rest and is allowed nothing by mouth after midnight.

The psychologic preparation of the patient is also important. He should know that he will be isolated and will receive only the minimum of care necessary while the radium is in place. If the patient understands this and why it is necessary, he will not be likely to think that he is being neglected. Reassurance of the nurse's interest and stopping by the door frequently will help to relieve the patient's anxiety.

When the patient is returned to the unit, he is placed in a room by himself, and a sign is placed on the bed and door indicating that the patient is receiving radiotherapy. The patient should be instructed to lie quietly to avoid any displacement of the radium. The vital signs are checked at frequent intervals until they are stable, and the temperature, pulse, and respiration are checked every 4 hours unless directed otherwise. When radium is placed in the cervix, the patient is positioned with the head and chest fairly low. The patient should be turned frequently and encouraged to breathe deeply. The legs should be held close together and straight, and the patient should be carefully rolled to the side in turning. No perineal care is given while radium is in place in the cervix.

The patient may have a Foley catheter inserted into the bladder to prevent distention, and it should be checked at intervals to ascertain that it is draining properly. Patients should be watched for any bleeding and leaking of urine around a Foley catheter, and the radiologist should be notified if such complications occur. The patient should use the bedpan for bowel evacuation and should be instructed not to strain. The contents of the bedpan should be inspected carefully before the nurse disposes of them. All emesis, clothing, and bed linens are inspected before they are removed from the unit. Dark threads are attached to the radium and brought to the outside, where they are fastened to the skin with adhesive tape. The patient should be cautioned to avoid any pulling on the threads, and they should be counted every 8 hours and a record made on the patient's chart. If any radium becomes dislodged, the radiologist should be notified immediately.

The nurse should encourage the patient to drink fluids freely and discourage talking when radium is placed in the mouth.

The radiologist calculates the dose of radium necessary to destroy cancer cells, and the exact hour that the radium is to be removed is noted on the patient's chart and may be noted on a tag that is placed on the patient's wrist. The radiologist should be notified at least 30 minutes before the hour of removal, and a tray with the necessary equipment should be at the patient's bedside. After removal of the radium the patient should be given a warm cleansing bath and made comfortable, and the bed should be changed.

Self-protection. There are three main factors that determine the amount of radiation the nurse will receive while caring for the patient. First, the amount of time spent with the patient should be the absolute minimum required for whatever care is necessary. The nurse should plan the care of the patient so that not more than 1 hour a day will be spent with the patient while the radium is in place. When radium is placed in the pelvic area, close contact with the area should not exceed more than 15 minutes a day. However, nursing care should be planned so that good care is given without the nurse presenting a hurried appearance. Second, the nurse should understand that as the distance from the source of radiation (the patient) is increased, there is a corresponding decrease in the amount of radiation exposure. Visitors should be discouraged and may be prohibited in some hospitals. However, a telephone at the patient's bedside will help him to keep in touch with his family. Third, shielding must be considered for self-protection. Various materials, such as a lead sheet, can be placed between the nurse and the patient to absorb the radiation.

When radium has been placed in the pelvic area, a drawsheet placed on the operating room table under the patient may be used to lift him from the table onto the stretcher and from the stretcher onto his bed, thus avoiding close contact. Walking at the head rather than at the side of the stretcher while transferring the patient also reduces exposure. On discharge of the patient the equipment and utensils in the room are not radioactive and require only the routine cleaning.

Radioactive isotopes

Radioactive isotopes can be used for the treatment of cancer as well as in diagnostic procedures. The cobalt-60 unit has become a common source of radiation therapy. The radioisotope is enclosed in a shielded unit, and rays are emitted when required through a shutter. Large doses of radiation can be given to a greater depth with fewer side effects in this way; also it is more economical than other forms of radiation. Care of the patient receiving cobalt-60 radiation is the same as for those patients having x-ray therapy.[17] Cobalt-60 can also be placed in a container and applied directly to the skin. Liquid solutions of radioactive material can be placed in applicators similar to those containing radium and be used in the treatment of malignancies in cavities of the body, such as the bladder. Some radioisotopes are available in the form of needles that can be implanted in the tumor, and occasionally radioisotope solutions can be injected directly into the tumor tissue.[7]

Numerous factors in the use of radioactive isotopes must be taken into consideration in evaluating their possible hazards. These include the form of the material, whether it is sealed or unsealed, the time it takes to lose its radioactivity, the amount given, the method of administration, its behavior in the body, and the kind of ray it emits.

The nursing care of patients receiving radioactive isotopes requires some understanding of radioactive materials and is not a task for the amateur. The nurse participating in the care of patients who are receiving isotope therapy should be familiar with the instructions for their care and the precautions for self-protection.

Care during radiation procedures

The nurse may be working in hospital areas that involve some contact with radioactive substances, with diagnostic and therapeutic x-ray procedures, or with caring for patients who are receiving some form of radiotherapy. The nurse should be aware of the potential dangers from radioactive materials, but when proper safety measures are employed, the nurse need have no fear. The radiologist is responsible for giving specific instructions and for assuring the safety of personnel as well as the safety of the patient.

Radiation accumulates in a person's body over his lifetime. Exactly how much radiation a person can receive without danger is not known positively, but it has been estimated to be about 5 roentgens in 12 months. The nurse should understand that each time a dental or chest x-ray examination is being done there is exposure to minute amounts of radiation. In caring for patients who are receiving radiotherapy the importance of self-protection cannot be overemphasized.

The cumulative effects from radiation may involve damage to the skin and bone marrow. White blood cells are highly sensitive to radiation and may be destroyed; overexposure of the eyes to radiation may result in the development of cataracts. The lungs may be damaged, and congenital malformation may result from radiation if it is applied to the fetus in utero between the second and sixth weeks of gestation. Delayed manifestations include increased susceptibility to cancer at sites previously exposed to radiation and changes in the genes, which carry the traits of inheritance. Through the development of new machines, methods for developing x-ray films, and procedures for immobilization of patients, many hazards have been eliminated; however, all dangers will never be competely eliminated.

Chemotherapy

Cancer is a disease involving cells, and much of present cancer research is directed toward finding chemicals that will control the growth and multiplication of malignant cells. Much has been learned about the growth rate of cells, and based on this information survival rates have been increased through chemotherapy for some forms of cancer. Drugs do not cure cancer, but new methods of treatment with drugs have led to the destruction of cancer cells at a rate faster than that at which they can multiply, thereby allowing normal cells

to recover. Drugs may be used in combination with surgery or radiotherapy.

A new technique in the use of drugs involves a schedule of administering the drug at intervals to achieve a selective toxicity. This technique is called *pulsing therapy,* and its basic purpose is to provide a rest period for normal cells before the cancer cells can grow back to their original base line. The technique of perfusion has been in use for some time. It may be regional, in which the tumor area is isolated from the general circulation and an extracorporeal circulation to the isolated tumor area is established. This method necessitates passing the returning venous blood through an oxygenator and then returning it to the artery.[6] In intra-arterial chemotherapy the drug is placed in an artery supplying the tumor area and given under pressure. The tumor receives the full strength of the drug, and the drug is thus weakened before it reaches the general circulation. Not every tumor can be treated by perfusion. Cancer of the colon-rectum, lungs, and breast is not usually treated by drugs unless other methods have failed.

Drugs used in the treatment of cancer are alkylating agents such as nitrogen mustards, which act as poisons to the cells. Antimetabolites such as methotrexate, 6-mercaptopurine, 5-fluorouracil, and cytosine arabinoside resemble certain essential constituents of normal cell metabolism and are therefore taken up by the cell. Other drugs include both male and female sex hormones, cortisone, and vinblastine and vincristine, which are derived from the periwinkle plant. Some antibiotics have been developed that are effective anticancer drugs.[14]

When the patient is receiving chemotherapy, the nurse should be aware of the potential dangers and the toxic symptoms that may occur. Damage may occur to blood cells, bone marrow, and lymph nodes. Bleeding from the mouth and dry, cracked lips may occur. Nausea, vomiting, diarrhea, and loss of appetite occur with some drugs. Aplastic anemia is not an unusual complication among patients being treated with anticancer drugs. The use of reverse isolation in units such as the "life island," a plastic bubble, or vertical air (laminar) flow units provides a germ-free environment for the patient and has been shown to reduce the incidence of infection.[12] The nursing care of the patient in the isolator is demanding and elaborate. The nurse who is caring for the patient who is receiving chemotherapy should report observation of untoward symptoms and should avoid any specific discussion with the patient concerning his treatment or the drug that he may be receiving.

Emotional care

One of the most important aspects of care of the patient with cancer is psychologic support. Many times this is more important than the physical care of the patient. In a recent study of emotional reactions to cancer, anxiety was the most common response and depression was the second response. Many patients suffered from feelings of guilt and saw their illness as a punishment for their own past deeds. Overt anger was also a common behavior pattern in cancer patients and usually was accompanied by acute anxiety.[13] Although they may not be verbalized, these feelings are close to the surface, and hope is the one indispensable aspect of treatment that must permeate all persons involved in the patient's care. Public education has gone far in making people more conscious of the seriousness of cancer, and although many patients may know consciously or unconsciously that the diagnosis is cancer, they still hope that a cure may be found. In the past many physicians believed that patients should not be told that they had cancer. Education has resulted in a greatly enlightened public. The modern communication media have been utilized to present fictional drama concerning cancer. These factors have helped bring about changes in the knowledge and understanding of cancer. It is believed that a majority of patients suspect or know that they have cancer without being told. The nurse should be aware of statements made by the patient indicating that he is looking for some confirmation of his belief. The patient may say, "I'm sure that I have cancer" or "Did the doctor tell you that I have cancer?" Answers to such statements and questions may not be easy to give. The individual's knowledge or understanding does not eradicate the emotional impact when he finds that he does have cancer. It has been suggested that the person with heart disease may discuss it with pride, but this is not the case with cancer. Cancer is a threat to survival, and most persons want to look forward to life, not death.

The patient with cancer is desperate for help, and he and his family will grasp at whatever offers the slightest ray of hope. The patient wants reassurance that something is being done. The nurse should be careful about giving the patient hope, since a false hope is more damaging to the patient than no hope at all. It is better to stress the progress and events of the day rather than refer to the future optimistically. A young woman with cancer of the cervix was dismissed from the hospital to her home but returned at intervals because of severe hemorrhage. Each time she was transfused with whole blood. On her final admission she felt secure that something was being done because she could see the blood being administered but did not know she was losing it as fast as it was being replaced.

The cancer patient is deserving of the kindest consideration, and the nurse who is gentle, efficient, and patient and who gives affectionate care may be giving emotional support. The ability to communicate with the cancer patient does not always involve the spoken word. A soothing back rub, change of position, or refreshing drink may be more meaningful to the patient than any verbal conversation.

While caring for the patient, the nurse should avoid using the term *cancer* or discussing any drugs or methods of treatment. Members of the patient's family often need emotional support as well as the patient, and they may question the nurse concerning other methods of treatment. They may wonder why some other patient has received a different form of treatment. It is best for the nurse to avoid any specific or authoritative answers and to refer such questions to the physician. Giving emotional support to the family may mean providing a blanket or a pillow at night or getting a cup of hot coffee or tea or a report from surgery that the patient is all right and doing well. The nurse can help the patient by advising the physician of the patient's fears, apprehensions, and special problems. The patient with cancer, perhaps more than patients with other conditions, appreciates visits from the hospital chaplain or the minister of his faith. The nurse can be helpful in arranging for such visits. The nurse should always remember that many patients with cancer are cured but should avoid discussing the possibility of cure with the patient.

When everything has been done for the patient that is humanly possible, and the physician has terminated therapeutic measures, the nurse should remember that nursing care continues with the same gentle, affectionate devotion to the physical comfort and emotional support of the patient and his family.

Complications and emergencies

The most common emergency occurring in the care of patients with cancer is hemorrhage, which may result from sloughing of tissue after radiation therapy, from extension of the malignant tumor into blood vessels, from decay of tissue, or as a postoperative complication. Denuded areas of the skin or mucous membrane may develop secondary infections, which may be more painful than the cancer. Such areas may give rise to unpleasant odors that cause embarrassment to the patient. These areas should be kept clean with irrigations such as physiologic saline solution or with wet dressings, using a solution ordered by the physician. Hemorrhage occurring about the head and neck may necessitate ligation of blood vessels; however, the patient should be kept quiet with sedation, and pressure should be applied at the site of bleeding. Hemorrhage from the uterus is usually treated by packing. In case of hemorrhage the patient is in some degree of shock and receives the same treatment as patients with postoperative hemorrhage, as reviewed in Chapter 9.

REHABILITATION

Rehabilitation of the patient with cancer is an obligation of those responsible for his care. The patient is confronted with unique problems that are seldom experienced by patients with other diseases. The patient may have a permanent colostomy or a permanent tracheostomy, with loss of voice, or he may have a ureterostomy. The thought of facing life with the loss of these normal functions may be overwhelming to the patient. If mutilating surgery is to be performed, the patient should know prior to the surgery what to expect and should be assured that he will be cared for and taught self-care so that he will be able to lead a normal life. Patients often receive help and encouragement when given the opportunity to meet and talk with a person who has had a similar kind of surgery. The patient who is to have a laryngectomy should be visited by the speech therapist, who can explain how he will be taught to speak again. As soon as desirable after surgery the patient should be permitted to assist with procedures; he should be able to assume complete management of the tracheostomy care, suctioning, colostomy irrigations, oral irrigations, or gastrostomy feedings before leaving the hospital. The patient who has had a mastectomy should be taught arm exercises. All patients with cancer should remain ambulatory and perform their daily activities of self-care as long as possible. Many will be able to do so until the last stages of their terminal illness. Although prognosis may be poor, with only a few months remaining, many patients return to their normal work for a period of weeks or months.

All patients should be encouraged to participate in diversional activities and interests, and the recreational therapist can provide much assistance. A referral system should make it possible for the public health nurse to visit the patient before he leaves the hospital. Such a visit will reassure the patient of a genuine interest in his welfare, and supervision by the public health nurse in the home will provide continuity of care between the hospital and the home.

Many cancer patients prefer to be in their own homes. The extension of home-care programs makes it possible for nursing care to be given in the home by visiting nurses, public health nurses, or public health nursing assistants. The patient has the advantage of being with family and friends amid familiar surroundings that tend to boost his morale. In addition, there is the economic advantage of reduced hospital costs.

Summary outline

1. Cancer deaths in United States exceeded only by deaths from heart disease
   A. Largest number of cancers occur in three areas of body
      1. Lungs
      2. Colon-rectum
      3. Breast
   B. Lung cancer in men increasing at alarming rate
      1. Estimated number of deaths in 1974: 59,900 men and 15,500 women
      2. Survival rate of 7% for 5 years after diagnosis
   C. Cancer of large intestine and rectum kills 48,800 each year
      1. Small increase in survival rates over past two decades
      2. Sigmoidoscopic examination could discover 75%
      3. Digital examination could discover 50%
   D. Cancer of breast common in women 40 to 45 years of age
      1. Estimated new cases in 1974: 90,000, with 33,000 deaths
      2. If diagnosed early, 85% will survive for 5 years
      3. If diagnosis delayed, less than half will survive 5 years
2. Cancer research—in fiscal year of 1973-1974 U.S. Congress appropriated $500 million for National Cancer Institute
   A. Grants and contracts awarded to organizations whose work contributes to prevention, detection, diagnosis, and treatment
   B. Objective of cancer research is control of cancer in humans
   C. Progress is measured by
      1. Increased knowledge about malignant disease
      2. Identification and control of factors related to cause and prevention
      3. Improvement in detection, diagnosis, and treatment
   D. Cancer—large group of diseases characterized by abnormal, unrestricted cell division
   E. Causative theories
      1. Error in developing embryo, for example, Wilms' tumor
      2. Precancerous conditions include polyps of the rectum, solitary lumps in breast, black pigmented moles
      3. Chronic irritation includes bladder stones, chronic infections, parasitic infestations, sun's rays, smoking, atmospheric pollution
      4. Viruses can cause cancer in some animals, related to leukemia in humans; area of most research
      5. Inherited tendency
      6. Chance mutation
      7. Genes capable of uncontrolled cell division may be present in all cells; cancerous cells may be produced in human body constantly
      8. Strengthening the body's immune system may help destroy malignant tissue
   F. Progress has been made
      1. Acute lymphocytic leukemia survival rate increased from 40% to 50%
      2. Significant advances in chemotherapy, surgery, irradiation, or combinations of these techniques
3. Prevention and control
   A. First symptoms of cancer are insidious
   B. Prompt diagnosis and treatment could save 50% of all cancer victims; currently one out of three survive
   C. Establishment of laboratories for tissue examination
   D. Cancer clinics for examination, diagnosis, and treatment for cancer
   E. Cancer-detection centers for examination of apparently well persons
   F. Health examinations now include diagnostic tests as Pap smears and proctoscopic examinations
   G. American Cancer Society, Inc.
      1. Contributes money for research
      2. Provides information for public through printed material
      3. Contributes to improvement of patient care through institutes for nurses
      4. Local branches provide dressings, drugs, and transportation
   H. Metropolitan Life Insurance Company and John Hancock Life Insurance Company provide free pamphlets on cancer
   I. American National Red Cross and church groups provide volunteer service in many ways
   J. Role of the nurse
      1. Help to educate the public regarding seven danger signals of cancer
      2. Answer questions simply and directly
      3. Encourage persons to seek medical attention when symptoms appear
      4. Encourage regular health examinations
      5. Know basic pathophysiology of cancer and diagnostic and treatment methods
4. Characteristics of tumors
   A. Carcinomas the most common form and arise from epithelial cells
   B. Sarcomas occur less frequently than carcinomas and arise from connective tissue
   C. Carcinomas and sarcomas are solid tumors and are considered systemic diseases
   D. Other forms of cancer that are considered generalized diseases include
      1. Leukemias
      2. Lymphomas
      3. Multiple myeloma (bone cancer)
   E. Neoplasms are new growths of abnormal tissue
   F. Benign tumors do not spread and are usually harmless
      1. Adenoma

2. Angioma
3. Chondroma
4. Fibroma
5. Lipoma
6. Myoma
7. Nevus
8. Osteoma
9. Papilloma
G. Malignant tumors are capable of continued growth, which will compress, invade, and destroy normal tissue
H. Metastasis occurs when malignant cells break away from original sites and are transported by blood or lymph to new sites where they grow and multiply
I. Cancer spreads by
1. Direct extension into adjacent tissue
2. Permeation along lymphatic vessels
3. Embolism through lymphatic or blood vessels
4. Diffusion or seeding within a body cavity

5. Symptoms
May not occur during early stages, but if these danger signs exist longer than 2 weeks, they should be investigated
A. Any unusual bleeding or discharge
B. Lump or thickening in breast or elsewhere
C. Any sore that does not heal
D. Any change in bowel or bladder habits
E. Hoarseness or cough that persists
F. Indigestion or difficulty in swallowing
G. Any change in wart or mole

6. Diagnostic tests and procedures
A. Papanicolaou smear test studies cells that body sheds; if cancer cells are present, cancer cells are shed
1. Malignant conditions can be diagnosed before symptoms are apparent
2. Can be effectively used to study cells shed from stomach, esophagus, lung, colon, bladder, discharge from breasts, and secretions from cervix
3. Preparation for Pap smear of cervix
a. Test not done during menstrual period
b. Douches avoided for several hours prior to test
c. Tub bath or coitus avoided for 24 hours
B. Breast self-examination should be done once a month by all women over 35 years of age
C. Biopsy—surgical removal of tissue for microscopic examination
D. Phosphatase acid test useful in diagnosing metastasizing cancer of prostate
E. Mammography
1. X-ray film of breast without radiopaque medium
2. Recommended for women with the following:
a. Symptoms of any disease of breast
b. History of breast biopsy
c. History of breast cancer in family
d. Mastectomy of one breast

e. Large, pendulous breasts, which make palpation difficult
f. Persistent morbid fear of cancer
g. When adenocarcinoma is suspected, but exact site is undetermined
F. Thermography
1. Technique to locate hot and cold areas on skin over breast by use of infrared scanner to detect tumors
G. Xerography
H. Breast self-examination
I. Biopsy of small amount of tissue from suspicious lesion
J. Proctoscopic and sigmoidoscopic examination to visualize lower 10 inches of colon and rectum
K. Barium enema used when physician wishes to visualize colon above sigmoid
L. Gastrointestinal series (GI series) is study of upper gastrointestinal tract
M. Radioisotope studies used for scanning organs for pathology through use of radioisotopes, which emit rays of energy; patient is not considered radioactive after test

7. Treatment
A. Surgery
B. Radiation
C. Chemotherapy

8. Surgery may be preventive, diagnostic, curative, or palliative
A. Research in progress to increase chances of cure by surgery
1. Use of antibiotics to decrease spread during surgery
2. Combination therapy with drug administration and radiation
3. Cryosurgery destroys tumors by freezing with liquid nitrogen
B. Preoperative and postoperative care of patient with cancer essentially the same as care for other surgical patients

9. Radiotherapy
Radioactive materials sometimes combined with chemotherapy or surgery
A. X rays are electromagnetic waves similar to heat and light waves
1. Penetrate most substances and alter photographic plates producing an image on film
2. Used to visualize body cavities, organs, and bones
3. Fluoroscopy used to visualize internal structures by x rays
4. Nursing precautions
a. Wear lead apron and gloves when assisting with test
b. Avoid contact with beam of radiation
5. Principle of radiation for treatment of cancer is to give large enough doses to destroy cancer cells but not destroy normal tissue
6. X rays can be used for external applications or to penetrate into deeper tissues and organs

7. High-intensity x-ray machines now permit rays to be focused on internal tumors with minimal effect on adjacent tissues
8. Patient and his surroundings are not made radioactive
9. Nursing considerations
   a. New patients need much assurance and support
   b. Nausea, vomiting, and diarrhea may occur; patient's nutritional status must be maintained
   c. Indelible ink used to outline area receiving radiation; markings should not be washed off
   d. Ointments, powders, or deodorants should not be used unless approved by radiation department
   e. Skin may become red, dry, and may slough—should not be referred to as a burn

B. Radium and radon are radioactive materials that produce penetrating rays
   1. Prepared in needles, tubes, capsules, applicators, and molds
   2. Form used determined by area to be treated
   3. Removed by radiologist at exact time specified
   4. Radon is gas given off by radium as it slowly disintegrates
      a. Sealed in glass tubes or gold seeds
      b. Left as foreign body
      c. Becomes harmless in a few weeks
   5. Patient who is to receive radium is prepared in same manner as surgical patients
   6. Postoperative care of patient receiving radium requires that patient and all who have contact with him be protected from radiation; nurse should be familiar with instructions for care of such patients
   7. Psychologic preparation of patient important
   8. Self-protection for nurse
      a. Time should be kept to the absolute minimum necessary
      b. Distance—the farther away nurse remains from the source of radiation the less radiation will be received
      c. Shielding will absorb radiation

C. Radioactive isotopes
   1. Cobalt-60 unit has become common source of radiation therapy; patient care same as for those receiving x-ray therapy
   2. Radioisotopes can be placed in containers and implanted at site of tumor; patients then become source of radiation
   3. Institutions using radioactive isotopes must have trained personnel and adequate safety equipment
   4. Nurse assisting with care of patients receiving treatment with radioisotopes must understand instructions for their care and nurse's self-protection

10. Care during radiation procedures
    A. Radiation cumulative during person's lifetime
    B. Exact amount one can receive without danger unknown
    C. Two most important measures for self-protection are time and distance
    D. Cumulative effects may cause damage to skin and bone marrow
    E. Lungs may be damaged
    F. Malformation of fetus in utero may result from exposure between second and sixth weeks of gestation
    G. Overexposure of eyes to radiation may cause cataracts
    H. Increases susceptibility to cancer at sites previously exposed to radiation
    I. Changes in genes that carry traits of inheritance

11. Chemotherapy
    A. Cancer a disease of cells
    B. Research being done to find chemicals that will control growth and multiplication of malignant cells
    C. Techniques of treatment with drugs
       1. Pulsing therapy—schedule of administering drugs at intervals to achieve selected toxicity
       2. Perfusion
          a. Regional
          b. Intra-arterial
    D. Classification of drugs used in treatment of cancer
       1. Alkylating agents
       2. Antimetabolites
       3. Sex hormones
       4. Cortisone
       5. Derivatives of periwinkle plant
       6. Some antibiotics
    E. Nurse must be aware of potential dangers and toxic effects of drugs
    F. Aplastic anemia often a complication
       1. Use of "life island" to provide germ-free environment reduces incidence of infection
       2. Nursing care demanding and elaborate

12. Emotional care of patient sometimes more important than physical care
    A. Common reactions to diagnosis of cancer are anxiety, depression, guilt feelings, and anger
    B. Education has resulted in greatly enlightened public
    C. Many patients suspect or know that they have cancer without being told
       1. Patient may be looking for confirmation of suspicions
       2. Knowledge and understanding does not eradicate emotional impact
    D. Patient with cancer is desperate for help; needs to feel that something is being done
    E. Nurse should give emotional support through gentle, efficient, patient, and affectionate nursing care

F. Avoid using word *cancer* or *cure* when working with patient
G. Patient's family also need emotional support
H. Patient with cancer, more than other patients, appreciates visits from hospital chaplain or minister of his faith

13. Complications and emergencies
Most common emergency is hemorrhage
A. May result from several causes
1. Sloughing of tissue after radiation
2. Extension of malignant tumor into blood vessels
3. Decay of tissue
4. Postoperative complication
B. Denuded areas may develop secondary infection and give rise to unpleasant odors
C. Methods of controlling hemorrhage comprise:
1. Direct pressure over area of bleeding
2. Ligation of blood vessels
3. Packing uterus, if bleeding from that cavity
4. Administering sedation to keep patient quiet
5. Treatment for shock
6. Transfusion with whole blood

14. Rehabilitation
Obligation of those responsible for patient's care; problems of many patients with cancer are unique
A. Patient should participate in care as soon as possible and assume responsibility for all care before leaving hospital
B. Patient should remain ambulatory as long as condition permits; may return to work if able
C. Referral system using services of public health nurse provides continuity in patient's care and indicates active interest in him
D. Patient should be encouraged to take part in diversional and recreational activities

Review questions

1. What is the most common site of cancer among women between 40 and 45 years of age?
a. breast
2. When new cancer sites are formed from an original site, what is the process called?
a. metastasis
3. What is a test used to detect uterine cancer?
a. pap smear
4. What is the term for the surgical removal of a small amount of tissue for examination?
a. biopsy
5. When a radiopaque substance is used for examination of the colon and the rectum, what is it called?
a. Ba enema
6. What are the three methods used for the treatment of cancer?
a. radiation
b. surgical removal
c. chemotherapy

7. Discuss what information about nursing care may be given to a patient who is to receive radium for uterine cancer.
8. How can the nurse help in the prevention and control of cancer? education
9. Name three factors that must be considered for self-protection when caring for a patient with a radioactive implant.
a.
b.
c.
10. Discuss three leading theories concerning the cause of cancer.
11. Discuss how you may provide emotional support to the family of a cancer patient.
12. In which organ of the body has there been an alarming rate of increase in cancer?
a. lung

Films

1. Prescription: roses (29 min., color, sound, 16 mm.), Office of Information, Cancer Control Program, Department of Health, Education, and Welfare, Public Health Service, 4040 North Fairfax Drive, Arlington, Va. 22203. Attempts to illustrate comprehensive patient care; portrays events that occur in a hospital during admission, diagnosis, and surgery of a patient with breast cancer and the anxiety of the patient when she finds that she has cancer. May be small rental fee for film. Reports indicate it is excellent and may be well worth the fee.
2. Mammography—diagnosis, the normal breast and nonmalignant disease—TFR-1179 (50 min., sound, black and white, 16 mm.), Media Resources Branch, National Medical Audiovisual Center (Annex), Station K, Atlanta, Ga. 30324. Deals with x-ray interpretation of the sound and diseased breast, with emphasis on malignancy and common benign conditions.
3. Cancer chemotherapy (21 min., sound, color, 16 mm., 8 mm.), American Cancer Society, Inc., any local or state branch. Demonstrates the action of drugs used in the treatment of cancer, their indications, contraindications, and side effects.
4. From one cell (13 min., sound, color, 16 mm.), American Cancer Society, Inc., any local or state branch. Pictures cancer growth with time-lapse sequences of normal and abnormal living tissue.
5. Psychological aspects of the nurse-patient relationship in cancer (22 min., sound, black and white, 16 mm., 8 mm.), American Cancer Society, Inc., any local or state branch. Discusses the emotional reactions of patients to cancer, and deals with the interaction of the nurse and patient and the nurse's role in assisting family members.
6. Radiation therapy in the management of cancer (25 min., sound, color, 16 mm., 8 mm.), American Cancer Society, Inc., any local or state branch. Discusses low, medium, and high energy sources of radiation. Advantages of each

are presented and related to the type, location, and size of the tumor.

7. The embattled cell (21½ min., sound, color, 16 mm., 8 mm.), American Cancer Society, Inc., any local or state branch. Informative film showing cancer cells growing in time-lapse photography. Shows the body's defense mechanisms in action.

8. Surgical regional chemotherapy (22 min., sound, color, 16 mm.), Baxter Laboratories, Inc., 6301 Lincoln Ave., Morton Grove, Ill., 60053. Procedure for regional perfusion treatment for cancer, including new procedures.

References

1. Ackerman, Lauren V., and del Regato, Juan A.: Cancer: diagnosis, treatment, and prognosis, ed. 4, St. Louis, 1970, The C. V. Mosby Co.

2. American Cancer Society, Inc.: A cancer sourcebook for nurses, New York, 1963, American Cancer Society, Inc.

3. American Cancer Society, Inc.: '74 Cancer facts and figures, New York, 1973, American Cancer Society, Inc.

4. Appendix, the budget of the United States Government, fiscal year 1974, Washington, D. C., 1974, Government Printing Office.

5. Beland, Irene L.: Clinical nursing: pathophysiological and psychosocial approaches, ed. 3, New York, 1975, The Macmillan Co.

6. Bouchard, Rosemary, and Owens, Norma F.: Nursing care of the cancer patient, ed. 2, St. Louis, 1972, The C. V. Mosby Co.

7. Brunner, Lillian Sholtis, and Suddarth, Doris Smith: Textbook of medical-surgical nursing, ed. 3, Philadelphia, 1975, J. B. Lippincott Co.

8. Egan, Robert L.: Mammography, American Journal of Nursing **66:**108-111, Jan., 1966.

9. French, Ruth M.: The nurse's guide to diagnostic procedures, ed. 3, New York, 1971, McGraw-Hill Book Co.

10. Haberman, J. D.: Present status of mammary thermography, Cancer **18:**315-321, Nov.-Dec., 1968.

11. Isler, Charlotte: Radiation therapy, the nurse and the patient, RN **34:**48-51, March, 1971.

12. Isler, Charlotte: The cancer nurses. How the specialists are doing it, RN **35:**28+, Feb., 1972.

13. Peck, Arthur: Emotional reactions to having cancer, Ca **22:**5, Sept.-Oct., 1972.

14. Rodman, Morton J.: Anticancer chemotherapy, RN **35:**45-48, Feb., 1972.

15. Shafer, Kathleen N., Sawyer, Janet R., McCluskey, Audrey M., Beck, Edna L., and Phipps, Wilma J.: Medical-surgical nursing, ed. 6, St. Louis, 1975, The C. V. Mosby Co.

16. Silverstein, Melvin J., and Morton, Donald L.: Cancer immunotherapy, American Journal of Nursing **73:**1178-1181, July, 1973.

17. U. S. Department of Health, Education, and Welfare: Treating cancer, Publication no. 72-210, Washington, D. C., 1972, Government Printing Office.

CHAPTER 6

Nursing the patient with prolonged illness

KEY WORDS

A.A.R.P.
chronic disease
CircOlectric bed
collagenase (ABC)
   ointment
debridement
decubitus ulcer
exacerbation
flotation
Homemaker Service

hyperbaric oxygen
isometric exercise
Meals on Wheels
necrosis
prognosis
remission
shearlings
stasis

What is prolonged illness and what is not prolonged illness? During the life-span of each individual from birth to death a normal process of growth and development occurs. For most individuals this is an orderly process with certain physiologic and psychologic changes occurring throughout the life cycle. These normal changes do not in themselves constitute illness. An individual by reason of age and the normal changes that occur may become a resident of a nursing home (p. 126). However, this should not be construed to mean long-term illness.

For some persons something occurs at some period along the way that sidetracks or interrupts the normal pattern of growth and development. It may be a congenital disorder caused by defective genes or malformation in utero, a serious accident causing a partial or complete paralysis, or a disease such as cancer for which there is no cure. Therefore any person whose physiologic or psychologic condition is compromised to such an extent that he is partially or totally dependent on others for care may be said to have a chronic disorder and to require long-term care.

The following terms often associated with prolonged illness should be understood by the nurse.

chronic disease A condition that involves structure or function or both and may be expected to continue over an extended period of time.
convalescence A period of recovery after an acute illness or surgical procedure.
exacerbation A return or increase of symptoms of a disease.
extended care Care of the patient during the intermediate period when he no longer requires

intensive hospital care but is not yet well enough to go home.

remission Relief of symptoms of a disease and temporary improvement.

terminal illness A disease from which the patient is not expected to recover.

FACTORS RELATED TO CHRONIC DISEASE

Chronic disease does not always mean that the person is ill, and the person requiring long-term care may not have a chronic disease. However, in some situations prolonged illness is caused by a chronic disease.

There is considerable overlapping of the various states of illness. The patient with a chronic disease may develop an acute illness, such as the diabetic patient who develops an acute respiratory infection. The respiratory infection may lead to pneumonia, and the patient may become terminally ill. The child with leukemia may be acutely ill but with treatment may have a remission and appear well. However, eventually he will have an exacerbation and will become terminally ill. Some patients with a chronic disease do not succumb from the disease itself but from some acute illness; however, the chronic disease may be a predisposing factor. Other patients die as the result of the chronic disease, as in cancer. Some patients have more than one chronic disease at the same time, such as a patient with arthritis who also has hypertension. Chronic illness may strike with unexpected tragedy. A patient undergoing a simple surgical procedure may suddenly go into cardiac arrest. Unless there is immediate restoration of the cardiac function the brain may be deprived of oxygen, and the patient will suffer irreversible brain damage.

Considering all the factors just mentioned, the nurse can see that preparation to care for a wide variety of patients with differing states of illness is necessary. Each will have special problems that must be handled on an individual basis.

Age

Chronic disease is no respecter of persons. It may be found among young and old, rich and poor. Frequently, prolonged illness is associated with elderly persons, and although more than 75% of persons

in the United States who are 65 years of age or older have one or more chronic diseases, approximately 20% of persons with chronic disease are under 17 years of age, and more than 30% are between 17 and 24 years of age. It can be seen that chronic disease and prolonged illness affects a large segment of youth.

Psychosocial factors

When any condition compromises the physical health of an individual, his psychologic behavior will also be affected. The physiologic and psychologic factors cannot be separated, and therefore the whole patient must be considered. The patient must be considered in relation to society. Modern society through urbanization, industrialization, and technologic progress has created an environment whereby the quality of health has been compromised. Although environmental factors may not destroy life, they may destroy the quality of life.[3]

The problem of environmental air pollution has become serious in some urban areas, and it has been predicted that it will become worse in the future. The way in which air pollution may contribute to the development of chronic disease is not completely understood at this time, but the way in which it affects persons with serious heart disease and chronic obstructive pulmonary disease is well known (p. 206). When the index of air pollution is high, persons with chronic respiratory disease may experience an acute exacerbation of the condition.

When chronic disease renders an individual unemployable, society loses that individual's services, and his financial loss may reduce him to the poverty level and require him to seek public assistance. Physical disability causes loss of the individual's sense of worth and dignity. Those with religious orientation often find personal satisfaction in attending church. The individual may have membership in various community social groups, or he may be active and hold office on committees. In these activities he has status and feelings of belonging. Chronic long-term illness deprives the individual of the stimulation and feeling of social acceptance, and he may react toward society with hostility and

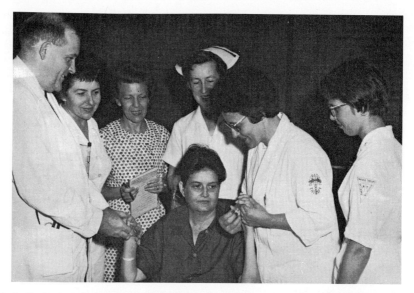

Fig. 6-1. Preparing the patient for discharge is a team responsibility at Eugene Talmadge Memorial Hospital. The physician, nurse, medical social worker, laboratory technician, occupational therapist, and physical therapist all contribute toward meeting the needs of each individual patient. (Courtesy Eugene Talmadge Memorial Hospital, Augusta, Ga.)

anger. Various kinds of emotional behavior may be anticipated when an individual is reduced to partial or total dependency. He may be irritable and make unreasonable demands on those caring for him. He may also experience feelings of loneliness and become depressed and uncommunicative. The loss of bodily function and financial resources together with dependency and social neglect may lead the individual to self-destruction. This is especially true of the chronically ill aged, but it may occur at any age.

PREVENTION AND CONTROL OF CHRONIC DISEASE

Significant progress has been made in preventing some diseases that frequently resulted in chronic disease in the past. Treatment for sore throat caused by hemolytic streptococci may prevent rheumatic fever and subsequently rheumatic heart disease. Immunization of infants against diphtheria prevents the disease and the complicating heart disease. The rubella vaccine presently being given to children is designed to protect the child and the pregnant woman who might contract the disease from the child. By preventing the disease in the pregnant woman, possible

deafness, heart disease, and mental retardation in the offspring may be avoided. Congenital syphilis can be prevented by treatment of the infected pregnant woman.

Although they may not be curable, several chronic diseases can be controlled. Among these are diabetes mellitus, vitamin-deficiency diseases, some parasitic infections, epilepsy, and myasthenia gravis. There is also evidence that the drug levodopa (L-dopa) may relieve symptoms in Parkinson's disease in some persons.

At the present time little can be done to prevent or control many chronic diseases. Although progress is being made, cancer cannot be prevented. Some patients may be cured, but many can expect only a short period of survival. Other diseases include hypertension, arteriosclerosis, nephritis, mental illness, and obstructive pulmonary disease. It has been fairly well confirmed that smoking aggravates or contributes to some chronic diseases. There is some evidence accumulating that the hallucinogenic agents such as LSD may result in malformed offspring of mothers using the drug.

As life expectancy in the United States has increased, so has the number of elderly persons and the incidence of chronic disease. Many disorders of older persons are termed degenerative diseases. Some are specifically related to changes occurring during the normal aging process. Most of these diseases are well advanced before they produce significant symptoms, by which time they have often progressed so far that therapy is no longer effective. Examples of such disorders include vascular diseases, disorders of the urinary system, liver disease, arthritis, heart disease, and chronic bronchitis. Most degenerative diseases tend to be progressive. Some progress slowly over a period of years, whereas others progress to a particular stage, after which there is no further change. Just as all persons do not age at the same rate, so all degenerative diseases do not progress at the same rate or exhibit the same degree of severity; they vary from person to person.

PROLONGED ILLNESS AND THE FAMILY

Long-term illness always affects the family; for some it is a major catastrophy, whereas for others it is accepted as a part of life. Long-term care usually means adjustment for members of the family. It may require rearrangement of the home facilities to provide room and bath for the individual. If it is necessary to secure outside help with the care of the patient, additional responsibility and adjustment may be necessary. A child may have to leave school to help out with the family finances. In some areas the public health nurse is available to visit the home and instruct a member of the family in the person's care and to return for supervision of the care. It may be impossible to care for the individual at home, and he is placed in a nursing home, convalescent facility, or mental hospital if he has a psychosis.

Economically, extended illness may drain the financial resources of the family; hospitalization insurance may be completely utilized and illness and unemployment benefits used up. Chronic disease such as cancer, in which periodic admissions to the hospital are necessary, may not only consume life savings but also may result in loss of a home and reduction of the family to complete dependency. The person with an acute illness realizes that it is temporary

and knows that when his health returns, he can deal with problems realistically. The patient with a prolonged illness becomes discouraged and depressed; fear and anxiety are his constant companions, and he may believe that he is losing his grasp on life. Studies indicate that a high percentage of families receiving some form of public assistance have one or more persons in the home suffering from chronic disease.

HOME-CARE PROGRAMS

Some persons must be cared for in the hospital because of the nature of their illnesses, but many may be cared for in their homes under planned home-care programs. Some patients may not be ready to be returned to their homes and may be transferred to an intermediate facility (extended care), where medical and nursing care is sufficient to provide for the patient's continued convalescence.

Various types of home-care programs have existed for years, including those provided by voluntary visiting nursing associations, many of which are still in operation. During the past 15 years other home-care plans have been developed. In some areas a modified plan for home care has been developed by Blue Cross for patients who are covered by Blue Cross hospital insurance. Persons who are 65 years of age and older may be eligible for care under the Social Security Act. Amendments to the Social Security Act of 1935 provide for care in an extended care facility or at home. The extended care facility must meet certain requirements established under Medicare and must provide skilled nursing care and medical supervision. Medical insurance provides up to 100 days of care in an extended care facility. When visiting nurse services are available, Medicare will pay for 100 home visits a year. The home-care plan covers only part-time nursing care but also includes speech therapy, physical and occupational therapy, and medical social services. Medical supplies are covered, but no drugs are included. Changes are constantly being made in services covered, and the patient or his family should be advised to visit their nearest Social Security office to secure the most current information. Additional programs to supplement home care such as Homemaker Service and Meals on

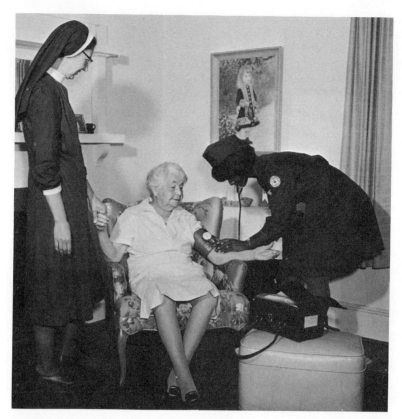

Fig. 6-2. Public health assistants help provide home care for chronically ill patients.

Wheels are available in some areas, primarily in metropolitan areas.

In recent years group hospital programs have been developed under the American Association of Retired Persons (A.A.R.P.). Individual members of the association who are 55 years of age and older may secure any of a variety of hospital and medical care programs at a moderate cost.

Advantages. Home care removes the patient from the hospital environment where he is constantly confronted with sickness and death. It provides increased freedom and fosters greater do-it-yourself care. It may permit a mother to manage the affairs of the home. The patient is returned to an environment where he is among family and friends, those who care for and love him. When the patient is properly conditioned, home care may promote well behavior rather than sick behavior. It relieves the family of the heavy burden of hospital costs.

Disadvantages. Patients who have been hospitalized for long periods of time often develop feelings of dependency and are unable to make the adjustment to home care. They may believe that because of their incapacitation their role in home life has changed and become depressed and morbid. Depending on their disability, they may be unable to return to their traditional patterns of living, and although some will accept their situations and strive to be "good patients," others will be resentful and demanding of family members or may try to exert control by acting completely helpless. Although the family may have agreed to the home-care plan, they may find that the burden of meeting the patient's physical and emotional needs is more than they can endure.[4]

SPECIFIC ASPECTS OF NURSING CARE

Specific diseases will be reviewed in their appropriate sections; however, special problems are encountered in caring for many

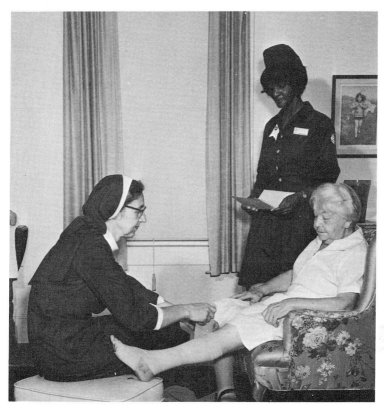

Fig. 6-3. Nurses provide care to patients in their homes.

patients with long-term illness. Caring for these patients is not always pleasant. The nurse must have the capacity to feel for the person being cared for, must avoid emotional ties, but must be able to bring to the patient something that will break the monotony of the humdrum existence he so often experiences.

Bed rest. Long periods of bed rest may be especially hazardous for the older patient. If the patient is permitted out of bed, he should be up several times a day. If the patient is required to remain in bed, his position must be changed at regular intervals to avoid stagnation of the normal flow of blood. The patient confined to bed may easily develop circulatory stasis in the lower extremities, which contributes to clot formation. Body weight should be evenly distributed, and support should be provided with pillows, trochanter rolls, and a footboard. Prolonged bed rest affects nearly all body systems.

The CircOlectric bed is an electrically operated bed (Fig. 6-4) that permits easy turning of the patient from the supine to the prone position, or it may place him in a standing position. There is a removable section that provides for easy use of the bedpan. The flexibility of the bed makes it possible to position the patient to relieve pressure on areas where the skin may break down. In the standing position it assists the patient in getting into a chair and contributes to the achievement of ambulation and rehabilitation.

Urinary incontinence. A major problem associated with long-term illness may be keeping the patient dry. There are many factors that contribute to urinary incontinence, but whatever the cause, it results in embarrassment for the patient and causes social withdrawal. Systematic habits of both bladder and bowel function are important, and a planned program of bladder training may be instituted with permission of the physician. (See Chapter 15.) If the patient is ambulatory, he may be

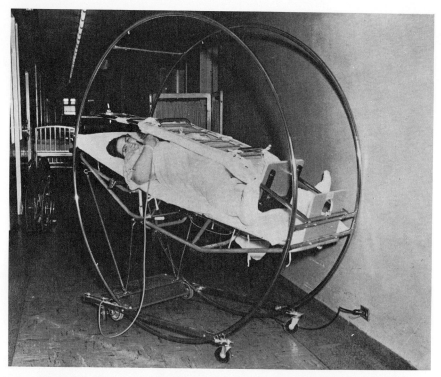

Fig. 6-4. CircOlectric bed simplifies turning the patient and facilitates early ambulation. The bed may be operated by the patient and may be tilted to a standing position. (Courtesy Orthopedic Frame Co., Kalamazoo, Mich.)

taken to the bathroom or may be permitted to use a bedside commode. The psychologic effect of being able to utilize the facilities to which he is accustomed and of being in a normal position often corrects the problem (Fig. 6-5). Skin care is a must for the incontinent patient if decubiti are to be prevented. However, all chronically ill patients should receive careful perineal care at regular intervals. Meticulous perineal care for both male and female patients cannot be compromised if urinary tract infection is to be controlled and odors are to be prevented. Many medical-surgical patients are able to provide this care for themselves. However, a large number of patients with long-term chronic illnesses are unable to do so. This then becomes just as much a nursing care responsibility as is giving a medication. It is suggested that the nurse wear disposable gloves and use cotton balls and an antiseptic such as benzalkonium chloride (Zephiran) solution 1:1000 to cleanse the area, using the same technique as that for

catheterization.[6] Disposable underpads that are waterproof and medicated to prevent skin irritation and odors are available commercially. They may be obtained in several sizes. In the home a suitable substitute can be made from several layers of newspapers covered with clean cloths.

Indwelling catheters. Infection of the urinary tract is most common among patients with indwelling catheters and continuous bladder drainage. The care of catheters is reviewed in Chapter 15. Carelessness in maintaining aseptic technique during catheterization and irrigating procedures is an important factor in the occurrence of infection.

Decubitus ulcers. Necrotic ulcers may be a cause of considerable discomfort for the patient and may require costly nursing time and dressings. Decubitus ulcers commonly occur over areas of the body in which bones are near the surface of the skin and where there is little muscle and fat between the bone and the skin. Pressure over these

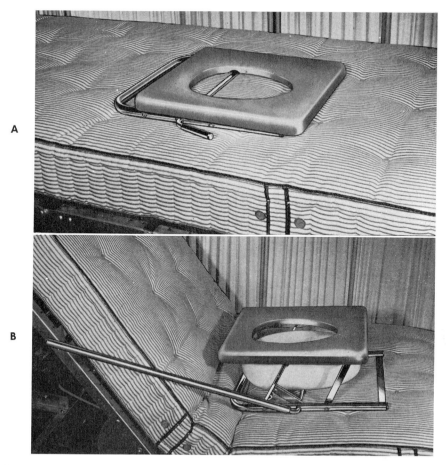

Fig. 6-5. Pan-Aid is a simple, comfortable, and safe device for patients confined to bed. It facilitates urinary continence and bowel training. With the pan laying flat, as shown in **A,** roll the patient onto the Pan-Aid. **B,** Elevate the head of the bed and elevate the Pan-Aid with the lever; slip the pan into place. (Courtesy R. D. Grant Co., Cleveland, Ohio.)

areas cuts off the blood supply and deprives the area of nutrition. When the skin is broken, there is rapid destruction of the underlying tissues. The ulcer becomes infected, frequently with *Escherichia coli* (p. 68). Any patient who must be on prolonged bed rest is likely to develop decubitus ulcers unless they receive expert care. Malnourished, debilitated, and emaciated individuals are especially susceptible when on bed rest. Urinary and fecal incontinence, moisture from perspiration, together with poor skin hygiene are contributing factors.[14]

Prevention. The cost of caring for one patient with a decubitus ulcer has been estimated to be from $2000 to $10,000. In spite of preventive measures, they continue to occur, and curative measures have left much to be desired. Researchers have worked diligently to discover a safe way to prevent this painful and costly complication. Prevention basically depends on the amount of nursing care necessary to protect areas most susceptible to breakdown. There is no substitute for conscientious nursing care. Nursing procedures of importance include (1) a dry, unwrinkled surface, (2) freedom from irritating substances such as crumbs in the bed, (3) frequent change of position, and (4) frequent massage of threatened areas. The old method of using doughnuts and rubber rings is discouraged because these devices create rings of pres-

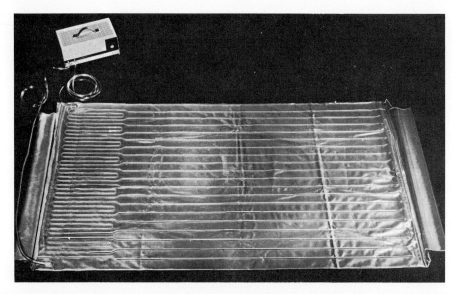

Fig. 6-6. Airmass alternating pressure pad is an adjunct to good nursing care in preventing decubitus ulcers. (Courtesy R. D. Grant Co., Cleveland, Ohio.)

sure, which further restrict circulation. Preventing decubitus ulcers in long-term and elderly patients requires intensive nursing care and is not an easy task. Ulcers may occur quickly from only slight pressure; this is especially true with elderly persons. Frequently, patients entering hospitals and nursing homes have large necrotic ulcers when admitted.

The free circulation of air stimulates the peripheral circulation of blood, and the bedding may be elevated over a bed cradle to allow free flow of air. The judicious and proper use of various devices as adjuncts to nursing care is helpful in preventing decubitus ulcers, but should never be used to replace good nursing care.

The CircOlectric bed, mentioned previously, permits easy, smooth, and frequent change of position. The fact that this may be accomplished by the patient or by one nurse not only is important to economy in nursing time but also permits frequently inspection of pressure areas and treatment with a minimum of effort.

The Airmass alternating pressure pad (Fig. 6-6) is designed as a nursing aid. It is essentially a pneumatic mattress with air cells running up and down its entire length. The air cells empty and fill so that when part of the cells are empty, others

are filled; thus no part of the body is under pressure longer than 90 seconds. The nurse should explain the procedure for using the pad and its purpose before placing the patient on the pad. Care should be taken not to puncture it with pins when fastening the bell signal or tubes to the sheet.

Shearlings are often used to prevent decubitus ulcers in patients confined to bed. The skin is placed over the drawsheet under the patient and will usually reach from the shoulders down to the buttocks of the average patient. They are made in sizes to fit other parts of the body such as the heel as well as in the large size. If they are used for incontinent patients, it is necessary to provide more than one skin to allow time for laundering. To maintain the sheepskin in good condition, proper laundering is essential. Instructions for laundering may be obtained from the address below.*

Elbows and heels may be protected by using sponge rubber cups (Fig. 6-7).

A new approach has been achieved by a device known as the Stryker flotation pad with Spence Gel (Fig. 6-8). A PolyVent mattress is placed on top of the regular

---

*Division of Products Development and Technical Services, The Wool Bureau, Inc., 360 Lexington Ave., New York, N. Y. 10017.

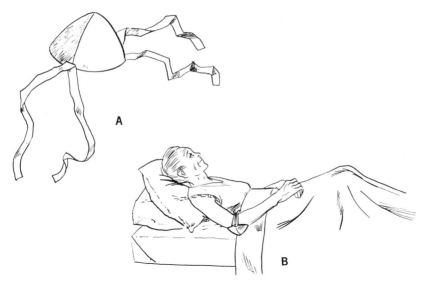

Fig. 6-7. Elbows and heels may be protected from friction by the use of sponge rubber cups made from bra padding purchased from the dime store. Twill tape is sewed to them, **A,** and the tape can then be tied about the part to keep the cups in place, **B.**

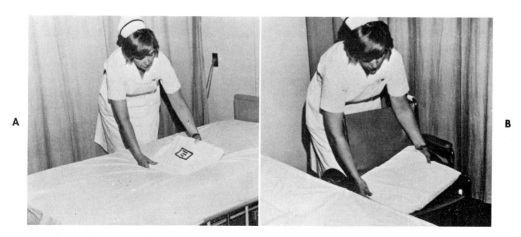

Fig. 6-8. Flotation pad. **A,** Pad centered over polyvent mattress covered with a sheet. **B,** Pad may be transferred to the chair when the patient is sitting up. (Courtesy Stryker Corp., Kalamazoo, Mich.)

Don't cover Gel c̄ sheet!

mattress and is covered with a sheet. The flotation pad is placed on top of the sheet, and the patient is positioned on the pad. The pad is constructed of a delicate material called Spence Gel and is covered by a thin elastic membrane to protect the gel. The pad may be cleaned with soap and water or a mild antiseptic, or it may be autoclaved. Research studies using the Stryker flotation pad have produced excellent results in preventing decubitus ulcers.[10, 13]

Continued research has led to other types of flotation therapy for both prevention and treatment of decubitus ulcers. The Jobst Hydro-Float bed employs the principle of hydrostatic buoyancy, which results in a state of semiweightlessness. The Hydro-Float bed is a complete flotation unit that utilizes hydraulic power. By the simple

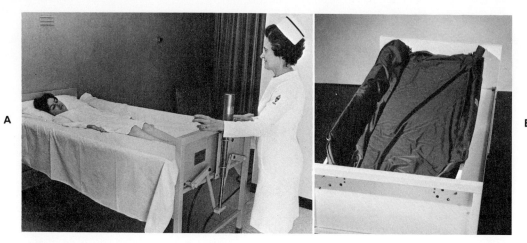

Fig. 6-9. A, Hydro-Float bed is easily placed in operation by one nurse. **B,** Hydro-Float bed minimizes pressure, which is equally distributed and remains constant. The bed requires little maintenance and saves nursing time. (Courtesy Jobst Institute, Inc., Toledo, Ohio.)

closing of one valve and opening of another the patient may be placed in flotation; the reverse procedure removes the patient from flotation for nursing care. When the patient is placed in flotation, pressure is evenly distributed over the greatest possible contact surface of the body. A pressure of approximately 8 mm. Hg is maintained over the entire surface of the body. A healthy flow of blood that prevents formation of pressure sores and permits those already present to heal is maintained (Fig. 6-9). Flotation pads are also available as wheelchair cushions, commode pads, and bed pads, all of which utilize the same principle of hydrostatic buoyancy.

Flotation has also been achieved in a water bed. The bed is simple in design, consisting of a foam rubber frame that is the same length and width of a standard hospital mattress. The frame fits over the hospital bed but is deeper than the mattress and is hollowed out. A plastic bladder partially filled with water is placed in the hollowed-out part and provides uniform support for the patient's body without concentrating pressure over any weight-bearing area of the body. It has been shown that when the patient is placed in the water bed, frequent turning is not required.[5] A type of water bed has been developed for home use and is available on the commercial market.

Treatment. The physician should prescribe treatment for decubitus ulcers just as he would for any other condition. It is the responsibility of the nurse to report the condition to the physician. Care is extremely difficult, and many methods of treatment have been tried with varying results.

The present trend in the treatment of decubitus ulcers appears to be toward some form of flotation therapy that will equalize pressure over the entire body area, rather than concentrate it over bony pressure areas. Although some flotation devices are somewhat expensive at the present time, others are available at a reasonable cost. In cases of large necrotic ulcers that fail to respond to treatment by any method, debridement and surgical closure are frequently considered.

As the search for satisfactory treatment of decubitus ulcers continues, several new methods are being used with some success. An enzymatic ointment (collagenase ABC ointment) has been developed for use as a debriding agent. Several precautions are necessary when using the ointment: (1) detergents and agents containing hexachlorophene must not be used, (2) soaks or preparations containing metals should be avoided, and (3) normal skin must be protected to avoid irritation and maceration. Prior to application of the ointment the lesion is cleaned with physiologic saline solution, and as much loose debris is removed as possible. If bacterial infection is present, it must be treated before the ointment is used. The ointment is applied directly to the lesion with a tongue blade, or it may be spread on gauze and applied to a superficial ulcer. The dressing is changed daily and any excess ointment removed before applying a new dressing.[1]

A method using hyperbaric oxygen has also been developed. The use of hyperbaric oxygen means exposing the area to oxygen at a pressure greater than atmospheric pressure. Special chambers have been developed that enclose only the lesion being treated. The necrotic ulcer is exposed to the oxygen daily for an average of 4 to 6 hours.[14]

Based on the technique of using hyperbaric oxygen for treating decubitus ulcers, an enterprising licensed practical nurse has developed a method of exposing decubitus ulcers to ordinary oxygen under slight pressure. By using plastic bags and equipment readily available, the area to be treated can be exposed to the oxygen. The results of the experiment appear to be rewarding.[7]

The nurse must remember that oxygen is an explosive gas, and when it is used, strict precautions must be followed.

Exercise. Exercise for the patient confined to bed is for the purpose of maintaining normal functioning of healthy muscles. In a well person muscle tone is maintained because the muscle fibers are constantly being stimulated. When a person is confined to bed, muscle fibers receive little or no stimulation, and the muscles lose their tone, become soft, and atrophy. The muscles that help to support a person in an upright position are the ones most likely to suffer, that is, those of the legs, back, hips, and neck.[8] Skeletal muscles lose their strength quickly, which is estimated to be about 5% a day. Passive exercise will help to prevent contracture of the joints but will have no effect on the muscles. A program of isometric exercises can be performed by nearly all patients, and when they are taught by the physical therapist, the patient can do them without nursing assistance.[2] "The physician indicates the amount of activity for the patient, but beyond this it is the nurse's responsibility to plan a program of exercise appropriate for the patient's capabilities."* The patient who lies quietly in bed with no exercise is predisposed to complications that involve most body systems. When the patient can sit up in a chair, support and gentle rocking in a rocking chair help to provide some muscle stimulation. If the patient must be totally confined to a bed, a side-lying position provides more muscle stimulation than does a supine or prone position.[8] The physician should be consulted regarding patients with arthritis and heart disease such as congestive failure before starting any exercise program.

Pain. Pain is something that cannot be defined by anyone except the person experiencing it. Since it is subjective, it is interpreted from different professional and cultural points of view; for example, Italian people place greater emphasis on the pain that they experience, Jewish people are more concerned about the cause of the pain, and physicians may believe that their professional ability is being questioned by the patient if they cannot relieve or eradicate the cause of the pain. It is the role of the physician to try to eliminate the pain by eliminating its cause. If eliminating the cause is impossible, the physician attempts to relieve the pain so that the person can tolerate it. There are two general types of pain: (1) skin pain, which causes a person to react quickly, and (2) deep pain, which may be described as an aching pain. Pain may be excruciating, or it may be so mild that it is almost unnoticeable. Some parts of the body are more sensitive to pain than are other parts. Superficial wounds are more painful than deep wounds, and organs such as the kidneys and the liver are almost insensitive to pain. Chronic pain may be a concomitant of some chronic and degenerative diseases such as cancer and arthritis.

Dr. Bonica of the University of Washington believes that the most disabling illness in the United States is chronic pain and that there is no reliable estimate of the number of persons who suffer from persistent inescapable pain.[9] Patients react dif-

---

*Kelly, Mary M.: Exercises for bedfast patients, American Journal of Nursing **66:**2209-2212, Oct., 1966.

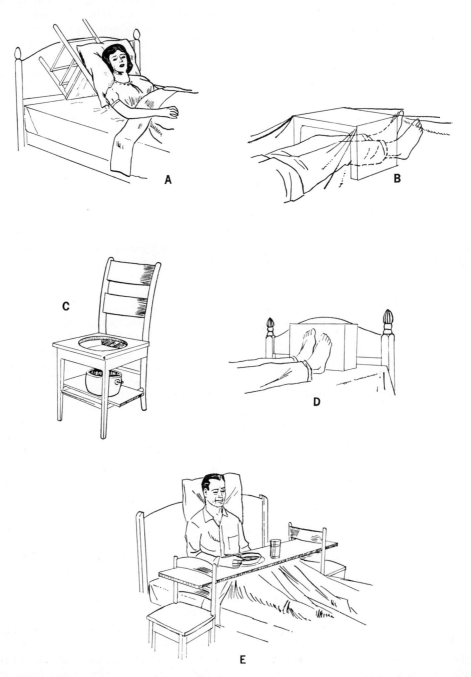

Fig. 6-10. Simple, homemade devices may be used to provide comfort for the patient with long-term illness. **A,** A chair may be used for a backrest. **B,** An ordinary cardboard box cut to fit over an extremity will prevent discomfort from weight of covers. **C,** A kitchen chair may be converted into a bedside commode. **D,** A box placed at the foot of the bed prevents foot drop. **E,** A board across two kitchen chairs serves as an overbed table.

ferently to pain, but whether mild or severe, it is always real to the person experiencing it. The nurse may observe various behavior indicators of pain such as facial expression, position assumed, tenseness, or clenching of the teeth or hands. The pain is subjective—it cannot be seen; therefore, the nurse should report only what is seen or what the patient describes. Patients in pain do not respond normally; talking and noise may only serve to intensify the pain. The nurse should remember that the patient may know the best way to be moved with the least pain. Supporting joints, proper placement of pillows, gentle massage of an aching part, tightening a sheet, adjusting room temperature, or providing encouragement may help mitigate the pain. When analgesics are ordered, it is often best to administer them before pain becomes too severe.[11]

Injections. Patients with protracted illness, whether in the home or in the hospital, frequently require the administration of drugs by subcutaneous or intramuscular routes. Among the most common drugs needed are narcotics for the relief of pain, especially in certain terminal illnesses. Although many persons with diabetes administer their own insulin, the nurse will have to administer it to some persons. Vitamin B_{12} and liver extract may be ordered for patients with primary anemia, and some patients may be receiving antibiotics. Edema occurs in some patients with heart or kidney disease, and nurses should remember not to inject drugs into edematous tissue. Basic nursing for the exact technique of injections should be reviewed, and the nurse should understand the desired results of the drug as well as the toxic signs that must always be anticipated.

Dressings. Numerous and varied dressings are frequently required by patients with chronic disease. In addition to dressings, soaks and irrigations are often needed. Patients with terminal cancer may require many dressings, as will patients with diabetic gangrene, varicose ulcers, and syphilitic gummas, which are chronic types of wounds requiring dressings. Often severely burned patients require dressings over a period of months.

Dental care. Care of the patient with prolonged illness should include dental care

and oral hygiene. When patients are unable to brush their teeth themselves, the nurse should assume the responsibility as part of good nursing care. Teeth should be brushed at night and in the morning and partial dentures removed for cleaning. Lack of oral hygiene leads to odors, bad taste, and tooth decay, accompanied by inflammation and bleeding gums. Poorly fitting dentures may cause irritation and sore gums, and unless they are removed and cleaned, they become unhygienic. Disorders commonly found in patients with prolonged illness include trench mouth (Vincent's angina) and abscessed teeth. If possible, patients should be taken to the dentist for care. In some large cities there are dentists who provide dental care for patients in their homes.

Rehabilitation. Rehabilitation of the chronically ill person requires a team effort. The patient needs to be constantly confronted with his abilities rather than his disabilities (Fig. 6-10). The nurse contributes to the total rehabilitation of the individual by helping the patient from bed to chair, assisting him to walk, and teaching him to administer his own insulin or to irrigate a colostomy and change the dressing. Persons with irreversible chronic illness are too often forgotten by society. It should be remembered that they want to have self-respect, some interest in life, and a feeling that they are loved and wanted. To help the chronically ill person achieve fulfillment of his own personal needs the nurse must believe in the dignity and worth of the individual, no matter how old or how sick he may be. All who have contact with any person with prolonged illness should seek to inspire and motivate the patient to greater independence and self-care and to help provide or create a climate of social acceptance and communication.[12] (See Chapter 10.)

Summary outline

1. Chronic illness is any condition in which the physiologic and psychologic condition causes partial or total dependency
2. Terms frequently associated with long-term illness
   A. Chronic disease—disorder involving structure and/or function that may be expected to continue over an extended period of time
   B. Convalescence—period of recovery after illness or surgical procedure

C. Exacerbation—return or increase of symptoms of disease

D. Extended care—care of patient during intermediate period when he no longer requires intensive hospital care but is not well enough to go home

E. Remission—relief of symptoms of disease and temporary improvement

F. Terminal illness—disease from which patient is not expected to recover

3. Factors related to chronic disease
There is considerable overlapping of various states of illness
A. Chronic disease may be predisposing factor in other illness
B. More than one chronic disease may exist in same person at same time
C. Each patient with chronic illness must be handled on individual basis

4. Age factors—chronic disease no respecter of persons
A. Seventy-five percent of persons with chronic illness are over 65 years of age
B. Twenty percent of patients with chronic disease are under 17 years of age
C. Over 30% of the chronically ill are between 17 and 24 years of age

5. Psychosocial factors
A. Any physical condition that affects health will affect psychologic behavior
B. Patient must be considered in relation to society
C. Environmental air pollution affects some persons with chronic illness
D. Physical disability causes loss of individual's sense of worth and dignity
E. Chronic illness deprives person of stimulation and feeling of social acceptance
F. Emotional behavior is to be anticipated
G. Psychosocial factors may lead to self-destruction

6. Prevention and control of chronic disease
Significant progress in preventing some diseases that caused chronic illness in the past
A. Prevention of
1. Rheumatic fever and rheumatic heart disease resulting from sore throat caused by hemolytic streptococci
2. Heart disease resulting from diphtheria
3. Deafness, heart disease, and mental retardation through immunization against rubella
4. Congenital syphilis through treatment of infected pregnant women
B. Chronic illness that can be controlled but not cured
1. Diabetes mellitus
2. Some parasitic infections
3. Epilepsy
4. Vitamin-deficiency diseases
5. Myasthenia gravis
6. Parkinson's disease
C. Diseases for which there is little prevention or control
1. Cancer
2. Hypertension

3. Arteriosclerosis
4. Nephritis
5. Mental illness
6. Chronic obstructive pulmonary disease
D. Personal factors
1. Cigarette smoking
2. Hallucinogenic agents
E. Chronic disease increased because of increase in number of older persons
1. Degenerative diseases may be related to normal aging process
a. Most tend to be progressive
b. All do not progress at same rate and may vary in different individuals

7. Prolonged illness and family
A. Viewed by some as major catastrophe and and accepted by others as part of life
B. Requires adjustment for members of family
1. Rearrangement of home
2. Readjustment and responsibility when outside help is needed
3. Child may have to stop school
4. Public health nurse may teach and supervise member of family in care of patient
5. It may not be possible to care for patient in home
C. Extended illness drains financial resources
1. Hospital insurance used up
2. Illness and unemployment benefits exhausted
3. Life savings completely used
4. May reduce family to complete dependency
D. Patient becomes discouraged and depressed
1. Develops feelings of fear and anxiety
2. May feel he is losing grasp on life

8. Home-care programs
Some patients must be cared for in hospital because of the nature of their illnesses
A. Voluntary visiting nursing associations
B. Blue Cross hospital insurance programs
C. Social Security benefits
1. In extended care facility
2. In home
D. Group hospitalization under A.A.R.P.
E. Supplementary programs to home care
1. Homemaker Services
2. Meals on Wheels
F. Advantages
1. Removes patient from hospital environment
2. Fosters do-it-yourself care
3. Permits mother to direct activities of home
4. Patient among family and friends
5. Promotes well behavior rather than sick behavior
6. Relieves family of heavy burden of hospitalization
G. Disadvantages
1. Patient develops feeling of dependency and is unable to adjust
2. May become depressed and morbid
3. May become demanding and resentful
4. May try to control situation by acting helpless

5. Family may find burden of care too much for them
9. Specific aspects of nursing care
    A. Bed rest may be hazardous for elderly persons
        1. Position must be changed frequently
        2. Body weight should be evenly distributed and supported with pillows, trochanter rolls, and footboards
    B. Urinary incontinence—major problem in care of patients with chronic disease
        1. Systematic habits are important
        2. Bladder training with physician's permission
        3. Take patient to bathroom whenever possible
        4. Meticulous perineal care to avoid urinary tract infection and odors
    C. Indwelling catheters—increased likelihood of urinary tract infection is more common in patients with indwelling catheters and constant bladder drainage
    D. Decubitus ulcers
        1. Cause discomfort for patient
        2. Occur over areas where bones are near surface with little muscle and fat
        3. Contributing factors
            a. Person malnourished, debilitated, and emaciated
            b. Urinary and fecal incontinence
            c. Moisture from perspiration
            d. Poor skin hygiene
        4. Prevention
            a. Estimated cost to be from $2000 to $10,000
            b. Prevention based on amount of nursing care to protect susceptible areas
            c. Dry, unwrinkled bed surface
            d. Freedom from irritating substances in bed
            e. Frequent change of position
            f. Massage of threatened areas
            g. Avoid use of doughnuts and rubber rings
        5. Devices that augment nursing care
            a. CircOlectric bed
            b. Airmass alternating pressure pad
            c. Shearlings
            d. Stryker flotation pad
            e. Jobst Hydro-Float bed
            f. Water bed
        6. Treatment
            a. Enzymatic ointment (collagenase ABC ointment)
            b. Hyperbaric oxygen
            c. Oxygen under slight pressure by use of plastic bags
            d. Surgical debridment and skin closure
    E. Exercises to maintain normal functioning of healthy muscles
        1. Isometric exercises
        2. Gentle rocking of patient in rocking chair provides some muscle stimulation
        3. Side-lying position when in bed
    F. Pain
        1. General types of pain
            a. Skin pain
            b. Deep pain
        2. Observing patient with pain
            a. Facial expression
            b. Position assumed
            c. Tenseness
            d. Clenching teeth and hands
        3. Talking and noise may intensify pain
        4. Measures to help mitigate pain
            a. Let patient decide how to move to cause less pain
            b. Support joints
            c. Proper placement of pillows
            d. Massage of aching part
            e. Tightening of sheet
            f. Adjusting room temperature
            g. Provide encouragement
            h. Use of analgesics
    G. Injections, administered by subcutaneous or intramuscular routes, required for many patients with chronic disease
    H. Dressings required for patients with chronic ulcers, severe burns, and other conditions
    I. Dental care
        1. To prevent odors, bad taste, and tooth decay
        2. Common disorders are trench mouth and abscessed teeth
        3. Patients should be taken to dentist if possible
    J. Rehabilitation
        1. Team effort required
        2. Emphasis on abilities rather than on disabilities
        3. Inspire and motivate to greater independence
        4. Provide or create climate of social acceptance and communication

Review questions

1. What is the term for a temporary relief of symptoms?
    a. *remission*
2. How would you define a chronic disease?
    a. *incurable - long lasting - debilitating*
3. What emotional problems may be anticipated in a patient with a chronic disease?
    a. *depression*
    b. *anger*
    c. *fear*
    d. *dependency*
    e.
4. List three advantages of home care for a chronically ill person.
    a. *financially less burdensome*
    b. *among loved ones*
    c. *familiar surroundings*
5. List two disadvantages of home care for a chronically ill person.
    a. *lack of trained personnel*
    b. "   " *medical equipment*
6. What is a major complication of prolonged bed rest?
    a. *stasis & decubitus*
7. What are three methods of treating decubitus ulcers?

a. *hyperbaric O₂*
b. *surgical closure*
c. *H₂O bed-flotation mattress*

8. Why is the older method of using cotton doughnuts and rubber rings not recommended?
   a. *added pressure to parts*
9. What bacterial organism may cause infection of a decubitus ulcer?
   a. *E. coli*
10. What observations would you make if a patient reports pain?
   a. *redness*
   b. *swelling*
   c. *expression*
   d. *position*

Films

1. A short way home—M-1454-X (12 to 15 min., sound, color, 16 mm.), Media Resources Branch, National Medical Audiovisual Center (Annex), Station K, Atlanta, Ga. 30324. Portrays home health services with emphasis on home care; shows a variety of patients receiving services in the home and the team activities in providing such care.
2. Dental care for the chronically ill and the aged—Mis-704 (19 min., sound, color, 16 mm.), Media Resources Branch, National Medical Audiovisual Center (Annex), Station K, Atlanta, Ga. 30324. Shows how dental care can be provided for chronically ill, aged, bedridden, and nonambulatory patients in the home.
3. Techniques for maintenance of range of motion—F-1471-X (19 min., color film slides, 89 frames, 35 mm.), Media Resources Branch, National Medical Audiovisual Center (Annex), Station K, Atlanta, Ga. 30324. Demonstrates various kinds of passive exercise that can be used for any patient confined to bed for a prolonged period of time.

References

1. Barrett, Daniel, Jr., and Klibanski, Aron: Collagenase debridement, American Journal of Nursing 73:849-851, May, 1973.
2. Brower, Phyllis, and Hicks, Dorothy: Maintaining muscle function in patients on bed rest, American Journal of Nursing 72:1250-1253, July, 1972.
3. Dubos, René: The crisis of man in his environment, Journal of the American Association of University Women 62:164-167, May, 1969.
4. Field, Minna: Patients are people—a medical-surgical approach to prolonged illness, ed. 3, New York, 1967, Columbia University Press.
5. Flotation therapy, The Journal of Practical Nursing 19:29-31, Feb., 1969.
6. Gibbs, Gertrude E.: Perineal care of the incapacitated patient, American Journal of Nursing 69:124-125, Jan., 1969.
7. Hoffmiller, Mary: Oxygen therapy—its use in chronic skin ulcers, The Journal of Practical Nursing 23:20-23, May, 1973.
8. Kinnaird, Leah S.: Preserving skeletal muscle tone in inactive patients, American Journal of Nursing 69:2662-2663, Dec., 1969.
9. Pain, Washington, D. C., 1968, Government Printing Office.
10. Robertson, Caroline E.: Gel pillow helps prevent pressure sores, The Canadian Nurse 67:44-46, Oct., 1971.
11. Smith, Dorothy W., and Germain, Carol P. Hanley: Care of the adult patient, ed. 4, Philadelphia, 1975, J. B. Lippincott Co.
12. Soller, Genevieve R.: The aging patient, American Journal of Nursing 62:114-117, Nov., 1962.
13. Spence, Wayman R., Burke, Richard D., and Rae, James W.: Gel support for prevention of pressure necrosis, reprinted by the Stryker Corporation from a report presented June 28, 1966, to the American Medical Association, Chicago.
14. Torelli, Michael: Topical hyperbaric oxygen for decubitus ulcers, American Journal of Nursing 73:494-496, March, 1973.

CHAPTER 7

The dying patient and death

KEY WORDS

acceptance
anger
bargaining
bereavement
catastrophic
circumvent
denial
depression
deprivation
dignity
electroencephalograph
euthanasia
expertise
grief

hemodialysis
homicide
irreversible
living will
phobia
priority
psychosomatic
stigma
suicide
thanatology
transplantation

From the earliest records to the present day, men have known that they would die. They spend much of their lives in preparation for the time when they will die. The individual secures life insurance to provide for his family when he is gone. He provides for the unpaid principal on his home. He seeks education and income sufficient to accumulate an estate to pass on to his heirs. He desires offspring so that his name will continue. He builds living monuments to himself in the form of foundations, scholarships, art, literature, and technology so that he will not be forgotten after death. He prepares a will and arranges for a burial lot and in some instances has been known to write his own obituary. Although men do not know the day or the hour when they will die, they know that death will come and make elaborate preparation for it while at the same time living as if it will never happen to them.

Death has permeated much of the religious music throughout the ages, imploring people to be ready and offering comfort to those who remain.

> Sunset and evening star,
>   and one clear call for me!
> And may there be no moaning of the bar
>   when I put out to sea.
> *Alfred Tennyson, 1889*

Death, sorrow, and grief is told in some of the modern music of the twentieth century. In opera, tragic death with sorrow and mourning brings the audience closer to the realization of their own eventual death. In literature, fiction and nonfiction death may be a central theme.

The poet writes of death:

> Garlands upon his grave
> and flowers upon his hearse,
> and to the tender hearts and brave
> The tribute of this verse.
>
> *Longfellow, 1874*

On radio and television, fantasy and reality of death, with its sorrow, grief, and mourning constantly remind that death comes to all regardless of age, sex, race, religion, or social and economic status. The fact cannot be altered, and each person knows it.

SCIENTIFIC RESEARCH

Than-a-to is a combining form meaning death, and *thanatology* means the study of death by scientific methods.[5] It is necessary to understand how the physiologic and psychologic factors surrounding death affect the individual. Many of the physiologic processes are well known, and the physician can predict death with reasonable accuracy. However, the psychologic impact of impending death on the patient is less understood.

Although death is the culmination of living, it has been shrouded in mystery through the ages. Until the last two decades few persons have been fearless enough to write or even talk about death and dying. Recently numerous research studies have been initiated, and many articles have been published in professional publications; in fact, many books on death and dying are appearing. At this time few specific conclusions have emerged, and most scientists agree that much more research is needed.

As each person moves toward his own death, he views the experience and accepts death in his own way. Therefore there is no specific pattern applicable to all persons. Through the scientific study of death and dying it is hoped to gain insight that will aid physicians, nurses, and others in caring for and understanding the fatally ill person and in providing support for the family.

CAUSE OF DEATH

Death results from many different causes. The largest number of deaths are caused by disease, and heart disease and malignant disorders cause more deaths than other diseases. Some persons may have prolonged lingering illness before death occurs, whereas others may experience sudden death. Many children formerly died from infectious diseases, but medical research and active immunization programs have prevented most of these deaths. Accidents on the highway, at home, in industry, and on the farm claim thousands of lives every year. Other deaths may result from catastrophic occurrences. Whereas many accidents cause instant death with no time to prepare for the event, injured persons may die later as the result of the accident. Death may also occur from acts of violence. When one person kills another person, it is called *homicide;* when an individual takes his own life, it is called *suicide* (p. 113).

Many persons die every year from the ingestion of poisons or lethal doses of drugs. Such deaths may be accidental, as in children who ingest poison substances or medicines. Overdoses of drugs may be taken deliberately to cause death.

The fetus may die in utero, or the infant may be stillborn; some infants who are born alive die soon after birth. At the other end of the continuum are elderly persons, most of whom have various chronic diseases that may cause their death. Some elderly persons die with no cause known. Lay persons often attribute such deaths to "natural causes." There is no such thing as death from a natural cause. Such a statement implies that there is a predetermined time for an elderly person to die. Actually death may have been caused by disease for which he failed or refused to secure medical care.[13]

Certain deaths such as suicide or highway accidents caused by intoxication with alcohol are often looked on as a stigma. It is not unusual for the victim's family to attribute death to a heart attack.

The nurse may now realize that death results from many different conditions and situations. Death also may occur at any point along the continuum from fetal life to extreme age. Whatever the cause, death is inevitable at some time in the life of each individual.

Few persons can predict the time of their own death. There are some recorded instances in which a person has indicated when death would occur, but most occur among elderly persons who realize that because of their age they may not live long. Sometimes their predictions are associated with members of the family who died at a specific age. When the individual reaches that age, he predicts that he will die as members of his family did.[15]

WHEN DOES DEATH OCCUR?

The question of when death occurs is highly controversial. A diagnosis of death is usually made when there is an absence of heartbeat and cessation of respiration. These signs as the only criteria for determining death were questioned when the first transplantation of a human heart was accomplished in 1967. Physicians who were interested in organ transplants believed that a new definition should be found. The principle reason for this is that the organ from a donor must be removed as quickly as possible after death. A question that has not been resolved concerns whether a person is actually dead even though the heart may still be beating.

In an effort to answer the question, "When is death?" physicians employed the electroencephalograph to measure brain activity. They believe that the absence of brain activity, even though the heart is still beating, indicates that death has taken place. Based on this assumption several new definitions have been proposed.

In 1968, Healey and Harvey[14] defined death as "the irreversible cessation of (1) total cerebral function, (2) spontaneous function of the respiratory system, and (3) cessation of the circulatory system." Christian Barnard believed that a person may be considered dead when (1) the heart shows no electrical activity for 5 minutes, (2) no spontaneous respiration, and (3) the absence of reflexes.[14] Recently a large medical center has stated that most physicians accept a definition based on the absence of brain waves.

A noted lawyer speaking at a conference of the Euthanasia Foundation stated that any definition as to "When is death?" is a complicated legal problem.[14] A question that remains unanswered concerns exactly when the brain may be considered dead.

The use of the electroencephalograph in determining when a person is dead will probably be used only in medical centers where organ transplants are performed. In most hospitals physicians will determine death by the traditional methods, absence of heartbeat, and cessation of respiratory function. This determination is a medical responsibility, and nurses should not assume this function.

DEATH WITH DIGNITY

Death with dignity means that an incurably ill, dying patient will be allowed to die without prolonging life by extraordinary measures. This is also called *passive euthanasia* and means withholding any form of treatment that would continue life. When a patient's life is terminated by methods other than natural death, it is called *positive euthanasia*. Suicide is an example of voluntary euthanasia.

These are new concepts in a society where death and dying has been a taboo subject. The question of death with dignity or any form of euthanasia gives rise to many emotional and controversial issues with varied interpretations.[1] A noted clergyman has stated that passive euthanasia is practiced throughout all hospitals. He believes that the quality of life is what is important, and when there is no chance for a person's life to be meaningful, that person is already dead.[3] However, not everyone will agree with this philosophy.

Technology has made available sophisticated equipment to prolong life. Medical science has developed drugs and devised ways to prolong life and relieve suffering. The locale of the dying person has been transferred from the home to the modern hospital, where he may have the benefit of the scientific equipment. However, with even the finest facilities the patient finds himself in a lonely friendless world, surrounded by endless mechanical equipment and with personnel who are impersonal concerning what happens to him.[10] It is still true that the function of the modern hospital is to save life, not to end it. Social change has not only provided the means to save life but has also brought a change in the philosophy of the hospital. Some physicians are finding that the idealistic and moralistic philosophy engendered by the Hippocratic oath is giving way to a more realistic belief in purposeful survival.

If saving a life does not provide for the life to be a meaningful one, what efforts should be made to save it? This is the problem encountered by many physicians and hospitals. Thus the question of using extraordinary means to prolong life of a hopelessly terminally ill patient becomes entangled in a web of ethical, religious, legal, moral, and idealistic problems.

To circumvent the issues involved in prolonging the life of the dying patient the Euthanasia Educational Fund, Inc., prepared the "living will." The document directs the patient's physician to let him die if his condition is irreversible. It is believed by some persons that the living will does not solve all of the questions concerning the dying patient and may actually create problems.[2] The living will may also be interpreted as voluntary and indirect euthanasia.

In August of 1972 a Senate Special Committee on Aging held a hearing for the purpose of developing priorities in dealing with terminal illness and the related questions. After 3 days of hearings it was agreed that there are no easy answers to such an emotional and controversial issue.[2]

It is the responsibility of the physician to determine when heroic measures should be initiated and when they should be terminated. The nurse is not responsible for these decisions; however, in a crisis situation the nurse may find it necessary to make a decision to save a patient's life.[6]

The comfort of the dying patient precludes the use of any measure that will contribute to his comfort and safety and allay his emotional fears. If the use of oxygen relieves labored respiration, it should not be considered a heroic measure. However, administering a new expensive drug that can in no way alter the fatal outcome must be considered an unnecessary procedure.

PRIORITIES

Who will live and who is destined to die? These are questions facing many patients, families, and physicians. Medical science has made it possible to perform surgical procedures unheard of a decade ago. Anesthesia, drugs, and the expertise of well-trained nurses contribute to the medical revolution. The scientist has perfected complicated equipment. Some will have the benefit of living because of these medical and technologic advances, whereas others for various reasons will be denied the right to live. For example, some persons with failing renal function may be selected for hemodialysis in a medical center or in the home. Some of these persons will be kept alive and eventually receive a kidney transplant. Facilities, equipment, and donors are not available for all. Thus the physician must determine who will benefit most. The ultimate decision will mean that some will live and some will die. The same selective process may determine which patient may benefit from open heart surgery and which patient because of certain factors will not have surgery and will face certain death.

Nurses must understand why such decisions are made and must be prepared psychologically to accept them. In such situations the emotional support of the patient and his family should be uppermost in the nurse's mind.

FEAR OF DYING AND DEATH

The noted psychoanalyst Sigmund Freud believed that it was impossible for man to even imagine his own death.[4] Fear in many forms has always accompanied mortal existence. In some persons fear is so persistent and serious that it becomes a phobia. Fear exists from almost the moment of birth. A child may fear to go into a dark room, a father may fear the loss of his job, and a mother may fear mutilating surgery. Fears of this nature are unrelated to the fear of dying, but they do indicate the human ability to live with and overcome fear.

It is believed that there is a difference between the fear of dying and the fear of death. Fear of dying is usually present when the health of the individual is so compromised that there is a distinct possibility that he may die. This fear may lead the person to seek and/or accept extraordinary measures to prolong and prevent death. When all measures fail to preserve life and death is imminent, the person fears death. This fear concerns the physical cessation of vital functions and what will happen when mortal life ceases. The fear of dying may also be related to sociologic factors, frequently overlooked, which are often of primary importance to the dying patient.

Although research into fear of dying is limited, there is some indication that not all persons fear dying. Kastenbaum and Aisenberg[8] report that fear and anxiety may be found in the dying patient but that depression is far more common. The patient with severe, painful physical symptoms may be more anxious, whereas the patient who is aware of his terminal condition may experience a greater degree of depression.

There are many variables related to the fear of dying, including age, social status, educational and occupational background, serious chronic disease, and the mental condition of the individual. The aged person who has undergone biologic changes characteristic of his age group appears to show less fear of dying than younger persons. Jager and Simmons[7] report that elderly persons rarely refer to dying or to death and seem to accept death as the inevitable outcome because of their age. They also found that when one person died in a ward of elderly persons, the others accepted the loss with no significant emotion.

Death means the end of everything that the person has held dear and enjoyed throughout life. Although he mourns his loss, his fears are primarily related to the unknown. What happens after death? Is there an afterlife? Is death a painful experience? What happens to the body after death? One person expressed that his fear of mutilation by the living creatures of the soil was a thought that he could not bear. The person who has a religious background and who has a firm belief in an afterlife may experience less fear of death. A person may have fear about what will happen to his family and the grief and sorrow that his death will cause. As death nears, most fears subside. As mentioned previously, when the psychologic and social factors have been resolved, this contributes to the calmness of death. Kübler Ross[9] found that when there is opportunity for communication, counseling, and resolution of problems, death can be more easily accepted.

EMOTIONAL ATTITUDES TOWARD DEATH

Observation of terminally ill patients has seemed to indicate that a patient may exhibit several well-defined attitudes toward his illness and approaching death. Not all persons accept this concept. It is also known that not all patients exhibit behavior characteristics of each stage. There may also be variation in the sequence of behavioral attitudes exhibited by the patient. These behavior patterns have been variously identified as denial, anger, bargaining, depression, and acceptance.[9]

Denial. Denial is not confined to the patient. It is found among members of the patient's family and the medical and nursing staff. Kübler-Ross[9] found that physicians denied having terminally ill patients on the hospital wards. Others have found that physicians avoid dying patients and refuse to answer their questions. Jager and Simmons[7] report that hospital policies frequently prevent nurses from discussing terminal illness with patients and that they tend to follow the practice of physicians. When the patient is unable to face the diagnosis of a serious disease, he denies its existence. Denial becomes a defense mechanism to protect the individual from thoughts that he is unable to accept. He denies the diagnosis, being certain that the physician has made a mistake. Denial may lead the patient to one or more physicians or to a large medical center, always hoping to find that a mistake has been made. For example, Mrs. A. was found to have inoperable carcinoma. As soon as she was able to travel, she entered a large medical center where she died before being able to return home. Mr. B. was found to have gastric cancer. His wife denied the accuracy of the diagnosis and refused to allow it to be mentioned to other members of the family.

Anger. Although the patient is not ready to accept his terminal illness, he may become angry. His anger is not directed toward physicians and nurses but toward his illness. He angrily asks, "Why couldn't it be someone else? Why should it be me?" His anger causes him to become complaining and difficult to care for. He finds everything to be wrong and nothing right.

Bargaining. Anger may subside, and the patient begins to think how he can buy time. His first approach may be to God. He asks for an extension of time and may promise God that he will lead a better life.

He may request a visit from the chaplain, seeking his intervention with God. He may implore the physician to tell him exactly how much time he has—always just enough time to accomplish some favorite activity or just to be alive.

Depression. Depression is marked by loss and grief. As the ravages of disease and illness begin to take their toll and the patient becomes weaker, he finds that he cannot deny his illness any longer. He becomes sad, he may cry, he may show less interest in visits from family and friends, and he withdraws and may become uncommunicative.

Acceptance. The final stage is one of acceptance. It is not one of active acceptance but passive acceptance because he is too weak to fight any longer. He longs for quiet and sleep and does not want to be disturbed by his friends. Although the family may have gone through the same stages as the patient, they also now accept the finality of the illness.[5]

Although these five stages may or may not be observed, hope never ends. Throughout terminal illness the patient never loses hope that some new drug, treatment, or medical discovery will alter the outcome of his illness.

Grief and bereavement

Grief is a severe emotional reaction to loss. The loss may be of material possessions, of self-identity, or of some body function or part. Separation from loved ones as in war or incarceration may cause one to grieve. Death of a close relative or friend may cause intense emotional behavior.

The dying patient may grieve because he is losing his life and the meaningful experiences of the past and the separation from those he loves. However, when the patient dies, there is nothing more that can be done for him. Attention is then focused on the significance of the death and what it means to others and to society.

Death always means bereavement, and persons most directly affected are the close family such as husband, wife, parents, or a child. More distant members of the family group may also mourn the loss of the relative. Nurses who have had long association in the care of the terminal patient may grieve

over his death. Studies of bereavement indicate that a wide range of behavior patterns may accompany grief. Some individuals are able to accept the crisis situation and appear to have the emotional stability and techniques to adjust to the loss, whereas others may develop psychosomatic complaints. There are studies indicating that in some instances pathologic conditions have developed after the loss of a close relative.

According to the United States census, the number of widows far exceed the number of widowers, and it has been estimated that by 1990 there will be 1000 widows for each 675 widowers. Women who lose their husbands are especially vulnerable to bereavement because of its consequences. It has been shown that an elderly woman who loses her husband may not experience the same problems associated with bereavement as a younger widow, her age being the mitigating factor. To maintain self-respect and self-identity is of paramount importance for the younger widow. The loss of the mate invariably means deprivation. Socially she may no longer have the same status and play the same role as when her husband lived. Often there is a loss of economic security and the standard of living that she formerly has been accustomed to. A widow may be reduced to poverty level or may be required to seek employment to support herself and a family. She is deprived of her husband's companionship and may find herself in a world of loneliness. She may experience sexual frustration and be left with the responsibility of rearing a family. According to Parkes,[12] when there is loss, there is also deprivation. The individual is most acutely aware of loss at the time of death and may not think about deprivation until some time later. However, deprivation invariably follows loss.

Parkes has indicated that grieving is a psychologic process with three distinct phases. After death of the individual the survivor may be numb with grief. It is at this time that the grieving family is surrounded by friends and sympathizers. After the burial rites have been completed and details taken care of the grieving person usually finds himself alone, and the second phase of grieving begins. The grief-stricken person begins to realize the loss and to mourn for the deceased. Although the person may continue to mourn and grieve, he will enter the last phase of the process—depression. It is during the phase of depression that most psychosomatic complaints may occur.

Many variables affect the grieving process, and there is no clear-cut pattern that can be applied to every individual. For some persons the period of grief may be only a few weeks, whereas for others it may last more than a year. The process may vary if the death is sudden and unexpected or if it occurs after a prolonged terminal illness. The death of a child may cause more intense grief than the death of an aged person. Emotional support and help that the nurse may provide to the grieving person will be discussed in the next section.

NURSING CARE OF THE TERMINAL AND DYING PATIENT

Earlier in this chapter attention has been focused on death as a normal event in the mortal life of all persons. Some of the current concepts in the changing social philosophy concerning terminal illness have been explored. It has been pointed out that some of these ideas are highly controversial and not accepted by all. In certain instances the role of the nurse in contrast to the responsibility of the physician has been delineated.

The responsibility of the nurse in the care of the terminal and dying patient is first to herself or himself, then to the patient, and finally to the patient's family. Since the family is so intimately related to the patient during terminal illness, it is difficult to separate them. After the patient's death the family becomes the primary concern.

Most of the literature documents the fact that nurses avoid the dying patient. It has been rationalized that the reason is because the dying patient reminds the nurse of her or his own death.[11] Schoenberg[13] believes that there are three factors relevant to the nursing care of the dying patient. First, the educational system fails to teach the student nurse how to care for the dying patient. Second, the system of medical practice in the hospital is one of nonin-

volvement. This philosophy prevents the nurse from providing more than the basic elements of care. Third, the nurse does not receive the emotional support necessary to work through personal feelings and to develop a philosophy about the care of the dying patient.

The nursing care of the terminally ill patient comprises physical and psychologic factors and their social implications. Terminal illness has been defined on p. 95. Terminal illness does not mean that the patient is facing immediate death. Many illnesses from which the patient is not expected to recover are marked by long remissions, punctuated by exacerbations at infrequent intervals, for example, leukemia, Hodgkin's disease, and cancer. Eventually there will be a final admission to the hospital.

During admissions to the hospital the nurse should come to know the patient—learn about his social and cultural background, his religious orientation, and personal problems that are of particular concern to him. The nurse should try to gain some insight into the patient's feelings and acceptance of his illness. Some patients may know their diagnosis and prognosis, whereas others may not have been given the information but appear to know. The patient may create situations hoping to get confirmation from the nurse. The nurse should be aware of this possibility and be prepared to handle it carefully. It is especially important that the nurse know what the physician has told the patient and his family.

If staffing patterns permit, the same nurse should be assigned to care for the patient on each admission. When this is possible, the patient develops a feeling of trust, security, and confidence. When the patient is admitted for the last time, the personal relationship that has been established may help to bridge the gap between living and dying.

As previously stated, a patient faces death in his own way. Some persons prefer to be left alone, whereas others may wish the presence of the nurse or a close relative. In most instances the patient does not want to feel that he has been abandoned. Frequent visits to the patient's room, a softly placed hand on the patient's shoulder, and a kindly spoken word conveys to the patient that he is not alone. The tendency to darken the room should be avoided. Lights should not be glaring, but normal light should be provided. The patient should be placed in an area where he can hear nurses moving about and thus feel that he is not alone.

The physical care of the patient must continue to the end. The patient may be unable to continue to perform for himself the care that was possible throughout his illness. Bathing, including perineal care, regular turning, skin care, support of dependent parts, and oral care must be given. Psychologically as well as medically the mouth has special meaning for the patient. Frequently during terminal illness the patient has neglected oral care. The membranes become dry and sore, and infection may be present causing mouth odor. The oral condition will interfere with speech and swallowing. When dentures cannot be worn, drooling will occur. Pathogenic organisms and oral secretions may cause stomatitis and maceration of tissues around the mouth. These conditions may cause the patient actual pain.[13] Oral care should be given at regular intervals and be sufficient to keep the tissues clean and free from odor. This care is especially important when oral cancer is present.

During terminal illness the nurse may expect that the patient will exhibit various kinds of emotional behavior. Whatever the behavior, the nurse must be willing to accept it. If the patient cries, the nurse should let him cry. The nurse should not tell him not to cry and that everything will be better after a while. If the patient is demanding and angry, it is important to understand that the behavior is not directed toward the nurse, who should not avoid the patient because of the behavior. Kindness will convey to the patient that the nurse accepts the behavior and will not forsake him.

A one-to-one relationship, that is, the nurse to the patient, should be maintained, keeping all channels of communication open at all times. The nurse should listen to what the patient says; ideas that the nurse may have should not be projected on the patient. It should be remembered that the dying patient is not interested in what the nurse thinks. When the nurse listens to the patient, it will be possible to identify what problems are of concern of him. They may be beyond the nurse's ability to solve; however, the social worker, hospital chaplain, or psychiatrist may be called to help the patient.

The nurse should remember that some religions teach that there is a life after death, and the dying patient may have a strong abiding faith in this belief which may often comfort the patient during the lingering hours preceding death. The patient's religious philosophy should be supported regardless of the nurse's own belief. Prayer by the hospital chaplain often provides emotional support for the patient and his family.

The patient may make accusations and display anger toward the family. The nurse must be able to provide emotional support for the family and interpret the patient's behavior to them. As previously reviewed, grief is a normal reaction to loss through death. Crying is to be expected. The family should be provided with a quiet place where they may be by themselves. It may be comforting to them if the nurse or the chaplain remains with them.

Sometimes feelings of guilt may cause the family to criticize the hospital and the care given to the patient; others may feel that everything possible has been done for the deceased person. Before the body is removed the family should have the opportunity to view the body in private if they wish to do so. After removal of the body, the nurse should assist the family in gathering the patient's belongings. The way in which the articles are handled may convey to the family the nurse's concern for their feelings. Escorting the family to their car with a kind word of encouragement is also helpful.

Each hospital has its own policies for care after death, varying with the hospital's size and location. The legal requirements concerning autopsy and interstate movement of the body may dictate some of the policies. Most morticians prefer to receive the body as soon after death as possible. In some instances the body may be placed in the hospital morgue. Nurses should become familiar with the policies and procedures of the hospital where they are employed.

SOCIETY AND DEATH

Almost all deaths touch society in some way. Society attaches labels to patients with certain kinds of disease. A diagnosis of cancer conveys to the patient, to his family, and to society a picture of prolonged, painful, and terminal illness. Society may not view other diseases in the same way, although they may be equally serious. Society also considers death according to the worth of the individual to society. An adolescent with a promising career ahead will be considered as a greater social loss than an elderly person who has lived a full life. The death of a noted artist or composer will make the headlines of the leading newspaper so that all society may mourn the loss.

Sudden death, as in acute myocardial infarction or in an emergency, may have a profound effect on society. An outstanding educator is drowned, a young physician is killed in a plane crash, a nurse is killed in an automobile accident, and a father is killed in an industrial accident—each of these situations have one thing in common, the loss of valuable service to society. There is also the monetary loss. In each case the lifetime income of the individual has been lost.

Societal problems are created each time a violent death occurs. Man-hours of work in investigation, autopsy, criminal laboratory examinations, and lengthy court litigation are often followed by years of incarceration. Society must pay the costs through public taxation.

When the breadwinner is killed or dies leaving a family, society may have to assume responsibility for the family. Governmental programs in the form of public relief and aid to dependent children are the result of public taxation.

In many areas land is becoming scarce for cemeteries, and new ways are being sought to care for the dead. Social change is bringing change to the inner cities, and mortuaries tend to move to residential suburbs. The transfer of the establishment often gives rise to controversy among residents of the area.

Although society may mourn the loss of the individual, the effects are often far reaching and long term and may touch every individual in society.

SOME GUIDELINES FOR THE CARE OF THE DYING PATIENT AND HIS FAMILY

1. The responsibility of the nurse is to provide nursing care for the patient so that his passage from mortal life to death will be as easy as possible.
2. Relief from the emotional problems as well as the physical suffering should be provided by any person who may be best able to help the patient.
3. The nurse should assess what the loss means to members of the patient's family, and those most vulnerable to grief should be given special attention to enable them to accept the loss with peace and calm.
4. Some members of the patient's family may be more susceptible to grief than other members. These persons may benefit from counseling and treatment.
5. To maintain self-esteem and dignity the patient should be permitted to make as many decisions concerning his nursing care and treatment as are compatible with his condition.
6. All channels of communication should be kept open.
7. Frequently, nonprofessional persons may be more important than professional personnel and have the compassion and understanding necessary to help the patient in his final hours.
8. The team includes all of the persons who may help to provide total patient care.
9. Decisions concerning some of the newer concepts such as the use of heroic measures to prolong life, or death with dignity, are the responsibility of the physician. However, this decision should be shared with the team and the patient's family.
10. Although the physician is concerned about the death of the patient, the family should be aware that the physician is also concerned about his own death.
11. Bereavement caused by the illness and death of a loved one may cause feelings of guilt. The members of the team should be available to provide service for these persons.

12. The ritualistic practices of some cultures may weaken the person's ability to adjust to bereavement. However, in some situations the presence and support afforded by others may be of benefit to the bereaved person.
13. Grief and bereavement may be minimized when the person seeks the opportunity and directs his energies into productive activities.*

Summary outline

1. The living prepare for the time when they will die
   A. Life insurance
   B. For unpaid principal on home
   C. Accumulates an estate
   D. Builds monuments so he will not be forgotten after death
      1. Foundations
      2. Scholarships
      3. Art and literature
      4. Technology
   E. Prepares a will
   F. Arranges for burial site
   G. May write own obituary
2. Death told in music, literature, radio, television
   A. Religious music
   B. Popular music
   C. Opera
   D. Literature and poetry
3. Scientific research
   Thanatology is study of death by scientific methods
4. Causes of death
   A. Disease
   B. Accidents
   C. Homicide
   D. Suicide
   E. Fetal and neonatal death
5. When does death occur?
   This is controversial question
   A. Traditional method
      1. Absence of heartbeat
      2. Cessation of respiratory function
   B. Electroencephalograph to measure brain activity
   C. Other suggestions for definition
      1. Healey and Harvey
      2. Christian Barnard
   D. When is death? This is complicated legal question
6. Death with dignity
   A. Passive euthanasia
   B. Positive euthanasia
   C. Use of extraordinary measures to prolong

life involves ethical, religious, legal, moral, and idealistic problems
   D. Living will—may be interpreted as voluntary, indirect euthanasia
   E. To use or not to use measures to prolong life is responsibility of physician
7. Priorities
   Selective process in determining who will benefit most from modern surgical and technologic procedures
   A. Hemodialysis
   B. Kidney transplant
   C. Open heart surgery
   D. Nurse needs to understand physician's decision
8. Fear of dying and death
   A. Biologic, psychologic, and social factors are important
   B. Anxiety related to pain
   C. Depression more common when patient is aware of terminal illness
   D. Many variables related to fear of dying
   E. Fear of death related to fear of unknown
      1. Communication, counseling, and resolution of problems contribute to acceptance of death
9. Emotional attitudes toward death; there may be variation in patient's behavior pattern
   A. Denial
   B. Anger
   C. Bargaining
   D. Depression
   E. Acceptance
10. Grief and bereavement—severe emotional reaction to loss
    A. Material possessions
    B. Self-identity
    C. Body function or part
    D. Separation
    E. Bereavement and deprivation for family members
    F. Grieving is a psychologic process
       1. Phases
          a. Numb with grief
          b. Mourning loss
          c. Depression
          d. Some may develop psychosomatic illness
    G. Many variables affect grieving process
11. Nursing care of terminal and dying patient
    A. Responsibilities of nurse
       1. To self—developing a philosophy
       2. To patient
       3. To family
          a. Primary concern after patient's death
    B. Factors relevant to nursing care of dying patient
       1. Educational system fails to teach student how to care for dying patient
       2. Hospital promotes noninvolvement
       3. Nurse does not receive emotional support that helps development of philosophy about care of dying patient
    C. Nursing care
       1. Physical factors

*Adapted from Kutscher, Austin H.: Anticipatory grief, death and bereavement (a continuum), In Kutscher, Austin, and Goldberg, Michael: Caring for the dying patient and his family, New York, 1973, Health Sciences Publishing Corp.

Statements	Strongly agree	Agree	Uncertain	Opposed	Strongly opposed
1. A 28-year-old man has been unconscious for 1 year after an injury. Any further efforts to keep him alive should be terminated.					
2. A 75-year-old woman was seriously injured in an accident. She was irrational and in pain. She probably will die. The physician ordered a drug that you knew would end her life. The nurse should not administer the drug.					
3. The number of elderly persons is increasing. Many are in institutions with no chance for a meaningful life. Positive euthanasia is the answer to the problem.					
4. The nursing care of an unconscious stroke patient is demanding, and therefore it would be better if he died.					
5. Each person should have the right to die if that is what he wants.					
6. Every person with a terminal illness should be told his diagnosis and prognosis.					

    2. Psychologic factors
    3. Social implications
D. Nurse should learn about patient during admissions
    1. Important for same nurse to care for patient on each admission
E. Physical care
    1. Bathing, including perineal care
    2. Regular turning
    3. Skin care
    4. Support of dependent parts
    5. Oral care
F. Patient may exhibit emotional behavior
    1. Crying
    2. Demanding
    3. Anger
G. Keep channels of communication open
H. The family
    1. Provide emotional support
    2. Interpret patient's emotional behavior
    3. Provide quiet place where family may be alone
    4. Family may have feelings of guilt
    5. Family may be critical of hospital and nursing care
    6. Assist family to gather patient's personal belongings
    7. Escort family to car
I. Policies for care after death
J. Society and death
    1. Attaches labels to certain diseases
    2. Death considered according to worth of individual to society

    3. Loss of service
    4. Loss of lifetime earnings
    5. Violent death costs society through taxation
    6. Financial assistance to family when breadwinner dies
    7. Scarcity of land for cemeteries
    8. Transfer of mortuaries to suburban areas

Several statements related to death are listed at the top of the page. There are five possible responses to show how you feel about the statement. Read each statement carefully, think about it, and when you have decided how you feel about the suggested solution, place a check (✓) in the column under the choice that best indicates your feeling. There are no right or wrong answers.

Films

1. Death (43 min., sound, black and white, 16 mm., rental $35.00), Film-makers Library, Inc., 290 West End Ave., New York, N. Y. 10023. Film is a portrait of a 52-year-old man dying with cancer. Studies the response of the family, hospital personnel, and other patients. Film is a reminder of mortality of human beings and the need to live freely.
2. How could I not be among you? (28 min., sound, color, 16 mm., rental $35.00), The

Eccentric Circle Cinema Workshop, P. O. Box 1481, Evanston, Ill., 60204. Describes a poet with leukemia who has 6 months to live. It is the portrait about the agony, hope, terror, and faith of a young man during his final days. The film forces viewers to examine their own feelings about death.
3. To die today (50 min., sound, black and white, 16 mm., rental $35.00), Film-makers Library, Inc., 290 West End Ave., New York, N. Y. 10023. Focuses on the work of Dr. Elizabeth Kübler Ross while she is a professor of psychiatry at Chicago's Billings Hospital. Shows interviews with dying patients and reviews the five stages of dying, her work with students, physicians, and nurses, theology, and psychology.
4. You see, I've had a life (30 min., sound, black and white, 16 mm., rental $24.00), The Eccentric Circle Cinema Workshop, P. O. Box 1481, Evanston, Ill., 60204. The story of a 14-year-old boy with leukemia. Shows remissions and exacerbations with readmission to the hospital. The family seeks to share the realities of the illness with Paul and to face the experience with him.

References

1. Death with dignity, editorial, The Journal of Practical Nursing **22**:13, Nov., 1972.
2. Death with dignity, American Association of Retired Persons, News Bulletin **13**:1, Sept., 1972.
3. Fletcher, Joseph: Ethics and euthanasia, American Journal of Nursing **73**:670-675, April, 1973.
4. Freud and death, New York, Newsweek, May 17, 1972.
5. Gullo, Steph Viton: Thanatology: the study of death and the care of the dying, Bedside Nurse **5**:11-14, May, 1972.
6. Hershey, Nathan: On the question of prolonging life, American Journal of Nursing **71**:521-522, March, 1971.
7. Jager, Dorothea, and Simmons, Leo W.: The aged ill, New York, 1970, Appleton-Century-Crofts.
8. Kastenbaum, Robert, and Aisenberg, Ruth B.: The psychology of death, New York, 1972, Springer Publishing Co., Inc.
9. Kübler Ross, Elizabeth: On death and dying, New York, 1970, The Macmillan Co.
10. May, Rollo, editor: Existential psychology, New York, 1967, Random House, Inc.
11. Mervyn, Frances: The right of dying patients in hospitals, American Journal of Nursing **71**:1988-1990, Oct., 1971.
12. Parkes, Colin Murray: Bereavement, New York, 1972, International Universities Press.
13. Schoenberg, Bernard, Carr, Arthur C., Peretz, David, and Kutscher, Austin C., editors: Psychosocial aspects of terminal care, New York, 1972, Columbia University Press.
14. The right to die with dignity, New York, 1971, The Euthanasia Educational Fund, Inc.
15. Weisman, Avery D.: On dying and denying, New York, 1972, Behavioral Publications.

CHAPTER 8

Nursing the geriatric patient

KEY WORDS

bath itch *~dryness of skin - severe itching*
biopsychosocial *itching*
disengagement *problems of aging*
geriatrics *specialty*
gerontology *aged*
kyphosis *humpback - same thing - new term*
lordosis *opposite - inward curvature of the spine*
Medicare
osteoporosis
physical, emotional & social relationship

pathologic *presence of a disease*
prostatic hypertrophy *enlargement of the prostate*
pyogenic *pus producing*
retirement *unemployment by reason of age !*
senescence *becoming old*
senility *old age + physical & mental changes*

curvature of the lumbar spine

detachment of oneself from other persons or responsibilities .

federal program - hospital & medical care for over 65 age group

demineralization or absorption of minerals from the bone - chronic & common in women past menopause

TERMINOLOGY

Terms associated with the process of growing old include geriatrics, senescence, and senility.

Geriatrics. The term *geriatrics* has been described as follows:

"Geriatrics is concerned with the care of the older person. The practice of geriatrics places emphasis on prevention of disabilities intensified by the aging process; treatment of the patient with special attention to the needs created by the aging process; and restoration of the person to a level consistent with the limitation imposed by the aging process."*

Senescence. Senescence represents the last stage in the life cycle. It is preceded by the process of growth and development during which the individual attains maturity; then a gradual decline begins. Senescence is not a pathologic condition but, rather, a normal biologic process.

Senility. Senile and *senility* are terms that are gradually decreasing in use. They indicate that an individual by reason of age has a weak mind. Pathologic changes may occur in the brain causing what is commonly referred to as "senile psychosis." The mind is a function of the brain that enables a person to make decisions, to remember, to experience feelings of various emotions, to reason, and to be orientated within his environment. An aged person's mind may function well within these areas, and any decline may be a normal biologic process.

---

*Nursing concerns in health insurance for the aged, American Journal of Nursing **65**:120-121, Sept., 1965.

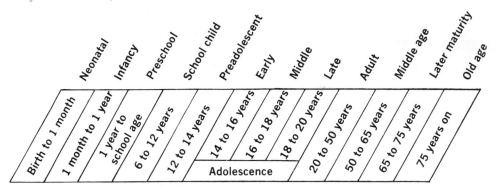

Fig. 8-1. The span of life is continuous but has been divided into periods, each presenting different needs and problems. The geriatric patient is near the end of the continuum and has his own special needs and problems.

POPULATION CHANGE

It has been stated that the elderly comprise the fastest growing minority group in the United States. In 1900 only 3% of the population were 65 years of age or older. As of January 1, 1973, there were 21.2 million or 10.1% of the population who were 65 years of age or older. This represents an increase of 9.9% since January 1, 1968. During the same period persons under 15 years of age declined by 4.3%.[24]

The number of women surviving as compared to men increased. In 1940 the number of women and men was approximately the same. According to the 1970 census there were 3.2 million more women 65 years or older than men.

Geographically there has been a gradual shifting in locale of the elderly. During the decade of 1960 500,000 elderly persons left the northern states, whereas the southern states gained 450,000 persons. The number of elderly persons in Florida is 50% above the national average. New York state has 2 million elderly persons, with the state of California only slightly less.[26]

During 1972 the overall population of the United States increased by only 0.78%, the smallest growth rate since 1936. This is credited to a decrease in the birth rate.[24]

What do these few statistics mean to the nurse and the nursing profession? There are significant changes at the extremes of the continuum. There will be fewer babies to care for and an increasing number of elderly persons needing the expertise of

nurses trained in geriatric care (Fig. 8-1). There will be many more women than men to care for, and the need for nurses to care for the elderly will vary with the distribution of the aged. It can be predicted with reasonable accuracy that this trend will continue for many decades. Nurses should avail themselves of every opportunity to increase their understanding and skill in meeting the nursing needs of elderly persons.

PROGRESS AND RESEARCH

It may be said that since 1961, when the first White House Conference on Aging was held, there has been a new awakening to the needs of the elderly. Although many recommendations were formulated and submitted to this conference, one of the most important was the eventual enactment of legislation establishing Medicare and the Older Americans Act.[19]

Benefits under Medicare became available July 1, 1966. Some changes have been made in the original act; however, millions of older Americans have received and are continuing to receive hospital and medical care under its provisions. The Older Americans Act became law in 1965. Since then, numerous changes and amendments have been made, and some parts have been completely rewritten. Certain parts of the act are administered by the federal government through the Department of Health, Education, and Welfare, whereas other parts are implemented by state and local agencies. The act covers a wide range of services to the elderly. In 1973 the Older Americans Comprehensive Services Amendments were passed by Congress, extending the range of services through 1975. A total expenditure of $543.6 million was authorized under their provisions.[17]

Special emphasis has been placed on meeting nutritional needs of elderly persons. In March, 1972, $250 million was approved for a 2-year period to provide hot meals for persons 60 years of age and over.[27] In the same year the National project FIND was initiated, and 50,000 volunteers participated in an effort to locate elderly persons eligible to receive food stamps and surplus food.

Numerous programs are funded under various parts of the Older Americans Act. Among these programs are homemaker services, home health aides, foster grandparents program, employment referrals, housing, health screening, research and demonstration programs, and training programs in the field of aging.

The Social Security Act of 1965 and its subsequent amendments provide monthly benefits for elderly persons. Periodic increases in benefits have been granted to cover increased living costs. Along with the Social Security benefit the ceiling on earned income has been raised without loss of the monthly benefit. This makes it possible for elderly persons to continue part-time work.

Many universities and medical centers have opened research centers to study the biologic and psychologic factors related to aging. The sixteenth such center to be opened was the Ethel Percy Andrus Gerontology Center at the University of Southern California, which was dedicated in February, 1973. The center immediately announced the beginning of a 3-year research study, which would be the most comprehensive study of aging ever undertaken.[22]

Although many older persons have searched for the "fountain of youth," none has ever found it. Studies on aging have led one group of researchers to the use of a drug that they believe could extend the life of a person many more years.

Although tremendous strides have been made to provide a better life for millions of elderly Americans in the United States, not all are receiving these benefits. Many communities have active ongoing programs, whereas other communities lag far behind with little interest in improving the life of the elderly.

RETIREMENT AND AGING

Retirement is conceived as the time in a person's life when he has reached the peak of his productive years. It is the time when he leaves his job and enters into another phase of life. With the increasing number of persons who have reached 65 years of age there is also an increase in the number of retired persons.

During the early history of the United States when the economy was rural and agricultural, there was little concern about retirement. The individual worked well into his later years, and even when he was advanced in age, there were always chores that kept him occupied.

In the twentieth century the older worker is pressured into retirement to provide jobs for the young. A new concept has been developing that suggests retirement as a reward for labor, a dividend of time earned after years of work, and the opportunity to do every day what one wants to do.[29]

Most individuals think of retirement when they reach 65 years of age. For many the social system has made 65 years a mandatory retirement age. For some, retirement is optional, but only a few are financially able to retire at an early age. Although some persons may be required to retire early because of health problems, most think of themselves as in good health at 65 years of age and want the freedom of being able to choose to work or retire.[22] The older worker finds that hunting for a new job after retirement is difficult. The Age Discrimination in Employment Act of 1967, Public Law 90-202, is designed to protect persons between 40 and 65 years of age from discrimination in hiring, discharge, and other conditions of employment solely on the basis of age. However, long years of social policy and discrimination are not easily corrected by law.[29] The worker who finds personal satisfaction in his job, personal identity, the stimulation of his co-workers, and the feeling of being useful finds that these personal satisfactions are gone when he retires. Some persons will create new patterns for life and develop new social roles that will provide satisfying experiences, whereas others will settle back into a life of apathy, accepting the role of consumer, although financial resources for that role may be limited.

Women in the labor force also will be faced with the problem of retirement. For many women retirement is not as traumatic as it may be for men. The woman may have been engaged in church, club, or community activities. She may view retirement as the opportunity to increase her social and community interests. However, some women may devote all of their time to their work and isolate themselves from others and from social activities. For these persons adjustment to retirement may be difficult.

The basic needs of the retired older worker are to feel financially secure, to be useful, to form new associations and interact with people, to maintain a sense of dignity and self-respect, and to feel needed and wanted in society. The fulfillment of these needs begins in the middle years of life by careful planning for the future.

SOCIOECONOMIC AND CULTURAL FACTORS

Many variations exist in the cultural patterns of different groups of people as well as within families at different periods. In early Oriental cultures the older members of society were revered and called the "wise ones." In primitive cultures the elderly persons were the source for information and knowledge. They always knew where to find food and water, and they traveled with the tribe. When they became too feeble to travel and could not be cared for, they accepted death.[14] In the early culture of the United States the older citizens were important. They were consulted about the political and educational affairs of the community. They were respected because of the knowledge that they had acquired during their life. An elderly woman said, "Everything is different now; only the sun, the moon and the stars are the same." The present-day American culture is youth oriented, and the elderly occupy a lower position and possess lower prestige. They may look back with feelings of nostalgia to a time when there was

solidarity of the family unit and youth showed respect and devotion to the aged members of the family.

The social system forces the individual into retirement at a time in life when it is more difficult to make decisions than at an earlier age. For many, financial resources are limited and the individual is forced to make critical decisions and adjustments. One of the most pressing problems is housing. Frequently the home is located in the central city, and city planning, slum clearance, and urban renewal may force persons to give up the homes to which they are attached. Often abrupt changes are made without consideration of individual differences and needs. Lifetime patterns are not easily changed and must be evaluated in terms of what they mean to the individual.

Mrs. H., an 80-year-old widow, was persuaded to sell the farm on which she had lived and move into a small house built for her by her daughter. To the daughter this seemed the sensible thing to do. Mrs. H. had always owned land, but now she lived on land owned by someone else. One day Mrs. H. went out and bought a farm, which she in turn leased. She had not consulted her daughter, but now she could live happily in her daughter's house, since she was once more a landowner.

Mrs. S., an 83-year-old widow, lived in two small basement rooms of a house in a textile mill village. The public health nurse was appalled at the lack of sanitation and sought ways to place Mrs. S. in a clean, comfortable room. When Mrs. S. was approached with the suggestion, her reply was, "All I want is to be left alone with my things."

Under the Federal Housing Act, funds have been made available for construction of housing units for the aged. However, the problems of relocating elderly persons are often overwhelming. Many cities and towns have secured funds for urban renewal, and frequently elderly persons are required to give up their homes and to readjust their lifelong patterns of living. The disruption causes anxiety and feelings of hostility.

Mrs. C. had lived for 46 years in the home that had been her parents. However, when urban renewal came, Mrs. C. had to move. In reference to her new home Mrs. C. said, "I like it quite well, but it's very inconvenient. You see, I was right there in town. Out here I have to call a taxi every time, and I don't always have the money."

Mrs. F. had lived in her old home for 34 years. She said, "Now it's plum gone." Speaking of her new home, she said, "It's not what I want. I have no praise for urban renewal. It's lying and stealing and anything else they can do to get your money."

Homes in urban renewal areas frequently belong to elderly persons whose income has declined over the years. They are no longer financially able to make necessary repairs, and gradual deterioration occurs. Not all elderly persons are confronted with this problem; some are retired professional, executive, or business people who have been able to maintain their homes because of sufficient financial resources.

NURSING HOMES

Many elderly persons have no place to go when they can no longer care for themselves. Although some elderly persons may wish to live with their children, others are forced by economic or health reasons to do so. Often the plan is not mutually acceptable to the children or the elderly family member. For many of these persons the nursing home is the only place for them. However, according to one study, 50% of the nursing home residents could be cared for in their own homes.[13]

Statistics indicate that more than 23,000 nursing homes are in operation, with 1 million beds and 500,000 employees. The United States government contributes annually over $1 billion to nursing homes.[13] Late in 1971 a statement concerning some policies and procedures in nursing homes was read into the Congressional Record of the Ninety-second Congress. The statement included mention of the widespread use of tranquilizers and sedatives administered to patients to keep them quiet. In 1972 the general accounting office of the United States indicated that 40% of all drugs used under Medicaid were tranquilizers and sedatives.[13, 16]

A beginning to upgrade nursing homes was made in 1970, when federal legislation provided that no nursing home may receive federal funds after July 1, 1970, unless the state in which it is licensed has established a program for licensing nursing home administrators.[12] A report in 1973 stated that of 7000 nursing homes certified for Medicare patients, 500 had either withdrawn or been decertified because of failure to meet federal standards for patient care and safety.[4] Additional efforts to upgrade nursing homes and the nursing care of patients resulted in a series of seminars for nursing home administrators and medical directors to define responsibilities.[9, 28] In addition, a program to train nursing home inspectors was implemented.[18]

Nursing homes approved for Medicare require that the personnel maintain nursing care plans for each patient. Plans should be based on the immediate and long-term needs of the patient. As in the general hospital, they should reflect the thinking of the entire nursing home staff.[30]

In recent years several serious fires have occurred in nursing homes and retirement institutions, with considerable loss of life. This has led many states and communities to make changes in their present building codes and fire regulations to prevent such disasters.

The average nursing home patient differs little from most other persons of the same chronologic age. In addition to the normal degenerative changes, many have chronic diseases and may be malnourished and debilitated. The nursing care must be individualized according to the individual's particular needs. Some patients will be ambulatory and be able to provide much of their own care, others will need assistance with personal hygiene, and some must have total patient care. The patient's psychologic needs should be met, reassuring him of his personal worth and seeking to maintain a sense of dignity and self-respect.

Many nurses are employed in nursing homes, and they may be questioned concerning the selection of a suitable nursing home. The nurse should be familiar with the accepted standards for a good nursing home and be able to contribute toward choosing a suitable place for an elderly person.

ALTERNATIVES TO INSTITUTIONAL CARE

Home care. If the patient is to be cared for in his own home, the family and the community must provide the necessary services. Most elderly persons prefer to remain in their own home and are happier when they can do so. Each person must be carefully evaluated medically and socially for home care. When the person's potential for self-care has been determined, a program is planned for him. Many of the services under the Older Americans Act such as meals, transportation to physicians or clinics, home health aides, and homemaker service as well as visits by the public health nurse or visiting nurse may be needed. "Home care can preserve the elderly person's independence, dignity, and identity—precious human qualities that are often lost when the elderly person is placed in an institution."*

Day hospital. Experimental programs for the care of the aged are being tried in both the United States and in Canada. The objective is to prevent or delay admission to an institution and to promote independence. Individuals must be ambulatory; however, the patient may be permitted to use a walker or a cane. Emergency care is available if needed. A kitchen may be available for retraining and motivation. Transportation is provided, and a noon meal is provided in a cafeteria. Each person is encouraged to participate in group activities and in various crafts. A team approach is used with a physician, nurse, dietitian, psychiatrist, and occupational therapist. Patients are evaluated as to progress and may become sufficiently independent to maintain themselves at home. Thus some leave the program and others are admitted.[5, 6]

Foster home. The care of the elderly in a foster home has not been successful. The concept that an elderly person will be a happier person in a home environment and be able to share in family relationships has not developed as conceived. Disadvantages have centered around the lack of medical care and the fact that the foster home is operated for profit.

Other services. The extended care facility provides stort-term, intermediate and convalescent care. It may be part of a general hospital or be operated as an independent institution. Its function is to provide care after an acute illness until the person is able to return home.

A variety of community outpatient services are available in many communities. These include mental health clinics, physi-

cal therapy, dental clinics, speech clinics, and a variety of social services.[2]

BIOPSYCHOSOCIAL FACTORS

The biologic process of aging causes physiologic changes in the total human organism. Changes usually develop slowly, and many persons consider themselves to be in good health. Although declines varies among individuals, most elderly persons complain of physical symptoms that should be given medical attention. While proclaiming good health, the individual may have poor nutrition, be in need of dental care or dentures, need glasses, have problems of constipation, be in need of a hearing aid, or be dehydrated. In addition, many elderly persons have pathologic conditions that require hospital, medical, and nursing care. Frequently the stress situations related to the psychosocial problems affect the physical condition of the individual.

Most elderly persons become aware of the shortness of time. They become concerned about changes in their body and their loss of strength or the presence of disease. Some persons have had a lifetime of frustrations, and the grief after the loss of a spouse and close friends may cause the person to question continued existence. The individual may progress into a state of depression and prefer self-destruction to continuation of life. With the increased incidence of geriatric suicide the nurse caring for elderly patients should be alert to warning signs. The person who expresses a desire to die or makes threats of suicide should not be taken lightly.[20] It is during such periods of loneliness and depression that the individual needs emotional support. Some communities have volunteers who make regular visits to elderly persons or make frequent telephone calls. An 85-year-old woman who has lost all of her family lives alone in her home. She often says, "I wish the Lord would take me, no one calls me and I just sit here alone for days."

Many of the concepts held concerning psychosocial factors in old age have never been proved and are now being questioned.[11] It is only recently that research, although limited, has enabled society to learn some of the factors that affect the social life and attitudes of elderly persons.

*From Connecticut testing home care plan for the aged, Aging 223:8, May, 1973.

It has been stated that chronologic age may be unrelated to old age. Throughout this text the individual is emphasized. Elderly people are individuals and must be treated as such. It has been suggested that older persons represent a "subculture." Society has fostered such a culture through community programs that tend to segregate older persons, such as senior citizens and golden age groups and day care centers. These programs take older persons out of the mainstream of society and provide little opportunity for interaction with younger persons. Thus elderly persons develop a feeling of alienation and become conscious of their age, identifying themselves with others of the same age group. They find that they are unable to control and adapt to their external environment. The result of this process is called *disengagement*, which is characterized by feelings of loneliness, social isolation, and the desire for solitude apart from the social system.

It is generally believed that individuals who were well adjusted and able to meet problems and make adaptations during their younger years are better prepared to face problems with advancing years. When elderly people are confronted with a situation that they do not have the resources to deal with, they become frustrated and develop feelings of anxiety, fear, and helplessness. It is at such times that a one-to-one relationship with another person may be helpful.[8]

Levine[11] conducted research on a small group of people and found that disengagement, in which social relationships are severed or altered, is an inevitable process of aging. As nonpathologic physical changes occur, it appears that the need for social interaction also declines. However, there are variations among individuals in the degree of disengagement. In the sample studied by Levine it was found that elderly persons preferred solitary, unstructured, and nonobligatory activities rather than group or club activities. It is suggested that society should study and reevaluate the beliefs it holds about the needs of the aging person. Disengagement from society and the desire for a static, tranquil, and self-centered life may be part of the normal aging process.[11]

MENTAL HEALTH

Many elderly persons are dependent on others for part or all of their care. Dependency results in loss of dignity, self-esteem, and lowered morale. When disease and illness are superimposed on normal deterioration, adaptation is difficult for the individual.

Maintaining mental health in the older person does not mean doing for him but rather doing with him. A large number of elderly citizens want something to do and want to feel that they are useful. Many are ambulatory and able to remain in their own homes, where they are happier. For some this is not possible. Older people have problems, and no matter how small the problem may appear to others it may be extremely important to the older individual. A community counseling service should be available where the person may have privacy, quiet, and an unhurried atmosphere to talk over problems.

The dependency that elderly persons experience may give rise to feelings of resentment toward family, friends, or those trying to help. They may become demanding, tend to magnify normal aches and pains, and complain of loss of sleep and of various digestive disturbances. Many elderly persons are seen in clinics and physician's offices with exaggerated complaints and trivial conditions. It must be remembered that older persons have many adjustments to make at a period of their lives when they tolerate stress situations poorly. In 1969 Morris Fishbean wrote, "I feel that anxiety underlies all senile symptoms, and causes them. In old age you have more anxiety-evoking situations and fewer anxiety-reducing opportunities; that formula in itself could account for senility or emotional breakdown in the aging."* Following are some of the adjustments that the older person may have to make:

1. Death of a spouse
2. Retirement and reduced income
3. Disengagement and alienation of family and friends
4. Identification with an older age group
5. Adjusting to depleted physical energy and a gradually deteriorating body

---

*From Medical World News, May 16, 1969.

The older person is confronted with fears of illness, physical suffering, helplessness, and death. Disengagement and chronic disease or illness result in low morale, but when meaningful friendships exist, even when the health of the individual is poor, he is less likely to suffer from low morale. These are times when the mental health clinic can provide emotional support and give the individual a feeling of friendship, warmth, and a sense of personal worth.

There is a wide range of activities designed to keep older persons in the mainstream of life and in contact with society. Some of these activities operate under the Older Americans Act and others through local community programs. The success of a mental health program for the elderly depends on a social consciousness within the community that is oriented toward mental health.

The following activities are in operation in many communities throughout the United States:

Volunteer service activities

Foster grandparents' program

Employment service for the elderly

Tours and trips to sporting events, night clubs, and political meetings

Hand crafts and bazaars

Square dances

Free bus transportation in some communities, enabling older people to be more independent

Making doll clothes and dressing dolls for social agencies

Woodwork such as constructing children's chairs, bird houses, etc.

Collecting many varied items

Educational classes for elderly persons in a few universities

The nurse can be an innovator of new ideas and can be a source of inspiration, not only to individuals but to the community in the development of an ongoing mental health program for its elderly population.

PATHOPHYSIOLOGY OF AGING

Aging is a nonpathologic process. However, pathologic conditions may occur as a complication of aging. After a person has reached maturity a gradual aging of all body tissues and organs begins. By the time a person has reached 70 years of age the aging process may be well advanced. The rate and extent of aging varies among individuals, and the rate at which various organs age may also vary. Although there is considerable variation among individuals and within the same person, the years of physiologic decline are often long and protracted.

Cardiovascular system. Biophysiologic aging may be partly caused by the normal wear and tear on the body over the years. The heart pumps blood out into the vast network of arteries 72 times a minute, 24 hours a day, and 365 days a year for year after year. As the years go by and as a person ages, changes occur in the cardiovascular system. There is a decrease in the ability of the heart to perform its normal function. Less blood is pumped out to the organs and tissues of the body, with a decrease in oxygen and nutrients to the tissues. As a result, the organs of the body are no longer able to function as they did at an earlier period in life.

Endocrine system. From 45 to 50 years of age the functions of the endocrine system decline. After climacteric the female *(menopause)* breast, vaginal mucosa, uterus, and ovaries and the male prostate gland undergo change and begin to atrophy.

Sensory system. In the sensory system changes affect vision, hearing, sense of pain, and ability to adapt to darkness. These changes may occur so gradually that the individual may not be aware of them. Changes in the middle and inner ear may result in some loss of balance and sense of body position or may cause dizziness.

Integumentary system. The skin and its appendages slowly age. The epidermis becomes thinner, and there is less secretion from the sebaceous glands. The skin may become dry, and pigmented spots occur on the face and back of the hands. Wrinkling of skin is caused by loss of subcutaneous fat and a decrease in water content of the skin. The nails become thick, hard, and brittle, leading to cracking and splitting. The hair becomes dry and loses its pigmentation, and hair in the axillary and pubic areas become scanty.[3]

Musculoskeletal system. Aging of the musculoskeletal system affects bones, joints, muscles, and their attachments. The bones become porous and on x-ray examination appear spongy, which is caused by the loss of calcium in the bone structure. The intervertebral disks lose water and elasticity of the connective tissue, causing the individual to lose height. The person tends to bow forward, and kyphosis of the thoracic vertebrae and lordosis of the lumbar vertebrae occur. The contour of the chest cage is changed, predisposing the person to respiratory disease. Changes occur in the joints, especially the weight-bearing joints such as knees, hips, and vertebrae. The changes are partly caused by the years of wear and tear, a decreased blood supply, inadequate nutrition, and a decrease in ambulation as aging occurs. Cartilage and tendons become weakened, and muscles become soft and flabby. All of these changes contribute to the likelihood of falls resulting in fractures.

Nervous system. The nervous system is affected by the loss of brain cells, few if any of which are replaced. There is a decrease in cells of the nerve fibers, causing a decrease in the speed of response. There is a decline in memory for recent events, although the person may have a vivid memory for events that occurred in childhood and young adulthood.

Digestive system. Changes occur in the gastrointestinal system with age. There is a decrease in gastric secretions and a slowing of peristaltic action. This may lead to various digestive complaints. There is a loss of the sense of smell and taste, which tends to decrease the appetite and the desire for food. An individual may complain that food does not taste the same or is not as good. Many elderly persons are poorly nourished because of food problems. The lack of teeth or dentures may cause a person to eat only soft foods that require little mastication. Some psychiatrists relate eating habits of elderly persons to the kind of behavior exhibited by them.

Urinary system. The kidneys lose part of their normal functional capacity because of decreased blood supply. Urine is more concentrated because of decreased fluid intake. Many elderly persons have some urinary incontinence and often find it necessary to go to the bathroom during the night.

NURSING THE ELDERLY

The care of the elderly includes those procedures designed to protect the person from injury, provide comfort, improve nutrition, maintain personal hygiene, and provide care during illness and convalesence.

Preventing injury. The National Safety Council reported in 1971 that 28,000 persons who were 65 years of age or older died as a result of accidental injury; 17,000 accidental deaths occurred in persons 75 years of age or older. One half of these accidents were caused by falls that led to terminal complications.

Since most falls occur in the home, precaution should be taken to protect elderly persons. Scatter rugs should not be used unless they are secured by rubber mats beneath them. Children's toys left on the floor and furniture moved to unfamiliar places may be responsible for a fall. Rubber mats should be placed in bathtubs and support provided to assist persons stepping from the tub (Fig. 8-2).

Night lights and lights in bathrooms and on stairs should be left on at night, and increased illumination should be provided in the evening. Elderly persons are susceptible to accidents on streets and highways at dusk or in the evening; to avoid such accidents an elderly person should be accompanied, should carry a flashlight, and should have reflectorized material attached to clothing.

Providing comfort. Elderly persons may be burned more easily than younger persons because their pain receptors do not respond as readily. For this reason bed socks, a bed jacket, or an extra blanket are preferable to a heating pad or hot-water bottle. Elderly persons often need extra clothing or wraps. The feet may be cold because of circulatory changes. Care should be taken so that electric fans or air conditioners do not blow directly on the patient, or he is not placed in a draft.

Short rest periods of 15 or 20 minutes after meals will be of greater value than long naps that may interfere with sleep at night. Older people frequently complain of sleepless nights and on such occasions may get up and walk about the house. Many times they try to follow the same pattern of retiring as they did when

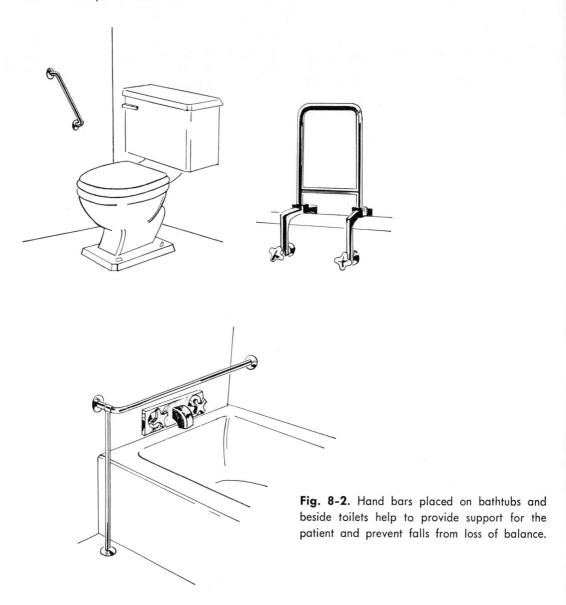

Fig. 8-2. Hand bars placed on bathtubs and beside toilets help to provide support for the patient and prevent falls from loss of balance.

younger, when more sleep was required. Providing evening entertainment such as television will help to keep the person up later, and he will be able to sleep well and to awaken refreshed.

Meeting nutritional needs. The dietary patterns of the elderly may be affected by the following factors:

1. Reduced income
2. Inadequacy of cooking facilities
3. Loneliness and having to eat alone
4. Physical inability to prepare food
5. Decreased gastric secretion and slowing of digestion
6. Loss of teeth or poorly fitting dentures
7. Living too far from a market and lack of delivery service

As a group, elderly people appear to be highly susceptible to malnutrition. In senescence the metabolic processes decrease from 10% to 30%, physical activity decreases, and the individual needs fewer calories. However, if appetite fails, the individual will become malnourished.[15] Some elderly persons are obese and continue to follow dietary patterns of overeating, particularly of eating rich foods.

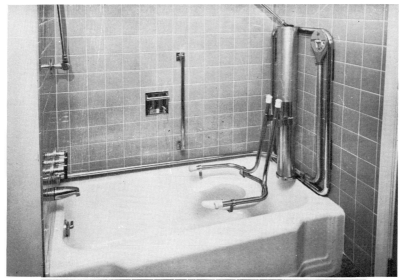

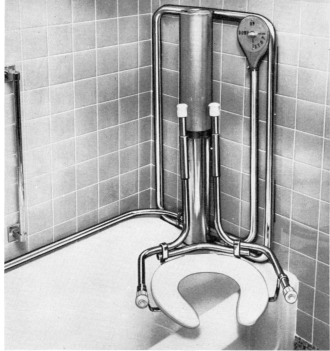

Fig. 8-3. Bathe-A-Lift offers a safe method of assisting an elderly patient into and out of a bathtub without risking the possibility of a fall. It may be used in the hospital or home. (Courtesy R. D. Grant Co., Cleveland, Ohio.)

They, too, may be undernourished, not in calories but in dietary essentials.

The diet should include all of the nutritional requirements, that is, carbohydrates, fats, proteins, vitamins, minerals, and water. Because of reduced physical activity and a decline in the metabolic activity, elderly persons need fewer calories than when they were younger. Caloric needs must be evaluated individually. Men may require more calories than women, and some persons are more active than others and expend more energy, which requires more calories. It has been suggested that there should be a reduction in calories of 7% to 8% every 10 years after a person has reached 25 years of age.[31]

The diet should include the following four basic food groups:

1. Meat, fish, poultry, and eggs
2. Milk
3. Fruits and vegetables
4. Breads and cereals

The basic food groups apply to all persons regardless of age, with the calories adjusted through smaller or larger servings. There is some evidence that proper utilization of food in the body depends on all nutrients being present at approximately the same time. The frequency and the amount of food served is also important, and it is recommended that the daily food requirement be divided into six small feedings. Vitamin and mineral supplements should be used only on the advice of the physician. Whenever possible, the individual should eat with the family, and food should be prepared the way the person likes it and served attractively. It is wise to allow the elderly person some participation in meal planning, but he should not be allowed to dominate the selection of food.

Personal hygiene. Daily baths result in excessive dryness and scaling of the skin, often accompanied by itching. Frequent bathing with inadequate rinsing may cause a form of dermatitis known as *bath itch*. It usually occurs along the shins but may spread over the body, confining the person to bed. The individual may be rendered uncomfortable from burning and itching of the affected parts. Complete baths should be reduced to one or two a week, using a superfatted soap, followed by careful rinsing and drying. The bath should be prepared by someone in the home who will assist the person into and out of the tub (Fig. 8-3). An elderly person should not be permitted to be alone in a locked bathroom. A chained door guard may be used on the inside of the door. This allows a person to slip his hand in and open the door if necessary.

Because of diminished activity of oil glands, the hair should be shampooed about once a month. Shampoos containing alcohol should be avoided because of their drying effect.

Care of the feet is important. In the home warm soaks with thorough drying, particularly between the toes, followed by massage with baby oil or lanolin will prevent excessive drying. A member of the family or the nurse should trim the nails. If financial resources permit, the individual may be taken to a podiatrist for foot care. Visits may be scheduled at 4- to 6-week intervals. Corns, calluses, and infections require special care.

Although most elderly people have lost their teeth, some will have part or all of their teeth and others will have dentures. The loss of teeth and presence of dental caries or poorly fitting dentures affect the person's general health by interfering with dietary needs. Normal shrinking of the gums exposes the soft parts of the tooth structure, which are more sensitive to injury. Improperly fitting dentures may cause the gums to become sore. Regular gum massage will stimulate circulation and help to keep gums healthy. For those who have their own teeth regular visits to the dentist are necessary. Teeth should be brushed after meals with a mild dentifrice and a soft-bristle brush, and dentures should be brushed after each meal.

Sluggishness of the bowel may accompany aging; it is primarily the result of inactivity and faulty diet. When it occurs, it is not unusual for the person to resort to the use of some form of laxative that he has seen advertised or that a well-meaning friend or neighbor has told him about. Laxatives, as any other medication, should be prescribed by the physician. However, regularity of toilet habits should be encouraged, and when possible, diet should include some soft bulk to facilitate bowel evacuation. Simple measures such as prune juice at night or a glass of warm water with a little lemon juice before breakfast may be all that is required.

Some degree of urinary incontinence may occur because of normal anatomic changes or physiologic changes that result from aging. Whatever the cause, it may result in embarrassment for the individual. A medical examination should be sought to correct any condition that might contribute to the problem. There should be change of clothing as necessary to prevent odor.

The individual should be encouraged to maintain good personal hygiene and personal appearance with reference to hair and clothing. For many elderly persons some member of the family will have to help with or supervise care daily. The same principles of personal hygiene apply to the individual who may be hospitalized or in a nursing home or similar institution.

PATHOLOGIC COMPLICATIONS OF AGING

The elderly person is susceptible to most of the illnesses and diseases of younger persons. The elderly person may have lost his immunity to certain communicable diseases characteristic of childhood. In such a situation if he is exposed to a disease in which he has little or no immunity, he may contract the disease. Benign and malignant neoplasms and tuberculosis often occur in elderly persons. However, there are some pathologic conditions that occur as complications of the aging process. Most are chronic, and the individual may or may not require hospitalization. Some diseases may be acute and may progress to a fatal outcome.

Atherosclerosis and arteriosclerosis. Earlier in this chapter it was stated that changes occur in the heart and the vascular system. These changes begin early in life and progress over the years. Atherosclerosis is a form of arteriosclerosis, a condition in which the blood vessels lose their elasticity that is frequently spoken of as "hardening of the arteries." Atherosclerosis results from fatty deposits (plaques) that form in the intima of the blood vessels. These changes make it increasingly difficult for blood to flow through the vascular system. The flow of blood to the kidneys, brain, and lower extremities is often affected. The condition may become severe enough to cause serious disease of the heart and coronary arteries. As blood supply to the brain is diminished, mental confusion may occur. (See Chapter 13.)

Osteoporosis. The cause of osteoporosis has not been completely identified. Since one out of four women past menopause is affected, many researchers believe that it is related to the loss of the female hormone estrogen. Other factors that may contribute to the condition include immobilization and possible induction by the use of steroids.

Osteoporosis affects the vertebrae, the neck of the femur, and the pelvis and may affect the hands and wrists. The disorder develops slowly, and the first sign may be backache. As the disease progresses, the bones become porous and brittle, which is caused by loss of calcium. If untreated, spontaneous fractures may occur. Treatment consists of adequate doses of estrogen. Estrogen will not correct the condition but will help to prevent fractures. Other treatment includes the administration of calcium, fluoride, and recently calcitonin[23] (p. 368).

Vaginitis. After menopause there is a decrease in estrogens, with tissue changes about the vulva and vagina, a thinning of the epithelial cells, and the loss of normal vaginal acidity. Pyogenic organisms may easily gain entrance to the vagina, and a mild inflammation (atrophic senile vaginitis) may occur. The symptoms include a vaginal discharge that causes irritation and pruritus. Treatment consists of the administration of estrogen hormones, either orally or as a cream placed in the vagina. Treatment with estrogen changes the vaginal epithelium back to its premenopausal state and thus eliminates the infection[25] (p. 372).

Prostate gland. In many men who are over 50 years of age the prostate gland enlarges, resulting in benign prostatic hypertrophy, which may cause obstruction of the flow of urine. The individual may have frequency of urination, especially at night, and complete emptying of the bladder may not occur. Inflammation of the bladder often results. Difficulty in voiding increases, often accompanied by pain. Medical care and frequently surgery are necessary to correct the condition.

Pulmonary disorders. Because of changes in the contour of the chest cage, there is a decreased ventilatory capacity and a reduced ability to cough up secretions. Frequently pathogenic microorganisms take over, and hypostatic pneumonia may occur. This is especially true if the person is confined to bed. During periods when influenza is prevalent the death rate among elderly persons usually increases, caused by pneumonia complicating influenza. Many elderly persons suffer from chronic obstructive pulmonary disease, which often limits their activity. (See Chapter 11 for more information.)

Varicosities. The function of the veins is to return blood to the heart. To keep the blood flowing in the right direction valves are located along the vein. When the valves fail to operate normally, the flow of blood through the valve may be decreased, causing the vein to become dilated with stasis of the blood. The condition usually affects the lower extremities, and several factors may cause or contribute to varicose veins. The condition usually begins in middle life and unless corrected, usually by surgery, may cause pain and cramps in the legs. When the elderly person finds standing and ambulation difficult, the disorder may further complicate his ability to move about.

CARE OF THE HOSPITALIZED PATIENT

Nursing elderly patients with acute medical or surgical conditions is different in many respects from nursing younger persons. The normal degenerative changes that have occurred produce physiologic and psychologic patterns that would not be observed or would be less significant in younger persons.

Vital signs. Blood pressure is influenced by age, but the range of systolic pressure may be rather wide; however, the diastolic range is less wide. Any significant change in blood pressure should always be reported. The blood pressure of elderly persons may be affected by chronic disease or the stress situation of illness. In the elderly person a small change may be more important than it would be in a younger person. In an older person the pulse rate may be less significant than the volume and rhythm. The rate must be considered together with other symptoms and the patient's condition. It is not uncommon for the pulse in an elderly person to be intermittent, and patients who are receiving digitalis often exhibit changes in the normal rate and rhythm of the pulse. Most people over 70 years of age have premature beats, which occur sooner than expected in the rhythmical pattern. The

nurse should develop a sensitivity to what is felt and be able to report it accurately.

Sedation. Elderly patients often do not tolerate sedative drugs as well as do younger patients; after surgery smaller amounts of narcotics are generally required. Often changing the patient's position, giving a warm drink, or sitting with an anxious patient will be of greater value than administering a drug. When a hyponotic is administered to an elderly person at bedtime, it is important for the nurse to check on the patient frequently. Often the patient may become confused, try to get out of bed, and falls, causing a serious injury. When administering any medication to elderly persons, it is well not to use the term *drugs*, since many of them associate drugs with addiction.

Intake and output. Total fluid intake, including that used in foods, should be sufficient to produce 1500 ml. of urine in 24 hours. Since many older persons are dehydrated, fluids will often be retained until a physiologic balance has been established. A severely dehydrated patient may retain and absorb solution administered as an enema. Persuading an individual to take oral fluids is often a frustrating experience, and small amounts at frequent intervals will often be better accepted than a large amount at one time. When fluids are restricted because of a cardiac or other condition, the nurse should understand the amount permitted and calculate it carefully. In some conditions and postoperatively the physician may order the administration of solutions intravenously. An important factor in the administration of intravenous fluids to elderly persons is the rate of flow. Severe cardiac disturbance may result if fluids are administered too rapidly. Unless ordered otherwise by the physician, 1000 ml. of fluid should not be administered in less than 4 hours. Frequently elderly persons do not tolerate blood transfusions well. The blood should drip slowly, and the patient should be carefully observed during the procedure.

Careful records of intake and output should be maintained and accurate measurements made.

Ambulation and convalescence. Recovery from acute illness is often accompanied by chronic disease, which may affect the rate of recovery. Older people require longer periods for recovery than do younger persons, and their progress is slower. The older person should be out of bed as much as his condition permits to prevent complications. The process of ambulation should be slow and progressive, beginning by elevating the patient in bed. The next step is to have the patient sit on the side of the bed, and then sit up in a chair for 15 to 20 minutes beside the bed, taking a few steps, gradually lengthening the time up and the extent of walking. The patient should be observed for color, respiration, and pulse rate, and if faintness or dizziness occurs, he should be returned to bed. An elderly person out of bed for the first time should not be left alone. The patient will need a great deal of encouragement and support. The elderly patient undergoing surgery believes that he is going to die and is ready to give up. The will to live must be rekindled and kept alive by a sympathetic understanding nurse.

When caring for elderly patients in the hospital or in the home, the nurse should speak clearly and distinctly and be sure that the patient understands. This is especially important when giving medications or treatments, since the individual often responds to a name that is not his own.

When working with elderly patients in the hospital or in the home, the nurse should not expect to make requests and secure a quick response. The patient may respond with "all right" or "in a minute." Directions should be given slowly, being certain that the patient understands. The patient may indicate that he understands, but action may be slow. He should not be hurried because he may become confused and be unable to respond.

Summary outline

1. Terminology
   A. Geriatrics *gerontology*
   B. Senescence
   C. Senility
2. Population change
   A. In United States 10.1% or 21.2 million persons 65 years or older
   B. Increase of 9.9% since January 1, 1968
   C. Census for 1970 showed 3.2 million more women 65 years older than men
   D. Gradual shifting of elderly from northern to southern states and far west

3. Progress and research
   A. First White House Conference on Aging in 1961
      1. Eventual enactment of legislation establishing Medicare and the Older Americans Act
         a. Benefits under Medicare became available July 1, 1966
         b. Older Americans Act became effective 1965
   B. Older Americans Comprehensive Services Amendments passed in 1973
      1. Extended services for elderly
   C. Special emphasis on nutritional needs of elderly
      1. Hot meals for persons 60 years or older
      2. National project FIND to locate persons eligible for food stamps and surplus food
   D. Numerous programs funded under Older Americans Act
   E. Social Security Act of 1965 provides monthly benefits for elderly persons
   F. Sixteen research centers open to study biologic and physiologic factors related to aging
4. Retirement and aging
   A. Older worker pressured into retirement to make room for younger person
   B. Age Discrimination in Employment Act of 1967
      1. Protects persons between 40 and 65 years from discrimination in hiring, discharge, or other conditions solely on basis of age
   C. Basic needs of retired worker
      1. Financial security
      2. To be useful
      3. To form new associations
      4. To maintain sense of dignity and self-respect
      5. To feel needed and wanted in society
   D. Planning for retirement should begin in middle years of life
5. Socioeconomic and cultural factors
   A. Oriental cultures—revered persons
   B. Primitive cultures—aged persons were storehouses for important information
   C. Early American culture—aged consulted about affairs of community
   D. Modern culture—youth oriented
   E. Social system forces person into retirement when it is difficult to make decisions
6. Nursing homes
   A. Estimated that 50% of nursing home residents could be cared for in own home
   B. More than 23,000 nursing homes in operation, with 1 million beds, and 500,000 employees
   C. United States government annually contributes over $1 billion to nursing homes
   D. In 1972 general accounting office indicated that 40% of all drugs used under Medicaid were tranquilizers and sedatives
   E. Upgrading of nursing homes

1. State to license nursing home administrators
2. Reports in 1973 indicate that 500 of 7000 nursing homes have been decertified or have withdrawn because of failure to meet federal nursing home standards
3. Seminars held for nursing home administrators and medical directors
4. Training of nursing home inspectors
5. Maintenance of nursing care plans for every patient
6. Improvement in building codes and fire regulations
   F. Alternatives to institutional care
   1. Home care
   2. Day hospital
   3. Foster home
   4. Extended care facility
   5. Community outpatient services
      a. Mental health clinics
      b. Physical therapy services
      c. Dental clinics
      d. Speech clinics
      f. Social services
7. Biopsychosocial factors
   A. Aging causes physiologic changes in total human organism
   B. Stress situations related to psychosocial problems may affect physical condition
   C. Increased incidence of geriatric suicide
   1. Nurse should be alert to warning signs
   D. Society fosters subculture
   1. Elderly person develops feelings of alienation and disengagement
   E. Mental health
   1. Need for community counseling service for elderly
   2. Anxiety may be cause of emotional breakdown
   3. Adjustments to be made by elderly
      a. Death of spouse
      b. Retirement and reduced income
      c. Disengagement and alienation of family and friends
      d. Identification with older age group
      e. Adjustment to depleted energy and gradually deteriorating body
   4. Activities to keep elderly person in mainstream of life
8. Pathophysiology of aging
   A. Aging is nonpathologic process
   B. Pathologic conditions may occur as complications of aging
   C. Variation in rate and extent of aging
   D. Cardiovascular system
   1. Normal wear and tear on system over years
      a. Decrease in functional ability of heart
      b. Less blood pumped out of heart
      c. Decrease in oxygen and nutrients to tissues and other organs of body
   E. Endocrine system—function declines
   1. Atrophy of breasts, vaginal mucosa, uterus, ovaries, and prostate gland

F. Sensory system
   1. Changes affect vision, hearing, sense of pain, and ability to adapt to darkness
   2. Loss of balance and sense of body position
G. Integumentary system
   1. Affects skin and appendages
      a. Skin becomes dry, thinner, pigmented, and wrinkled
      b. Nails become dry, thick, and brittle
      c. Hair dries, loses pigmentation, and decrease of hair in axilla and pubis
H. Musculoskeletal system—affects bones, joints, muscles, and their attachments
   1. Loss of calcium in bone structure
   2. Atrophy of intervertebral disks
      a. Changes contour of chest cage
   3. Changes in weight-bearing joints
   4. Cartilage and tendons become weakened
   5. Muscles become soft and flabby
I. Nervous system
   1. Loss of brain cells—few replaced
   2. Loss of cells in nerve fibers
      a. Decrease in speed of response
      b. Decrease in memory for recent events
J. Digestive system
   1. Decrease in gastric secretions
   2. Slowing of peristalsis
   3. Decrease in sense of taste and smell
K. Urinary system
   1. Decrease in blood supply to kidneys with some loss of function
   2. Urinary incontinence may occur
9. Nursing the elderly
   Care designed to protect from injury, provide comfort, improve nutrition, maintain personal hygiene, and care during illness
   A. Preventing injury
   1. In 1971, 28,000 persons 65 years of age and older died as result of accidental injuries
   2. Avoid use of scatter rugs in home
   3. Use rubber mats in bathtub
   4. Avoid moving furniture to unfamiliar places
   5. Night lights in bathroom, stairs, increased illumination in evening
   6. Accompany elderly person on street at dusk or in evening, carry flashlight, and use reflectorized material on clothing
   B. Providing comfort
   1. Use bed socks, bed jacket, or extra blanket at night
   2. Avoid use of hot-water bottle or heating pad to prevent burns
   3. Provide extra clothing or wraps
   4. Do not place person in draft or where electric fans and air conditioners blow on them
   5. Short rest periods after meals
   6. Provide evening entertainment
   C. Meeting nutritional needs
   1. Diet may be affected by

a. Reduced income
b. Inadequacy of cooking facilities
c. Loneliness and having to eat alone
d. Physical inability to prepare food
e. Decrease of gastric secretions and slowing of digestion
f. Loss of teeth or poorly fitting dentures
g. Living too far from market and lack of delivery service

2. Metabolic process decreases 10% to 30%
3. Reduce calories after 25 years of age
4. Diet should include four basic food groups

D. Personal hygiene
1. Reduction of complete baths and shampooing of hair
2. Foot care by member of family or podiatrist
3. Brushing of teeth or dentures and regular visits to dentist
4. Laxatives should be prescribed by physician
5. Care if urinary incontinence occurs
6. Encourage to maintain good personal appearance

10. Pathologic complications of aging
A. Atherosclerosis and arteriosclerosis
B. Osteoporosis
C. Vaginitis (senile)
D. Prostate gland (benign prostatic hypertrophy)
E. Pulmonary disorders
1. Hypostatic pneumonia
2. Increase in death rate during epidemics of influenza
F. Varicosities

11. Care of hospitalized patient
A. Vital signs
1. Blood pressure influenced by age; small changes may be important in aged person
2. Pulse rate must be considered with other symptoms
B. Sedation—elderly do not tolerate sedatives as well as do younger persons
C. Intake and output—intake should be sufficient to produce 1500 ml. of urine in 24 hours
1. Intravenous fluids must be administered slowly to prevent cardiac difficulties
D. Ambulation and convalescence—older person requires longer periods for convalescence; progress is slower
1. Ambulation should be gradual
2. Speak clearly and distinctly to patient
3. Give directions slowly and be sure that patient understands

Review questions

1. According to the 1970 census, was the number of women compared to the number of men found to be:
a. Decreasing
b. Remaining the same
c. Increasing

2. What two pieces of federal legislation was enacted after the first White House Conference on Aging?
a. *medicare*
b. *Older Americans Act*

3. What is the most important need of the retired older person?
a. *financial security*

4. List three services that should be provided on an outpatient basis.
a. *mental health clinics*
b. *dental care*
c. *physical therapy*

5. List four basic food groups that should be included in the diet of older persons.
a. *meat - eggs - fish - poultry*
b. *milk*
c. *fruit - veg*
d. *cereal - bread*

6. Why should intravenous fluids run slowly when being administered to an elderly person?
a. *the heart has decreased function*

7. What condition is caused by a loss of calcium in the bones of older persons?
a. *osteoporosis*

8. List several activities that may contribute to the mental health of older individuals.
a. *educational classes*
b. *employment services*
c. *craft classes, tours,*

9. List four normal physiologic changes that you may expect in an older person.
a. *muscles weaken*
b. *skin becomes thin & flabby*
c. *decreased appetite*
d. *osteoporosis, lordosis, kyphosis*

10. Frequent bathing of an elderly person may lead to a form of dermatitis commonly called:
a. *bath itch*

Films

1. Ready for Edna—MIS-962 (29½ min., sound, black and white, 16 mm.), Media Resources Branch, National Medical Audiovisual Center (Annex), Station K, Atlanta, Ga. 30324. Deals with old age. Edna, who is widowed, has had a mild stroke and is recovering. Edna is trying to rebuild her life, physically and emotionally; the film shows the community services required to help her. New developments in health services are described.

2. There is a way—MIS-738 (35 min., sound, black and white, 16 mm.), Media Resources Branch, National Medical Audiovisual Center (Annex), Station K, Atlanta, Ga. 30324. Deals with a method of treating the incontinent patient, the patient unable to control the bowels and bladder. Presents a training program for such patients. Explains physiology of normal bowel and bladder functions and emphasizes importance of creating proper emotional environment.

3. Environmental health aspects of nursing homes—MIS-667 (14 min., sound, color, 16 mm.), Media Resources Branch, National Medical Audiovisual Center (Annex), Station K, Atlanta, Ga. 30324. Presents specific and environmental health factors significant in nursing, home facilities. Accident and fire prevention, food sanitation, lighting, furnishings, and decorations included.

References

1. Accidents to the aging claim 28,000 lives in 1971, disable another 800,000, Aging **219:** 14, Jan., 1973.
2. Butler, Robert N., and Lewis, Myrna I.: Aging and mental health, St. Louis, 1973, The C. V. Mosby Co.
3. Cahn, Milton, W.: The skin from infancy to old age, American Journal of Nursing **60:**993-996, July, 1960.
4. Callender, Marie: National approach to long-term care, Nursing Outlook **21:**22-24, Jan., 1973.
5. Cooper, Shirley: A day hospital for elderly persons, The Canadian Nurse **66:**41-43, Jan., 1973.
6. Day hospital for aged, The Journal of Practical Nursing **23:**11, May, 1973.
7. Elwood, Thomas W.: Old age and the quality of life, Health Services Reports **87:**919-931, Dec., 1972.
8. Evans, Frances M. C.: Visiting older people: a learning experience, Nursing Outlook **17:**20-22, March, 1969.
9. Kernodle, John R.: Toward a brighter future for nursing homes, Health Services Reports **88:**316-319, April, 1973.
10. Larson, Laura G.: How to select a nursing home, American Journal of Nursing **69:**1034-1037, May, 1969.
11. Levine, Rhoda L.: Disengagement in the elderly—its causes and effects, Nursing Outlook **17:**28-30, Oct., 1969.
12. Licensing examination for nursing home operators, Public Health Reports **84:**473, May, 1969.
13. Long-term care of the aged, Proceedings and Debates of the 92nd Congress, 1st sess., Congressional record, Washington, D. C., Nov. 22, 1971.
14. Mead, Margaret: New thoughts on old people, Practical Nursing **11:**12-13, Jan., 1961.
15. Mitchell, Helen S., et al.: Cooper's nutrition in health and disease, ed. 15, Philadelphia, 1968, J. B. Lippincott Co.
16. Moss, Frank E.: Is the quality of care adequate in nursing homes? Has the tranquilizer replaced TLC? Bedside Nurse **5:**11-16, Sept., 1972.
17. National project FIND seeks elderly eligible for food program, Aging **214:**4, Aug., 1972.
18. Nursing home surveyors are trained under HSMHA contracts, Health Services Reports **87:**817, Nov., 1972.
19. Ornstein, Sheldon: Objectives—a national policy on aging, American Journal of Nursing **71:**960-963, May, 1971.
20. Poulos, Jean: The geriatric suicide, Bedside Nurse **4:**24-26, July, 1971.
21. Shafer, Kathleen N., Sawyer, Janet R., McCluskey, Audrey M., Beck, Edna L., and Phipps, Wilma J.: Medical-surgical nursing, ed. 6, St. Louis, 1975, The C. V. Mosby Co.
22. Shock, Nathan W.: The biologists' view of aging, Modern Maturity **16:**25-26, June-July, 1973.
23. Soika, Cynthia Vaugham: Combating osteoporosis, American Journal of Nursing **73:** 1193-1197, July, 1973.
24. Population gains in the United States and Canada, Statistical Bulletin, New York, April, 1973, Metropolitan Life Insurance Co.
25. Taylor, E. Stewart: Essentials of gynecology, ed. 4, Philadelphia, 1969, Lea & Febiger.
26. The Public Health Conference on Records and Statistics meeting jointly with the National Conference on Mental Health Statistics, Health Services Reports **87:**708-715, Oct., 1972.
27. Title 111 nutrition plans funded for $200 million, Aging **226:**5, Aug., 1973.
28. Training medical directors of nursing homes, Health Services Reports **88:**476-477, May, 1973.
29. Transition a guide to retirement, Washington, D. C., 1972, Government Printing Office.
30. Tysenhouse, Phyllis: Care plans for nursing home patients, Nursing Outlook **20:**169-172, March, 1972.
31. Williams, Sue Rodwell: Nutrition and diet therapy, ed. 2, St. Louis, 1973, The C. V. Mosby Co.

CHAPTER 9

Preoperative and postoperative nursing care of the patient

KEY WORDS

ambulation *walking*
anesthesia
anesthesiologist *a dr.*
atelectasis
crisis
cutdown
dehiscence *separation of*
dehydration *surgical incision*
depilatory cream
electrolytes
embolism *clot in lung*

evisceration
flatulence *gas*
hypostatic pneumonia
hypothermia *lowered body temp.*
infiltration
intravenous therapy
thrombosis *blood clot in vein*
Trendelenburg position *head lower than feet*

Modern surgery has alleviated many diseases that have crippled or killed past generations. Surgery is a planned alteration of physiologic processes within the body in an attempt to arrest or eliminate disease or illness. The meaning of surgery varies with each individual; however, it is generally a frightening experience to even the best prepared person. Surgery entails an invasion of one's most intimate privacy, and faith in physicians and other health care workers is necessary to assist in a time of dependency and need.[5]

The nursing care of surgical patients is a step-by-step process, beginning when the patient is admitted to the hospital and terminating when recovery is complete and he returns to his normal routine of living. The nurse who is assigned the care of surgical patients will need to have a broad understanding of individual reactions to the surgical procedure. The fear and anxiety felt by each patient and the nonverbal expressions of fear must be understood. Freedom of communication must be maintained between the nurse and the patient, between the patient and his surgeon, and between the patient's family and the surgeon. The patient's anxieties must be communicated to the physician. The nurse must possess a wide range of technical skills as well as a keen sense of critical observation. The line between safety and danger in the care of many surgical patients, especially older patients, may be a narrow one. However, the alert nurse will recognize early signs of impending trouble and report them so that preventive measures may be taken.

The objective of surgical nursing is to prepare the patient mentally and physically for surgery and to assist him to full recovery in the shortest time possible with the least discomfort that his condition permits.

ADMISSION OF THE PATIENT

Surgical patients may be admitted to the hospital in emergency situations, suffering from traumatic injuries received in an accident or a condition requiring immediate surgery, such as acute appendicitis. Most patients are admitted by prearranged plans made by the patient's surgeon. The patient may be admitted several days prior to anticipated surgery, during which time he may undergo a series of tests and studies. The patient who is admitted in an emergency situation may be taken directly to the operating room with limited preparation. Other patients are usually exposed to a series of routine procedures designed to determine the patient's immediate physical condition and to prepare him for the surgical procedure.

The nurse should be ready to receive the patient at the time of admission, and a friendly, interested, and unhurried attitude will help to make the patient feel secure and believe that he is in good hands. The nurse should be alert to any fears or apprehensions expressed by the patient and transmit such information to the surgeon. The patient and his family should be encouraged to communicate freely with the physician.

A complete history, including previous illnesses, accidents, or surgery, and a history of the present illness, its symptoms, duration, and related information, are secured from the patient. In the case of children and aged persons, members of the patient's family may be helpful in supplying information. The physician, assisted by the nurse, will examine the patient. (See a textbook on basic nursing for the procedure.) Often a number of laboratory examinations may be completed prior to admission, including urinalysis, a complete blood count, and determination of hemoglobin, bleeding time, clotting time, and hematocrit. In some cases a blood glucose test or electrocardiogram may be ordered. Many hospitals automatically require a chest x-ray examination of each patient admitted to the hospital.

The physician will evaluate the patient's nutritional status with reference to dehydration and malnutrition. When severe vomiting and diarrhea have occurred, there may be an electrolyte imbalance and a protein and vitamin deficiency that will result in decreased resistance to infection and delayed wound healing. If hemorrhage or slow bleeding has occurred, there may be a decrease in hemoglobin and red blood cells. It may be necessary to transfuse the patient with whole blood or to administer electrolytes and vitamins intravenously before performing surgery.

PREOPERATIVE ORDERS

The evening before surgery the physician will write the preoperative orders for the patient. Hospitals and physicians will vary in the kind of peoperative preparation desired; however, certain routine procedures are fairly uniform.

Diet. The patient is allowed a light diet the evening before surgery and is permitted to have water until midnight. If surgery is not to take place until late in the day and does not involve the gastrointestinal tract, the patient may be given a light breakfast and may be allowed water up to 8 hours before surgery. The nurse is responsible for removing the water from the patient's room and identifying the room and bed to avoid error.

Enema. Most surgical patients are given an enema preoperatively; however, the procedure is not uniform. The enema may consist of soapsuds, saline, or tap water. There is increasing use of commercially prepared enemas such as the Phospho-Soda enema, which is more comfortable for the patient. The reasons for administering a preoperative enema are as follows:

1. To remove feces from the intestine prior to surgery of the gastrointestinal tract
2. To relieve the patient of postoperative pain that might be caused by straining to have a bowel movement after abdominal surgery
3. To avoid an impaction postoperatively
4. To avoid exertion or the tendency to strain after certain kinds of surgery such as eye surgery

5. For the psychologic effect when the patient may fear having a bowel movement while under anesthesia[10]

In most cases bowel elimination does not occur until 2 or 3 days after surgery. The nurse should be sure that all enema solution is returned, and failure to achieve results should be reported to the physician.

Skin preparation. The evening before surgery the skin about the site of operation is prepared. Procedures vary, but the basic objective is to render the area as free of bacteria as possible and to cleanse it as thoroughly as possible without injury to the skin. In some hospitals a member of the operating room staff is responsible for this procedure. Some surgeons prefer that the skin preparation be done in the operating room on the day of surgery. The nurse should be familiar with the policy of the hospital or the physician and should secure instruction concerning the area to be prepared before beginning the procedure. Any dressings are removed, and adhesive tape may be removed from the skin with ether or benzene. Procedures among hospitals vary, but two basic principles should be kept in mind: (1) soap inactivates ammonium compounds (p. 49) and (2) preparations containing hexachlorophene act slowly and may be inactivated by the use of alcohol or soap. Common skin antiseptics are 70% ethyl or isoprophyl alcohol, Zephiran 1:750, iodine 1% or 2% in 70% alcohol, and hexachlorophene.[5] A skin antiseptic called polyvinylpyrrolidone-iodine complex (PVP-I), or povidone-iodine (p. 49), is effective for preoperative cleansing of the skin. Although more expensive, depilatory creams have been found to be effective in removing hair from the operative site. They avoid the risk of possible cuts, nicks, and abrasions and are more comfortable for the patient, especially for an apprehensive patient. The cream is spread onto the skin with a tongue blade or the gloved hand. It should be about ¼ inch thick and should remain on the skin for 10 minutes. It is then removed with a tongue blade or with moistened sponges, and the skin is washed with soap and water and patted dry. The nurse should be aware that some persons may be sensitive to the preparation used.[3]

Several commercial companies provide prepackaged, sterilized trays for skin preparation. Each tray contains all the equipment needed and assures the patient of individual supplies. In preparation for abdominal surgery special attention must be given to the umbilicus. Hair is removed from the area with a sharp, sterilized razor and new blades. The nurse must be careful to avoid cutting, nicking, or scratching the skin, since such cuts may become sites of infection. If the skin is injured, the surgeon may refuse to perform the surgery. Caution must be used in shaving around moles or warts, and any skin eruption must be reported. In shaving areas such as the axilla and pubic area the nurse may clip the long hair first to make shaving easier.

Care should be taken not to expose or embarrass the patient, and he should be left dry and comfortable after the procedure. Skin preparation for the male patient is usually done by the orderly or the physician.

Psychologic preparation. Preparation for surgery should begin as soon as the patient is told that an operation is necessary. Much can be done to alleviate fears prior to admission as well as during hospitalization. Fear of the unknown can produce much anxiety. The amount of information given to the patient should depend on his ability to comprehend what is told to him. The nurse should be able to explain the general meaning of x-ray procedures, laboratory tests, medications, and nursing procedures. Often the nurse will discuss the operative procedure with the patient and explain what can be expected postoperatively. *fear of anesthesia*

Fear of disability, or possible death, is frequent. The nurse should encourage the patient to talk about his fears. Usually patients will be more willing to express their feelings if they have established a good relationship with a member of the nursing team. Any misconceptions can be dispelled, and the patient can be encouraged to have faith in his physician and modern surgical techniques. Sometimes it is helpful to have the patient talk with other patients who have had similar surgery. The patient's family should be included in any discussions or explanations whenever possible. They should be encouraged to understand

*Prep.:
redress;
finances
family relations
Prognosis*

Be a good "listener"

the anxiety the patient faces and to visit often.

Many patients are placed in intensive care units after extensive surgical procedures. Electronic monitoring equipment may be frightening to the patient unless he is given a simple explanation of how it is used to contribute to his nursing care. The patient's family often believes that the patient is in a critical condition when he is placed in the intensive care unit. They should be given the same information the patient is given. Explanation concerning the patient's care can often be given during visiting hours when the family is present, thus saving the nurse's time.[6]

Exercises. Postoperative care will be facilitated if the patient is taught and allowed to practice deep breathing, coughing, and exercises prior to surgery. He may be taught how to turn himself in bed and should be told the reasons why these procedures are important. He should be assured that the nurse will assist him after the surgery until he is able to perform the exercises alone.

Sedation. A barbiturate such as pentobarbital (Nembutal) or secobarbital (Seconal) is usually ordered by the physician to be given at bedtime the evening before surgery to ensure adequate sleep and rest. After administration of the sedative the patient should be instructed to call a nurse rather than get out of bed alone, since he sometimes experiences confusion after the administration of barbiturates. In the case of elderly persons, side rails should be placed on the bed, and the patient should be observed at frequent intervals. All urine voided during the night should be measured and recorded on the patient's chart.

OPERATIVE DAY

On the operative day, visiting should be limited to some member of the family who is permitted to see the patient before he goes to surgery. However, the patient should be allowed to rest and should be kept as quiet as possible. He should be reassured, and his questions or those of his family should be answered. If the patient shows signs of undue anxiety or apprehension, it should be reported.

Time should be allowed for personal

hygiene such as bathing, oral care, and shaving. The vital signs—temperature, pulse, respiration, and blood pressure—are checked and recorded. Any elevation of temperature must be reported immediately. All pins and combs are removed from the hair, and long hair is placed in two braids. The hair may then be covered with a cotton cap or wrapped in a towel. Dentures and removable bridges should be removed and placed in a container marked with the patient's name, then put in a safe place to avoid loss or damage.

Procedures vary among anesthesiologists, but frequently the anesthetist prefers that all makeup be removed before the patient goes to surgery. Any reduction of oxygen to the tissues may be observed in the lips, face, and nail beds, or it may be detected by the color of the blood at the operative site. Some anesthetists believe that the removal of nail polish is unnecessary because the hands are covered with sterile drapes and are not accessible, and others have suggested that colored nail polish be removed from only a couple of fingers.

Valuables such as money and jewelry should be listed in the patient's presence, sealed in an envelope, and locked up or given to a responsible member of the family. The nurse should be familiar with the policy of the hospital concerning the care of valuables and should use every precaution to protect the patient's personal property. Often considerable sentiment is attached to the wedding ring, and the patient may be allowed to wear it; however, it should be tied with a small piece of bandage and secured about the patient's wrist to avoid loss. Religious medals should be securely fastened to the wrist with a bit of tape or bandage.

A hospital gown that ties in the back is put onto the patient, and some hospitals require that leggins made of muslin be put onto the patient. The patient should be encouraged to void, and the amount should be measured and recorded on the patient's chart. Inability to void should be reported to the physician. Depending on the type of surgery, the patient's age, and his condition, the physician may order a retention catheter inserted into the urinary bladder preoperatively. The physician may also order a gastric tube inserted preoperatively. The surgeon may request that the patient's legs be wrapped with elastic bandages. The purpose is to prevent thrombophlebitis. The leg should be wrapped with 4-inch bandage, beginning at the ankle and ending at the midthigh.

Preoperative medications, which are ordered by the anesthesiologist, are usually administered hypodermically. The purpose of preoperative medications is to help the patient accept anesthesia more easily and to provide for a smoother induction. Preoperative medications fall into three groups: (1) agents that relax, relieve apprehension, and decrease metabolic rates; (2) those that reduce secretions in the respiratory tract, minimize spasm of the larynx, and help maintain a clear airway; and (3) those that relieve apprehension, produce a sedative effect, and help prevent vomiting during anesthesia and in the immediate postoperative period[6] (Table 9-1). Preoperative medications are ordered individually for each patient, and the anesthetist will consider the patient's age, general condition, other medications such as insulin that the patient may be receiving, and the anesthetizing agent to be used. The medication is ordered to be administered at a specific hour, and it is important that the nurse give the medication on time so that its maximum effect is reached during induction of anesthesia. If for any reason the medication is not administered as directed, the anesthetist should be notified so that adjustment may be made. After administration of the preoperative medication the patient should be instructed to remain in bed, and the nurse should provide a quiet environment so that the patient may rest. The hospital may require that identification be attached to the patient's wrist, including such information as the patient's name, room number, medication given, hour administered, and signature of the nurse.

Just prior to being transported to the operating room the patient should empty his bladder and the time should be noted. Vital signs should be taken and recorded.

The nurse should check the chart carefully to be sure that all reports such as laboratory reports of blood and urine have been recorded and that a signed operative permit is attached to the chart. Operative permits should be signed prior to administration of medications. All preoperative medications and procedures should be accurately charted before the patient goes to

Table 9-1. Preoperative medications

Group I
  Provide relaxation
  Relieve apprehension
  Lower metabolic rate
	Barbiturates
	  Pentobarbital sodium (Nembutal sodium)
	  Secobarbital sodium (Seconal sodium) *Valium also used.*
	Narcotics
	  Morphine sulfate
	  Meperidine hydrochloride (Demerol)
	  Methadone hydrochloride (Methadon, Adanon, Dolophine hydrochlorides)
	  Alphaprodine hydrochloride (Nisentil)
	  Levorphanol tartrate (Levo-Dromaran) *Innovar — used occ. (narcotic + tranquilizer) less nausea + vomiting po*

Group II
  Reduce secretions
  Minimize spasm
  Maintain clear airway
	Belladonna derivatives
	  Atropine *most used*
	  Scopolamine

Group III
  Reduce apprehension
  Produce sedative effect
  Reduce possibility of vomiting
	Tranquilizing agents
	  Chlorpromazine (Thorazine)
	  Promethazine hydrochloride (Phenergan)

the operating room, and a new physician's order sheet should be attached to the record.

The patient may be transferred to the operating room in his own bed or by stretcher. He should be moved carefully and with as little confusion as possible. The patient should be protected from drafts and exposure with cotton blankets and should be made comfortable with a small pillow under his head. The nurse should accompany the patient and remain with him until relieved by a member of the operating room staff. The patient's record is given to the operating room nurse, who is also advised verbally of the patient's name and any significant problem existing at the moment.

ANESTHESIA

Most patients have some fear of anesthesia and frequently ask the nurse questions concerning the kind of anesthetic they will receive. The nurse should tell the patient that the kind of anesthetic is planned for him individually by his physician and will be the kind best suited for him. The nurse may tell the patient that the anesthetic will be administered by a physician or a nurse who has had special training. The anesthesiologist's preoperative visit to the patient's room promotes confidence and helps to relieve anxiety.

An anesthesiologist is a physician who specializes in the selection and administration of anesthesia and assumes responsibility for the extrasurgical care of the patient in the operating room and recovery room.

A nurse anesthetist is a professional nurse who has received postgraduate training in the administration of anesthetics and who functions under the responsibility of the operating surgeon.

Some hospitals have anesthetizing rooms in which the patient is anesthetized; when the surgeon is ready, the patient is wheeled into the operating room. When patients are taken directly to the operating room, all the nurses should remember that the patient is in a strange and sometimes frightening environment. There should be no bright lights or unnecessary noise and talking.

The kind of anesthetic administered to the patient may affect his postoperative condition and his return to consciousness, and a brief description of some anesthetizing agents will help the nurse assess the patient's condition and anticipate his needs postoperatively.

Types

Anesthesia is classified as general or conductive, with conductive anesthesia further differentiated as local or regional. When the surgeon wishes all sensations in the entire body to be suspended temporarily, the patient is given a general anesthetic. When only a part of the body is involved, the patient may be given a conductive anesthetic, which may be local or regional. General anesthetics include drugs that are administered by inhalation.

Inhalation anesthesia. Drugs used in inhalation anesthesia may be in the form of liquids that vaporize, with the patient inhaling the vapor. Examples are ether and chloroform. Inhalation drugs are also in the form of gases such as nitrous oxide, ethylene, and cyclopropane. All drugs used in inhalation anesthesia are administered in combination with oxygen or air by a mask or through an intubation tube that is inserted into the trachea or bronchi. Ether is one of the oldest and safest anesthetizing agents but is explosive. Ether is irritating to the respiratory passages and may produce nausea and vomiting; the nurse must exercise care to avoid the aspiration of vomitus by the patient. The patient given ether is much slower to regain consciousness.

A number of other drugs are being used, including halothane (Fluothane), a liquid that vaporizes. Induction is fairly rapid, and the patient usually regains consciousness fairly quickly. Little or no nausea or vomiting occurs; and the drug is nonexplosive, but since the drug has no prolonged analgesic effect, the patient will complain of pain and will be restless and apprehensive. The nurse will have to give close attention to these patients, since they often become difficult to keep quiet. The nurse should be alert for respiratory difficulty or change in the blood pressure. The depth of sedation and the length of the surgical procedure are factors that affect the time necessary to regain consciousness. After the administration of all these drugs the nurse must observe the patient for respiratory obstruction and hypotension. Hypotension is especially common after the use of cyclopropane and ether.

Intravenous drugs. Drugs given intravenously are not anesthetics but adjuncts to anesthesia. They are always administered in combination with drugs producing inhalation anesthesia such as nitrous oxide gas and oxygen. The drugs used are short-acting barbiturates that produce unconsciousness in 30 seconds. The most common drugs in use are thiopental (Pentothal) sodium and thiamylal (Surital) sodium. When large amounts have been given, the patient will not return to consciousness quickly. The patient must be watched carefully for laryngeal spasm, which may be indicated by retraction of the soft tissues about the neck muscles, severe cyanosis, and restlessness. The anesthesiologist should be notified immediately if these symptoms appear. However, a safeguard is checking to be sure the airway is kept clear. All vital signs must be checked frequently and carefully and any significant change reported.

Muscle relaxants. Curare and succinylcholine chloride (Anectine) are powerful muscle-relaxant drugs that are often administered to increase relaxation of abdominal muscles during surgery. Both drugs may cause respiratory difficulty, and the patient should be watched extremely carefully.

Rectal anesthesia. Partial anesthesia is produced by injecting tribromoethanol (Avertin) fluid into the rectum; however, it is not used frequently, since it is difficult to control its absorption from the rectum and colon. Also, a pseudoanesthesia may be induced by rectal thiopental sodium, and true anesthesia may be induced by rectal ether. Soon after injection the patient falls into a deep sleep. Often this type of anesthesia is used for children, and the dosage is based on body weight. Therefore weight should be taken carefully and recorded preoperatively. Postoperatively the patient must be watched for respiratory difficulty, and blood pressure must be checked frequently because hypotension may occur.

Spinal anesthesia. A solution of a local anesthetic drug may be injected into the subarachnoid space, which contains cerebrospinal fluid. The drug anesthetizes nerves as they leave the spinal cord. The method of injection is the same as that for any spinal puncture. Under this type of anesthesia the patient may remain awake; therefore it is necessary to avoid any careless conversation that may be misinterpreted by the patient. During the operation the patient may be aware of pressure or pulling sensations but no pain. After spinal anesthesia the patient must be kept flat in bed for several hours. Vital signs, especially blood pressure, should be watched because hypotension may occur. Sensations to the anesthetized part do not return immediately, and careful positioning of the patient is important to prevent later discomfort. Placing the patient in the Trendelenburg position is contraindicated unless ordered by the physician. The patient may have severe headache, which is thought to be due to leakage of spinal fluid from the puncture site. The headache often lasts for several days, possibly weeks. The physician will probably order pain-relieving drugs to keep the patient as comfortable as possible.

Analgesic blocks. Analgesic blocks are used to inhibit nerve impulses to various parts of the body. A local anesthetic drug is injected in and around nerves, resulting in anesthesia of the area supplied by the particular nerves. Several different drugs may be used, including procaine hydrochloride, tetracaine hydrochloride (Pontocaine), and lidocaine (Xylocaine). Local anesthesia may be used for operations in which tissue is incised, for example in the removal of a small breast tumor, or a solution of the drug may be used to anesthetize a region, for example the lower abdomen and perineum (caudal block) in obstetrics. Since all drugs used for local anesthesia are potentially toxic, the patient should be carefully observed for signs of itching of the skin, twitching, convulsions, cyanosis, nausea, and vomiting; also, blood pressure, pulse, and respiration should be carefully checked. The patient is conscious but may be drowsy if a sedative has been administered prior to the operative procedure.

Tranquilizers. A large number of tranquilizing drugs are on the market under various trade names and are often used as preanesthetic sedatives. They tend to reduce tension and anxiety, and some may produce a small degree of muscle relaxation. Some have antiemetic effects and may be used to reduce vomiting during anesthesia or postoperatively. The commonly used drugs include promethazine (Phenergan), chlorpromazine (Thorazine), promazine hydrochloride (Sparine), triflupromazine hydrochloride (Vesprin), thiethylperazine (Torecan), and others. When used for surgical patients, these drugs may produce undesirable side effects such as hypotension and drowsiness. If these drugs are given with a narcotic, oversedation and increased sleepiness are dangers to consider.

Induced hypothermia. Hypothermia in itself is not a type of anesthesia, but rather a means of decreasing oxygen demand and consumption during anesthesia and surgery so that circulation may be compromised or interrupted to make possible or facilitate surgery in vital areas. The procedure consists of slowly lowering the body temperature to between 82° and 86° F. Dangers and problems exist in lowering the temperature and also in rewarming the body after surgery. Specially trained nurses are required, and continuous care and observation are necessary. The use of hypothermia is increasing in many types of surgery and in conditions in which the patient has a very high temperature. Techniques used to induce hypothermia include placing the patient in a tub of ice water or covering the patient with a blanket containing coils through which ice water circulates. In regional hypo-

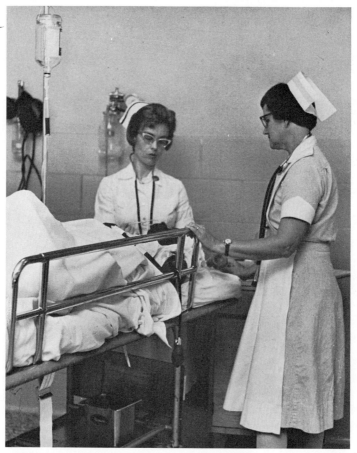

In O.R.
circulating nurse
scrub nurse
technician (OR)
surgeon
anesthesiologist
patient

Fig. 9-1. Modern recovery room provides skilled nursing care for patients recovering from anesthesia. (Courtesy Memorial Hospital of Chatham County, Savannah, Ga.)

thermia an extremity such as a leg is packed in ice and deliberately frozen so that surgery, usually amputation, may be performed without anesthesia. This procedure is useful in treating patients who are poor risks, but it requires much work, constant observation, and extremely close coordination in the operating room. There are many nursing responsibilities in the care of patients undergoing hypothermia, such as the administration of intravenous fluids, intake and output, filling ice packs, giving oral care and eye irrigations, turning and positioning the patient, and replacing and assembling equipment.

RECOVERY ROOM CARE

It must be stressed that the patient recovering from anesthesia cannot be left alone and has to be watched constantly. Many hospitals maintain facilities for the immediate postoperative care of the patient, and the patient is transferred from the operating room to the recovery unit on a specially designed bed or stretcher. The recovery room is generally located near the operating rooms and is equipped with the necessary supplies, drugs, and equipment for care in any emergency that might arise. The recovery room is considered a part of the surgical suite and is under the supervision of the anesthesiologist. Nurses who care for patients recovering from anesthesia should accept their responsibility seriously, realizing that this is the most critical period for the surgical patient. (See Fig. 9-1.)

The anesthesiologist accompanies the patient from the operating room to the recovery room and advises the nurses of the patient's condition and any special problems that may require care or attention. The anesthesiologist will make sure that the airway is clear and that vital signs are satisfactory before leaving the patient. The patient should be protected by side rails on the bed, which may be padded to avoid injuring a restless patient. The patient should be moved as carefully as possible. Anesthetics are stored in the body during surgery, and until they are eliminated every movement of the patient, such as from operating table to stretcher or bed, riding in elevators, or wheeling around corners in corridors, may

cause serious changes in the vital signs.[8] The patient should be protected with warm cotton blankets.

Airway. The immediate responsibility of the nurse is to make certain that the airway is clear and that it remains clear. The patient should be turned and placed in the Sims' position with the head flat to allow for drainage of blood or mucus from the mouth. When it is not possible to turn the patient, his head should be turned to the side. If increased secretions obstruct the respiratory passages, they are aspirated with a catheter attached to suction. If the suction is on, the catheter must be pinched while it is being inserted to prevent damage to the mucous membrane (p. 196). If secretions have been removed, but evidence of respiratory difficulty is still present, the nurse's thumbs and fingers should be placed at the angle of the jaw on both sides and the jaw should be pushed forward (Fig. 9-2). The tongue may be grasped with a piece of gauze and pulled forward. If these measures do not relieve the difficulty, the anesthesiologist should be called. Often the anesthesiologist leaves a plastic, rubber, or metal airway in place that is not removed until the patient shows signs of regaining consciousness (Fig. 9-3). The respiratory rate should be checked at frequent intervals; shallow, quiet, and slow respirations may be an early sign of respiratory difficulty. The movement of air in and out of the lungs can be felt by holding the hand near the patient's mouth. Respiratory rates of 30 or above or below 16 should alert the nurse to difficulty.

Circulation. Blood pressure and pulse should be taken at 15-minute intervals for

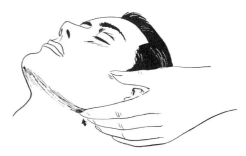

Fig. 9-2. Method of pushing the jaw forward to relieve respiratory difficulty.

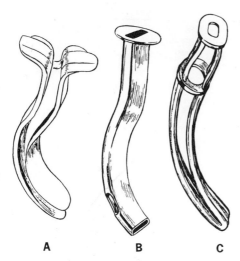

Fig. 9-3. Artifical airways. **A,** Plastic airway. **B,** Rubber airway. **C,** Metal airway.

at least 2 hours, then every 30 minutes for 2 hours. A drop in blood pressure may occur after certain types of anesthesia, the administration of muscle-relaxing drugs, or the use of some tranquilizing drugs. It may also occur as the result of moving the patient or of unrelieved pain. If any noticeable drop occurs, the anesthesiologist should be notified. A critical systolic pressure must be determined for each patient individually. The pulse should be checked for rate, rhythm, and volume. A drop in blood pressure and a weak, rapid, thready pulse with a cool, moist skin may indicate severe bleeding, and the physician should be notified immediately. Treatment is based on the cause, and the physician will order the appropriate procedures. (See the discussion on the treatment of severe bleeding later in this chapter.)

Dressings. The nurse must check dressings every 15 minutes for evidence of drainage or bleeding. If bright red blood appears on the dressing, it should be observed frequently to see if it spreads; the surgeon should be notified if there is any increase.

Suction siphonage. All drainage tubes are connected to the appropriate type of drainage. Gastric tubes are connected to suction siphonage, which is always placed on low pressure.

Drainage. After mastectomy, radical neck surgery, and gallbladder surgery the physician may order tubes connected to drainage; urinary drainage tubes are connected to the proper drainage container. If a catheter is used after thoracotomy, it is connected to underwater drainage. Under no circumstances may the drainage bottle be removed from the floor. Urinary drainage bottles must not be lifted above the level of the bed.

Physician's orders. The nurse should check the physician's orders for any procedures or medications, such as administration of intravenous fluids or blood, and carry out all orders.

Relief of pain. As the patient begins to wake up, he will complain of pain. Patients who are extremely apprehensive before surgery may evidence pain early in the postoperative period. Before giving pain-relieving drugs, the nurse should consider the length of time since the preoperative sedatives were administered, the type and action of the anesthetizing agent used, the status of vital signs, the age of the patient, and the preoperative emotional state. Whenever any question arises concerning the administration of a narcotic, the physician should be consulted.

Voiding. The patient should be encouraged to void while still in the recovery room. With the return to full consciousness and the awareness of pain, the patient becomes tense, and voiding may become difficult; however, he may be able to void voluntarily before painful stimuli cause tension.

Transfer to patient's room. The length of time the patient remains in the recovery room will be determined by his immediate postoperative condition. When the vital signs are stabilized and the patient has regained consciousness, he may be transferred to his room. The patient may be considered conscious when he responds to his name and is oriented to time and place. The patient is accompanied to his room by the nurse, who reports his condition and any problems encountered.

INTENSIVE CARE UNIT (ICU)

The evolution of the intensive care unit began early in the 1960s. Nearly all units were in large metropolitan hospitals. Dur-

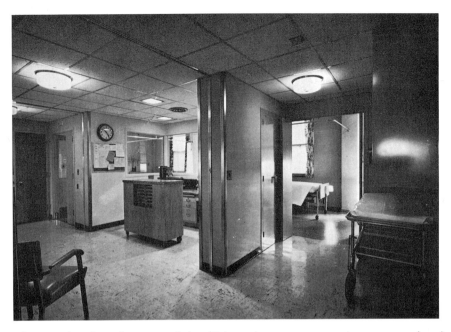

Fig. 9-4. Modern intensive care unit in which continuous expert nursing care may be given to specified medical or surgical patients who are critically ill. (Courtesy Community Hospital, Battle Creek, Mich.)

ing this decade the number increased so that now even the small rural hospitals have a few beds set aside for the care of critically ill patients. The nurse-patient ratio has been kept low, and nurses have been given extensive training to prepare them to provide expert nursing care and to meet any emergency that might arise. Today the number of beds has increased, and the numbers and kinds of patients admitted to ICU have also increased. A patient is admitted to ICU because he is in need of intensive nursing and medical care, which it is assumed cannot be given on the regular clinical units (Fig. 9-4). According to one author,[11] all nursing, whether in ICU or on the clinical unit, should be practiced as intensive nursing care. Burrell and Burrell[2] believe that a large number of diseases and disorders are a potential threat to the life of the individual and that when vital processes are compromised, intensive nursing and medical care may maintain those processes until the inner resources of the human body can effectively take control.

Many of the larger hospitals have discovered that the increasing number of pa-tients whose lives may be saved cannot be cared for adequately in a single unit. The trend is developing toward establishing separate intensive care units for specific kinds of patients, that is, burn units, shock units, coronary care units, respiratory care units, neurosurgical units, pediatric care units, and renal care units. Nurses assigned to each unit will be highly trained as clinical specialists in their particular area. However, this trend is not accepted by all hospitals, and most of the smaller ones will continue to care for patients in a single unit.

Nursing personnel in the ICU should include the head nurse who is responsible for the nursing care given to all patients. The head nurse organizes and plans the work, assigns duties, and supervises all personnel in the unit. Nurses, nursing aides, orderlies, and inhalation therapists may participate in patient care in the ICU. The head nurse is responsible for seeing that all equipment is in working order and that all drugs, supplies, and emergency equipment are always available. The action of drugs administered to a patient, the route for administration of each one, and its dosage, effect, contraindications, and side effects must be understood. Emergencies must be anticipated and appropriate action taken before the physician arrives. Intravenous infusions and oxygen must be started, and the patient may be defibrillated if the nurse is trained in this procedure in the event of ventricular fibrillation. The nurse may also set up and record an electrocardiogram, carry out closed-chest massage, and use a respirator when respiratory assistance is needed. The nurse may give general nursing care and may assign such nursing care to others in the unit. ICU nursing is individualized nursing care and is much more than sitting at a desk in front of a monitor.

A trained inhalation therapist should be a member of the ICU team. This specialist has become increasingly important in helping to maintain inhalation equipment and its proper functioning and in the proper administration of various types of respiratory therapy by continuously monitoring ventilators and supervising the administration of oxygen or aerosol therapy.

The ICU is frequently the scene of crisis situations, and personnel must be able to use good judgment and make accurate decisions quickly in any emergency. They must be able to encourage and support the patient with a warm feeling and a devoted attitude. They must be able to meet with members of the patient's family and convey to them their interest in the patient, the necessity of certain procedures, and how they help the patient.[1]

Visitors are strictly limited in the ICU. Usually only close members of the family are permitted to visit for not more than 5 minutes at a time. All extraneous diversions such as flowers, radios, televisions, telephones, and food are prohibited. When the patient's condition improves so that continuous care is no longer needed, he is transferred to a room on a clinical unit.

CONTINUING POSTOPERATIVE CARE

The continued postoperative care of the patient is directed toward the prevention of complications, rehabilitation, and a return to normal living. Elderly or confused patients should be protected by side rails on the bed. A member of the family should be permitted to see the patient as soon

as he returns to his room and in some instances may be allowed to remain with the patient.

Comfort measures. A pillow may be placed under the patient's head, and the head of the bed may be slightly raised. Since the patient is sensitive to temperature changes, care should be taken to avoid chilling by exposure to drafts; electric fans or air conditioners should not blow directly onto the patient. The patient's skin may feel cool, and he may complain of being cold. This is because of air-conditioned operating and recovery rooms. The patient may be covered with a blanket until his skin is warm and dry, after which the blanket should be removed to prevent overheating. The patient who becomes too warm will be restless, and excessive perspiration will result in the loss of body fluids and important electrolytes.

Oral care should be given and the face and hands washed. The back should be bathed and may be rubbed with alcohol. The patient is turned onto the side in the Sims' position, with a pillow placed to the back to give support. A small pillow or towel rolled and placed in a piece of stockinette may be tucked under the abdomen to support sagging abdominal muscles. If intake of water is not permitted, the lips should be moistened with cool water at intervals. The room should be well ventilated and free from unnecessary noise.

Turning. The patient should be turned regularly every 2 hours from side to side until he is ambulatory. Turning is essential to prevent respiratory complications and thrombus formation.

Intravenous therapy. Veins provide an excellent route for the administration of fluids that the patient may need preoperatively, during surgery, or postoperatively. The patient may be admitted with a fluid and electrolyte imbalance that must be corrected prior to surgery. Often intravenous fluids are begun the day before surgery to ensure that the patient is well hydrated; this will help to minimize the effects of fluid loss during surgery. With every surgical procedure there is a loss of fluid and electrolytes through bleeding and drainage. Postoperatively these losses can also occur from excessive perspiration, rapid breathing, and vomiting. Rather large amounts of fluids can be given quickly to replace losses through intravenous infusion.

Fluids are introduced into veins through plastic or metal needles or through plastic catheters inserted either through metal needles or by means of a cutdown. The latter is a minor surgical procedure where a small incision is made into the vein. The catheters are then anchored to the skin with a small piece of gauze under the hub of the needle and tapes. A bottle or plastic bag filled with solution and an intravenous infusion set should have been prepared prior to the procedure and connected to the needle or catheter after being firmly anchored in place. The fluid is then started and proper flow rate established.

Many kinds of solutions can be administered, depending on the needs of the individual patient. In general there are three basic solutions that are commonly used. Hydrating solutions are administered when the patient is dehydrated, and kidney function is stimulated as a result. These solutions usually contain carbohydrates (sugars) in water or saline. The carbohydrate is metabolized, and the water is free to be absorbed by cells or eliminated; 5% dextrose in water is an example. Balanced, or maintenance, solutions provide water, electrolytes, and carbohydrates and are effective for patients who must be maintained on intravenous solutions for a period of time; Butler's solution is an example. Replacement solutions are used primarily to replenish losses from the gastrointestinal tract occurring from vomiting, suction, fistulas, ostomies, and diarrhea. These solutions do not hydrate the patient; lactated Ringer's solution is an example.[4]

It is the nurse's responsibility to observe the patient who is receiving intravenous fluids. The rate of flow is ordered, and the number of drops per minute must be regulated. The injection site should be watched for swelling, which indicates that the needle has slipped out of the vein and is entering the soft tissues. If the bottle of solution is lowered below the patient, blood should appear in the tubing. If blood does not appear, the in-travenous fluid has infiltrated. Often a patient will complain of burning pain at the site if the needle has left the vein. When infiltration occurs, the intravenous infusion should be removed and restarted in another area.

Complications can occur from intravenous injections. Nurses should be continuously alert for symptoms of respiratory distress and increased venous pressure. Shortness of breath, increased respirations, coughing, increased blood pressure, a bounding pulse, and distended veins can be symptoms of circulatory overload. If infusions continue, pulmonary edema can result. Thrombophlebitis is a common complication in which the vein becomes inflamed and a clot forms. Redness and edema occurs at the injection site, and the patient will complain of pain along the vein. When this occurs, the intravenous infusion should be discontinued and warm, moist compresses applied to reduce pain and stimulate healing. Air embolism occurs occasionally when substantial amounts of air enter the blood through an improperly running infusion. The apparatus should be checked frequently and the infusion should be stopped or solution changed before the bottle and tubing are empty. This will prevent air from entering the vein. Sudden vascular collapse can occur from air embolism, with symptoms of shock and loss of consciousness. Other abnormal reactions are nausea, vomiting, increased pulse rate, and chills. If these occur, the infusion is stopped and the physician called. Other signs and symptoms may occur that are related to the patient's surgery.

Coughing and deep breathing. The purpose of having the patient breathe deeply and cough is to remove mucus and other secretions that accumulated in the respiratory passages during anesthesia and to facilitate expansion of the lungs. When the patient has been taught breathing and coughing exercises preoperatively and understands their importance, the nurse will find that the procedures are accomplished more readily and thoroughly. Many hospitals use techniques such as blowing up balloons, breathing in and out of paper bags or long tubes with the nose pinched, and blowing into "blow bottles" partially filled with water to provide resistance to the blowing process. All of these techniques stimulate deep breathing, and the patient is then encouraged to cough. Coughing should be deep and should result in expectorating the mass of mucus from the respiratory passages. Better results may be obtained if the patient is placed in a sitting position and the nurse assists him by splinting the incision with a folded towel. If the patient is unable to cough up mucus, and secretions accumulate in the respiratory passages, they should be removed by suctioning. Patients who have surgery of the brain, of the spinal cord, or on the eyes should not be permitted to cough.

Voiding. The physician may have written an order for the patient to be catheterized every 8 hours if he is unable to void, or a longer period may be permitted. The nurse should be aware of the danger of urinary tract infection even under aseptic conditions and should use every means to have the patient void voluntarily. The patient should be encouraged to void at frequent intervals, and in some instances the male patient may be permitted to stand at the bedside with the assistance of the orderly. After some types of surgery the patient may be allowed to use a bedside commode or walk to the bathroom. Adequate hydration of the patient through intravenous fluids or forcing fluids by mouth when permitted will facilitate voiding. Running water while the patient is attempting to void, placing the patient's hands in warm water, or pouring warm water over the genital area may help. The patient should be catheterized only when the bladder is distended and palpable above the pubis and he complains of distress. Records should be maintained of all urine voided. (See Chapter 15.)

Bowel function. After surgery of the gastrointestinal tract, peristalsis is temporarily absent and usually does not return for approximately 48 hours. The patient's expulsion of flatus or spontaneous movement of the bowels indicates that normal peristalsis has returned. Bowel sounds may be heard through the abdomen with a stethoscope, and the nurse should question the patient concerning the passing of gas. Cathartics are not usually administered to surgical patients, and they are not encouraged to have bowel evacuation for several days after surgery. Elderly patients who are accustomed to having a daily bowel movement often become worried and do not understand the seeming lack of concern on the part of the nurse.

Exercises. Unless contraindicated, exercises should be started as soon after surgery as possible or by the end of the first postoperative day. This is especially important if early ambulation is to be delayed. Exercises stimulate circulation, prevent venous stasis, prevent contractures and loss of function, and facilitate recovery. Parts to be exercised include the fingers, hands, arms, and feet and may include abdominal and gluteal muscles. At first the exercises should be passive, but after a day of two the patient should participate actively with little assistance from the nurse. Pillows should not be placed under the patient's knees, and the knee gatch of the bed should not be elevated. The practice of letting the patient sit on the side of the bed and dangle his legs is discouraged. All these procedures cause pressure on veins and contribute to clot formation.[10]

Diet. Most surgical patients are not given food until peristalsis returns, since it may result in nausea, vomiting, and the formation of gas. They may be allowed sips of cool water (ice cubes moisten the mucous membrane and may help to prevent nausea), and they are usually given intravenous fluids. Patients having surgery other than on the gastrointestinal tract may be allowed a soft or regular diet soon after surgery. However, most patients do not feel like eating and may need encouragement. Liquids such as fruit juices, tea, and water are generally desired by the patient and are better tolerated than are solids.

Tubes. When the patient has a retention catheter in the urinary bladder or a gastric tube such as a Levin tube, the nurse must check it frequently to be sure it is draining properly. If periodic irrigations with physiologic saline solution have been ordered by the physician, the procedure should be carried out regularly, as described in a textbook on basic nursing. All drainage from the tube is measured and recorded on the patient's chart.

Dressings. Dressings should be observed at intervals for bleeding or drainage. The nurse should not change a dressing unless it has been ordered by the physician. If drainage soaks through the dressing, it may be reinforced with additional dressings until an order has been secured for changing. All dressing of wounds must be carried out under strict surgical asepsis. Most hospitals have routine procedures for dressing wounds that have been approved by the surgical staff. These procedures, including types of dressings and equipment used, will vary among hospitals and surgeons. Some hospitals have dressing rooms in which a nurse changes all dressings. Some types of dressings such as those used for severe burns or plastic surgery may be changed by the surgeon, and the patient may be given a light anesthetic for the procedure. When frequent changing of dressings is necessary as a result of draining wounds, Montgomery straps may be employed to avoid the repeated use of adhesive tape on the skin. Abdominal binders are usually worn to support the incision while the patient is up. On clean incised wounds the dressing is usually not changed until the sutures are removed, and by the time the patient leaves the hospital no dressing is required.

Ambulation. Most surgical patients are allowed out of bed on the first or second postoperative day. Patients who have had anesthesia should be subjected only to slow, gradual changes in posture in the process of getting out of bed; if at any time faintness or nausea is experienced, they should return to the last previous comfortable position and remain for a few minutes before trying to rise again. Early ambulation facilitates the normal functioning of all body organs and systems, thereby reducing the danger of postoperative complications. The type of surgery and the condition of the patient will determine when ambulation may be started and the extent of walking permitted. Ambulation means walking, not sitting in a chair; however, it should be a gradual process and should not tire the patient. Some elderly persons may need to be elevated to a sitting position in bed before they are allowed out of bed. When allowed out of bed, they should be assisted by the nurse, and only a few steps may be sufficient at first. Ambulation permits the patient to be independent and self-sufficient and to carry out most self-care activities. It decreases feelings of helplessness, shortens the hospital stay, and enables the patient to regain strength more readily.

POSTOPERATIVE COMPLAINTS

Pain. Pain is a subjective symptom indicating physical or emotional distress, which varies widely among individuals and races. Regardless of the circumstances, the nurse should remember that pain is always real to the person experiencing it and that efforts should be made toward its relief.

Pain is usually associated with anxiety. The patient may verbally complain of discomfort, or the pain may be manifested in other ways. Facial expressions are an excellent indication of pain, for example, clenched teeth, wrinkled forehead, widely open or tightly shut eyes, and grimacing. Often a patient will groan, whine, cry, gasp, or cry out. Body movements can also indicate the presence of pain, for example, muscle tension, immobilization of a part or of the whole body, kicking, tossing and turning, and rubbing. Observation of these symptoms can help the nurse and physician to assess the level of pain and provide adequate relief. Often patients are unaware that they may have a pain medication or are reluctant to ask.[7]

The patient's first complaints of pain occur early in the postoperative period and are usually the result of the traumatic effects of the surgery. When a patient complains of pain, the nurse should note the location of the pain, ask whether it is constant or intermittent, and ask whether it is a sharp, dull, or burning sensation. This information should be recorded on the patient's chart and communicated to the charge nurse and physician. The early administration of a pain-relieving drug such as morphine, meperidine hydrochloride (Demerol), or anileridine (Leritine) will often provide relief for several hours and permit restful, quiet sleep. Pain resulting from the surgical procedure should diminish after the first 24 hours; however, pain may be experienced from other causes such as abdominal distention, urinary retention, and casts that are too tight, consequently pressing on a nerve. Headache sometimes results from spinal anesthesia, and patients having abdominal surgery will experience pain when coughing deeply. The apprehensive and nervous patient may complain of more pain than the calm, passive individual. Elderly patients tolerate more pain than do younger persons, and obese persons often need larger amounts of drugs to relieve pain. Whatever the cause of pain, the nurse should make every effort to relieve it and to make the patient comfortable. Changing the patient's position, washing the face and hands, rubbing the back with alcohol, applying a cold cloth to the forehead, or just sitting with the patient will provide relief and decrease the need for drugs. Before giving a narcotic for pain, the nurse should remember that drugs are not substitutes for good nursing care. Drugs such as morphine depress respiration and should not be given when the respiration is compromised; also, narcotics should not be given when the blood pressure is below what has been established at normal for the patient or if the blood pressure is unstable, since it may contribute to shock. Narcotics should not be given just before getting the patient out of bed. It should also be remembered that continued use of narcotics may lead to addiction. When the patient complains of pain and is being given a narcotic, the nurse should be sure that the patient has been made comfortable before administering the drug, then the patient should be told that the medication is for pain. Nursing care can then be given when the patient is receiving the most benefit from the medication. The psychologic effect of knowing that something is being done relieves anxiety and tension and contributes to relaxation and the effectiveness of the drug. The nurse should remember that when a narcotic has been given to an elderly person, he must be closely observed.[10]

Nausea and vomiting. Postoperative nausea and vomiting may be the result of any one of several causes, including the anesthetic, sensitivity to drugs, surgical manipulation, or serious postoperative complications. Patients who have experienced considerable preoperative vomiting and who fear vomiting postoperatively may be more inclined to do so. Often a gastric tube attached to suction siphonage is left in place for 24 to 48 hours to keep the stomach empty and to reduce the incidence of nausea and vomiting. Nausea and vomiting resulting from anesthesia should not last longer than 8 hours. When vomiting appears to be the result of drugs, the physician will usually change the medication order. Most postoperative vomiting is mild and self-limiting, requiring little treatment; however, several drugs belonging to the group known as phenothiazines may have an antiemetic effect for some patients and are often ordered by the physician. Some of these include thiethylperazine (Torecan), promazine hydrochloride (Sparine), promethazine hydrochloride (Phenergan), and perphenazine (Trilafon). If the patient is premitted to have fluids by mouth, sips of hot tea with lemon, ginger ale, or cola drinks may be given to relieve nausea. Persistent vomiting may be serious because it results in loss of body fluids and electrolytes.

Retention of urine. An overdistended bladder may cause the patient considerable discomfort and actual pain. Patients having surgery of the rectum, pelvis, or lower abdomen commonly have difficulty voiding. When the nurse has exhausted all measures designed to help the patient void, he should be catheterized under strict surgical asepsis. Because continued inability to void will result in loss of bladder tone, the physician may order a retention catheter inserted until the patient's condition improves. (See Chapter 15.)

Abdominal distention. Abdominal distention occurs as the result of an accumulation of gas in the stomach and intestines; it occurs to some extent in most surgical patients, giving rise to what is referred to as "gas pains." Because of the temporary loss of peristalsis, gas is not moved through the intestinal tract, accumulating in the greatest amount in the large intestine. The cause for the accumulation of gas in the intestinal tract is not clearly understood; however, the nurse should know that it has no relationship to gas anesthesia. Severe abdominal distention may interfere with respiratory function, making the patient uncomfortable. Measures to provide relief include the use of a well-lubricated rectal tube, which should be inserted just past the internal sphincter. The tube should not be left in longer than 30 minutes, but it may be used every 3 to 4 hours if it provides relief. The free end of the tube should be placed in an emesis basin or wrapped in a disposable diaper. The surgeon may order a Levin tube inserted into the stomach and attached to suction to prevent the stomach from becoming dilated with gas and to prevent paralysis of the intestines (paralytic ileus), which may be serious. A small low enema or one of the carminative enemas such as milk and molasses may be ordered. Drugs that stimulate peristalsis, for example, vasopressin (Pitressin) and neostigmine bromide (Prostigmin), are sometimes ordered. Early ambulation and the return to a regular diet generally prevent or reduce the amount of distention.

POSTOPERATIVE COMPLICATIONS

The incidence of postoperative complications has been reduced through more careful preoperative preparation for surgery, improved surgical procedures, and improved postoperative care. However, several postoperative complications continue to occur and probably always will to some extent. The most serious complications are hemorrhage, surgical shock, respiratory conditions, thrombosis and embolism, wound infection, and dehiscence and evisceration.

Hemorrhage. Blood loss may occur during the surgical procedure in the operating room or after the surgery has been completed and the patient has been returned to his room. The surgeon will evaluate the amount of blood loss during surgery, and if the loss has been great enough, will order the patient transfused with whole blood. Secondary hemorrhage may result from an untied blood vessel or the slipping of a ligature. It may involve a capillary, vein, or artery and may be external or internal (into a body cavity or organ). All hemorrhage creates an emergency situation requiring that immediate steps be taken to control bleeding and restore blood volume.

The nurse should be conscientious about inspecting the dressing for evidence of bleeding from the wound. A small amount of oozing may be controlled by placing a sterile dressing over the site and applying a pressure bandage. If an extremity is involved, the part may be elevated. When bleeding is internal, the patient will be returned to the operating room so that the wound can be opened. The nurse should be alert to the symptoms that may indicate internal bleeding. Early detection is important to prevent damage to cells, vital organs, or even death.

The patient may be restless and appear apprehensive. The skin is pale, moist, and cool, and the pulse becomes rapid and weak; the respiratory rate increases, and the temperature becomes subnormal. The patient will complain of thirst, the respiration will become gasping in character as bleeding continues, and the blood pressure will fall. In addition to blood on dressings, external evidence of hemorrhage may be observed such as blood in vomitus, in urine, or from the lungs (hemoptysis). Patients receiving anticoagulant drugs should always be watched for bleeding into the skin or from a body orifice. The nurse should remain calm and reassure the patient while carrying out emergency measures until the surgeon arrives. The head should be kept low, the patient should be kept quiet, through sedation if necessary, and oxygen should be administered.

Surgical shock. Causes of surgical shock include trauma to the tissues, hemorrhage, and anesthesia. A number of physiologic changes occur that give rise to a characteristic set of symptoms. An alert nurse may be able to recognize the early symptoms, which include an increased pulse and respiratory rate, skin that appears pale and become moist from perspiration, and decreasing urinary output (oliguria). Although the blood pressure may be normal at this time, it will begin to fall, indicating a decreased blood volume. Unless treatment is started immediately, complete circulatory collapse may occur. Oxygen should be given by nasal catheter or mask to supply as much as possible for absorption in the lungs. If shock results from blood loss, the blood volume must be restored with whole blood, plasma, or dextran. If blood is not immediately available, 5% glucose in dis-

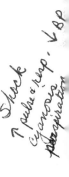

tilled water or physiologic saline solution may be given intravenously. The trunk is kept flat, but the legs may be elevated. The Trendelenburg position should be avoided, since it may further depress the respiration. Extremes of heat and cold should be avoided. The blood pressure, pulse, and respiration should be checked at frequent intervals and recorded. In certain types of shock the physician may order drugs that dilate or constrict the blood vessels, depending on the results desired. The nurse should reassure the patient and should not leave him alone until the vital signs have become stable.

Respiratory conditions. Many respiratory complications can be prevented through careful postoperative care. Those patients who have respiratory disease preoperatively are most likely to develop complications after surgery. The nurse should observe the patient preoperatively for coryza, coughing, or sneezing and report such symptoms to the physician. The most frequent complications are bronchopneumonia, hypostatic pneumonia, bronchitis, pleurisy, and atelectasis. (See Chapter 11.) Maintaining a clear airway, instructing the patient to breathe deeply and cough, regular turning, placing the patient in Fowler's position, and encouraging early ambulation are nursing procedures designed to prevent respiratory complications.

Thrombosis and embolism. Several factors contribute to the formation of a thrombus (blood clot) in the vein. The complication is most common in middle-aged persons who are required to be on a schedule of bed rest. Other predisposing factors include tight abdominal binders, injury or pressure to veins occurring in the operating room at the time of surgery, decreased respiration and blood pressure, or any condition that results in the decreased flow of blood through the veins. The nurse is an important person in both the prevention and detection of thrombosis or pulmonary embolism (fragment of a clot lodged in the lung). Postoperative exercises, early ambulation, and frequent change of position are nursing functions that aid in preventing complications. (See Chapter 13 for more information.)

Wound infection. Problems related to wound infection caused by the staphylococcus organism and the dressing of wounds were reviewed in Chapter 4. Clean incised wounds should heal without infection if they are uncontaminated.

Dehiscence and evisceration. Dehiscence and evisceration may result from infection, abdominal distention, coughing, and poor nutrition. They are caused by the sloughing out of sutures before healing takes place. In dehiscense some or all of the sutures may give way, causing the edges of the skin to separate. When evisceration occurs, the incision suddenly opens up and the intestines are released to the outside. The patient may state that he felt as if something gave way, and inspection of the dressing reveals a clear pink drainage. The wound should be covered with a sterile dressing or a sterile towel and held loosely in place with a binder. The surgeon should be notified immediately. The nurse should remain calm and reassure the patient. The patient should be placed in a low Fowler's position, and food or fluids should be withheld until he is seen by the physician. If the patient is to be taken to the operating room for closure of the wound, he should be moved in his own bed.[9]

Summary outline

1. Surgery
   A. Planned alteration of physiologic processes within the body in an attempt to arrest or eliminate disease
   B. Frightening experience
   C. Means invasion of privacy
   D. Need for faith in physician and others in time of dependency
2. Role of nurse
   A. Technical and observational skills needed
   B. Maintain communications between patient and physician, nurse and family
   C. Understand fear and anxiety and means of expression
3. Admission of patient
   Patient may be admitted by prearranged plan or in emergency situation
   A. Physical examination
      1. Complete history, clinical examination, and laboratory tests and examinations
      2. Evaluation of nutritional status and need for blood transfusion, electrolytes, or vitamins
4. Preoperative orders
   Vary among hospitals and physicians
   A. Diet
      1. Light diet allowed evening before surgery

2. No water or fluids allowed after midnight
3. Light breakfast and water up to 8 hours before surgery allowed when surgery scheduled for late in day

B. Enema—warm soapsuds, saline, or tap water enema usually given on evening before surgery
1. Reasons for giving enema
   a. To remove feces from intestine prior to surgery
   b. To relieve postoperative pain caused by straining to evacuate bowel
   c. To avoid impaction postoperatively
   d. To avoid exertion or tendency to strain after some kinds of surgery such as eye surgery
   e. For psychologic effect if patient fears having stool during anesthesia

C. Skin preparation
Purpose—to cleanse skin and render it as free from bacteria as possible
1. Hair removed with sharp razor, avoiding injury to skin
2. Use of antiseptics to cleanse skin
3. Depilatory creams—effective in removing hair
   a. Avoids risk of cuts, nicks, and abrasions
   b. More comfortable for patient
   c. Patient may be sensitive to preparation
4. Responsibility of nurse to secure instructions before beginning procedure

D. Psychologic preparation
1. Should begin as soon as patient is told of need for surgery
2. Fear of the unknown; patient should be given information according to ability to comprehend
3. Fear of disability or death
   a. Encourage patient to talk about fears
   b. Dispel misconceptions
   c. Encourage faith in physician and modern surgery
4. Include family in discussions and explanations

E. Patient taught exercises to be performed postoperatively, such as those for deep breathing and coughing

F. Hypnotic for sleep and rest usually ordered, to be administered at bedtime

G. Measurement and recording of all urine voided during night

5. Operative day
Patient kept as quiet as possible
A. Procedures to be completed before patient goes to surgery
1. Allow time for personal hygiene
2. Check and record all vital signs
3. Remove pins and combs from hair; braid long hair and cover with cotton cap or towel
4. Remove dentures and removable bridges
5. List valuables and lock in approved place
6. Place hospital gown and leggins on patient
7. Insert retention catheter or Levin tube if ordered
8. Wrap legs with elastic bandage if ordered
9. Administer preoperative medication as ordered
   a. Purpose of preoperative medication
      (1) To relax, relieve apprehension, and decrease metabolic rate
      (2) To reduce secretions in respiratory tract, minimize spasm of larynx, and help maintain clear airway
      (3) To relieve apprehension, produce sedative effect, and help prevent vomiting during anesthesia and immediate postoperative period
10. Place identification on patient's wrist
11. Instruct patient to remain in bed and to rest
12. Have patient void; measure and record amount
13. Check chart for signed operative permit and laboratory reports of all tests; add new physician's order sheet

B. Patient may be transported to operating room in own bed or by stretcher
1. Protect patient from drafts with cotton blankets
2. Remain with patient until relieved by operating room nurse

6. Anesthesia
Special anesthesia room available in some hospitals
A. Anesthesiologist—physician who specializes in selection and administration of anesthesia and assumes responsibility for extrasurgical care of patient in operating and recovery rooms
B. Nurse anesthetist—professional nurse with postgraduate training in administration of anesthetics; functions under responsibility of operating surgeon
C. Operating room technician—may be a person with training in operating room nursing
D. Kind of anesthesia administered to patient may affect postoperative care

7. Types of anesthesia
General anesthetics used when all body sensations are to be suspended; conductive anesthetics used when only part of body involved (local or regional)
A. Inhalation anesthesia—liquids or gases used such as ether, chloroform, halothane (Fluothane), nitrous oxide, or cyclopropane
1. Ether—irritating to respiratory tract,

may produce nausea and vomiting, patient slow in regaining consciousness; has wide margin of safety but is explosive

2. Halothane—induction fairly rapid, patient regains consciousness quickly, produces little nausea or vomiting, is not explosive; patient should be watched for irregularities in heartbeat
3. Cyclopropane—rapid induction, rapid recovery, little nausea and vomiting, explosive, no analgesic effect; patient will complain of pain early, will be restless and apprehensive; watch for respiratory difficulty

B. Intravenous drugs—consist of barbiturates; administered with inhalant drugs
1. Thiopental (Pentothal) sodium and thiamylal (Surital) sodium produce unconsciousness rapidly
2. Large amounts make patient slow to regain consciousness
3. Watch for spasm of larynx
4. Check vital signs carefully

C. Muscle relaxants—increase relaxation of abdominal muscles during surgery
1. Patient should be watched for respiratory difficulty

D. Rectal anesthesia—tribromoethanol (Avertin) solution or rectal ether injected into rectum; patient falls into deep sleep
1. Difficult to control absorption
2. Often used for children with dosage based on body weight
3. Watch patient for hypotension and respiratory difficulty

E. Spinal anesthesia—solution of local anesthetic injected into subarachnoid space; patient remains awake
1. Keep patient flat in bed
2. Watch vital signs because hypotension may occur
3. Severe headache may last for several days
4. Trendelenburg position contraindicated unless ordered by physician

F. Analgesic blocks—inhibit nerve impulses to various parts of body; many drugs available for local anesthesia, all capable of producing toxic symptoms
1. Check vital signs carefully
2. Watch for itching of skin, twitching, or convulsions, cyanosis, nausea, and vomiting
3. Patient is conscious but may be drowsy if sedative has been given

G. Tranquilizers—may be used as preanesthetic sedative to relieve tension and anxiety; some have antiemetic effect
1. May produce hypotension and drowsiness
2. May result in oversedation if given with narcotic

H. Induced hypothermia—lowering body temperature to between 82° and 86° F.

1. Specially trained nurses required
2. Care is continuous

8. Recovery room care
Patient must be moved as carefully as possible to avoid serious changes in vital signs; patient recovering from anesthesia must be watched constantly and never left alone

A. Immediate responsibility of nurse to provide and maintain clear airway
1. Place patient in Sims' position with head flat
2. Suction secretions from respiratory passages
3. Plastic, rubber, or metal airway may be left in mouth
4. Check respiratory rate frequently; movement of air in and out of lungs felt by holding hand near patient's mouth

B. Circulation
1. Blood pressure and pulse taken every 15 minutes for 2 hours, then every 30 minutes for 2 hours
2. Critical systolic pressure determined for individual patient
3. Drop in blood pressure, weak rapid pulse, and cool moist skin may indicate hemorrhage

C. Check dressings every 15 minutes for evidence of bleeding

D. Connect all tubes to proper drainage or suction

E. Check and carry out all physician's orders

F. Relief of pain—evaluate factors regarding preoperative sedation, anesthetic, age, vital signs, and emotional state before giving narcotic

G. Encourage patient to void

H. Accompany patient to room; patient considered conscious when responds to name and is oriented to time and place

9. Intensive care unit (ICU)
A. Increase in number of units and in number and kind of patients
B. Trend in some large hospitals toward individual units for special kinds of patients
C. ICU personnel may include head nurse and other persons
D. Increasing importance of inhalation therapist as member of ICU team
E. Good judgment and quick accurate decisions necessary in crisis situations
F. When condition permits, patient transferred to clinical unit

10. Continuing postoperative care
Care directed toward preventing complications, rehabilitation, and return to normal living

A. Comfort measures
1. Place pillow under patient's head and raise head of bed slightly
2. Give oral care; wash face, hands, and and back; rub back with alcohol
3. Place in Sims' position with pillow at back for support
4. Moisten lips with cool water

5. Provide well-ventilated, quiet environment
6. Remove blanket when patient's skin is warm and dry to prevent overheating
B. Patient should be turned every 2 hours from side to side to prevent respiratory complications and thrombus formation
C. Intravenous therapy
   1. Losses of fluids and electrolytes occur from bleeding, drainage, excessive perspiration, rapid breathing, and vomiting
   2. Fluids introduced by needles or catheters
   3. Solutions
      a. Hydrating solutions administered for dehydration and to stimulate kidney function
      b. Balanced solutions used for intravenous maintenance over period of time
      c. Replacement solutions used primarily to replenish losses from gastrointestinal tract
   4. Nurse's responsibility
      a. Observe patient
      b. Regulate flow
      c. Check for infiltration
   5. Complications
      a. Circulatory overload
      b. Thrombophlebitis
      c. Air embolism
      d. Systemic symptoms
D. Deep breathing and coughing encouraged to remove mucus accumulated in respiratory passages during anesthesia
   1. Place patient in sitting position when possible; assist patient by splinting incision with folded towel
   2. Patients with brain, spinal cord, and eye surgery should not cough
E. Use all means to assist patient to void voluntarily
   1. Adequate hydration and forcing fluids facilitate voiding
   2. Catheterize only when bladder distended and palpable above pubis and patient complains of distress
F. Bowel evacuation—temporary absence of peristalsis exists for approximately 48 hours after surgery
   1. Expulsion of flatus or spontaneous bowel evacuation indicates return of peristalsis
   2. Cathartics not usually given to surgical patients
G. Exercises—to stimulate circulation, prevent contractures and loss of function, prevent venous stasis, and facilitate recovery
   1. Begin by end of first postoperative day
   2. Pillows should not be placed under knees, knee gatch should not be raised, and patient should not dangle legs while sitting on side of bed to prevent pressure on veins
H. Diet—food usually not given until peristalsis returns

1. Give sips of cool water or ice cubes in mouth
2. Liquids such as fruit juices, tea, and water tolerated better than solids
3. Encourage patient to eat
I. Tubes and catheters—retention urinary catheters with continuous drainage and Levin tube must be checked frequently for proper drainage
   1. Irrigate tubes according to physican's order
   2. Measure and record all drainage
J. Dressings—observe for bleeding and drainage
   1. May be reinforced if necessary
   2. Change only on physician's order
   3. Observe strict aseptic technique when changing dressing
   4. Montgomery straps for frequently changed dressings; avoid adhesive tape on skin
   5. Abdominal binder applied when patient up
K. Ambulation—means walking, not sitting; may be permitted on first or second day; should be gradual
   1. Some patients elevated in bed
   2. Slow, gradual change in posture necessary for patients who have had anesthesia
   3. Observe patient for dizziness, faintness, or hypotension
   4. Ambulation permits patient to be independent and self-sufficient
11. Postoperative complaints
A. Pain—varies among individuals and races
   1. Pain usually associated with anxiety
   2. Manifested by verbal complaints, facial expressions, body movements
   3. Pain in first 24 hours due to traumatic effects of surgery; should diminish
   4. Note location and nature of pain
   5. Other causes—abdominal distention, retention of urine, pressure on nerves from tight casts, headache from spinal anesthesia or from nervousness and apprehension
   6. Comfort measures may relieve pain
   7. Whatever the cause, pain should always be relieved
   8. Precautions when administering narcotics
      a. Morphine depresses respiration and should not be given when respiration is compromised
      b. When blood pressure is unstable, narcotic may contribute to shock
      c. Narcotics should not be given before getting patient out of bed
      d. Continued use of narcotics may lead to addiction
      e. Observe elderly person closely after administering narcotic
   9. When person knows pain is being relieved, anxiety and tension are reduced,

and relaxation and effectiveness of drug are increased

B. Nausea and vomiting—may be result of several causes
1. Nausea from anesthesia usually subsides within 8 hours
2. Gastric tube attached to suction may be left in place several days; reduces nausea and vomiting by keeping stomach empty
3. Antiemetic drugs belonging to phenothiazine group may be administered
4. Persistent vomiting may indicate serious complication

C. Retention of urine—may cause considerable discomfort and pain
1. Continued inability to void may result in loss of bladder tone

D. Abdominal distention—result of accumulation of gas in stomach and intestines; may cause "gas pains"
1. Severe distention may interfere with respiratory function
2. May be relieved by insertion of well-lubricated rectal tube
3. Small saline or carminative enema may be ordered by physician
4. Drugs to stimulate peristalsis may be given
5. Early ambulation and regular diet prevent and reduce abdominal distention

12. Postoperative complications
Reduced through careful preoperative preparation, improved surgical procedures, and improved postoperative care
A. Hemorrhage
1. May result from surgical procedure
2. May result from untied blood vessel or slipping of ligature
3. May be external or internal; may involve capillary, vein, or artery
4. Dressings should be inspected frequently for evidence of bleeding
5. Pressure bandage or elevation of extremity may help control bleeding
6. Symptoms of internal hemorrhage
   a. Restlessness and apprehension
   b. Pale, moist, cool skin
   c. Weak, rapid, thready pulse
   d. Increased respiratory rate; gasping
   e. Subnormal temperature
   f. Thirst
   g. Falling blood pressure
7. Emergency treatment—notify physician
   a. Administer oxygen
   b. Keep head low
   c. Keep patient quiet
8. External symptoms of hemorrhage
   a. Blood on dressings
   b. Blood in vomitus
   c. Blood from lungs (hemoptysis)
   d. Bleeding into skin or body orifices, resulting from anticoagulant drugs

B. Surgical shock—caused by injury to tissues, anesthesia, or hemorrhage
1. Symptoms similar to those of hemorrhage
   a. Increased pulse and respiratory rates
   b. Pale, moist skin
   c. Falling blood pressure
   d. Oliguria
2. Treatment and care
   a. Administer oxygen by nasal catheter or mask
   b. Replace volume of circulating fluid
   c. Keep patient flat; elevate legs
   d. Check blood pressure and pulse at frequent intervals
   e. Physican may order drugs when indicated
   f. Stay with patient until vital signs are stable

C. Respiratory conditions—nurse should be alert to and report any signs of respiratory difficulty preoperatively
1. Preventive measures include maintaining clear airway, encouraging deep breathing and coughing, turning patient at frequent intervals, and early ambulation

D. Thombosis and embolism—occur most frequently in middle-aged persons
1. Contributing factors
   a. Prolonged bed rest
   b. Tight abdominal binders
   c. Injury or pressure on veins
   d. Decreased respiration and blood pressure
   e. Any condition resulting in slowing or decreasing flow of blood through veins
2. Preventive measures
   a. Postoperative exercises, frequent change of position, early ambulation

E. Wound infection—see Chapter 4

F. Dehiscence and evisceration
1. May result from infection, abdominal distention, coughing, and poor nutrition
2. Dehiscence when edges of skin separate
3. Evisceration when sutures give way, releasing intestines to outside
4. Cover wound with sterile dressing or towel and apply binder
5. Notify physican
6. Place patient in low Fowler's position and give no food or drink until physician sees patient
7. Remain calm and reassure patient

Review questions

1. Name two fears that patients may have prior to surgery.
   a. *death*
   b. *fear of the unknown*
2. How are general anesthetics usually administered?
   a. *inhalation*
3. List three observations the nurse should make while the patient is receiving intravenous therapy.
   a. *pulse rate*
   b. *IV flow rate*
   c. *watch site for infiltration (swelling)*

4. List five duties of the nurse in the recovery room.
   a. *maintain a clear airway*
   b. *circulation*
   c. *check dressings & vital signs*
   d. *drainage tubes*
   e. *relief from pain*
5. Why should blankets be removed from the postoperative patient as soon as he is warm?
   a. *to prevent loss of body fluid by perspiration*
6. List three procedures that may cause venous stasis in the postoperative patient.
   a. *failure to turn frequently*
   b. *lack of coughing & deep breathing*
   c. *pillow under knees*
7. Why should the nurse tell the patient when she is administering a narcotic for pain?
   a. *desired results are enhanced.*
8. List four signs that might indicate an internal hemorrhage after surgery.
   a. *restlessness & apprehension*
   b. *pulse ↑ & weak*
   c. *BP ↓*
   d. *skin pale, moist & cool*
9. List three conditions when a narcotic should not be administered to a postoperative patient.
   a. *↓ BP*
   b. *↓ respirations*
   c. *just before getting pt. OB.*
10. What are the three objectives of postoperative nursing care?
    a. *prevention of complications*
    b. *rehabilitation*
    c. *return to normal living*

Films

1. CS-1026 Intensive care in critical illness (29 min., sound, color, 16 mm.), Davis & Geck Film Library, American Cyanamid Co., 1 Casper St., Danbury, Conn. 06810. Outlines scope and development of intensive care and shows specific methods used in assessment and treatment of critically ill patients. There is a $5.00 service charge for 3-day use of film.
2. Intravenous fluid infusion—basic theory and practice (27 min., sound, color, 16 mm., no charge), Abbott Laboratories, Abbott Park, North Chicago, Ill. 60064. Basic information on fluid balance, cellular content and activity, chemical composition, electrolyte activity, decreases and increases of pH and its effect as a buffer system, compensation, and alkalosis and acidosis.
3. Surgical positioning—M-1654X (25 min., sound, color, 16 mm.), Media Resources Branch, National Medical Audiovisual Center (Annex), Station K, Atlanta, Ga. 30324. Shows established position and routine in operating room for every member of team. Demonstrates correct positioning of patient for all types of major surgery.
4. CS-755 Transporting the patient for surgery (18 min., sound, color, 16 mm.), Davis & Geck Film Library, American Cyanamid Co., 1 Casper St., Danbury, Conn. 06810. Stresses basic operating room principles as they apply to the transportation of the patient to and from the operating room. There is a $5.00 service charge for 3-day use of film.

References

1. Beal, John M., and Eckenhoff, James E., editors: Intensive care and recovery room care, Toronto, 1969, The Macmillan Co.
2. Burrell, Lenette O., and Burrell, Zeb L.: Intensive nursing care, ed. 2, St. Louis, 1973, The C. V. Mosby Co.
3. Ginsberg, Frances, Brunner, Lillian S., Cantlin, Vernita L., and Hurwitz, Alfred: A manual of operating room technology, Philadelphia, 1966, J. B. Lippincott Co.
4. Guide to fluid therapy, Morton Grove, Ill., 1971, Baxter Laboratories, Division of Travenol Laboratories, Inc.
5. LeMaitre, George D., and Finnegan, Janet A.: The patient in surgery, a guide for nurses, ed. 2, Philadelphia, 1970, W. B. Saunders Co.
6. Levine, Dale C., and Fiedler, June P.: Fears, facts, and fantasies about preoperative and postoperative care, Nursing Outlook 18:26-28, Feb., 1970.
7. McCaffery, Margo: Nursing management of the patient with pain, Philadelphia, 1972, J. B. Lippincott Co.
8. Mickley, Barbara B.: Psychologic hazards of position changes in the anesthetized patient, American Journal of Nursing 69:2606-2611, Dec., 1969.
9. Shafer, Kathleen N., Sawyer, Janet R., McCluskey, Audrey M., Beck, Edna L., and Phipps, Wilma J.: Medical-surgical nursing, ed. 6, St. Louis, 1975, The C. V. Mosby Co.
10. Smith, Dorothy W., Germain, Carol P. Hanley, and Gips, Claudia D.: Care of the adult patient, ed. 3, Philadelphia, 1971, J. B. Lippincott Co.
11. Zachoche, Donna, and Brown, Lillian E.: Intensive care nursing: specialism, junior doctoring, or just nursing? American Journal of Nursing 69:2370-2374, Nov., 1969.

CHAPTER 10

Rehabilitation in nursing

KEY WORDS

adaptation
ADL
amputee
body image
brace
conical
continuity
contractures
demineralization

exacerbation
gait
hemiplegia
motivation
prognosis
prosthesis
prosthetist
regression
rehabilitation
therapist

The concept of rehabilitation is broad and farreaching and is a fundamental process in providing total patient care. Many definitions and interpretations of this process exist; however, most definitions of rehabilitation have some commonalities. Basically, rehabilitation is a process of assisting individuals after a disabling event has occurred. It is most often associated with serious physical or mental disabilities, although recently the need for rehabilitation has been identified when any major event occurs that alters a person's previous way of life. Some disabling events may be minor and the need for rehabilitation limited. Others may require extensive rehabilitation that involves many facets of a person's life. Depending on the type of disability, the physical, mental, vocational, social, and economic aspects of a person's life may be altered.

Most authorities on rehabilitation believe that one of the most important concepts is that the individual should be restored to the ability of which he is capable.[17] The rehabilitation process must help patients to live the most productive life possible with limited dependence on others. The individual must be motivated to achieve these goals, or rehabilitation will be unsuccessful or incomplete. The following situation exemplifies what rehabilitation means. Thirty years ago Mr. J. would have looked forward to spending the rest of his life in a wheelchair, without legs, dependent on public support and charity. However, restoration of physical function has restored his independence, self-sufficiency, and self-image.

Mr. J., 35 years of age, is married and the father of five children. One day while at work he was driving his pick-up truck along a rain-slicked expressway when without warning a large truck suddenly crossed the highway and crashed into his vehicle. Mr. J. was rushed by ambulance to a hospital, where his condition was considered serious. Both legs were so badly injured that above-knee amputation was necessary. Today Mr. J. has been fitted with artificial legs and is learning how to walk with them. He is being trained for a new kind of work. He is enthusiastic and anxious to progress with ambulation. He is optimistic and ready to proceed with his training and is looking forward to complete independence and being able to care for his famly.

The nurse will care for acutely ill patients, chronically ill patients, geriatric patients, and children and adults with various physical and mental handicaps. Some of these persons will be in the hospital, some in the home, and others in various types of institutions, but all will need help in some form. "In place of the classical emphasis on disease, diagnosis and therapeutic procedure, the rehabilitation model stresses restoration of normal function, prognosis, and adjustment and retraining."[*] To restore a handicapped individual to a useful life the whole person must be considered. The handicapped person is a social being, and as a member of society his social image is that of a whole body. When a person loses a leg or arm or when a body function is altered as in a colostomy, he no longer feels he is a whole person, and his social image and self-concept are changed. He now realizes that he is different and never will be the same again. He begins to wonder how his family, friends, members of his social groups, and neighbors feel about him and if he will be accepted by them. He begins to wonder how the economic security that he had planned for his family will be affected. Gradually, as fear, worry, anxiety, and apprehension increase, he loses his self-confidence, self-esteem, and independence and may become depressed and discouraged.

The nurse must be sensitive to the needs of these patients and must have an attitude of optimism, hopefulness, and inspiration that will motivate the patient to make the most satisfactory adjustment in becoming a useful, self-sufficient member of the society in which he must spend the remainder of his life. Nurses must orient

their thinking concerning the patient and rehabilitation to include any condition that interfers with the individual's previous way of life. The following example shows how rehabilitation may affect the daily life of a handicapped person.

Mr. B., 65 years of age, suffered a severe accident that caused a complete paralysis of the lower extremities and left the upper extremities in a weakened condition. When Mr. B. was able, he was transferred to a rehabilitation center where he spent 4 months learning the activities of daily living (ADL). Mr. B. is now at home, and although confined to a wheelchair, he provides nearly all his personal care. With assistance Mr. B. gets into and out of the car, attends church, and frequently goes to public eating places for meals. The family recently purchased an organ, believing that finger exercises would strengthen Mr. B.'s hands and arms. It was discovered that he possessed an unusual and unique musical ability; in a few weeks he had mastered the organ. What had seemed like a hopeless situation has become one in which Mr. B. has a feeling of personal worth, dignity, and self-esteem.

Although rehabilitation is most often associated with serious physical or mental handicaps, it extends far beyond these areas. Nurses practice rehabilitation when they avoid placing pillows under the knees or raising the knee gatch of the bed of the surgical patient, thus preventing venous stasis, when they teach diabetic patients to administer their own insulin, or when they assist elderly persons in ambulation.

To be free of physical handicap is the wish of every person. The first question frequently asked by a mother after the birth of her baby is, "Is he all right?" The mother, hoping so much for a physically perfect baby, may question the nurse, fearing that something is being kept from her.

Modern medical science has made it possible for persons to live without an anatomically intact body, but so far it has been unable to prevent the thousands of birth defects, the crippling conditions of chronic disease, and the mutilating conditions resulting from highway accidents. The necessity for comprehensive rehabilitation services is greater now than at any other period and is likely to increase during the coming years.

POSITIVE RESULTS OF REHABILITATION

It is not enough to say that there are a given number of stroke patients, cardiac

---

[*]From Wessen, Albert F.: Medical vs rehabilitation roles, Rehabilitation Record 6:5-6, May-June, 1965.

patients, or blind and deaf persons who are in need of rehabilitation. The important question is, "What has been accomplished?" It is not possible to enumerate all the accomplishments; in fact, it is doubtful if they are all known. Following are a few of the results of rehabilitation that have been made known.

In 1969 Howard Rusk[12] reported the following results of rehabilitation at the New York Medical Center:

> Stroke patients—3000 treated and 85% returned to normal life
> Paraplegics—8000 treated and 85% returned to active life after 120 days
> Quadriplegics—75% of those treated returned to active life

The United States Social and Rehabilitation Service reported that a record total of 326,138 disabled persons were vocationally rehabilitated during 1972. Since the program began in 1921, over 3 million handicapped people have been restored to gainful employment and are now leading productive lives as contributing members of society.[2] It has been documented that for every dollar spent in vocational rehabilitation service, $500 are returned in taxes paid by the disabled worker within 5 years.[14]

REHABILITATION TEAM

Any comprehensive program in rehabilitation requires a group of experts in various areas of restorative care, since no single profession can provide all the necessary services for a complete rehabilitation program. This group meets periodically to establish patient goals, evaluate individual programs, and institute program changes. The physician is directly involved with the diagnosis, evaluation, and treatment that the patient requires. The physical therapist performs therapeutic techniques ordered by the physician. Good working relationships must exist between the physical therapist and the patient, and often it is the physical therapist who provides the encouragement and support that motivates the patient's progress. The occupational therapist provides purposeful activity that will help to restore physical function. Often occupational therapy involves the exploration of new vocations for the patient in co-operation with the vocational therapist, who counsels, tests, evaluates, and provides for job retraining and job placement when applicable. The services of a psychiatrist are helpful when patients have difficulty adjusting emotionally to their disability. The psychiatrist diagnoses, evaluates, works with the patient, and guides other team members in planning a therapeutic program. The psychologist also may be involved in counseling the patient and in psychologic and vocational testing. The social worker provides a link between the patient, hospital, home, and community. Special emphasis is placed on adequate income, housing, transportation, recreation, and the interaction between the patient and family members.[14] Often the team will include speech therapists, dietitians, orthopedists, dentists, teachers, and members of other professions, depending on the type of disability. The cleft palate clinics that are operated by many states provide an example of active rehabilitation teams.

Outside of established rehabilitation centers the team usually consists of the physician, the nurse, the patient, and his family. The nurse who has a basic understanding of rehabilitation and whose philosophy includes the whole patient may be a key person in rehabilitation. The nurse will be entrusted with the care and rehabilitation of many patients. When caring for patients in homes or in nursing homes the nurse should seek the guidance of the physician. In many areas the nurse will be able to secure help and guidance from the public helath nurse or the visiting nurse. In some states a visiting public health physical therapist is a member of the health department.

REHABILITATION FACILITIES

The incidence of handicap and disability resulting from two world wars placed emphasis on the establishment of centers for rehabilitative treatment. In 1970 a total of 7000 rehabilitation facilities were in operation, in which thousands of handicapped persons were receiving medical, psychologic, social, and vocational services each year. Centers are operated by state vocational agencies, insurance companies, and other types of community agencies.[9] In 1954 the Vocational Rehabilitation Act was passed by the United States Congress. This law provided funds to state agencies for improvement and expansion of rehabilitation services. The primary objective of the Social and Rehabilitation Service (formerly called the Vocational Rehabilitation Department) is the education and training of persons for employment (Fig. 10-1). Many handicaps can be corrected, rendering the individual employable and economically independent and self-sufficient. A 50-year-old woman who was a widow was employed to care for an elderly patient in the home. She was unable to continue because of severe varicose veins. Through vocational rehabilitation she received medical care and hospitalization for vein stripping, thereby enabling her to continue with employment.

The services under the Social and Rehabilitation Service have been greatly expanded to cover many more types of handicaps. The developmental disabilities program now extends services to persons afflicted by mental retardation, cerebral palsy, epilepsy, and other neurologic disorders. A primary problem has been the shortage of trained persons. In an effort to overcome this problem the Social and Rehabilitation Service has provided grants to universities and certain institutions to train individuals in vocational rehabilitation. Medicare, administered by the Social Security Administration, now includes rehabilitative services for both hospitalized patients and those recuperating elsewhere. The Veterans Administration provides rehabilitation services for veterans.

Some public school systems operate special classes for children with cardiac disease and those in need of sight saving. There are schools for children who are blind and deaf, have cerebral palsy, or are mentally retarded. The National Foundation for Asthmatic Children operates a school in Tucson, Arizona. Through the expanding medium of educational television, many handicapped individuals are being served. Late in 1970 the public became concerned about the problems of chronic alcoholism and drug addiction. Centers, public and private, are being opened in many large cities to treat and rehabilitate these persons.

Federal and state governments are developing programs of research in mental

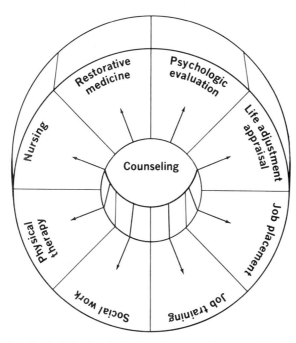

Fig. 10-1. Vocational rehabilitation is designed to provide comprehensive appraisal of the seriously disabled person and to assist him in becoming a self-supporting working citizen.

retardation. It is not only important to learn more about the causes of mental retardation but also to learn how many of the mentally retarded can be rehabilitated to lead normal, productive lives in the community. Physical and mental retardation is not the only area in which rehabilitative services are needed. Society has become aware of other kinds of sickness. Millions of persons are in need of rehabilitative services, such as the economically depressed, the elderly, migrant workers, juvenile offenders, children and young people who are addicted to drugs, and alcoholics. Some rehabilitative efforts are being made in these areas, but much remains to be done.

PHASES OF CARE

Patient care may be divided into several phases, or stages—the preventive phase, the period of acute illness, and recovery and rehabilitation.

Preventive phase. Emphasis should be placed on the *prevention* of disease and accidents. The protection of all susceptible individuals against those diseases for which positive immunizing agents are available is the first step. The crippling conditions of poliomyelitis have nearly been eliminated by administration of polio vaccine. Many of the chronic diseases could be avoided by early medical care, education, and supervision. Early diagnosis and treatment of certain forms of cancer result in cure, preventing the physical and psychologic impact of chronicity and terminal illness. Such preventive measures could enable individuals 65 years of age and older to be free from chronic disease and invalidism, making life a joy. The federal and state governments are initiating programs to prevent highway accidents and control air and water pollution, which have become major concerns in recent years.

Stage of acute illness. It is during acute illness that good nursing care is of the greatest importance. Rehabilitation begins the day the patient enters the hospital, and the nurse who recognizes the physical and psychologic needs of the individual patient and is able to meet them is practicing rehabilitative nursing. During this phase an effort may be made to classify the disability as temporary or permanent, and partial or complete; the cause of the disability will also be determined.[13] The physician makes the diagnosis and determines the course of treatment. Even at the earliest stages of a disability, realistic short-term and long-term goals should be established that reflect the patient's potential for rehabilitation. The nurse must utilize these goals in planning daily care for patients. Good nursing care will include maintenance of proper body alignment, prevention of decubiti, and keeping joints free so that they will not become bound by fibrous connective tissue.

Recovery and rehabilitation. The period of recovery is one of convalescence, which is a gradual process that may extend over a considerable period of time and be punctuated with one or more relapses. As soon as the acute phase of illness has passed, a careful evaluation of the disability should be made, and a program of therapy should be planned for the individual patient. If the nurse's concept of rehabilitation includes all patients, irrespective of disability, the nurse will guide many individuals with nondisabling illnesses in self-help activities and an early return to normal living. There is no time in the course of any illness when rehabilitation begins or ends. It should run concurrently with the illness, whether the illness is acute or chronic, temporary or permanent, disabling or nondisabling. Many more patients are being rehabilitated and returned to useful and productive lives than in the past. Research has contributed to rehabilitation through the development of new and improved prostheses, techniques, and methods. When rehabilitation procedures are begun early, immediate hope is given to the individual, mental depression and discouragement are avoided, and the disabling conditions resulting from prolonged bed rest may be prevented.[4]

It is not possible to restore all patients to productive lives; however, no matter how severe the mental or physical handicap the patient should not be allowed to believe that nothing is being done and that his condition is hopeless. Rusk believes that patients who suffer severe cardiac or brain damage or who have malignant hypertension probably will not benefit from rehabilitation efforts.[12]

Rehabilitation of the aged and chronically ill is likely to be long and tedious.

Often these persons suffer from low morale, lack of motivation, and discouragement. The nurse working with these individuals must understand their self-concepts and their feelings of dependency and isolation. Rehabilitation of the aged will require the services of the entire rehabilitative team and the cooperation of community agencies.

EMOTIONAL RESPONSES TO DISABILITY

Although a person may recuperate from a physical disability without complications, the extent of his rehabilitation depends on his psychologic or emotional acceptance of his condition. An amputee's stump may have healed and a prosthesis been fitted, but the patient is not considered rehabilitated if he has refused to care for the stump, wear the prosthesis, or attempt to become a self-reliant individual. Many factors can influence a person's ability to cope with a disabling event. A person born with a physical abnormality usually has less difficulty accepting his disability, since he has never perceived himself as a whole person and therefore does not have to adjust to a changed body image. If the disability is due to a traumatic accident, a more acute emotional reaction can be expected than that occurring from a slowly progressive disease.[17] The meaning of the loss of function that has occurred will vary with every person. Loss of an arm will usually affect a professional pianist more severely than a school teacher or chemist. Much depends on how the loss affects the patient's everyday life. Personality problems that develop after a disability usually occur as a result of the patient's personality characteristics prior to the injury. A person who can easily be made to feel inadequate prior to his injury will have more emotional stress after the injury.

The initial reaction to a physical injury is shock. The patient experiences disbelief, anxiety, and fear, which are considered part of the mourning process.[17] Loss of anything that is meaningful to the patient will produce a period of grief. During early stages of adjustment, depression and anger may be present. The patient may be unable to look at the change, attempting to deny its existence. Gradually the patient will begin to talk about the change, and often nurses are the first to be questioned

about the disability. The patient may ask to see the part and may seem both fascinated and revolted. Eventually the patient realizes that his life cannot be as it was before, and he will begin to examine the values he placed on conventional "normality." He realizes that the disability need not alter his entire life, and he begins to react more openly with others. Time is essential for this process of acceptance.[1]

Similar reactions occur with patients facing surgery or progressively deteriorating diseases. However, the surgical patient usually has time to begin adapting prior to surgery. Patients with chronic illness have time to adjust to each stage of their illness.

THE PATIENT'S FAMILY

The way the family feels about the patient with a severe handicap depends on how they felt about the patient before he was handicapped, his place in the family, the nature of the handicap, and the socioeconomic status of the family. During the acute phase of the condition the family will suffer from anxiety, apprehension, and fear. The family should be given emotional support, comfort, and all the information possible during this critical period. If the patient is the breadwinner, the spouse may be distressed about how medical and hospital bills will be paid or how to provide for the family. A serious handicap may mean social isolation for the family as well as the patient. To set an individual apart from other individuals means loneliness and depression. As soon as prognosis can be made, long-term goals should be established for the patient. The family should be given information about sources of help in rehabilitation and economic assistance. A social worker may help the family with plans, but often no social worker is available; therefore every nurse should be familiar with community agencies and with the sources of help for a family in trouble.

ROLE OF THE NURSE IN REHABILITATION

The nurse, as a member of the rehabilitation team, must assume a share of responsibility for guiding the patient toward health and independence. Many nurses will be working with the physician without the services of other persons who contribute

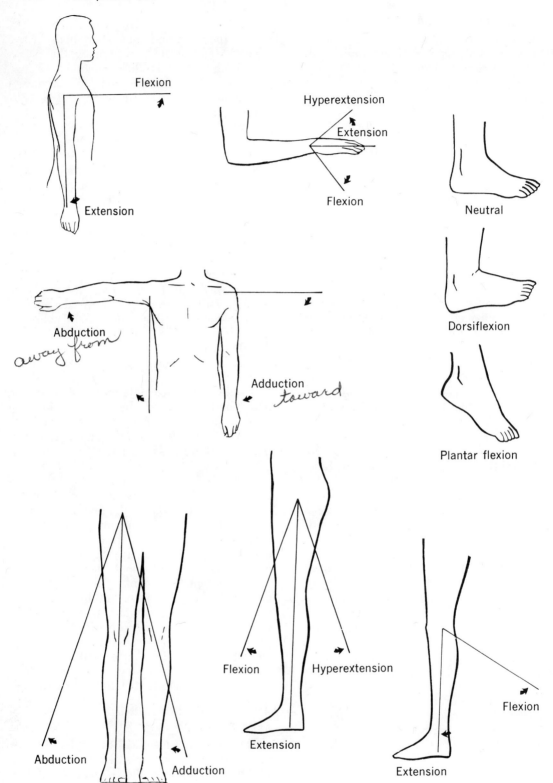

Fig. 10-2. Range of motion. The figures illustrate the methods of exercising joints to prevent contractures and to stimulate circulation.

to a comprehensive rehabilitation program. Therefore it is increasingly important for the nurse to be familiar with the local and state agencies that can provide services to the patient. Each patient must be accepted as an individual, and each will have his own special problems. The nurse should understand that the patient may go through several stages characterized by varying emotional reactions before being able to adapt and adjust to his illness or handicap. The nurse should not attempt to change the patient's life patterns but through listening and understanding him provide support while he moves toward adaptation and a new way of living.[3]

Prevention of deformities. The National Federation of Licensed Practical Nurses, Inc.,* has defined the role of the practical nurse in rehabilitation as one who "assists with rehabilitation of patients, according to the patient care plan, through:

1. Knowledge and application of the principles of prevention of deformities (e.g. the normal range of motion exercises, body mechanics and body alignments).
2. Encouragement of patients to help themselves within their own capabilities.
3. Awareness of and encouraging the fulfillment of the special aptitudes and interests of patients.
4. Utilizing community resources and facilities for continuing patient care."

One of the most important services that the nurse can render is to provide good nursing care. Many individuals are in hospitals, convalescent homes, and nursing homes with crippling conditions that could have been prevented with more adequate nursing care. The nurse is with the patient 24 hours a day and is the person who must be constantly aware of the patient's needs.[10]

In caring for patients, it is especially important for joints to be moved through their normal range of motion several times a day. The primary purpose of these exercises is to preserve the patient's present range of

motion and prevent deformities that might occur from inactivity (Fig. 10-2). Joints that should be exercised include the shoulders, elbows, hands, fingers, hips, knees, and ankles. Unless joints are exercised regularly, they will quickly develop fibrous connective tissue; this is particularly true of the older patient. Contractures, or shortening of muscle tissues, may occur as a result of immobility. Foot drop and hip flexion are the two most common disorders occurring from prolonged bed rest and can be prevented by range-of-motion exercises. For many patients exercise will be passive, in which the nurse exercises the joints without assistance from the patient. Passive exercise does three things for the patient: (1) it helps to keep the joints movable, (2) it promotes venous return and lymphatic flow, and (3) it helps prevent excessive demineralization of the bones. The extent to which the patient is exercised depends on (1) the physician's orders, which will vary with each physician, (2) the physical condition of the patient, (3) the particular illness, and (4) the prognosis for recovery.[6]

Active exercises are ordered by the physician and are often carried out by the physical therapist. These exercises require the patient's participation in attempting to restore motion that has been lost.

In addition to exercises, good body alignment in either a sitting or lying position is important in preventing deformities and skin breakdown. While in a lying or supine position, legs and feet should be kept in line with the torso of the body, and an adjustable footboard that extends above the toes should be used to help prevent foot drop and keep covers off the feet. Heels should be kept free from pressure, with toes pointing toward the ceiling. Hip flexion should be avoided, and rolled towels or trochanter rolls can be placed along the outside of a limb to prevent outward rotation of the hip and limb. Arms should be flexed at the elbow, and hand rolls can be used to maintain a functional position and prevent wrist drop if paralysis is present. In a side-lying position good alignment should be maintained. The patient's top leg may be flexed, brought forward, and supported by pillows, and the arm should be supported in a flexed position. Patients

---

*From Statement of functions and qualifications of the licensed practical nurse, New York, April, 1972, National Federation of Licensed Practical Nurses, Inc.

need to be turned regularly every 1 or 2 hours and should be encouraged to turn themselves even more often if possible. Variations in positioning will depend on the patient's condition and diagnosis. A sagging bed makes it difficult to maintain good body alignment, and a board placed between the springs and mattress will help to provide firmness.

Patients should be out of bed as much as possible, depending on their condition; this is especially true of older patients. Moving from bed to chair provides activity for muscles that otherwise would receive little exercise and also provides for better ventilation of the lungs by helping to prevent the accumulation of fluid at the base of the lung. The longer the handicapped person remains in bed the more his self-confidence declines, and the more he dreads the responsibilities of becoming a self-reliant individual.

Much can be accomplished in bladder and bowel training for the incontinent patient, but before such training is started it should be discussed with the physician and his permission secured. Procedures for bladder training will be found in Chapter 15.

Motivation. Motivation means moving the patient to act for himself. The nurse is with the patient 24 hours a day and thus can help create within him the desire for independence and self-sufficiency. The patient needs constant encouragement and emphasis on his physical capabilities. The nurse must realize that there will be regressions as the patient moves toward independence. When the patient is unsuccessful in his efforts, he may feel "what's the use," and frustration and depression result. It is then that the nurse should stress what has been accomplished, no matter how small, and encourage the patient to believe in his own ability.

The nurse will encounter patients who may have received maximum benefit from rehabilitation, but in whom only partial recovery has been achieved. An understanding approach to these patients is extremely important, since they may be resentful and have periods of depression. A cheerful attitude stressing what the patient can do may help to bridge the feelings of rejection and antagonism.

The nurse must be constantly alert to the emotional problems of the patient and must provide opportunity for him to express his feelings. The nurse should understand that the patient's emotional reaction to the handicap may lead to frustration and psychologic blocks. This is particularly true of the aphasic patient. The nurse should learn to assess the patient's level of comprehension and his ability to participate in rehabilitation.

Teaching. The nurse assumes a major role in teaching the patient self-care activities. The program must be planned for the individual patient and must be realistic in relation to his handicap. The present concept of rehabilitation is doing things with the patient, not for him, and working with him, rather than on him. The patient needs to be reminded that he can do many things for himself, and the nurse should emphasize those things that the patient can do rather than what he cannot do. Some patients will tire easily and will need frequent rest periods. In teaching and helping the patient to learn an activity, he should not be hurried but should be allowed to work at his own pace. In helping the patient to achieve his goal of independence, many problems will develop, and extreme patience will be needed by the nurse and all other persons, including the family, who may be working with him.

The activities of daily living include all the functions that a person uses in everyday life. Normally a person may use the right hand for eating, brushing teeth, and writing. When a person finds that his right arm is paralyzed or if he loses his right hand, new ways of performing these activities must be found. The Institute of Physical Medicine and Rehabilitation, New York Medical Center, has prepared an inventory of activities under four categories: (1) activities that involve self-care, (2) those involved in ambulation and traveling, (3) activities for which use of the hands is required, and (4) special therapy such as speech.[14] Such an inventory can be helpful in assessing the patient's progress. The objective of teaching the patient how to care for himself is to make him an independent person. Learning self-care activities cannot be hurried, and each activity or movement must be practiced over and over. To teach the patient the nurse must avoid helping him. After giving instruction, the nurse must let the patient do the work.[13]

A basic principle of teaching-learning is progressing from the simple to the complex. Simple activities should be taught first and each mastered before a new one is begun. The patient will become discouraged many times and will need constant encouragement; even the slightest progress should be noted. Patients with certain types of handicaps may show greater improvement when they work in groups, since a small element of competition exists. Activities that involve ambulation, balance, standing, and crutch walking may be taught by the physical therapist, but the nurse will be expected to substitute for the physical therapist much of the time.

Because of the patient's disability, much of the day will be unfilled time, and keeping the patient busy is an important factor in rehabilitation. The occupational therapist provides opportunity for patients to learn handicrafts and skills or to renew some that they did know. However, the nurse is likely to be the only person to provide some recreational activity for the handicapped patient. There are books available for example, one by Marion R. Spear,[16] that contain a large number of suggestions for making things with readily available materials.

Continuity. There must be continuity between the care the patient receives in the hospital and the care that he receives in the home, as well as continuity in the care given by all members of the rehabilitation team. The patient must be taught one way of performing an activity and his practice centered on a single method. If the patient is taught different ways, he will become confused, frustrated, and discouraged. The nurse can assist each therapist who is working with the patient by observing and reporting progress or the lack of progress. The nurse will be able to report to the therapist any significant problems that arise in connection with the activities being practiced by the patient. If the patient is to leave the ward for therapy, it is important that the nurse see that the appointment is kept promptly and that the patient is in a presentable condition. As progress is made, the patient may be held responsible for his own preparation and keeping his appointments with little or no help from the nurse.

PROSTHESES

A prosthesis is an artificial substitute for some part of the body. The most common types of prostheses are artificial legs, arms, eyes, and breasts. Prostheses for amputees must be fitted for the individual patient, and they are adapted to the weight and size of the patient. They are made of various types of materials; however, those made of plastic material are light in weight, easy to keep clean, and do not absorb body odors. Prostheses for legs are held in place by pelvic belts, waistbands, or suction cups. Temporary prostheses for above- and below-the-knee amputations can be fitted immediately following surgery. These prostheses are made of casting materials contoured to the amputation stump and provide a rigid dressing that controls bleeding and swelling postoperatively. A temporary peg, or pylon, and foot are attached to the cast, which allows the patient to dangle and stand with aid within a few days after surgery. There are many advantages to this procedure. The patient is more active, muscle activity and circulation are stimulated, and the process of physical rehabilitation begins immediately. An upright position soon after surgery encourages the patient and helps him to adjust to his altered body image.

Research is being done to develop improved prostheses for extremities and improved methods of stump care. Immediate postsurgical filling of the prosthesis after the application of a rigid dressing is an approach being used for the arm amputee.[8] Small prostheses called *rocker pegs* have been used for children who are bilateral amputees. These permit early balance and ambulation.[11] The amputee is confronted not only with a physical problem but also with social, vocational, and psychologic problems and requires the services of the entire rehabilitation team and a skilled prosthetist.

When healing is underway, the stump must be molded to a conical shape to fit into the prosthesis. Compression bandages are generally used for this purpose. However, elastic stump-shrinking socks are also used and often are more desirable, since the art of wrapping the stump is difficult to achieve. Careful washing of the stump is important, and bandages should be removed and rewrapped several times a day. When the prosthesis arrives and the patient begins to wear it, the patient and the family should be instructed in care of the stump and the appliance. Not all patients are suitable candidates for an artificial extremity, and numerous factors with careful evaluation of the individual patient have to be considered.

If the appliance has joints, lint and dirt should be removed regularly (at least once a week) and a small amount of oil applied to the joint. Joints should be inspected for loose or worn screws and replacements made promptly. Shoes should be kept in good repair and should have rubber heels. The leather parts can be washed with warm water and saddle soap and then polished.[15]

Artificial eyes are made of glass or plastic and are painted by a skilled artist to match the patient's other eye. Eyes made of glass are heavier than those made of plastic and are easily broken if dropped, whereas those made of plastic, although lighter, are less durable and may be scratched unless care is taken. The prosthesis may be used as soon as the socket is healed, which may be from 3 to 6 weeks after surgery. When the eye is removed before the patient retires, it should be carefully cleansed with physiologic saline solution and may be kept in it when not in use.[15] The patient will have to be taught how to remove and insert the prosthesis; he may be nervous at first but will soon master the technique and develop skill and confidence. When a patient with an eye prosthesis is admitted to the hospital, the nurse should realize that he has his own method of caring for the eye and should supply whatever equipment he needs and should not try to change his methods.

Patients having a mastectomy should be advised concerning the various types of prostheses that are available, and if possible, the selection should be made before the patient leaves the hospital. Some prostheses are made of sponge rubber, some are filled with fluid, and others are filled with air. Whichever type the patient selects, it should be comfortable and should conform to her size and weight. When the prosthesis is worn, it should be covered with a well-fitting brassiere.[15] (See Chapter 16.)

BRACES

The overall purpose of using braces is to restore the individual to normal living. Specifically, they may be used to support the body weight, to limit involuntary movement of the body, and to prevent and correct deformities. Braces may be of the short leg or long leg type and may have attachments, depending on the purpose for which they are used. Braces usually consist of a steel frame with joints, hinges, and straps; belts are used to secure them in place. Braces are generally attached to the heel of the shoe. An inside lining protects the body from friction.

Proper care of the appliance should be taught the patient and should be emphasized. All locks should be opened weekly and lint and dirt removed. A drop of machine oil should be placed in each joint and any excess wiped away, since any oil left on leather will cause deterioration. The leather parts may be washed with warm water and saddle soap, then dried and polished. The brace should be checked at intervals to be sure it is keeping the part in good position. Shoes should be kept in good repair and should have rubber heels. Knee pads are part of the brace and should be worn with it. The skin should be inspected daily for discoloration, bruises, abrasions, or evidence of friction. Children who wear braces during their growth periods should have them checked at intervals by the physician, and any change indicated should be made promptly. A brace too small for a growing child may do more harm than good.

Braces may be used to support the torso and should be applied with the patient lying down with the body in good alignment. A cotton shirt worn beneath the brace helps to absorb perspiration and body odors and contributes to its comfort.

Preparing the patient for braces is no less important than preparing him for any other artificial aid. The patient needs to be prepared physically through range-of-motion and other exercise and proper position in bed. To be prepared psychologically the patient should understand why the braces are necessary, how they will help him, and how to care for them. Unless the patient is prepared for the aid, he may resent it and develop negative attitudes, in which case its value may be minimized. Young persons may be concerned with the cosmetic effect and must be given the chance to express their feelings.[5]

CRUTCHES

Crutches are devices for individuals who, because of their handicaps, must learn to walk again (Fig. 10-3). They may be used temporarily or permanently, but in either case the nurse has an important function in helping to prepare the patient for crutch walking. As soon as the physician determines that the patient has improved sufficiently, exercises should be started to strengthen the muscle groups involved in the use of crutches. These include the muscles of the arms, shoulders, chest, and back. Various types of exercises may be started while the patient is in bed, using such equipment as a trapeze placed overhead or a rope fastened to a pulley at the foot of the bed. The patient can be taught how to do push-ups by placing his palms flat on the bed, or sawed-off crutches can be used in the bed. During the patient's confinement to bed the legs should be put through the full range of motion several times a day. Before beginning to stand, the patient should be taught and should be able to move himself from the bed to the chair. Standing and balance are important prerequisites to ambulation. Many older people have a poor sense of balance and coordination. They may be fearful and find it difficult to strengthen muscles prior to walking; therefore the nurse will need to have a great deal of patience in working with them.[7] Ideally, parallel bars should be used when helping the patient to stand and balance himself; however, two beds

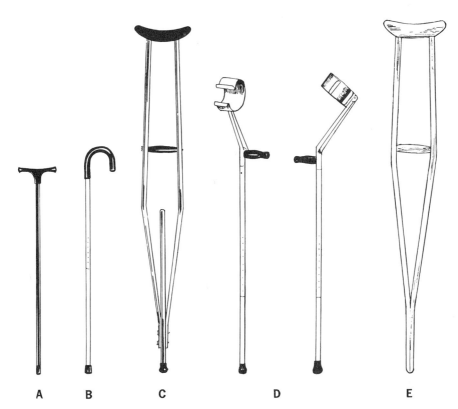

Fig. 10-3. Types of crutches and canes. **A,** Wooden T cane. **B,** Adjustable aluminum cane. **C,** Adjustable aluminum crutch. **D,** Adjustable aluminum Canadian crutch. **E,** Nonadjustable wooden crutch available in various lengths.

placed end to end will achieve the same results. The physical therapist usually assists the patient with standing and balance during his initial attempts to walk with crutches. In many places it will be the responsibility of the physician and the nurse.

Important points to be considered in crutch walking (Fig. 10-4) include the following:

1. The patient should be measured for crutches so that they will be the right size. They should have heavy rubber suction tips. The first crutches should be adjustable.
2. Padding of the axillary bar is generally discouraged, since it encourages the patient to place weight or lean on it. By doing so the patient may devel-

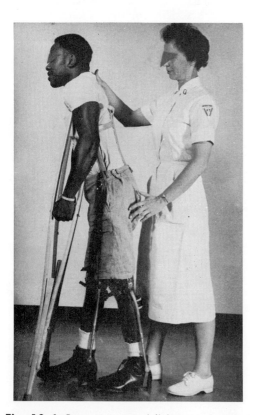

Fig. 10-4. Return to normal living requires that the patient learn how to maintain good body position while wearing braces and using crutches. The physical therapist assumes a major role in teaching and supervising the patient. (Courtesy Medical College of Georgia, Augusta, Ga.)

op a paralysis of the radial nerve (crutch paralysis). Crutches that are too long or too short may also cause crutch paralysis.

3. The patient should be taught from the beginning to maintain good posture. The head should be held high and straight with the pelvis over the feet.
4. Crutch walking must be taught, and several short lessons a day will be of more value to the patient than a long one resulting in fatigue.
5. When ambulation is begun, it is desirable to have an attendant in front of the patient and one behind him; however, they should not touch the patient.
6. Whether the patient is able to bear weight or shift weight will depend on the disability and the physician's order. Some patients, especially elderly patients, may learn to use a walker prior to using crutches.

Gait. There are several types of gait, and the type used will depend on the disability. The most common types of gait include four-point gait, two-point gait, and swing-to or swing-through gait (Fig. 10-5). In four-point gait the patient bears weight on both legs, and there are always three points of contact with the floor. This type of gait requires constant shifting. In two-point gait there are two points of contact with the floor. This method is similar to the four-point gait but faster. In swing-to gait the patient places the crutches ahead of him, then lifts his weight on the crutches and swings his body to the crutches. Swing-through gait is similar except that the patient lifts his weight and swings beyond the crutches. In three-point gait the weight is placed on the crutches and the unaffected leg. It may be used when partial weight bearing is permitted.

A patient who has been taught to use crutches should have mastered sufficient daily care activities to be independent when he leaves the hospital. He should also have been taught how to get up and down steps and into and out of cars.

If the patient is to learn to perform daily care activities successfully, many modifications and adaptations will be needed. A wide variety of devices are available to help the handicapped person. Others may

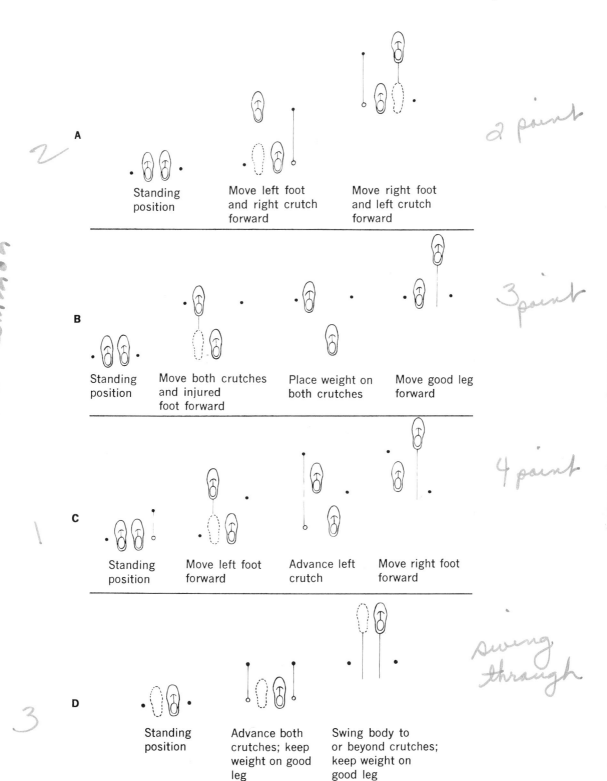

Fig. 10-5. Crutch walking. **A,** Two-point gait. **B,** Three-point gait. **C,** Four-point gait. **D,** Swing-to or swing-through gait.

be developed simply by the skill of an ingenious nurse or a member of the family. Following are some tools and procedures that may be used to assist the patient:

1. Sponge instead of washcloth for bathing
2. Sponge attached to a long handle with a pocket for soap
3. Loose clothing with large armholes
4. Front closing for clothing with grippers rather than buttons
5. Neckties already tied
6. Elastic shoelaces and long-handled shoe horns
7. Suction cups or sponge rubber mats for dishes
8. Runways constructed for wheelchairs
9. Hand rails
10. Wheelchair or ordinary chair with seat cut to fit over toilet
11. Lavatories and electric outlets placed at a height easily reached by the patient
12. Eating utensils such as silverware with padded or curved handles, glass holders, and plate guards
13. Food arranged clockwise on the plate and tray for the blind patient

• • •

Rehabilitation is a tremendous challenge to all nurses. The saving of lives and the increase in the life-span can have little meaning to the crippled and handicapped person unless he can believe that he is a respected member of the society in which he lives. With understanding, patience, sympathy, and perseverance, the nurse can assist the patient in the realization of independent living.

Summary outline

1. Concept of rehabilitation
   A. Broad and far reaching
   B. Many definitions and interpretations exist
   C. Process of assisting persons after disabling event has occurred
   D. Usually associated with serious physical or mental disabilities
   E. Now associated with any event that alters individual's previous way of life
   F. Physical, mental, vocational, social, and economic aspects of person's life may be altered
   G. Individuals should be restored to ability of which they are capable
   H. Individual must be motivated, or rehabilitation will be unsuccessful or incomplete
   I. Nurse must develop sensitivity to patient's needs
   J. Need to recognize patient as member of society whose social image is that of a whole body
2. Positive results of rehabilitation
   A. Stroke—3000 treated, 85% returned to normal living
   B. Paraplegia—8000 treated, 85% returned to normal living
   C. Quadriplegia—75% of those treated returned to active life
   D. Social and Rehabilitation Service reports 326,138 persons vocationally rehabilitated in 1972
3. Rehabilitation team
   A. Includes group of experts in various areas of restorative care
   B. Team members may include physician, physical therapist, occupational therapist, vocational therapist, psychiatrist, psychologist, social worker, speech therapist, dietitian, orthopedist, dentist, teacher, and nurse
   C. Nurse in home or nursing home must seek guidance of physician
4. Rehabilitation facilities
   A. In 1970 there were 7000 facilities providing medical, psychologic, social, and vocational services
   B. Government agencies
      1. Social and Rehabilitation Service—primary function is rendering individual vocationally employable
      2. Medicare provides rehabilitative services for hospitalized and home-bound patients through Social Security Administration
      3. Veterans Administration provides services for veterans
   C. Many public schools maintain classes for children who are blind, deaf, mentally retarded, asthmatic, or who have cerebral palsy
   D. Some schools for children with cardiac conditions or those who need sight conservation
   E. Millions of persons with other kinds of sickness need rehabilitation but are not being cared for at present
      1. Economically depressed
      2. Elderly
      3. Migrant workers
      4. Juvenile offenders
      5. Drug addicts
      6. Alcoholics
5. Phases of care
   May be divided into three periods—preventive phase, stage of acute illness, and period of recovery and rehabilitation
   A. Preventive phase
      1. First step is widespread use of available immunization agents

2. Early medical care, education, and supervision could prevent many diseases from becoming chronic

B. Stage of acute illness—good nursing care of greatest importance during this period
   1. Rehabilitation begins when person enters hospital
   2. Classification of disability
      a. Duration—temporary or permanent
      b. Extent—partial or complete
      c. Cause
   3. Objectives of good nursing care during this period
      a. Maintaining proper body alignment
      b. Preventing decubitus ulcers
      c. Keeping joints free by proper exercise
   4. Rehabilitation should run concurrently will illness; whether acute or chronic, temporary or permanent, disabling or nondisabling

C. Recovery and rehabilitation
   1. Convalescence is gradual process and may extend over long period of time
   2. Any plan of therapy must be for individual patient

D. All patients cannot be restored to productive life
   1. Severe cardiac damage
   2. Severe brain damage
   3. Malignant hypertension

E. Rehabilitation of elderly and chronically ill may be long and tedious
   1. Nurse must understand patient's self-concept and feelings of dependency and isolation

6. Emotional responses to disability
   A. Extent of rehabilitation depends on individual's psychologic acceptance of his condition
   B. Those born with disabilities usually have less difficulty accepting their condition
   C. Traumatic accidents produce more severe emotional reactions
   D. Meaning of loss will vary with every person
   E. Personality problems usually are result of patient's personality characteristics prior to disability
   F. Initial reactions to physical injury are shock, disbelief, anxiety, and fear
   G. Loss of anything that is meaningful to patient will produce period of grief
   H. Depression, anger, and denial may be present
   I. Gradually values are examined and limitation put in perspective
   J. Time is essential for acceptance

7. The patient's family
   A. During acute phase, family needs emotional support and comfort
   B. Should be given all information possible
   C. Should be given information about sources for rehabilitation services and economic assistance
   D. Social worker or nurse should be familiar with community agencies that can help

8. Role of nurse in rehabilitation
   A. May not have services of persons other than physician
   B. Important that nurse be familiar with local and state agencies that may help patient
   C. Nurse should not try to change patient's life patterns but should provide support
   D. Prevention of deformities
      1. Passive exercise
         a. Helps keep joints movable
         b. Promotes venous return and lymphatic flow
         c. Helps prevent excessive demineralization of bones
      2. Extent of exercise depends on
         a. Physician's orders
         b. Physical condition of patient
         c. Specific illness
         d. Prognosis for recovery
      3. Active exercise
         a. Ordered by physician
         b. Require patient's participation
   E. Motivation means moving patient to act for himself
      1. Encourage and emphasize capabilities
      2. Stress accomplishment no matter how small
      3. Be alert to emotional problems
   F. Teaching should include doing things with patient, not for him
      1. Teaching patient to perform his own daily care activities will enable independence
         a. Teaching and learning cannot be hurried; let patient work at his own pace
         b. Progress from simple to complex activities
         c. Encourage repeated practice
         d. Instruct patient, but let him do work
         e. Be sure each activity is mastered before going on to next one
      2. Patient may need frequent rest periods
      3. Activities of daily living
         a. Self-care
         b. Ambulation and traveling
         c. Activities that require use of hands
         d. Special therapies such as speech
      4. Group activity provides stimulation and mild competition
      5. Activities such as standing, balance, and ambulation usually taught by physical therapist; often nurse must substitute
      6. Teach handicapped person recreational activities to fill unused time
   G. Continuity—care and teaching received by patient in hospital, at home and from other therapists should center on single method
      1. Patient should be taught one way to perform activities
      2. Assist therapist by reporting progress or lack of progress
      3. Interpret problems that arise in connection with plan of therapy

4. See that appointments off ward are kept promptly

9. Prostheses
Replacement of some part of body with artificial substitute
   A. Most common types of prostheses are those for legs, arms, eyes, and breast
   B. Temporary prostheses immediately after amputation of arm or leg are becoming common
   C. Artificial eye
      Made of glass or plastic and hand painted to match normal eye color
   D. Several types of breast prostheses are available, including sponge rubber, fluid filled, and air filled

10. Braces
Used to restore individual to normal living
    A. Support body weight
    B. Limit involuntary movements
    C. Prevent and correct deformities

11. Crutches
Devices for individuals who, because of handicaps, must learn to walk again
    A. Crutches may be used temporarily or permanently
    B. Strengthening of muscle groups used in crutch walking should begin while patient confined to bed; exercises involving arms, shoulders, chest, and back muscles should start as soon as physician believes patient has recovered sufficiently
    C. Prior to ambulation patient should be taught and be able to move himself from bed to chair
    D. Standing, balance, and ambulation are usually taught by physical therapist; however, nurse will have to substitute often
       1. Older people may have poor sense of balance and coordination; patience is therefore required in teaching them
    E. Important points in teaching crutch walking
       1. Patient should be measured correctly for crutches, which should have heavy rubber tips
       2. Padding of axillary rest is generally discouraged, since leaning or placing weight on it may cause radial nerve paralysis
       3. Good posture, head held high, and pelvis over feet should be emphasized from beginning
       4. Several short lessons a day are better than one long lesson causing fatigue
       5. When ambulation is begun, having one attendant in front of patient and another in back of patient is desirable
       6. Type of gait used will depend on type of handicap and physician's orders
    F. Most common types of gait
       1. Four-point gait—patient bearing weight on both feet and three points of contact with floor
       2. Two-point gait—two points of contact with floor

3. Swing-to gait—crutches are placed ahead of patient and with weight on crutches he swings his body to crutches
       4. Swing-through gait—patient places crutches as in 3, but swings body beyond crutches
       5. Three-point gait when partial weight bearing is permitted
    G. Patient walking with crutches should have mastered sufficient daily care activities to be independent
       1. Patient should be able to get up and down steps and in and out of cars
    H. Nurse should be familiar with devices that help handicapped individuals perform daily care activities

Review questions

1. List four persons who should be members of the rehabilitation team.
   a. DR
   b. NURSE
   c. Pt
   d. Pt. family
2. What is the name of the federal agency concerned with the education and training of handicapped persons?
   a. U.S. Social + Rehabilitation Servic
3. List three groups of persons whose needs are not being met by rehabilitation at present.
   a. Migrant workers
   b. Elderly
   c. Drug addicts
4. What are three kinds of physical disability that probably will not respond to rehabilitation?
   a. severe cardiac damage
   b. "   "   brain   "
   c. malignant hypertension
5. What are three benefits to be derived from passive exercise?
   a. keep joints movable
   b. promote venous return + lymp
   c. prevent bone demineralization
6. List four kinds of prostheses.
   a. arms
   b. legs
   c. eyes
   d. breast
7. List five activities of daily living that are required for self-care.
   a. walking
   b. speech
   c. hand use
   d.
   e.
8. What are three purposes for using braces?
   a. support body part
   b. limit invol body movements
   c. prevent + correct deformities
9. What are four types of gait that may be used with crutches?
   a. 2 point
   b. 3 "
   c. 4 "
   d. swing through

10. Explain three concepts basic to the rehabilitation process.

a. *preventing deformities*

b. *motivation*

c. *teaching*

Films

1. Basic positioning (11 min., color, 35 mm. filmstrip with 33½ record), A/V Publications Office, Kenny Rehabilitation Institute, 1800 Chicago Ave., Minneapolis, Minn. 55404. Demonstrates methods for preventing deformities through correct positioning techniques. Supine, side-lying, and prone positions are shown.
2. Della (12 min., sound, color, 16 mm.), A/V Publications Office, Kenny Rehabilitation Institute, 1800 Chicago Ave., Minneapolis, Minn. 55404. A 35-year-old deaf paraplegic is physically rehabilitated and reeducated in living with a handicap. Depicts her present independent mode of living and her influence on deaf children in her community.
3. Immediate prosthesis after amputation (40 min., sound, black and white, 16 mm.), Division of International Activities, Social and Rehabilitation Service, 330 C Street S.W., Washington, D. C. 20201. Describes the surgical and rehabilitation procedures used in fitting prosthesis to an amputee immediately after surgery. Film produced in Poland, where procedure was first used.
4. Linda (14 min., sound, black and white, 16 mm.), Rehabilitation Institute of Oregon, 2010 Northwest Kearney St., Portland, Ore. 97209. Tells the story of Linda, a paraplegic as a result of an automobile accident, her treatment at the hospital and rehabilitation institute, and her adjustment to home and school. Some of the film narrated by the orthopedic surgeon who cared for her.
5. No barrier (14 min., color, 16 mm., free loan), President's Committee on Employment of the Handicapped, Washington, D. C. 20210. Depicts the rewarding and satisfying life of a man who can neither speak nor hear. Shows a man's strong individuality in creating a place for himself in his community.
6. Physical rehabilitation in hemiplegia—M-1579X (40 min., sound, color, 16 mm.), Media Resources Branch, National Medical Audiovisual Center (Annex), Station K, Atlanta, Ga. 30324. Describes role of the physician, physical therapist, speech therapist, social worker, and nurse. Bed positioning, passive range-of-motion exercises, evaluation of muscle power, and wheelchair, standing, balancing, ambulation, and stair climbing practice.
7. Range of motion therapy (26 min., color, 16 min.), Markwin, Inc., 325 East 77th St., New York, N. Y. 10021. Shows why range-of-motion exercises will prevent contractures and bed sores and maintain joint mobility. Demonstrates the method and precautions to be taken. Film accompanied by illustrated booklet.
8. Voyage to hope (28 min., sound, color, 16 mm.), Saginaw County Hospital, 3340 Hospital Road, Saginaw, Mich. 48605. Follows two patients during illness and convalescence in a modern rehabilitation center. Occupational therapy, physical therapy, speech therapy, medical, psychologic, recreational, and public health services are all presented.

References

1. Carlson, Carolyn: Behavioral concepts and nursing intervention, Philadelphia, 1970, J. B. Lippincott Co.
2. Caseload statistics: state vocational rehabilitation agencies, 1972, Washington, D. C., 1973, Government Printing Office.
3. Crate, Marjorie A.: Nursing functions in adaptation to chronic illness, American Journal of Nursing **65**:72-76, Oct., 1965.
4. Elementary rehabilitation nursing care, Public Health Service Publication no. 1436, Washington, D. C., 1966, Government Printing Office.
5. Flaherty, Patricia T.: Braces: a primer for nurses, Minneapolis, 1968, American Rehabilitation Foundation.
6. Fuerst, Elinor V., Wolff, LuVerne, and Weitzel, Marlene H.: Fundamentals of nursing, ed. 5, Philadelphia, 1974, J. B. Lippincott Co.
7. Knocke, Lazelle: Crutch walking, American Journal of Nursing **61**:70-73, Oct., 1961.
8. Martin, Nancy: Rehabilitation of the upper extremity amputee, Nursing Outlook **18**:50-51, Feb., 1970.
9. Massie, William A., and Landry, Edward B.: Rehabilitation facilities—how safe? Rehabilitation Record **11**:1-5, March-April, 1970.
10. Matheney, Ruth V., Nolan, Breda T., Hogan, Alice E., and Griffin, Gerald J.: Fundamentals of patient-centered nursing, ed. 3, St. Louis, 1972, The C. V. Mosby Co.
11. Naylor, Arthur: Fractures and orthopaedic surgery for nurses and physiotherapists, Baltimore, 1968, The Williams & Wilkins Co.
12. News briefs, progress in rehabilitation cited at NLN meeting, Bedside Nurse **2**:14, March-April, 1969.
13. Price, Alice L.: The art, science and spirit of nursing, ed. 3, Philadelphia, 1965, W. B. Saunders Co.
14. Rusk, Howard A.: Rehabilitation medicine, ed. 3, St. Louis, 1971, The C. V. Mosby Co.
15. Shafer, Kathleen, Sawyer, Janet R., McCluskey, Audrey M., Beck, Edna L., and Phipps, Wilma J.: Medical-surgical nursing, ed. 6, St. Louis, 1975, The C. V. Mosby Co.
16. Spear, Marion R.: Keeping idle hands busy, Minneapolis, 1950, Burgess Publishing Co.
17. Stryker, Ruth Perin: Rehabilitative aspects of acute and chronic nursing care, Philadelphia, 1972, W. B. Saunders Co.

Part three

CHAPTER 11

Nursing the patient with diseases and disorders of the respiratory system

KEY WORDS

aerosol *fine spray for inhalation*
apnea *temp. absence of breathing*
asphyxia *suffocation*
asthma *bronchial disease / lung collapse*
atelectasis *bronchial tube inflammation*
bronchitis *bronchi inflam*
bronchoscopy
cyanosis *bluish skin — lack of O₂*
dyspnea *shortness of breath*
epistaxis *nosebleed*
extrinsic *coming from outside*
hemoptysis *hemorrhage from lungs, etc*
hypoxia *deficiency of O₂ in tissues*

intrinsic *coming from in*
laryngectomy *removal of larynx*
lobectomy *removal of lung lobe*
orthopnea *must sit up to breathe*
pleurisy *pleural inflammation*
pneumonectomy *lung removal*
pulmonary edema *l. ventricle heart failure*
pulmonary embolism *clotting in lung*
pulmonary emphysema *over distension of the alveoli*
spirometer *meas vital capacity*
thoracotomy *opening into thorax*
tonsillectomy *removal of tonsils*
tracheotomy *opening into trachea*

STRUCTURE AND FUNCTION OF THE RESPIRATORY SYSTEM

The respiratory system is a continuous series of passages beginning with the nasal cavities and terminating with the tiny alveoli in the lungs which make it possible for gases to be exchanged between the blood and the air. The upper respiratory system includes the nasal cavities, pharynx, larynx, and trachea. The nose transports, warms, and humidifies air going to and from the lungs. It filters air by bouncing molecules back and forth along its convoluted pathways, where impurities are trapped by nasal hair and moist mucous membranes. The nose also serves as the organ of smell. Both air and food pass through the pharynx; air then entering the larynx through the opened epiglottis, a "trap door" that shuts on swallowing. The larynx contains the vocal cords and is located at the upper end of the trachea. The trachea is supported by rings of cartilage and maintains an open passageway for air flow. Mucous membrane lines the entire upper respiratory tract, and many of its cells contain fine hairlike projections called *cilia*, which continually sweep toward the pharynx where the mucus and impurities are expectorated or swallowed.

The right and left bronchi, their subdivisions, and the lungs comprise the lower respiratory system. The trachea divides at its lower end, forming two bronchi that have a similar structure. The bronchi are lined with ciliated mucosa, and each enters a lung where they immediately divide and branch forming bronchioles. This structure resembles an inverted tree. Further branching produces microscopic alveolar ducts, which end in alveolar sacs containing many *alveoli.* The left lung is divided into two lobes, whereas the right lung has three lobes. The uppermost part of the lung is called the *apex,* and the lower part is the *base.* Inside each lung 300 million alveoli are interlaced in a network of capillaries. It is here that oxygen is transferred to the blood and carbon dioxide is removed from the blood to be eliminated from the body. The lungs are separated by a space called the *mediastinum.* The lower part of the system and a portion of the trachea are enclosed in a bony framework known as the thoracic cage. The thoracic cage is separated from the abdominal cavity by the diaphragm, which contracts to create a partial vacuum during inspiration and relaxes during expiration, permitting abdominal organs to push upward and help force air from the lungs. The thoracic cavity is lined with a serous membrane (pleura), and each lung is enclosed in a saclike structure of serous membrane, the cells of which secrete a clear, sticky fluid. The respiratory process is under the control of the respiratory center, located in the medulla of the brain.

The function of the respiratory system is the exchange of gases, which is accomplished through the process of respiration. Respiration is both external and internal. External respiration consists of the movement of oxygen into the lungs (inhalation) and the removal of carbon dioxide out of the lungs (exhalation). During the inhalation phase the alveoli become distended with oxygen, which passes through the permeable membranes of the alveoli and the capillaries, thus reaching the blood. Oxygen then combines with hemoglobin in the red blood cells and is transported by the circulatory system to the body cells. Internal respiration is the process by which the oxygen is transferred from the blood to the body cells, and the carbon dioxide is passed from the body cells to the blood to be eliminated from the body. Under normal conditions respiration is a regular rhythmic process, controlled by the respiratory center in the medulla of the brain and is mostly involuntary. Any condition that interferes with this normal function should be regarded as serious because if all oxygen is cut off, death will ensue in 4 to 6 minutes. The cells of the brain cannot be deprived of oxygen for more than 3 minutes without causing irreversible brain damage. Therefore restoration of respiratory function takes precedence over correction of any other condition.

ABNORMAL TYPES OF RESPIRATION

The nurse will care for many patients with respiratory difficulties and should become familiar with the most common deviations from normal respiration and understand their significance.

Dyspnea. When breathing becomes difficult and labored and requires considerable exertion on the part of the patient, he is said to be dyspneic. Dyspnea is a subjective symptom of respiratory difficulty. It may result from pain, pulmonary disease, anemia, heart failure, obstruction, or emotional factors. Characteristics of the condition include pallor, restlessness and anxiety, increased pulse and respiratory rates, or rattling sounds in the respiratory passages. When the patient is unable to breathe except in a sitting position, he is said to be orthopneic. Dyspnea is one of the most frightening symptoms for the patient and his family. The patient often feels that his life is threatened, and as he becomes more anxious, the dyspnea may increase. The nurse caring for the dyspneic patient should be calm, reassuring, and confident in manner.

Hypoxia. Hypoxia is a general term meaning that an insufficient supply of oxygen is available to the body tissues. Its causes are many and varied. Decreased oxygen in the environment, pulmonary diseases, inadequate transport of oxygen by the red blood cells or circulatory system, or tissue edema can all result in a decreased oxygen supply to all cells of the body. Hypoxia is a symptom of an underlying disease or disorder, and treatment is directed toward relieving the cause. The condition may be acute if the supply of oxygen is quickly reduced as in airway obstruction caused by a foreign object or in blockage by respiratory secretions. The signs and symptoms of hypoxia vary with the amount of oxygen lack and the underlying cause. Generally, early signs of hypoxia are changes in behavior, decreased

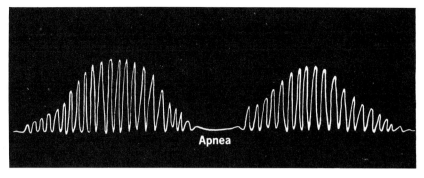

Fig. 11-1. Cheyne-Stokes respiration. Note the rhythmic pattern that repeats itself after a period of apnea.

judgment, drowsiness, lassitude, and head-ache. Occasionally patients will become restless and excited. As the condition progresses, shortness of breath, rapid pulse, blood pressure changes, nausea, delirium, convulsions, and coma can occur. Cyanosis is not an early sign of hypoxia and usually is not evident until the hypoxia is well advanced.

Apnea. Apnea is a temporary cessation of breathing. An increased respiratory rate may lead to an increase of oxygen in the blood and a decrease in carbon dioxide, and the apnea is a mechanism to compensate for the condition. Apnea is most frequently associated with Cheyne-Stokes respiration.

Cheyne-Stokes respiration. In the critically ill patient, Cheyne-Stokes respiration may be a sign of approaching death. The respiration follows an irregular rhythmic pattern, beginning with slow, shallow respirations that increase in depth and rapidity to a maximum, which is followed by a gradual decrease. A period of apnea lasting from 10 to 60 seconds follows, after which the respiratory pattern is repeated (Fig. 11-1).

Asphyxia or suffocation. When carbon dioxide increases in the tissues and oxygen is deficient, the patient may die from asphyxia. The condition may result from anything that cuts off the supply of oxygen, such as drowning, interference by foreign bodies, or the inhalation of smoke.

Cyanosis. Cyanosis is characterized by a bluish discoloration of the skin and mucous membrane. It results from a deficiency of oxygen in the blood and an increase in carbon dioxide. Cyanosis may occur sud-denly or develop gradually. It usually is present in dyspneic conditions and is associated with many cardiovascular disorders. In an emergency it is important to be sure that the airway is clear, and immediate medical care is indicated. The nurse should always report any evidence of cyanosis.

Hyperventilation. In the absence of disease, normal respiration provides the amount of oxygen necessary for the body cells and an orderly exchange of gases. In hyperventilation, inhalation is increased, with the amount of oxygen entering the alveoli in excess of the physiologic needs of the body. If continued, it may lead to changes in the circulation and upset the otherwise normal ventilatory process.

Hypoventilation. Hypoventilation is the opposite of hyperventilation and occurs when the amount of oxygen entering the alveoli is below that necessary to meet the body's gas exchange needs. It may be caused by any condition resulting from acute or chronic hypoxia.

DIAGNOSTIC TESTS AND PROCEDURES

Blood examinations. Routine blood examinations are usually ordered for patients with respiratory disease and include red blood cell count, white blood cell count, and hemoglobin determination. An abnormal increase in the number of white blood cells may indicate mobilization of the body's defenses against a respiratory infection, whereas a significant decrease of red blood cells and hemoglobin may be related to the oxygen-carrying power of the blood. Depending on the specific diagnosis of respiratory disease, the physician may order additional blood studies.

Blood gas studies. Studies of the partial pressure or tension of carbon dioxide and oxygen and determination of blood pH have become increasingly important in the diagnosis and treatment of patients with chronic lung disease. These blood gas studies determine how well the lungs are being ventilated and how well the gases are being exchanged in the body. Arterial blood is obtained through puncture of an artery, such as the femoral or radial artery, with a small needle or from a catheter previously placed into an artery.

Sputum examination. The examination of sputum is made by persons trained in laboratory methods, but the collection of the specimen is usually a nursing responsibility. Sputum consists of material coughed up from the lungs and may contain pathogenic and nonpathogenic organisms. If sputum is to be of diagnostic value, it must be collected in the correct manner. Specimens should be collected early in the morning so that they consist of the first sputum raised by deep coughing. Before collection the patient should rinse his mouth with clear water, after which he is encouraged to cough deeply and expectorate into a sterile container. If bottles are used, they should be closed with new corks or caps. The specimen should be properly labeled and sent immediately to the laboratory. Sputum collected more than 24 hours before laboratory examination may have no diagnostic value. When specimens are sent through the mail, specially prepared receptacles containing a preservative should be used.

The general appearance of sputum depends on the kind of substances and pathogenic organisms it contains. It is usually described as purulent, mucopurulent, bloody, serous, or frothy. Normally sputum is odorless, but in suppurative conditions of the lungs such as lung abscess, it may have a foul odor. Sputum examination using the Papanicolaou smear technique may be useful in detecting the presence of cancer cells. The amount, odor, and appearance of all sputum should always be recorded on the patient's record.

Pulmonary function tests. Pulmonary function tests are not diagnostic but may indicate the existence of some impairment of respiratory function and the necessity for additional investigation. There are four types of lung capacity that may be measured: (1) total capacity, (2) vital capacity, (3) inspiratory capacity, and (4) residual capacity.

Normal lung volumes and capacities are obtained by using a *spirometer,* which consists of an air-filled drum inverted over water. As the patient breathes in and out through a connecting mouthpiece and tube, the drum rises and falls and a graphic record *(spirogram)* is produced. A record of total lung capacity is obtained by asking the patient to take a breath, expanding the lungs to the greatest extent he can. The patient then exhales forcefully, expelling all the air possible, which is a measure of vital capacity. The largest volume of air inspired after a normal inspiration is a measure of inspiratory capacity, whereas residual capacity is tested by the amount of air retained in the lungs after a maximal expiration. In chronic obstructive pulmonary disease the volume of gas expired is usually decreased.[3] The nurse should relieve any apprehension that the patient may have by explaining that these procedures are breathing tests and that he will be asked to breathe into a small tube. Patient cooperation is important for securing accurate results.

Gastric washings. Some patients, including infants and small children, may have little sputum or be unable to expectorate it. When disease of the lungs is evident, particularly tuberculosis, the causative organism may be found in the stomach. It is believed that ciliary action may move sputum upward from the lungs to the larynx where it is swallowed. Gastric washings may also be found helpful in identifying cancer cells. When the patient is scheduled for a gastric washing, breakfast is withheld, and a gastric tube is passed through the nose into the stomach. A 30 or 50 ml. sterile glass syringe is attached to the tube, and by gentle aspiration the gastric contents are withdrawn and placed in a sterile container. The nurse should be sure the specimen is properly labeled and sent to the laboratory immediately.

X-ray and fluoroscope studies. X-ray examination of the chest is one of the most common of all x-ray procedures. It is ordered by the physician to detect disease of the chest or to follow the progress of a disease process. A small microfilm is used most often; if any abnormal condition is detected, a large film is taken. Many hospitals require routine chest x-ray films of all patients admitted. When chest x-ray films have been ordered for a hospitalized patient, the nurse should see that he wears a hospital gown tied in the back. Pins must not be used, and bras with metal hooks and any other article of clothing containing metal must be removed because the presence of metal will produce a shadow over the film. When x-ray films are taken in the outpatient clinic, the patient is instructed to strip to the waist and put on a gown tied in the back. Patients are transported to the x-ray department by stretcher or wheelchair and should be accompanied by an attendant. If the patient is too ill to be taken to the x-ray department, a portable x-ray machine may be taken to the patient's bedside; however, the preparation of the patient is the same. If the patient is receiving oxygen, it must be turned off during the x-ray examination.

Fluoroscopic x-ray examination is a screening procedure to detect any pathologic condition of the chest. It is also done to follow the course of barium through the esophagus into the stomach (p. 81). Patients should be told that they will be in darkness for a period of time but that there will be no discomfort involved. The preparation of the patient for fluoroscopic examination is the same as that for x-ray examination of the chest.

Bronchography and bronchoscopy. The bronchogram is an x-ray film of the lungs after a radiopaque substance has been instilled through the trachea into the bronchi and bronchioles. The examination enables the physician to visualize the bronchial tree for evidence of disease. The emotional preparation of the patient for bronchography or bronchoscopy is important. The procedures result in a certain amount of discomfort, and the apprehensive, fearful patient may cooperate poorly. Explaining to the patient what to expect and teaching him how to breathe during the procedure and how to relax will provide a greater feeling of security and help relieve anxiety.

The nurse should see that the teeth and mouth are thoroughly cleansed the evening before and again the morning of the examination. No food or fluid by mouth is allowed after midnight. Postural drainage may be ordered in the morning to remove any secretions that may have drained into the trachea or bronchi during the night. Special mouth care should be given after postural drainage, and dentures and bridges should be removed. A sedative in the form of one of the barbiturates is usually ordered for the patient. When the patient arrives in the x-ray department, a topical anesthetic is used to anesthetize the trachea, larynx, and bronchi, resulting in the loss of reflexes. A soluble radiopaque iodide is then instilled, and x-ray films are taken. When the patient returns to his room, postural drainage should be done to help drain the radiopaque substance from the lungs. No food or fluids should be given until the gag reflex has returned. This can be tested by tickling the back of the throat with a cotton swab.

The preparation of the patient for bronchoscopic examination is the same as that for bronchography. The bronchoscope is a long, rigid, hollow, lighted instrument that can be passed through the mouth into the trachea and major bronchi after a topical anesthetic has been administered. The room is darkened, and visualization of the bronchial tree is possible when light is reflected through the instrument. The examination is used to permit the physician to remove foreign bodies that have lodged in the bronchi, to suction secretions for laboratory examination, to observe the respiratory passageways for disease, and to obtain biopsy specimens. When the patient returns to his room, he should be positioned according to the physician's instructions. He should be encouraged to let secretions drain from his mouth and not swallow them and to try not to cough or talk. No food or fluids should be given until normal reflexes have returned. The patient should be watched carefully for respiratory difficulty, since edema of the larynx may occur. If a biopsy has been done, sputum may be tinged with blood for several days; however, the nurse should be alert for any unusual bleeding, and the physician should be notified immediately if such should occur.[16] If soreness of the throat and discomfort are prolonged, a mild analgesic such as aspirin may be ordered.

Thoracentesis. The removal of fluid from the pleural cavity may be done for diagnosis or for treatment. Fluid in the pleural cavity is often detected on x-ray examination; however, in some cases dyspnea may exist because of compression of the lung on the affected side. If the lung is compressed, a diminished expansion of the chest on the affected side with an increased expansion on the opposite side will be observed. Fluid in the pleural cavity may follow pneumonia, pleurisy, and tuberculosis. It may also occur in patients with cancer, heart disease, and kidney disease. When accumulation of fluid results from kidney disease or heart disease, both sides are usually affected, whereas only one side is involved in other disorders. When it occurs secondary to pneumonia, a pus formation may result (empyema); however, as a result of the present treatment with antibiotics and sulfonamide drugs, empyema rarely occurs.

When thoracentesis is to be done, the patient should be told about the procedure. The nurse should remember that what seems like a simple procedure may be frightening to the patient and that every means should be used to relieve the patient's anxiety. The procedure is usually carried out in the patient's room; the patient is in a sitting position with his head and arms resting on a pillow placed on the overbed table. Using aseptic technique, the skin is cleansed generally in the area of the eighth or ninth rib interspace, after which a local anesthetic is injected into the tissues. The patient must be cautioned not to move while the needle is being inserted to avoid damage to the lung or pleura. The primary function of the nurse is the observation of the patient during the procedure. The pulse and respiration should be checked several times, and the patient should be observed for any change in color or undue diaphoresis. Fluid withdrawn is observed for color, consistency, and amount and is recorded. In empyema the specimen is sent to the laboratory for bacterial diagnosis so that the appropriate antibiotic may be ordered.

Thoracotomy. A thoracotomy is a surgical opening into the thoracic cavity for the purpose of removing blood, pus, or air or to expedite reexpansion of a lung after accidental injury or surgery. A thoracotomy may be done to explore the thoracic cavity for evidence of disease, including cancer. If indicated, a biopsy may be done.

Patients having any type of open chest surgery are given endotracheal anesthesia. Anesthesia given in this way makes it possible to keep the unaffected lung expanded and functioning even when it is subjected to atmospheric pressure. Normally the pleural space contains a negative pressure, or subatmospheric pressure. The pressure within the lungs is normally that of atmospheric pressure. Inspiration causes the negative pressure in the pleural space to become even greater and creates a type of vacuum that "pulls" air into the lungs, expanding them. However, when the pleura is entered through surgery or trauma to the chest wall, atmospheric pressure enters the pleural space and the lung collapses. The negative pressure that kept the lungs expanded no longer exists. Therefore after chest surgery the patient will usually have one or more drainage tubes placed in the pleural cavity. The tubes permit the escape of air so that the lung will expand and allow for the drainage of fluid from the pleural space. Often one tube will be placed in the upper chest to remove air

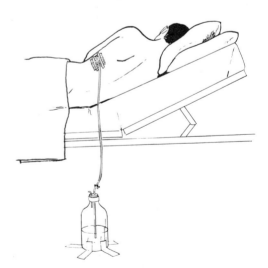

Fig. 11-2. Thoracotomy tube is connected to sterile closed drainage. Note the bottle fastened to the floor.

and another tube will be placed in a lower position to remove fluids. The chest catheters are then attached to a closed drainage system.

There are two basic types of closed chest drainage: gravity and suction drainage. Gravity drainage is accomplished by attaching the tubing leading from the chest to a long glass connecting tube that is inserted into a sterile drainage bottle containing sterile water. The glass tube is inserted below the water level, providing a

seal to prevent air from backing up into the pleural cavity. If the system is working correctly, the water in the long connecting tube will rise during inspiration and drop during expiration as air and fluid pass out into the water[15] (Fig. 11-2). The water level should be marked so that an accurate measurement of drainage may be made. The bottle is placed on the floor or below the level of the bed, and under no circumstances should it be lifted up, since this will allow fluid to drain back into the chest

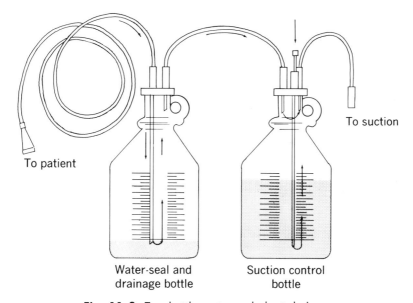

Water-seal and drainage bottle   Suction control bottle

Fig. 11-3. Two-bottle water-seal chest drainage.

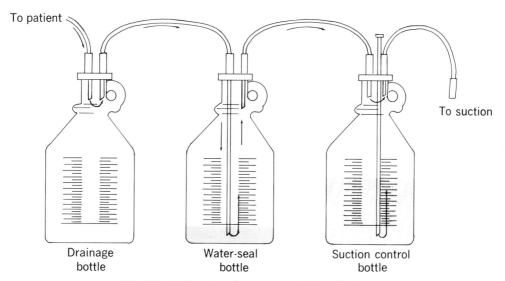

Drainage bottle   Water-seal bottle   Suction control bottle

Fig. 11-4. Three-bottle water-seal chest drainage.

cavity. If the bottle is placed on the floor, it should be secured with adhesive tape to prevent knocking it over. The entire system must be kept airtight. Occasionally two bottles may be used for gravity drainage, one accepting the drainage and the other supplying the water seal.

The application of suction may be necessary to reexpand the lung. Suction can be applied through the use of an electric pump or a wall suction outlet. Two-bottle or three-bottle drainage systems may be used. With a two-bottle system a suction control bottle is added to the water-seal and drainage bottle. The suction reaching the patient's chest is controlled by the length of the submerged tube in the suction control bottle (Fig. 11-3). The physician will order the amount of sterile water and the positioning of the tube in the suction control bottle. The submerged tube in the suction control bottle should bubble periodically as air is drawn in to reduce suction from the source. If this does not occur, assistance should be obtained at once. Three-bottle, water-seal drainage has a separate bottle for collecting drainage, with the second bottle providing the water-seal and the third bottle controlling suction[15] (Fig. 11-4).

The Pleur-evac is a sterile plastic disposable unit that provides water-seal drainage, using the principles incorporated in the three-bottle drainage system (Fig. 11-5). It can be hung from the bed or contained in a disposable floor stand.

A patient may have an air leak from the lungs from various causes. As the patient inhales, air is taken into the lungs, and small amounts of air may be released from a leak that escapes into the pleural cavity. Sometimes the patient may have a rather large air leak, and if there is no escape route for the air, he may develop a tension pneumothorax that could be fatal. For this reason the thoracotomy tubing should never be clamped, except as indicated later. The importance of not clamping tubing has been emphasized by von Hippel[20]: "For some unexplained reason nurses have always been taught to 'clamp chest tubes' if anything goes wrong. . . . It is well to insist on complete removal of all types of clamps from the vicinity of any patient with chest tubes to help avoid such a

catastrophe."[*] The catastrophe von Hippel refers to is pneumothorax, which could mean instant death of the patient. If the tubing should become disconnected or if the catheter should come out, the physician should be called without delay. However, von Hippel states that such a situation presents no immediate danger to the patient. When the patient has a pneumonectomy, the chest tubes remain clamped unless the surgeon orders otherwise.

The nurse should be familiar with the purpose for which the drainage is being used and the kind of drainage to expect. If the drainage contains excessive amounts of blood, the physician should be notified. Blood clots may form in the tubing, causing an obstruction; to prevent this from happening the tubing should be milked or stripped. Frequent checking is necessary to ascertain that the system remains airtight, that it is working correctly, and that the tubing does not become kinked when the patient is lying on his side. If a small pil-

---

[*]From von Hippel, Arndt: Chest tubes and chest bottles, Springfield, Ill., 1970, Charles C Thomas, Publisher.

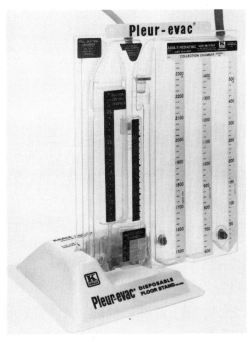

Fig. 11-5. Adult-pediatric, nonmetered Pleur-evac. (Courtesy DeKnatel, Inc., Queens Village, N. Y.)

low, folded towel, or rubber ring is placed under the chest when the patient is in a side-lying position, it will help to prevent obstruction of the tube.[16]

Tracheotomy. Tracheotomy is any endotracheal intubation in which an incision is made through the skin and tissues of the neck into the trachea that creates an artificial airway. Some confusion has arisen concerning the term *tracheostomy*, which is used by some physicians and nurses. It is evident that tracheotomy and tracheostomy are being used interchangeably to mean the same thing, and opinions differ widely on the accuracy of this practice. According to Egan,[8] the surgical procedure performed by the physician in creating the airway is a tracheotomy, after which a tracheostomy tube of the proper size is inserted. It should be noted that commercial distributors label tubing as tracheostomy tubes, indicating equipment and not procedure. Shafer[16] indicates that when a tracheotomy results in a permanent airway, as in a laryngectomy, a *tracheal stoma*, or *tracheostoma*, results, and the term used is *tracheostomy*. This interpretation is consistent with the medical definition—to provide with an opening or mouth. Similar procedures ending with the suffix *-ostomy* include colostomy and ileostomy, both of which are usually permanent.

A tracheotomy may be an elective procedure, or it may be performed in an emergency. If at all possible, it should be done in the operating room under strict aseptic technique. Indications for a tracheotomy include any condition in which respiration is compromised, such as blockage of the upper respiratory tract, respiratory failure, possibility of aspiration in the comatose patient, or a need for effective removal of excessive secretions. After the surgical procedure a tracheostomy tube is inserted into the opening and securely tied about the neck with cotton tape. A sterile gauze dressing (unfilled) covers the surgical wound around the tube (Fig. 11-6). The tracheostomy tube consists of three parts: the outer cannula, inner cannula, and obturator (Fig. 11-7). The obturator is used to guide the outer cannula through the surgical opening into the trachea, after which it is removed and the inner cannula inserted into the outer cannula and locked in place.

Cuffed tracheostomy tubes recently have come into use. These tubes are made of plastic material and have a cuff surrounding the middle portion of the tube that can be inflated with air (Fig. 11-8). The cuff prevents air from leaking around the

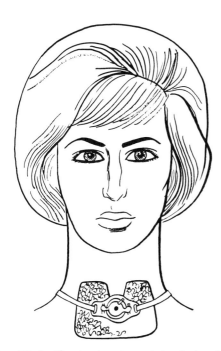

Fig. 11-6. The tracheostomy tube is in place and tied about the neck. The wound is protected with a sterile dressing.

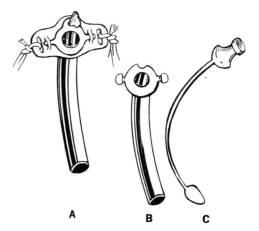

Fig. 11-7. Tracheostomy tube. **A,** Outer cannula. **B,** Inner cannula. **C,** Obturator.

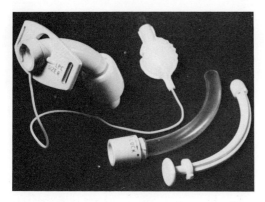

Fig. 11-8. Cuffed tracheostomy tube. (Courtesy Shiley Laboratories, Santa Ana, Calif.)

sides of the tube and holds the tube in place. Most cuffed tracheostomy tubes must be deflated regularly to decrease the effects of constant pressure on the tracheal mucosa. The use of these tubes provides a leak-proof system that is a definite advantage with mechanical ventilation (p. 199). They are available with or without inner cannulas.[15]

A primary nursing responsibility is the maintenance of a patent airway. A patient who has a newly formed tracheostomy will need frequent suctioning (p. 196). The inner cannula must be removed and cleaned frequently using sterile technique. If a form of mechanical ventilation is not used, a vaporizer may be used to keep secretions moist. Mid-Fowler's position provides comfort and facilitates breathing. Provisions must be made for the patient to communicate because he will be unable to speak. Patients are usually apprehensive and fear choking. The nurse must observe for complications, which may include apnea, cyanosis, shortness of breath, bleeding from the wound, and hypotension. Blood pressure should be taken prior to the surgical procedure and at intervals thereafter. An extra sterile tracheostomy set of the same size, a pair of scissors, and a tracheotomy dilator should be kept at the patient's bedside for emergency use in case the tube becomes displaced. Any patient having a tracheotomy should not be left alone for the first 24 hours after the insertion of the tube.

If a patient is to be discharged with a tracheostomy tube, he must be taught how to care for the tube himself. Suction equipment should be available at home. Persons who have a permanent tracheostomy must be told not to swim and to use caution when bathing so that water is not aspirated. Scarfs or collars worn about the opening should be made of porous material.

Whatever the purpose of a tracheotomy, whether it is temporary or permanent, the nurse should remember that the life of the patient depends on nursing skill in keeping the airway clear, since it is the only means by which the patient can breathe.

Endotracheal intubation. In endotracheal intubation a tube is passed by the physician through the nose or mouth into the trachea. This tube may also have an inflatable cuff, which holds the tube in place and prevents aspiration of substances from the upper respiratory tract. Usually a form of mechanical ventilation is then used to facilitate the patient's breathing. Endotracheal intubation is usually done as an emergency measure and seldom is left in place for more than 48 hours. If continued assistance is necessary after that time, a tracheotomy is then performed. The cuff of the endotracheal tube must also be deflated periodically to prevent damage to the trachea.[15]

SPECIFIC ASPECTS OF NURSING CARE

Any condition resulting in respiratory difficulty produces anxiety and apprehension for the patient and must be viewed as potentially serious. Respiratory embarrassment often results from oxygen deficiency, which may have several causes. The nurse should be familiar with the underlying condition responsible for the oxygen want. To meet the patient's oxygen needs the nurse must be able to recognize the signs of oxygen deficiency. Symptoms will depend on the degree of deficiency, and not all will appear in the patient. Some patients will exhibit restlessness and excitement, and there may be an increase in respiratory and pulse rates, headache, sighing and yawning, nausea and vomiting, and anorexia. Blood pressure may be normal, but as air hunger increases, the blood pressure will fall, cyanosis will appear, and twitching of muscles may occur. Since each patient must be treated individually, the nurse should have specific orders from the physican. However, it is the nurse's responsibility to execute the physician's orders with understanding, skill, and promptness.

Psychologic care. The inability of the patient to secure sufficient air is a frightening experience, particularly for children, and parents who may be anxious and apprehensive may pass their anxiety on to the child. When a patient's life is threatened, it is natural for the nurse to be anxious, but if anxiety in the patient or his family is going to be relieved, the nurse must be able to remain calm, unlike the nurse caring for a seriously ill patient who ran excitedly from the room into the hall, calling to another nurse, "Oh, I think my patient is dying!" Although the psychologic care of each patient depends on the patient's own feelings and the particular situation, the nurse who maintains a calm approach to the problem, has basic knowledge and ability to plan and organize patient care, and performs technical skills competently will set the stage for patient confidence and relief of anxiety.[13] When it is possible to explain procedures to the patient in simple terms that he can understand, it will contribute much to the relief of anxiety.

Coughing, suctioning, postural drainage, and percussion. These procedures are all designed for the same purpose, that is, to remove secretions and provide adequate ventilation of the lungs by maintaining a clear airway at all times. Increased secretions and sputum from the respiratory tract may cause mucus plugs to form, obstructing the passages and preventing free exchange of gases. Depending on the disease present and the condition of the patient, procedures must be instituted to remove secretions. For some patients deep productive coughing may be sufficient, whereas for others the nurse may be responsible for clearing the airway. Patients with hemoptysis should not be permitted to cough. When it is possible, the patient should be placed in a sitting position; if coughing is painful, the nurse should assist the patient by splinting the chest. Sputum should be collected in tissues and placed in paper bags pinned to the side of the bed. The patient should be taught to take a deep breath, hold it a second, and cough on expiration. Tissues should be folded and placed in the cupped hand. The nurse who handles sputum should wash the hands thoroughly after each encounter. Persistent shallow coughing is of no value and only tires the patient.

There are many cough medicines on the market. Some may be purchased over the counter in drugstores, whereas others require a physician's prescription. Cough medicines may be narcotic or nonnarcotic antitussives and are classified as demulcents, expectorants, or sedatives. The kind of cough remedy prescribed will depend on the condition for which it is needed and the result desired. Demulcents are protective and may be expected to relieve irritation of the throat by providing a soothing effect and protecting the mucous membrane from air. Demulcents are often found in gargles, lozenges, and syrups that contain various flavoring agents such as wild cherry. Some lozenges contain an analgesic that adds little, if anything, to its effectiveness. Expectorants act to increase or modify mucous secretions in the respiratory tract, making mucus less thick and therefore more easily expectorated. Among some of the expectorant drugs are syrup of ipecac, ammonium chloride, and iodide preparations. Sedative agents reduce coughing by depressing the cough reflex. They may contain a narcotic or barbiturate, which will also depress the respiratory center. Their use is usually limited to disorders involving extremely painful coughing. If an allergic factor is involved, an antihistaminic agent may be ordered. Often in an acute infection nasal congestion contributes to the patient's discomfort. Phenylephrine (Neo-Synephrine), ephedrine sulfate, or any of the numerous sprays and drops available may be ordered by the physician.[4]

When the patient is unable to cough, secretions may be removed by suctioning. When the patient is in respiratory distress because the airway is obstructed, the nurse may observe the following signs: an increase in pulse and respiratory rates, a harsh respiratory sound, restlessness, anxiety, pallor with cyanosis about the mouth, or generalized cyanosis.[9] If the distress is due to mucus obstructing the airway, the

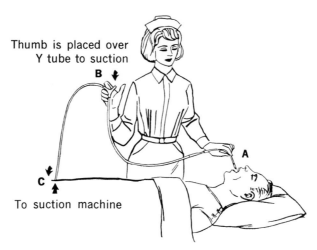

Thumb is placed over
Y tube to suction

To suction machine

Fig. 11-9. Suctioning. **A,** The suction catheter is being inserted. **B,** The thumb is placed over the Y tube for suction; note the thumb does not close the tube while the catheter is being inserted. **C,** The tubing is attached to the suction machine.

patient should be suctioned immediately, carefully, and thoroughly to relieve the symptoms and restore a patent airway. The procedure is to attach a whistle-tip catheter to tubing connected to an electric suction machine. If the patient is conscious, the procedure should be explained to him, and the nurse should use caution not to injure the mucous membrane. When the patient has an airway in the mouth or a tracheostomy tube, the suction catheter is inserted through the airway or tube. The most satisfactory method employs a Y tube, which is attached midway in the tubing and allows the nurse to have fingertip control of the suction (Fig. 11-9). When aspirating secretions, the nurse should maintain strict aseptic technique to prevent serious complications. Separate catheters must be used for nasal secretions and tracheobronchial secretions, and a sufficient number of catheters should be available to provide for sterilization between aspirations, or disposable catheters may be used. The whistle-tip catheter should be moist when inserted, and suction should not be applied until after insertion. The catheter is generally rotated while it is being withdrawn, and suction may be released by removing the finger from the Y tube valve. If possible, the patient should be placed in Fowler's position before beginning the procedure. Each suctioning should not exceed 10 seconds, and an interval of 3 minutes

should elapse before repeating the procedure. When suctioning through an airway or endotracheal or tracheostomy tube, the catheter should be inserted at least the length of the tube and not more than 4 to 8 inches into the trachea. The nurse should understand the physician's orders in regard to how far the catheter should be inserted. If it is necessary to aspirate secretions from the bronchi, the patient's head should be turned to the side opposite that of the bronchus to be aspirated, which allows for introduction of the catheter into the bronchus. Nurses should not aspirate the bronchi unless they have been taught and are supervised. Careful washing of the hands should precede and follow suctioning patients who have a tracheostomy.

Postural drainage is used to drain excessive secretions from the lungs, including pus from lung abscess and radiopaque substances used in x-ray examination of the lungs. Drainage is facilitated by placing the patient in a position that allows gravity to aid in the procedure. The position of the patient should be determined by the area of the lung to be drained. The upper lobes of the lung can best be drained in the sitting position, the lower lobes in a lying position. Positions vary, however, according to the patient's condition, strength, and respiratory function.[9] Gravity drainage of the lungs can be achieved in many ways

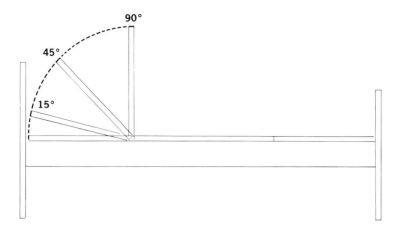

Fig. 11-10. Elevating the headrest of the Gatch bed an exact number of degrees.

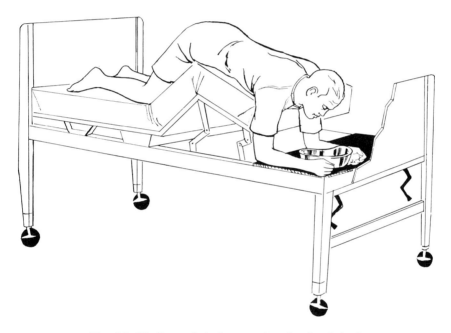

Fig. 11-11. Postural drainage, using the Gatch bed.

(Fig. 11-11). Usually younger patients can tolerate lowering of the head better than an elderly or debilitated patient. If possible, the mouth should be approximately 20 inches lower than the base of the lungs. Special beds and tables are available; however, the patient's own bed may be used, and whatever position is used, it should be one that provides good drainage. During the procedure the patient should be encouraged to cough deeply, and after his return to bed he may be expected to cough and expectorate large amounts of sputum.

One highly satisfactory method utilizes the Gatch bed (Fig. 11-10), in which the knee section is elevated as high as possible and the patient lies over the bend. A board is placed across the bed frame and protected with newspapers, thus providing a place for a receptacle for sputum and a place to rest the hands (Fig. 11-11). It has been found that the procedure is more effective when the patient has been taught and practices breathing with his diaphragm.

Elderly patients with hypertrophic arthritis may be unable to bend the body over the bed, and fairly satisfactory results may be obtained by elevating the foot of the bed. Postural drainage is often fatiguing for the debilitated patient, and he may be able to remain in the position for only a few minutes. However, with each effort he will experience less discomfort. The procedure should be supervised by the nurse and is best carried out midway between meals to prevent nausea and vomiting. The teeth should be brushed after the procedure, and an antiseptic mouthwash may be used if desired. The patient should be protected from chilling during the procedure and should be allowed to rest after returning to bed.

If the physician orders the drainage measured, it should be collected in a receptacle suitable for measuring. Color, amount, and consistency should be recorded on the patient's chart.

Percussion is a technique of rhythmically clapping and vibrating the chest wall over the involved area to help loosen mucus plugs and move them into the bronchi where they may be drained out or expectorated. It is performed with a cupped hand often in conjunction with postural drainage and is not painful.[9] Clapping and vibrating are not employed when there is danger of hemorrhage or if the patient complains of pain. The procedure should be performed by a nurse trained in the technique or the respiratory therapist.

Throat irrigations, steam inhalations, and aerosol therapy. Persons suffering from nasopharyngeal and bronchial infections often secure relief with warm throat irrigations. Physiologic saline solution at a temperature of 120° F. is commonly employed, and irrigations may be used several times a day. The application of heat to the irritated membranes promotes drainage of secretions, stimulates circulation, relieves pain and swelling, and relieves muscle spasm. The nurse may assist the patient with the procedure, or the patient may be taught to carry out the procedure under supervision. (Refer to a textbook on basic nursing.)

When the larynx and bronchi are involved or when infection extends into the sinuses, warm moist air in the form of steam inhalations may be ordered. Many hospitals use electric vaporizers, which are placed in the patient's room. Doors and windows should remain closed to provide the desired warmth and humidity. When electric kettles are used, the nurse should check at intervals to be sure they do not boil dry. If medicated inhalations are ordered, tincture of benzoin or tincture of benzoin with 1% menthol crystals in placed on a cotton ball or a piece of gauze, which is then placed in the cup at the end of the long spout so that steam flows over the medication. Precautions should be taken to place the vaporizer so that the patient will not be burned and bedding will not become wet. When vaporizers are used for croup tents, extreme caution must be taken to place them where the child will not be burned. Vaporizers used in the home must be placed where small children cannot pull them over onto themselves. Steam inhalations may be ordered continuously or for a specified period of time at intervals. They may also be used to provide warmth and moisture for patients with a tracheostomy.

The administration of antibiotics bronchodilators, mucolytic agents, and drugs such as epinephrine by nebulization is replacing some of the older methods of treating respiratory diseases. Penicillin is frequently administered in connection with oxygen under pressure. The nebulizer and atomizer are the same and operate in the same way. Squeezing the hand bulb on the atomizer forces air through the liquid, carrying with it a fine mist or spray. When oxygen under pressure is forced through the nebulizer containing penicillin, it carries fine particles of the penicillin into the respiratory tract. When oxygen is administered, it does not pass through the distilled water used for humidifying the oxygen but is connected directly from the oxygen gauge to an oxygen mask, and the gauge is set at 4 to 6 liters per minute. The oxygen may also be connected to a nebulizer placed in the patient's mouth. The patient should be instructed to place his finger over the open end of the tubing and inhale deeply, hold his breath for a second, remove his finger from the tubing, and exhale slowly through the nose. A Y tube may be placed in the tubing to allow for easy finger control. The procedure is repeated until all the medication has been used. The teeth should be brushed and the mouth rinsed after the procedure to prevent soreness.

Ultrasonic nebulizers are machines capable of atomizing cold sterile water into minute droplets through electronic vibrations, producing a type of mist therapy. The small droplets can be inhaled deeper into the lungs than can larger droplets, which tend to remain in the upper respiratory passageways. These nebulizers have been effective in administering highly humidified air or oxygen to patients with respiratory problems. Medications can also be administered, and some models mount on positive-pressure breathing devices and anesthesia machines.

Mechanical ventilation. Pulmonary ventilation is the process of taking oxygen into the lungs and releasing carbon dioxide. Under certain conditions the patient is unable to maintain optimum levels of arterial oxygen and carbon dioxide. When this occurs, the patient's survival is dependent on some type of mechanical assistance.

There are several conditions for which the patient may need ventilatory assistance. Among these disorders are poisoning from carbon monoxide or drugs, chronic obstructive pulmonary disease, respiratory failure, certain neuromuscular disorders, cardiac arrest, and pulmonary edema caused by ventricular failure. The kind of assistance needed by the patient is related to pressure, volume, and time. Therefore the various types of ventilators that are available are classified as (1) pressure cycled (Fig. 11-12) and (2) volume cycled (Fig. 11-13). The volume-cycled respirator may be preset as a time-cycled respirator.

The pressure-cycled ventilator is preset to provide a flow of air into the lungs until a desired pressure has been reached. The inhalation valve then closes automatically, and an expiratory valve opens and the patient exhales. At the end of expiration the entire process is repeated. The pressure-cycled ventilator may be used in two ways: (1) ventilation may be initiated by the patient for assisted breathing—intermittent positive-pressure breathing (IPPB); and (2) it may be set for self-cycling ventilation—intermittent positive-pressure ventilation (IPPV). The pressure-cycled ventilator operates on the basis of a predeter-

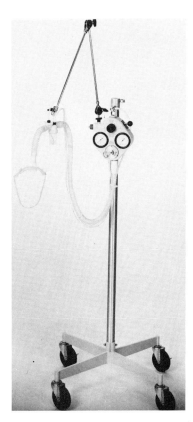

Fig. 11-12. Intermittent positive-pressure breathing (IPPB) therapy. (Courtesy Puritan Bennett Corporation, Kansas City, Mo.)

mined pressure, and the pressure cycle will not be completed until that pressure is reached. If there is any obstruction, such as mucus in the respiratory tract, the time for the pressure to be reached will be shortened. If there should be any malfunction of the machine such as a leak, the inhalation phase of the cycle will be prolonged.

The volume-cycled ventilator is set to deliver a predetermined volume of air into the lungs. When the volume of air has been reached, that phase of the cycle ends and the lungs are allowed to deflate. The entire cycle is then repeated. The volume-cycled ventilator may be set as a time-cycled ventilator in which the lungs will inflate and deflate on a predetermined time interval.

When mechanical ventilation is used, some form of humidity must be supplied to prevent drying of mucous membranes and thickening of respiratory secretions.

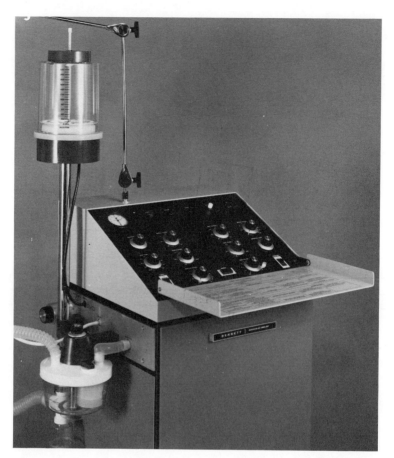

Fig. 11-13. Volume-cycled ventilation. (Courtesy Puritan Bennett Corporation, Kansas City, Mo.)

The volume-cycled ventilator is frequently used for seriously ill patients when the ability of the lungs to respond has been compromised.[6]

Patients receiving mechanical ventilation therapy must be carefully monitored and machines must be carefully set and changed to meet the changing needs of the patient. The patient may have a tracheostomy or an endotracheal tube with the machine attached to the tube. Tidal volume and blood gas studies are made as long as the patient is receiving ventilation therapy. When frequent studies are required, a catheter may be placed in the femoral artery to avoid frequent arterial punctures.

The nursing care of the patient receiving ventilation therapy includes positioning to provide for maximum breathing, turning the patient every hour, and carrying out passive range-of-motion exercises.

The patient should be observed for color, character of respirations, blood pressure, and pulse rate. All intake and output should be recorded. Suctioning of secretions may be necessary to prevent aspiration, and secretions should be observed for color, amount, and consistency. Specimens may be sent to the laboratory for cultures. Before administering sedatives or narcotics the blood pressure and pulse rate should be checked. If bronchodilating drugs or aerosols are administered, the patient should be observed for side effects or toxic signs. Adequate nutrition and fluid balance should be maintained. The nurse should provide emotional support and explanations of procedures and use of equipment if the patient is conscious.

Rotating tourniquets. The objective of the application and rotation of tourniquets is to decrease venous pressure and venous

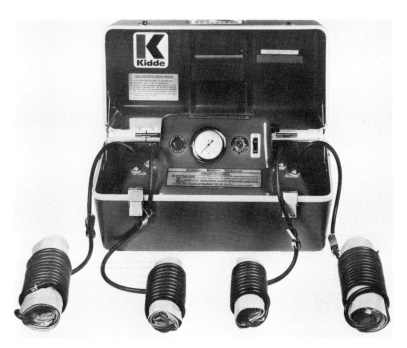

Fig. 11-14. Kidde automatic rotating tourniquet. (Courtesy Walter Kidde & Co., Inc., Belleville, N. J.)

return to the heart. This allows more blood to be pooled temporarily in the extremities and slows it return to the heart.

The physician orders the procedure and specifies the interval for rotation and the time that the procedure is to be continued. It then becomes the responsibility of the nurse to understand the technique of compression and release of the tourniquets and to recognize any complications should they occur.

When rotating tourniquets are ordered, any of the following methods may be used: (1) four blood pressure cuffs (if available), (2) the commercial automatic rotating tourniquet machine that is supplied with four pneumatic cuffs (Fig. 11-14), or (3) the use of four rubber tubes about 1 to 1½ inches in diameter and 2 feet in length. The tourniquets are placed on the distal third of the arm between the elbow and the shoulder and on the distal third of the thigh between the knee and the hip. One extremity is always left free. The tourniquets should be placed over the pajama sleeeves and legs, and a cotton pad or small towel may be used under the tourniquets. The tourniquet is secured with a slipknot and must not

be tight enough to obliterate the arterial pulse. Moving clockwise or counterclockwise, one tourniquet is removed at the prescribed interval, usually 15 minutes. The fourth tourniquet is applied first and then one is removed so that tourniquets are on three extremities at one time. The procedure continues for the time specified by the physician. When the tourniquets are discontinued they are removed one at a time, observing the same order and interval until all have been removed (Fig. 11-15). The nurse should maintain a time schedule at the bedside, so that the procedure may be carried out in the proper order.

If the patient is conscious, the procedure and its purpose should be explained to him. The blood pressure should be taken before beginning the procedure and at intervals during the procedure. The pulse should be taken after the application of each tourniquet. The tourniquet must be tight enough to occlude the venous flow but must not occlude the arterial flow. If the arterial flow is occluded, it may cause pulmonary embolism or phlebothrombosis (p. 210). When the procedure has been completed, the nurse should complete the patient's record with the following information: (1) the time the procedure was begun and ended, (2) the interval of rotation, (3) blood pressure and pulse readings, (4) any medications given, (5) urinary output, and (6) the patient's response to the procedure.

During the procedure the nurse should observe the patient for hypotension and any decreased urinary output. If they should occur, it should be reported immediately.

Oxygen therapy. The administration of oxygen is supportive treatment for patients in whom pulmonary ventilation is deficient. There are many methods now available for oxygen therapy. Some common types of equipment include catheters, masks, cannulas, and tents. Many hospitals have oxygen from a central source piped to wall outlets in the patient's room. When this is not available, tanks of compressed oxygen are used. Whichever source is used, provision must be made for humidification of the oxygen before it is delivered to the patient. There is no one best way to administer oxygen, and the decision to administer it, the amount, and the method depend on the purpose for which it is given. These are decisions to be made by the physician. The effectiveness of oxygen in the treatment of the patient depends on the pathologic process present. The physician will indicate the method by which oxygen is to be given and the number of liters per minute on the order

for oxygen. The nurse responsible for carrying out the order should act promptly and should remember that although oxygen may be beneficial, it may also be dangerous. Therefore when the patient is receiving oxygen he should be carefully observed.

Many patients and their families believe that oxygen is administered as a last resort. Although it is true that most patients receiving oxygen are seriously ill, the nurse should make every effort to reassure the patient and relieve the anxiety of the family. If the patient is conscious or even semiconscious, the nurse should explain the procedure to him, telling him that it will help him to breathe better and will make him more comfortable. If the patient is sick enough to receive oxygen, the method of administration should be such that he will receive the maximum benefit from it. To achieve this the nurse must be familiar with the equipment and know that it is in working order.

Oropharyngeal insufflation. From studies that have been made, oropharyngeal insufflation (commonly referred to as nasal oxygen) is the most efficient method of administering oxygen. The plastic transparent catheters are more comfortable for the patient, less irritating, and easier to clean than those made of rubber (Fig. 11-16). Several catheters should be available at the bedside so that the patient will not be without oxygen when the catheter is being cleaned or changed. The

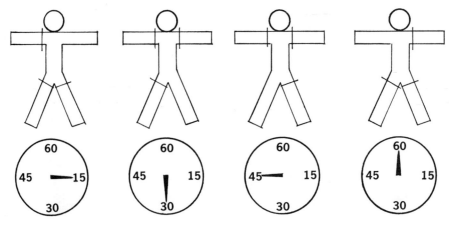

Fig. 11-15. Diagrammatic illustration of procedure for rotating tourniquets to reduce pulmonary edema. Note that the tourniquets are rotated clockwise each 15 minutes and that one extremity always remains free.

gauge should be set at the number of liters ordered by the physician and the oxygen allowed to flow through the catheter while it is being inserted. The catheter should be lubricated with a water-soluble jelly before it is introduced. Mineral oil should not be used because of the danger of the patient's aspirating the oil, which may cause pneumonia. After insertion the catheter should be taped to the forehead. Securing the catheter this way helps to prevent secretions from becoming encursted on the catheter and obstructing the flow of oxygen. It is recommended that a stop

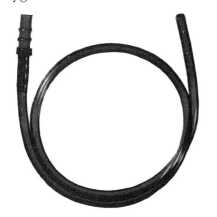

Fig. 11-16. Oxygen catheter. (Courtesy Becton, Dickinson & Co., Rutherford, N. J.)

be placed on the catheter near the nostril to prevent the catheter from slipping back into the esophagus, which might cause a serious complication (Fig. 11-17). Catheters should be changed ever 4 to 6 hours, or more often if necessary, alternating the nostrils. If disposable catheters are not used, catheters should be washed with warm soapy water and sterilized in a 1:1000 solution of benzalkonium chloride (Zephiran). The oxygen must be passed through distilled water, which acts as a humidifier, and most receptacles for water are marked to show the proper water level. The container should not be filled above the level indicated, or water will be sprayed into the patient's lungs. The oxygen must be turned off when the container is being refilled. (Refer to a textbook on basic nursing.)

Oxygen by mask. A well-fitting mask will give the desired concentration of oxygen; however, the size and shape of the patient's face may interfere with close fitting, and certain types of masks such as plastic do not mold easily to the contour of the face. There are several different types of masks available, including the nasal type, which covers only the nose, and the oronasal type, which covers both the nose and the mouth. Disposable plas-

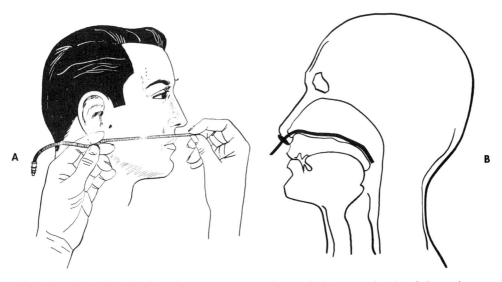

Fig. 11-17. Method for inserting an oxygen catheter. **A,** Measure the tip of the catheter from the end of the nose to the tragus of the ear and mark the place on the catheter with a small bit of adhesive tape. **B,** When the catheter is inserted and the length measured, the tip of the catheter should be just visible beside the soft palate in the throat.

tic masks are available in the oronasal type and are useful for patients with communicable disease. Their use saves time required in the cleaning, disinfection, and storage of other types of masks. A mask may be a rebreathing type, in which the patient rebreathes with each inspiration a portion of the air exhaled with the previous expiration, together with incoming oxygen. The mask may also be a nonbreathing type, in which the exhaled air escapes and a valve prevents it from being rebreathed. The Venturi mask is a disposable mask that provides for a mixture of air and oxygen in a constant concentration and eliminates any concentration of carbon dioxide.[8] The rebreathing mask is connected to a breathing bag, which the nurse should watch carefully, since the movement of the bag helps to indicate the efficiency of the system. If the bag collapses completely on inspiration, there may be too much leakage around the mask. The head strap should be adjusted to the position most comfortable for the patient, which is usually below the ears. All patients do not tolerate oxygen by mask equally well. The patient who is apprehensive or who has acute dyspnea may have a feeling of suffocation. Depending on the patient's condition, the mask should be removed and the face bathed and dried every 2 hours.

Oxygen by nasal cannula. The oxygen cannula is made of plastic and consists of two prongs that are placed in the nostrils and either a strap about the head or a plastic bow similar to the bow on glasses, which fits over the ear. The cannula will deliver a low concentration of oxygen, and if the patient breathes through the mouth, little benefit will be obtained from the oxygen. Proper placement of the prongs is important to avoid a direct stream of oxygen against the nasal mucosa, and despite correct positioning of the prongs, a greater degree of nasal drying occurs with this method. The double nasal cannula is used when an extremely low concentration of oxygen is needed, or it may be used as a placebo for its psychologic effect.

Oxygen by tent. There are many different types of oxygen tents, which, if properly humidified and cooled, may deliver oxygen in high concentrations. However,

many hospitals are limiting the use of oxygen tents for adult patients, since the concentration of oxygen is difficult to control. Successful results from oxygen therapy depend on uninterrupted administration. When oxygen tents must be entered often, the concentration falls rapidly and hypoxia may develop. Administration of oxygen by the other methods described largely prevents this occurrence. If a tent is used, it must be well tucked in, and a plastic or rubber sheet should cover the mattress to prevent the escape of oxygen through the mattress.

Oxygen precautions. Regardless of what method of oxygen administration is used, certain precautions must be adhered to when a patient is receiving oxygen. "No smoking" signs should be conspicuously displayed, and the patient and his visitors must understand that smoking is not permitted, since oxygen supports combustion. Electric appliances such as heating pads, razors, blankets, or call signals should not be used. The use of electric hot plates for hot compresses should be avoided. Although the practice is not uniform, it is recommended that equipment such as suction, x-ray, and electrocardiographic machines be used with extreme caution. When oxygen tanks are being used, they should be secured in such a way that they will not be tipped over. They should not be placed near lamps, radiators, or other heating devices.

Hyperbaric oxygen. The use of hyperbaric oxygen in the treatment of disease is still in the experimental stage. Not all authorities agree on its value; however, most agree that it may serve as an adjunct to other therapy. It has been reported that twenty-eight different conditions are being treated with hyperbaric oxygen, including cancer, in which it has been used as an adjunct to radiation therapy and perfusion with some of the new drugs.[11, 21] Researchers have also determined that there is danger of severe side effects from hyperbaric oxygen. Hyperbaric oxygenation is achieved by exposing the patient to pressure greater than normal atmospheric pressure. As a result, the amount of oxygen dissolved in the plasma is increased, causing an increase in the tissues of the body. Therapy is carried out in either small or large steel chambers in which the patient may enter alone or with staff members,[7] and all personnel involved are subjected to rigid physical examination and training.

NURSING THE PATIENT WITH DISEASES AND DISORDERS OF THE RESPIRATORY SYSTEM

Diseases of the respiratory system may result from many different causes, including infection, benign or malignant tumors, physical or chemical agents, allergy, senescence, and emotional factors. Specific symptoms will vary with the particular disease; however, characteristic of many diseases are coughing, with or without sputum, hemoptysis, dyspnea, cyanosis, and pain. Chest pain is usually related to breathing difficulty, since the pleura, lungs, and bronchi do not have nerves that transmit pain impulses. Respiratory diseases can be classified in many ways, but generally they fall into two groups: those that are not infectious and those that are infectious, which are caused by specific disease organisms.

Noninfectious respiratory conditions
Epistaxis

Nosebleed is rarely fatal or even serious, but it may cause the patient considerable anxiety. There are a number of causes of epistaxis. The nasal cavities are supplied by a fine network of blood capillaries, and anything that causes congestion of the nasal membrane may rupture a small capillary and result in bleeding. The condition may occur in persons with hypertension, cardiovascular disease, blood dyscrasias, and some communicable diseases. Epistaxis may also be caused by injury to the nose, picking, or forceful blowing. The cause should be determined by a careful examination, including laboratory tests.

Treatment and nursing care. Nursing procedures include placing the patient in Fowler's position with the head forward. The patient should be encouraged to let the blood drain from the nose, breathe through the mouth, and avoid swallowing the blood, since this may cause nausea and vomiting. The nostrils are then compressed tightly below the bone and held

for 10 minutes or longer. This procedure will control most cases of epistaxis. Other procedures include holding ice in the mouth, placing iced compresses over the nose, holding an ice collar to the throat, and spraying the nostrils with phenylephrine (Neo-Synephrine). If bleeding cannot be controlled, the physician should be called, and it may be necessary to pack the nose. Hemostatic agents such as Gelfoam, packing saturated with 1:1000 solution of epinephrine, petroleum gauze, and oxidized cellulose (Oxycel) are often used. In rare cases it may be necessary to cauterize the bleeding vessel.

Chronic obstructive pulmonary disease (COPD)

Diseases that interfere with ventilation cause psychologic, physical, and social problems for the individual. Fear, tension, frustration, and panic accompany these diseases. One of the most important aspects of medical and nursing care is the relief of anxiety. Inadequate ventilation causes a disturbance in the homeostasis of the body. Electrolyte balance is affected, changes occur in the extracellular fluid, and serious cardiac complications may occur. The constant shortness of breath, fatigue, and limitation of activity may cause retirement from gainful employment, limitation of social activities, and feelings of social isolation and depression. Chronic obstructive pulmonary diseases include emphysema, chronic bronchitis, asthma, and bronchiectasis, each of which may result in varying degrees of incapacitation for the individual.

Pulmonary emphysema

Pulmonary emphysema affects persons of all social and economic levels. It has been estimated that 10 million persons in the United States have emphysema and that one of every four wage earners who is past 45 years of age is disabled because of the disease. The disease is more common in men than in women, and reports indicate that most men past 70 years of age have destructive emphysema. The cause of emphysema is unknown; however, it is known that chronic bronchitis and asthma are frequently associated with emphysema. Research has indicated that cigarette smoking is the most important agent in the development of pulmonary emphysema.[19] Air pollution in heavily polluted and industrial areas, changes in temperature, and humidity appear to have an adverse effect on the disease.

Pathophysiology. In pulmonary emphysema the alveolar walls and capillaries are destroyed, resulting in a decreased area available for the exchange of gases between the bloodstream and the air. Chronic irritation to the bronchi, bronchioles, and alveoli causes an inflammation, with swelling and secretions. This process tends to narrow the lumen of the bronchioles, especially during expiration, and air becomes trapped in the alveoli. The alveoli become distended and as the process continues, they rupture or become scarred and thickened with loss of elasticity. Infections hasten the process. Expiration of air depends on the elasticity of the lungs. There is less muscular effort required during inspiration than during expiration. Because of the lost elasticity and the obstructed bronchioles, all of the inspired air cannot be forced out of the lungs. There is increased pressure in the alveoli, causing them to collapse. Distended air sacs (blebs) that occur on the surface of the lung may rupture and allow air to enter the pleural cavity, causing spontaneous pneumothorax. The pathologic changes cause a decrease in vital capacity and an increase in the residual volume of air retained in the lungs. Oxygenation of the arterial blood is decreased, and carbon dioxide tension of the arterial blood is increased. The retention of carbon dioxide in the blood may result in respiratory acidosis or carbon dioxide narcosis, stupor, and coma.

Dyspnea, chronic shortness of breath, hypoxia, and coughing with copious amounts of mucopurulent sputum are physiologic manifestations of the disease. Any emotional upset, exertion, or excitement increases the dyspnea and respiratory stress.

Treatment and nursing care. The most important factor in the treatment of patients with emphysema is prevention. The patient should be protected from respiratory infections, the occurrence of which intensify his breathing problems. Many physicians believe that an antibiotic should be administered to emphysema patients during the fall and winter months. Laboratory examination of sputum should be done to determine the specific bacteria present. Tetracycline or another broad-spectrum drug is usually given. The patient should be encouraged to secure influenza vaccine early in the fall. Since cigarette smoking is hazardous, every effort should be made to persuade the patient to discontinue the habit. The patient should avoid drafts and changes of temperature. Windows should be kept closed, and air conditioning is desirable. The patient should have a sleeping room and bath on the first floor if possible.[14] Treatment is palliative and is directed toward making breathing as easy as possible. Some patients do better in moderate climates with minimum temperature changes.

Coughing is the emphysema patient's first defense. Expectorants and high humidity will loosen secretions. Intermittent positive-pressure breathing treatments can humidify and administer medications deep into the lungs. Low, small, grunting coughs while the abdominal muscles are supported usually produces the best results. The patient may be taught to inhale by using his stomach muscles and exhale by blowing gently through pursed lips. Chest physical therapy such as percussion, vibrating, and postural drainage is often effective in removing secretions from affected lungs.[18]

Bronchodilators may be helpful for patients with bronchial obstruction. Ephedrine sulfate, 25 mg. orally, may be administered twice or three times a day. Other medications used include aminophylline preparations, which are administered in rectal suppositories. Isoproterenol hydrochloride in a 1:200 solution used in a nebulizer helps some patients. In patients in whom the bronchodilating drugs become ineffective, small doses of steroids may be given. Usually 5 to 10 mg. of prednisone given orally once a day may be ordered. If steroid therapy is continued, the patient must have an increased intake of potassium.[6] Intermittent positive-pressure breathing has provided considerable relief for some patients, and use of the rocking bed may help to make breathing easier.

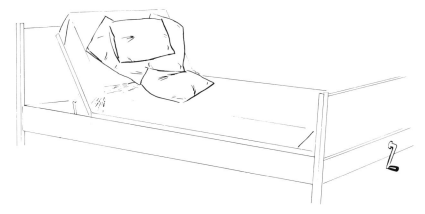

Fig. 11-18. When the head of the bed is elevated 45 degrees or more, pillows may be placed with one lengthwise along the back, one on each side at a diagonal position, and one crossways to support the head.

Because of the constant high level of carbon dioxide in the blood and tissues of the emphysema patient, his body has come to rely on low levels of oxygen as the main stimulus for respiration. Administering oxygen to such a patient would depress his respirations. If ordered, oxygen should not be administered except for brief periods under medical supervision. It should be started extremely slowly and the patient observed for restlessness, apprehension, flushed skin, shallow respirations, and stupor. The patient should also be observed for signs of right ventricular failure (cor pulmonale). The capillaries in the lungs have been destroyed by the disease process, and the heart has to work harder to pump blood through the diseased lungs. Edema of the feet and legs and distended neck veins may indicate the onset of right ventricular failure. Gastric ulcers also tend to occur in patients with emphysema, although the specific cause is unknown.

Physical therapy should be part of the patient's therapy program. Its purpose is to recondition and strengthen muscles that have become soft and flabby and have lost their tone because of inactivity. The patient should be encouraged to follow a graded program of daily exercise. The patient usually breathes most easily when sitting up. See Fig. 11-18 for placement of pillows. The patient may feel less well in the morning because secretions have collected in the lungs and bronchi during the night. A hot drink may help to loosen tenacious sputum so that it may be coughed up. By the end of the day the patient may feel completely exhausted. He should be encouraged to care for himself within the limits of his ability. The diet should be nourishing, eliminating gas-forming foods. The appetite may be poor, and several small attractive meals a day may be better than large meals. The taking of fluids should be encouraged to avoid the tendency toward dehydration. The nose and mouth should be kept clean, and all nursing care should be adapted to the needs of the individual patient. These needs will change as the disease progresses, and the physician, nurse, patient, and family must work together to plan a way of life for the patient.

Chronic bronchitis

Chronic bronchitis often occurs with pulmonary emphysema. In pulmonary emphysema it is possible to define pathologic changes in the lungs. In chronic bronchitis the changes are largely functional and cannot be observed on x-ray examination. However, physiologic findings in obstructive chronic bronchitis are similar to pulmonary emphysema. The incidence of chronic bronchitis is greater among persons who smoke cigarettes. Although other inhalants including air pollution may be contributing factors, it has been demonstrated that severe air pollution aggravates the disorder and may cause respiratory failure.

It is generally accepted that cigarette smoking is the primary etiologic factor in chronic bronchitis.

Pathophysiology. In chronic bronchitis there is an abnormal increase in the mucus-secreting cells of the bronchial epithelium and the mucus-secreting cells of the trachea. The goblet cells (so-called because of their shape) of the surface epithelium are increased. The bronchi become thickened, and fibrosis of the bronchioles with infiltration by inflammatory cells may occur. Chronic infection of the mucous membrane is usually present, and the sputum may contain a variety of pathogenic microorganisms. The normal function of the cilia is impaired so that they are unable to move secretions upward where they may be coughed up. Because of this, mucous secretions may form plugs in small bronchi, where they provide a media for infection.

The most common physiologic response in chronic bronchitis is a chronic persistent cough with large amounts of sticky, but fairly thin liquid mucus. In the presence of shortness of breath the vital capacity is reduced, and dyspnea, cyanosis, and wheezing occur. Severely debilitated patients may be unable to cough and clear the respiratory passages, and respiratory function is compromised.

Treatment and nursing care. The treatment is primarily directed toward a program of personal hygienic living. The patient should secure adequate sleep and rest, a well-balanced diet, and some recreational activity. He should be cautioned to avoid exposure to respiratory infections, dust, and other irritants. Work that requires the individual to be outside during cold or wet weather should be avoided. If change of employment is necessary, the patient may be referred to the Social and Rehabilitation Service.

The most effective single factor in treatment is to require that the patient stop smoking. Most methods of treatment including bronchodilators, intermittent positive-pressure breathing, nebulized agents, and oral medications have been shown to have limited effect on chronic bronchitis. However, some patients may think that they do provide some relief. Although antibiotics are often administered to prevent infection, the time to begin such therapy is debatable among physicians. When chronic bronchitis with obstruction of the airways has existed over a long period of time, the patient may develop respiratory failure and right ventricular failure.[2]

The nursing care of the hospitalized patient with chronic bronchitis is essentially the same as that for emphysema.

Asthma

Asthma can be classified as *extrinsic asthma*, meaning that it is caused by substance(s) outside the body; these substances are antigens to which the individual is hypersensitive. About half of all persons with asthma fall into this category. When it is impossible to determine any extrinsic factor, the disease is considered to be *intrinsic asthma*, or asthma resulting from internal causes. Most frequently intrinsic asthma is caused by chronic recurrent respiratory infection. There is no cure as such for asthma. About one in four persons who develop the disease in childhood will have a spontaneous recovery, and about an equal number will become progressively worse. Few adults with asthma have a spontaneous recovery, and most become progressively worse, with attacks lasting longer, becoming more frequent, and gradually becoming chronic. Most asthma in elderly persons is chronic and probably contributes to pulmonary emphysema.

Pathophysiology. In acute attacks of asthma the lumina of the small bronchi become narrow and edematous with spasm of the bronchial muscles. The mucus-secreting glands of the bronchi secrete a thick tenacious mucus, which obstructs the narrowed passages of the bronchi. Inspiration and expiration become difficult, and in an effort to get more air the patient uses the auxiliary muscles of respiration. More air is forced into the lungs than can be expelled, causing the lungs to increase in size. The vital capacity is decreased, whereas there is an increase in the residual volume of air. Because of the inadequate ventilation, cyanosis occurs. The heart is not affected, and the respiratory rate remains about normal. After the acute attack subsides the narrow lumen widens and the patient is able to cough and produce large amounts of thick stringy sputum. Although the lungs return to their normal size after an attack, continued episodes will lead to permanent impairment and emphysema.

The characteristic physiologic symptom of asthma is shortness of breath, accompanied by wheezing and coughing. The asthmatic attacks come in paroxysms, in which the patient breathes with a great deal of difficulty and in which it requires tremendous effort to get enough air into and out of the lungs. Respiratory rates are usually normal, but expirations are prolonged. As a result of the ventilation difficulty, the patient may become cyanotic, and in prolonged attacks, asphyxiation and death may occur. The patient generally perspires freely, the pulse may be weak, nausea and diarrhea may occur in children, and the patient may complain of pain in the chest caused by the respiratory effort. Children are more likely to have an elevation of temperature, which is often caused by some infection. The cough of persons with asthma is usually tight and dry in the beginning, but as the attack continues, there is thin mucous secretion that becomes copious, thick, and stringy and is expectorated with difficulty.[5]

Treatment and nursing care. Treatment and care of asthma is directed toward three factors: (1) relief of the immediate attack, (2) control of causal factors, and (3) general care of the patient.

Parents of asthmatic children may anticipate an approaching attack, and medication that provides sedation and bronchodilation should be given early. A combination of drugs such as short-acting barbiturate and ephedrine is frequently used. Adequate hydration should be provided by offering the child small drinks at frequent intervals. If the attack progresses, 0.1 to 0.2 ml. of a 1:1000 solution of epinephrine may be given subcutaneously. Adults with an attack of asthma may be given 0.3 to 0.5 ml. of epinephrine in a 1:1000 solution subcutaneously or intramuscularly. For long-lasting effects, epinephrine in oil in a 1:500 preparation may be ordered every 6 hours. Other drugs used in the treatment of an attack of asthma include ephedrine, 25 mg. every 4 hours, and a combination of ephedrine, aminophylline, and phenobarbital, 0.25 to 0.5 Gm., if the attack is not relieved with epinephrine. Tranquilizers

are frequently used, and terpin hydrate with codeine elixir, 5 ml. every 4 hours for coughing, may be administered. Many ambulatory patients benefit from nebulizers used with isoproterenol hydrochloride (Isuprel) or a similar drug. Intermittent positive-pressure breathing with oxygen or compressed air may be used as in other obstructive pulmonary diseases.[2]

The control of asthma depends on finding the cause and eliminating it. If the disease is due to extrinsic factors (allergy), identification of the offending allergen may be made through skin tests, and the patient can be desensitized (p. 533). If intrinsic factors are suspected, a thorough physical examination should be made to determine a source of infection, specific organisms, or other physicial factors.

Patients with asthma should be advised against smoking and should avoid exposure to cold wet weather. A program of personal hygiene, with sleep, rest, and breathing exercises, should be instituted. During an acute attack of asthma the nurse should make the patient as comfortable as possible, and the patient is often more comfortable and better able to breathe if he is in a sitting position. The overbed table may be prepared as for the cardiac patient (Chapter 13) and placed in front of the patient. Since the patient perspires profusely, clothing and bed linens should be changed frequently to keep him dry and prevent chilling. The use of a vaporizer helps loosen secretions so that they may be expectorated more easily. Dietary orders should be carried out, and the patient should be encouraged to take an adequate amount of fluids. If the fluid intake is inadequate, intravenous fluids may be ordered. Most attacks subside in 30 to 60 minutes, although they may continue for days or weeks.[16] The patient who has frequent attacks of asthma eventually becomes resistant to all forms of treatment and may develop what is called *status asthmaticus,* in which acute symptoms continue and a prolonged attack can cause exhaustion and death from heart failure. Repeated attacks of status asthmaticus can result in emphysema.

Severe attacks of asthma are frightening to all concerned, and it is at this time that the patient needs reassurance and support.

The nurse should understand that asthma in itself is rarely serious and should maintain a calm attitude while caring for the patient.

Bronchiectasis

Bronchiectasis is characterized by a permanent dilation of one or more of the bronchi from repeated infections. A single lobe of one lung or one or more lobes in both lungs may be affected. There is a tendency for the left lung to be involved more often than the right lung. However, in approximately 50% of patients both lungs are involved. The cause of the disease is unkown, and although some cases are believed to be congenital, most appear to result from chronic bronchitis and severe attacks of infectious respiratory diseases. It is primarily a disease of the young, often affecting persons 20 years of age or younger. In the early stages there may be no symptoms, but as the disease progresses, the most characteristic symptom is a productive cough. The cough is worse in the morning, and any change in position may produce a paroxysm of coughing. The cough produces large amounts of purulent sputum, which may be tinged with blood, and hemoptysis occurs in a large number of patients although it usually is not serious. As the disease gradually becomes worse, fever, chills, fatigue, loss of weight, clubbing of the fingers, and loss of appetite may occur. Diagnosis is made by x-ray examination (bronchography) and bronchoscopy. The only cure is surgical removal of the affected area (lobectomy). However, each patient must be carefully evaluated in relation to pulmonary function and prognosis, since not all patients are suitable candidates for such surgery.

Treatment and nursing care. Palliative treatment consists of measures to improve the general health such as adequate diet, rest, and prevention of respiratory infections. Cigarette smoking, alcohol, and excessive exercise should be avoided. Irritants from air pollution may contribute to recurrent episodes of acute respiratory infection. Sputum cultures often indicate the presence of specific microorganisms, and antibiotic therapy for the particular pathogen is administered. Postural drainage should be a part of the patient's daily routine, and moist inhalations may help to thin tena-

cious sputum and make it easier to raise. Many patients are treated on an outpatient basis, but in severe exacerbation the patient is often admitted to the hospital. The nurse should encourage and reassure the patient and assist him with postural drainage or other chest therapy. Mouth care must be given several times a day, and the use of an antiseptic mouthwash before meals may be desirable. The patient should be confined to bed rest, and the nurse should be constantly on the alert for obstruction of the airway by large plugs of mucus.

Pulmonary embolism and infarction

Pulmonary embolism occurs when a blood clot or other foreign matter becomes lodged in a branch of the pulmonary artery or arteriole. Pulmonary infarction is death of a portion of lung tissue due to an insufficient blood supply, and it often occurs as a result of pulmonary embolism. Usually clots arise as the result of poor venous circulation or thrombosis, break away from the vein in which they were formed, and are carried by the venous blood through the right side of the heart and into the capillary system of the lungs, where they become lodged. Pulmonary embolism may occur as a postoperative or postpartum complication or from bed rest. The seriousness of the condition depends on the size of the blood vessel affected. If a large vessel is occluded, death may occur instantly. The symptoms will also vary with the severity of the condition, but the most common sign is a sudden chest pain. There may be a productive cough with blood-tinged sputum, rapid shallow respiration, fever, increased pulse rate, and in severe cases cyanosis and shock. The nurse may be the first person to observe the signs and should be alerted when the patient says that he has a severe pain in his chest.

Treatment and nursing care. Treatment includes absolute bed rest and the administration of anticoagulant drugs such as heparin sodium, usually given intravenously for its immediate effect, and bishydroxycoumarin (Dicumarol), administered orally. The nurse must remember that when the patient is receiving anticoagulant therapy, prothrombin time must be tested daily. The patient's breathing will be assisted by a high Fowler's position, and nursing care is similar to that of a patient with a myocardial infarction (p. 274). The major factor in pulmonary embolism is prevention, and the nurse shares much of the responsibility. The postoperative nursing care out-·lined in Chapter 9 holds the key to prevention. In addition, many surgeons require patients having major surgery to wear elastic stockings while in bed after surgery, and some require that the legs be wrapped with elastic bandages preoperatively to prevent the pooling of blood in the superficial veins of the legs.

Pulmonary edema

Pulmonary edema is always a medical emergency. Although it is caused by cardiac failure, it is the pulmonary system that is affected. Because of the failure of the left side of the heart to pump blood through the body adequately, excessive amounts of blood collect in the left side of the heart, the pulmonary veins, and pulmonary capillaries. The increased pressure in the capillaries causes the serous portion of the blood to be pushed through the capillaries into the alveoli. Fluid rapidly reaches the bronchioles, and the patient begins to suffocate in his own secretions. This acute condition is ever present in patients with chronic heart disease but can follow cerebrovascular accidents, head trauma, rapid administration of intravenous fluids, and poisoning from barbiturates and narcotics.

The patient with pulmonary edema becomes cyanotic and dyspneic. The pulse is weak and rapid, and respirations become wheezy in character and sound moist with gurgling. The patient is unable to breathe unless sitting up. He develops a productive cough with frothy pink-tinged sputum. He may be covered with cold clammy perspiration and is restless and apprehensive.

Treatment and nursing care. Objectives of care for the patient in acute pulmonary edema are to achieve physical and mental rest, relieve hypoxia, decrease the venous return to the heart, and improve the function of the heart. The nurse should remain with the patient, and he should be placed in a high Fowler's position, or he may be allowed to remain in any position in which he is most comfortable. Physical and mental relaxation is most important. Morphine sulfate may be given in doses of 10 to 15

mg. intravenously at 30-minute intervals until about 40 to 60 mg. has been given. Morphine helps to relieve anxiety and apprehension and helps to achieve muscular relaxation. Since morphine is a respiratory depressant, the patient must be carefully observed; morphine is generally not given to patients with obstructive pulmonary disease. Oxygen is administered using a nonrebreathing mask or nasal catheter that will deliver up to 100% oxygen (p. 202). If the patient has not previously received digitalization, one of the following cardiac stimulants is administered intravenously: G-strophanthin (ouabain), deslanoside (Cedilanid-D), or digoxin (Lanoxin). Cardiac stimulants administered by the intravenous route must be given slowly, and continuous cardiographic monitoring should be maintained. A diuretic such as furosemide (Lasix) is administered intravenously. Drugs administered intravenously produce more rapid results than when administered orally. The nurse should observe the patient for any undesirable effects from intravenous administration. If pulmonary edema is mild, diuretics and digitalis may be administered orally.[6]

Rotating tourniquets may be ordered to reduce the venous pressure and the venous return of blood to the right side of the heart (p. 200). The use of intermittent positive-pressure breathing is controversial, and belief in its value is not shared by all physicians. However, many factors must be considered by the physician when treating this serious condition. The function of the nurse is to remain with the patient, remain calm, provide support for him, and assist the physician by careful observation of the patient and by promptly securing any supplies or equipment needed. In Chapter 8 attention was called to administering intravenous fluids slowly to elderly patients. This is especially important when the patient's cardiac reserve is poor. Too rapid administration may cause pulmonary edema by increasing venous pressure and venous return.

Atelectasis and pneumothorax

The conditions of atelectasis and pneumothorax (Fig. 11-19) result in collapse of the lung, but under different circumstances and for different reasons. Atelectasis occurs from blockage of air to a portion of

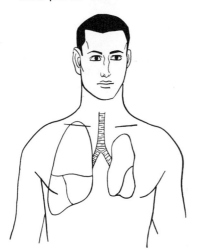

Fig. 11-19. Atelectasis, pneumothorax, and pneumoperitoneum all result in collapse of the lung.

the lung. It may occur from pressure against the lung due to air or fluid in the pleural cavity, tumors, enlarged heart, or any abdominal condition that pushes the diaphragm upward. It is a common postoperative complication when the patient breathes rapidly and shallowly to prevent pain from the surgical site. It may also result from an obstruction within one of the bronchi. A foreign body or a thick plug of mucus may completely occlude a bronchus, shutting off all air to a portion of the lung. As the air in the isolated part of the lung is absorbed by the capillaries and new air no longer enters, the part involved will then collapse. Treatment is removal of the obstruction by whatever means may be necessary.

Pneumothorax is a condition in which air fills the pleural space between the lung and the chest wall, and the lung consequently collapses. A common cause is the rupture of a bleb on the surface of the lung, which is a complication of emphysema. However, pneumothorax may occur during severe episodes of coughing in a patient with chronic respiratory disease. Chest injuries or wounds in which the membrane covering the lungs is torn allows air to escape into the pleural space. Spontaneous pneumothorax may occur without any known cause. A sharp sudden pain in the chest occurs, followed by dyspnea, diaphoresis, weak and rapid pulse, falling

blood pressure, and a lack of chest movement on the affected side; apprehension and shock sometimes follow. If the condition is not severe, the air may absorb or it may be aspirated with a needle, and a closed thoracotomy may be performed for some patients.

Treatment and nursing care. The care of the patient will depend to a large extent on the condition resulting in the collapse. Pain must be relieved and the patient made as comfortable as his condition will permit. The patient with spontaneous pneumothorax may be placed in a high Fowler's position and encouraged to breathe normally. The pulse and respiratory rates should be checked at frequent intervals and all exertion reduced to a minimum. X-ray films are usually taken to determine the amount of air in the chest cavity. Oxygen may be given and preparation made for a thoracentesis. A continuous flow of air into the pleural cavity may require closed-chest drainage.

Infectious respiratory conditions

An exceedingly large number of diseases of the respiratory tract are infectious and account for a great amount of illness. Most of these diseases, bacterial or viral in nature, find their way into the respiratory tract through breathing air saturated with the disease organism. Many infections follow a pattern, beginning with what appears to be a common cold but gradually involving all parts of the respiratory tract. A large number of infections of the lower respiratory tract have their beginnings with upper respiratory infection.

Pathophysiology. Invasion of the upper respiratory system by pathogenic microorganisms, usually viral, causes inflammation and edema of the mucous membranes. The mucus-secreting glands become hyperactive, producing large amounts of serous to mucopurulent exudate. The cervical lymph nodes enlarge and are tender. Air passages become occluded, causing impaired pulmonary ventilation. Respiratory rates increase in an effort to get more air to the lungs, and the heart works harder to supply the body's tissues with oxygen. The body mobilizes its forces to combat the invading pathogen, and leukocytosis occurs. The inflammatory condition of the mucous membranes causes the throat to become red, sore, and dry, the voice becomes hoarse, and there is a dry painful cough. The pathogen may invade the contiguous mucous membranes of the sinuses and the ears.

Acute coryza (common cold)

Acute coryza may be caused by one or several viruses. It is generally believed that the causative virus is constantly present in the upper respiratory tract and that a person's susceptibility may increase periodically from a wide variety of factors. Symptoms usually appear within 24 to 48 hours after exposure and may be transmitted to others several hours afterward. Symptoms include a chilly sensation, sneezing, and the nasal membranes feeling hot, dry, and congested. A slight throat irritation may occur, followed by a thin, serous nasal discharge. The nasal congestion causes pressure, which results in headache and tenderness of the cervical lymph nodes. If the infection remains uncomplicated, it generally subsides in approximately 1 week. If the nasal discharge becomes purulent, it is an indication that the infection is complicated by bacterial invasion.

Acute pharyngitis

Bacteria or viruses from acute coryza may extend to the pharynx, or pharyngitis may occur without prior evidence of a cold. The throat becomes inflamed and red, the tonsils and cervical lymph nodes become tender, and there may be a sensation of rawness and a dry cough. Chronic pharyngitis may occur from chronic infection of the sinuses or nasal mucosa and may not produce any significant symptoms. Acute pharyngitis usually responds to symptomatic treatment, with recovery occurring in about a week. If the condition is caused by one of several bacteria such as the hemolytic streptococcus, *Staphylococcus aureus*, or *Haemophilus influenzae*, symptoms may be more serious, and complications may occur.

Acute laryngitis

Acute laryngitis is generally secondary to other upper respiratory infections. The mucous membrane lining the larynx becomes inflamed, and the vocal cords be-come swollen. The disease is characterized by hoarseness or loss of voice and cough. Acute laryngitis sometimes occurs in children, especially at night (croup), and results in an alarming dyspnea that usually is not serious. The child should not be left alone. Often the attack can be relieved by warm, moist inhalations or for very young children, a croup tent. Although rare, a tracheotomy may be required in some cases. If it remains uncomplicated, acute laryngitis usually clears in a few days.

Tonsillitis

Acute follicular tonsillitis is an acute inflammation of the tonsils, often caused by streptococcus or staphylococcus bacteria. The throat is sore and painful, swallowing is difficult, and there is generalized aching of muscles with chills and an elevation of temperature. If tonsillitis is caused by the hemolytic streptococcus, the symptoms may be more severe, with nausea and vomiting and an increase in the leukocyte count. The primary concern is the prevention of complications such as rheumatic fever and nephritis. Repeated attacks of tonsillitis may require surgical removal of the tonsils.

Sinusitis

Sinusitis may be acute or may become chronic. It usually occurs as the result of other upper respiratory infections, and since mucous membranes of the nasal cavities are continuous with the sinuses, infection may be easily spread to the sinuses. Inflammation of the sinuses may occur from obstructions such as nasal polyps or from a deviated septum that blocks the drainage from the sinuses (p. 218). It may also be a complication of influenza or pneumonia. If an acute sinusitis is left untreated, it may become chronic or it may lead to more serious conditions such as meningitis, brain abscess, osteomyelitis, and septicemia. The primary symptom of sinusitis is pain, and its location is related to the sinus involved. When the maxillary sinus is affected, the pain occurs over the cheeks and may radiate downward to the teeth. Frontal sinus infection causes pain in and above the eyes. The bone over the affected sinus is usually sensitive to slight pressure, and puffiness over the area may be observed. Depending on the extent of the infection and the particular microorganism involved, the patient may have an elevation of temperature, nausea, and loss of appetite. When there is a continuous postnasal dripping into the back of the throat, coughing and soreness of the throat may result. Acute sinusitis causes discomfort and frequently results in loss in working time.[17]

Treatment and nursing care of upper respiratory infections

The treatment of upper respiratory infections is directed toward relief from the discomfort of symptoms and prevention of complications. Bed rest is desirable during the acute stage of the infection, and precautionary measures should be taken to prevent the spread of the infection to others. Nasal sprays, moist inhalations, hot saline gargles, throat irrigations, and aspirin provide symptomatic relief. Drugs should not be taken without a physician's order. At the present time antibiotics are not considered effective in respiratory infections of viral origin. Fluid intake should be increased, and if the temperature is elevated more than 1°, medical attention should be secured. When pharyngitis or laryngitis accompanies acute coryza, relief may be obtained by steam inhalations or an ice collar for the throat. If coughing is disturbing, an analgesic cough mixture or a mild sedative for rest at night may be ordered. When severe pharyngitis is present, the nurse should be alert to the possibility of dangerous complications. Temperature, pulse, and respiration should be checked every 4 hours unless otherwise ordered. The diet should be liquid or soft, with forcing of fluids. There should be daily bowel evacuation using enemas or mild laxatives if necessary. If the infection is caused by bacteria such as streptococci, the patient should be observed for skin rash, which might indicate scarlet fever. Blood cultures, white blood cell count, and urinalysis may be ordered. In bacterial infections there may be an elevation of the white blood cell count. When the larynx is involved, talking should be avoided or reduced. Antibiotic drugs may be ordered when the infection is caused by bacteria. Most patients with respiratory infections are more comfortable if they are placed in a low (15 degrees) Fowler's position, which provides for better drainage of secretions. A cool (68° to 70° F.) well-ventilated room with high humidity that is free from drafts provides a greater degree of comfort than an overheated room.

Influenza

There is a tendency for persons to associate certain repiratory symptoms with influenza, and one frequently hears the statement, "I have the flu." In reality most of these persons do not have true influenza but one of the respiratory infections just reviewed. Epidemics and pandemics of influenza have been known since the sixteenth century. The worst pandemic of modern times occurred in 1918 and 1919, when it was estimated that 20 million persons died, over half of these in the United States. It was during this epidemic that the disease was named *influenza*. In 1957 and 1958 a serious epidemic of influenza (Asian influenza) occurred, with more than 7000 deaths in the United States. The disease occurs in cycles, but there is evidence that variations of specific strains cause sporadic illness during nonepidemic years.

The disease is caused by a virus that has been identified and classified as type A, B, or C. Type D is now known as parainfluenza 1, and strains of A are known as A prime, or A_1 and A_2. In 1968, 1969, and extending into 1974, various parts of the world, including the United States, experienced a fairly mild form of influenza caused by a new strain of the A_2 virus, which has been called *A_2 Hong Kong–like virus*. The first symptoms of influenza occur with unbelievable rapidity, and the typical picture is one of chills, elevated temperature of from 102° to 104° F., severe aching of back, head, and extremities, sore throat, cough, considerable prostration, sneezing, coated tongue, and weakness. If the infection is uncomplicated, the acute period usually lasts from 3 to 5 days. Some cases do not follow the typical pattern but begin with gastrointestinal symptoms, bronchopneumonia, pleurisy, or sinusitis. Influenza is especially hazardous for elderly persons, and mortality rates from influenza-pneumonia generally rise sharply during an influenza epidemic.

Treatment and nursing care. The patient should remain on a regimen of bed rest during the acute phase and for 2 or 3 days after the temperature returns to normal. He should avoid overheated or cold rooms and should be protected against chilling. Analgesic and antipyretic drugs may be administered to relieve discomfort and reduce fever, and sedative cough mixtures may be given to relieve throat irritation. Fluid intake should be from 3000 to 5000 ml. a day. Humidity provided by steam inhalations helps to keep nasal passages clear and soothes inflamed membranes. The patient with influenza is uncomfortable and feels very ill; however, influenza alone usually is not serious. The danger lies in complications caused by streptococcus or staphylococcus bacteria. Bronchopneumonia is the most frequent complication, and very young, elderly, or debilitated persons are more likely to develop pneumonia.

It is recommended that persons with uncomplicated influenza remain at home on a regimen of bed rest. If admitted to the hospital, the patient runs the risk of acquiring a bacterial infection that could cause serious complications. It is well to remember that viral infections are self-limiting and that there is no drug that will cure them.

At the present time immunization for influenza is not recommended for healthy adults and children. Although its effectiveness may be limited, it is advised for persons of all ages who have debilitating diseases such as rheumatic heart disease, cardiovascular disorders, chronic broncho-pulmonary disease, and diabetes. The individual should be given one dose of the vaccine according to the manufacturer's directions. Local or mild systemic reactions occur in about half the persons receiving the vaccine. The vaccine should not be given to anyone who is hypersensitive to eggs.[12]

Acute bronchitis

Bronchitis is caused by inflammation of the bronchial tree and the trachea. As a rule, it is secondary to infection in the upper respiratory tract, but it may result from bronchial irritation caused by exposure to chemical agents or as a complica-

tion of communicable diseases such as measles. Acute bronchitis usually begins with hoarseness and cough, slight elevation in temperature, muscular aching, and headache. The cough may be dry and painful, but it gradually becomes productive. Bed rest is indicated as long as there is an elevation of temperature, and treatment should be directed toward preventing the extension of the infection. Either plain or medicated steam inhalations soothe irritated respiratory passages. Aerosol therapy may be given, and antibiotics may be ordered. Sedative or expectorant drugs may be ordered for the cough. If no complications occur, recovery may be expected in about a week.

Pneumonia

Pneumonia is a disease of the lungs caused by bacteria or any of several viral agents. It may occur in comatose or oversedated patients and in those whose pulmonary ventilation is inadequate. It may result from aspiration of infected secretions from the upper respiratory tract. Pneumonia may complicate certain viral diseases such as measles or influenza, and it may cause complications including empyema, septicemia, meningitis, and endocarditis. Most pneumonia is caused by *Diplococcus pneumoniae* (pneumococcus).

Pathophysiology. Infected secretions from the upper respiratory tract drain into the alveoli, where the normal defense mechanisms such as ciliary action and coughing are unable to remove them. An inflammatory process begins, and increased amounts of edema fluid are released in the area. The serous fluid moves easily into additional alveoli and bronchioles. As the process continues, less surface area is available for the absorption of oxygen and the release of carbon dioxide. Leukocytes and a few erythrocytes begin to accumulate in the affected alveoli, and the number increases until they eventually completely fill each alveolus, resulting in consolidation (Fig. 11-20, A). Phagocytosis begins in the consolidated alveolus, and the area is finally cleared. In the beginning only one lobe of the lung may be involved, but the infected edema fluid may spread to the bronchial tree of another

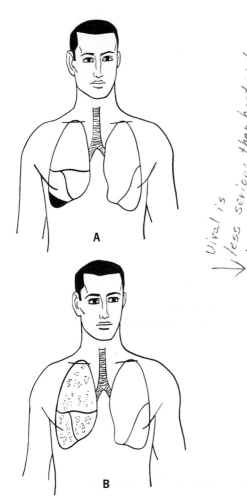

Fig. 11-20. A, Bacterial pneumonia may affect one or more lobes of the lung. **B,** Viral pneumonia appears as a patchy distribution throughout the lung.

lobe, setting up another infective process.[2, 6]

Symptoms may vary with the individual; however, the onset of bacterial pneumonia is usually sudden, with a severe chill and chest pain. This is followed by an elevation of temperature, which may be as high as 105° F., with increase in pulse and respiratory rates. The patient develops a cough, which may be painful and constant. At first the sputum may be clear or tinged with blood, but within 48 hours it develops a characteristic rusty appearance. The sputum is thick and tenacious and may be expectorated with difficulty; a suction machine should be available if

needed to help clear the airway. Leukocytosis is present, with the number of white blood cells from 20,000 to 30,000. The skin is hot and moist, the lips dry, and the tongue parched. Fever blisters (herpes simplex) appear about the lips and nose, and sordes may cover the tongue. Restlessness and delirium may accompany pneumonia and may forebode a crucial situation.

Pneumonia caused by a virus usually appears as a patchy infection throughout the lung (Fig. 11-20, *B*). The onset is slower and is characterized by chilly sensations or chills, fever, profuse sweating, aching, and a painful cough. The sputum is mucopurulent and may contain blood. The white blood cell count is normal. The temperature elevation generally runs an irregular course, varying widely even during the day, and may continue for as long as 3 weeks. Viral pneumonia is rarely fatal, and although the patient is extremely uncomfortable, the seriousness is less than that of bacterial pneumonia. However, these patients may require a longer period of convalescence.

Treatment and nursing care. Nursing care of the patient with pneumonia offers a real challenge to the nurse and is a major factor in the progress and prognosis of the illness. Pneumonia is debilitating and exhausting, and treatment and care are directed toward keeping the patient as comfortable as possible, planning care to avoid any unnecessary expenditure of energy, and using antibiotic and sulfonamide agents to assist the body's defenses and to overcome the infection. The type of antibiotic drug used will depend on the particular organism present and whether the organism remains sensitive to the drug. Sputum for diagnosis should be secured before treatment with the antibiotic is started. Meperidine (Demerol) is often used to relieve pain. Cough analgesics and increased humidity tend to relieve coughing. If the patient is cyanotic or dyspneic or if chest pain is sufficient to interfere with ventilation, oxygen may be ordered.

The patient's room should be well ventilated, with the temperature from 68° to 70° F., and free from drafts and should provide a restful, quiet environment. The patient should be positioned to provide for the greatest comfort and may be placed in a high, 90-degree Fowler's position or lying on the affected side. However, the position should be changed frequently. The nursing care plan should be made to provide nursing care with periods for uninterrupted rest. Visiting should be limited sharply during the acute period of the disease. Temperature, pulse, and respiration rates are checked every 4 hours, and blood pressure readings should be taken at least once a day. The diet usually consists of liquids, and the total fluid intake should be increased from 3000 to 4000 ml. a day. The patient may have to be encouraged to take food or fluids. If pneumonia occurs in a patient with cardiac disease, the nurse should determine if fluids and sodium are to be restricted. Intake and output records should be maintained. Intravenous fluids designed to maintain electrolyte balance may be ordered. Special mouth care will have to be given several times a day, using cold cream about the lips and to soften any crusts about the nares, but fever blisters should be kept dry.

Abdominal distention frequently accompanies pneumonia. Measures to relieve distress include the insertion of a rectal tube for a period no longer than 20 minutes, heat to the abdomen, or a small saline solution enema. Neostigmine bromide (Prostigmin) may be ordered if other measures fail. With decreased peristalsis a gastric tube may be inserted and attached to suction siphonage. The nurse should be alert to a fall in temperature with a weak rapid pulse, drop in blood pressure, increased cyanosis, and dyspnea. Bed rails should always be available, and if restlessness and delirium occur, the patient must be watched carefully and not left alone. Although the use of antibiotics has decreased the death rates from bacterial pneumonia, some patients succumb to the disease, and expert nursing care is therefore still essential.

Pneumonia caused by the staphylococcus bacteria should be isolated, and careful medical asepsis should be carried out. Pneumonia caused by other pathogens does not need to be isolated, but the nurse should be careful about handwashing and proper handling and disposal of sputum.

Pleurisy and empyema

Pleurisy results from inflammation of any part of the pleura. Several forms of the disease exist, which are referred to as dry pleurisy, wet pleurisy, or pleurisy with effusion, and empyema, which is characterized by pus formation. Although the disease may occur spontaneously, it is more likely to be a complication of pneumonia or tuberculosis. The disease has been less common since the development of antibiotic therapy. The first symptom may be a severe knifelike pain on inspiration, which may be referred to the shoulder or to the abdomen on the affected side. A cough, dyspnea, and vomiting may occur, and the patient may hold the abdomen with a boardlike rigidity.

Pleurisy with effusion is less dramatic than dry pleurisy, and the first symptom may be dyspnea, occurring when the accumulation of fluid in the pleural cavity has become large enough to compress the lung. The acuteness of the dyspnea is dependent on the size of the effusion; other symptoms are related to the cause and may include an elevation of temperature. If the fluid becomes purulent and empyema develops, the temperature may reach 105° F. with chills, profuse perspiration, and prostration.

Treatment and nursing care. The treatment of pleurisy depends on the type and stage of the disease and is directed toward removing the underlying cause through the administration of the appropriate antibiotic to combat the infection. If fluid is present in the pleural cavity, a thoracentesis may be done and the fluid aspirated, followed by the instillation of penicillin (p. 190). If the pleural fluid has become purulent and empyema has developed, adequate drainage and specific antibiotics must be provided. With antibiotic therapy the need for open thoracotomy has almost been eliminated. Patients with pleurisy are usually apprehensive and worried, and the nurse needs to be sympathetic and understanding. Good bedside nursing and providing as much comfort as possible in a quiet environment will do much to hasten recovery. The patient will be more comfortable if he lies on the affected side and turns toward the affected side when he coughs. Pain should be relieved, and generally the use of aspirin or dextropropoxyphene (Darvon) is sufficient. If dyspnea is severe, oxygen may be administered. Since pleurisy often follows a debilitating disease, diet is important. The diet should be one that is high in protein, calories, vitamins, and minerals; supplemental feedings may be helpful.

Obstruction of the respiratory system

Obstruction of the respiratory system may result from a deviated septum, nasal polyps, enlarged tonsils and adenoids, aspiration of foreign bodies, and laryngeal tumors.

Deviated septum

The nasal septum divides the two nasal cavities, and theoretically it should be straight; however, this is rarely true. There probably is some irregularity of the septum in most people, but unless it is great enough to obstruct breathing, they are unaware of the condition. During childhood children receive many injuries to the nose, including fractures, which often are not seen by a physician. If not cared for, these injuries may result in a bending of the septum to one side or the other, and if the deviation is severe, it will cause a partial blocking of the respiratory passageway on the side. When obstruction occurs, surgical correction is necessary.

Nasal polyps

A polyp is actually a small tumor attached to the mucous membrane of the nose. It may have been caused by a prolonged inflammation of the sinuses, and since it will obstruct free drainage of secretions, the inflammatory condition may be aggravated. Surgical removal may be necessary to relieve the inflammatory condition.

Submucous resection

Respiratory obstruction from a deviated septum or nasal polyps may be corrected by a surgical procedure called *submucous resection*. The procedure is performed while the patient is under local anesthesia, after administration of preoperative

sedation. After the procedure the nose will be packed for approximately 12 hours. If tampons are used, the strings should be fastened to the cheek with a bit of adhesive tape, and the patient should be instructed not to blow his nose. He is placed in a Fowler's position, and analgesics may be administered to relieve pain. Since the patient will be breathing through the mouth, he may be given chipped ice to help keep the mouth moist. Cold cream may be applied to the lips, and iced compresses may be applied over the nose. The patient should be observed for hemorrhage, indicated by expectoration of bright red blood, frequent swallowing, or increased flow of bright red blood through the packing. After removal of the packing the patient is allowed diet as desired and bathroom privileges. The patient should be told that he will lose his sense of smell for about 1 week.

Enlarged tonsils and adenoids

The pharyngeal tonsils (adenoids) are a mass of lymphoid tissue located at the back of the nose in the upper pharynx. The palatine tonsils are located on each side of the soft palate in the throat. These, too, are composed of lymphoid tissue. These tissues are normally larger in childhood, and under normal conditions removal is not considered necessary unless they become infected with bacteria and do not respond to conservative treatment. Occasionally they become extremely large, obstructing breathing through the nose, and the child is required to breathe through the mouth to get enough air. The tonsils may also obstruct the eustachian tube opening into the back of the throat and may cause some loss of hearing. It may become necessary to remove these lymphoid structures surgically to restore normal breathing and hearing.

Tonsillectomy. Although the tonsils are not a part of the respiratory system, their location may affect breathing. If they become infected, they may contribute to other respiratory infections. Tonsillectomy for an adult patient may be performed while he is under local anesthesia. On return from surgery the patient is placed in a Fowler's position. When a general anesthetic has been given, the patient should be placed on his side or abdomen with a pillow under his abdomen and his head hyperextended. Vital signs should be checked as for any postoperative patient. An ice collar is applied to the throat for relief of discomfort. The patient should be instructed not to cough or clear the throat, and talking should be discouraged for several hours. Postoperative hemorrhage should always be watched for, and care is directed toward its prevention. The patient should not be allowed to gargle the throat before healing begins, since this may dislodge the clot and produce bleeding. If nausea is not present and if there is no bleeding, water or chipped ice may be given. If temperature elevation occurs, the surgeon should be notified. A trace of blood is to be anticipated, but any unusual amount of bright red blood should be reported immediately. It should always be remembered that children may hemorrhage and swallow the blood, and it is a wise nurse who watches the pulse rate and blood pressure of children who have had tonsillectomies. Suction equipment and packing should be readily available for emergency.

Foreign bodies

Children are likely to put all sorts of small objects into their nose such as beans, peanuts, corn, and the like, which are sometimes aspirated into the lungs. If the object is visible, it can be removed with a pair of tweezers. If the object has lodged in the back of the nose or pharynx, the patient should be kept quiet and taken to a physician. Emergency treatment is necessary if foreign materials become lodged in the throat or trachea. If the object cannot be dislodged by the finger, an adult may be placed on his face, with the head lower than the feet, and slapped briskly between the shoulders. Children may be picked up by their heels and shaken. This often will cause the child to cough out the object.[16] Recently it has been discovered that standing behind the choking individual, placing arms around him below his rib cage, and quickly squeezing him (similar to a bear hug) will force residual air, and the foreign object out of the respiratory tract.

Aspirated foreign bodies are more likely to enter the right main bronchus, which is larger and in a more vertical position. If the object is small, coughing will occur with a slight dyspnea. Many times the aspiration of a foreign body creates an acute emergency, making prompt removal with a laryngoscope or bronchoscope necessary, and occasionally a tracheotomy may be required to prevent death. The nurse needs to approach the situation with calmness and efficiency in carrying out emergency orders. When foreign bodies are removed from the bronchus or lung, the child may be hospitalized, and it is important for the nurse to watch the vital signs. The throat may be sore, and steam inhalations may be ordered with sedative or analgesic drugs to relieve discomfort. The child is positioned on the side without a pillow.

Tumors of the respiratory system

Benign or malignant tumors may occur in any part of the respiratory system. Malignant tumors of the upper respiratory system are less common than are tumors in other parts of the body. Cancer of the larynx accounts for a small percentage of neoplasms. As with malignant tumors in other parts of the body, the cause of carcinoma of the larynx is unknown. What is known is that persons with laryngeal cancer are frequently heavy smokers. When the condition is diagnosed, early cure is possible. The disease is most common in men after 45 years of age.

The first symptom that may be observed is hoarseness of the voice, which will become progressively worse without treatment. If this symptom is neglected, metastasis to other structures will occur, and pain on swallowing or pain in the vicinity of the "Adam's apple" may radiate to the ear. Ultimately the airway will become obstructed, and dyspnea will occur. Carcinoma of the larynx is diagnosed by history and visual examination of the larynx with a laryngoscope. A biopsy is done for laboratory confirmation of the clinical findings. Depending on the location of the tumor and the extent of involvement, a partial or a total laryngectomy is performed.

Laryngectomy. Speech is the means whereby a person maintains personal and social relationships. Its loss is a threat to the individual's feelings of security, adequacy, and acceptance.[1] One of the most important decisions of a person's life is made when he consents to a total laryngectomy. When a total laryngectomy is performed, the larynx, the vocal cords, the thyroid cartilage, and the epiglottis are surgically removed. The trachea is sutured to the anterior surface of the neck as a permanent tracheostomy. Since the patient no longer breathes through the nose, he will have little sense of smell. The patient must be carefully prepared emotionally for the loss of normal speech and the change in normal breathing. The patient will have a host of personal problems, and nursing the patient through the difficult period of adjustment will require the skill and understanding of nurses and the help of family and friends. Preoperatively the patient should be given an explanation of the operation. This may be done by discussing with him the way in which normal speech is produced and how the operation will affect the production of normal speech. In addition he should be given some information about speech therapy and told that he will be taught to speak again.

After surgery the patient may be placed in the intensive care unit, since continuous nursing care should be provided for the first 48 hours or longer if necessary. If he is admitted directly to his room, it should be prepared to receive him after the surgery. The room should be warm

(approximately 80° F.) Vaporizers are often used to humidify the air. Equipment for caring for and cleaning a tracheostomy tube should be available, as well as a suction machine, tissue or gauze wipes, and pencil and paper or slate. Some surgeons do not insert a tracheostomy tube because the method of suturing keeps the wound open. If a tube is inserted, it is a laryngeal (laryngectomy) tube (Fig. 11-21), which is slightly larger in diameter and shorter than the ordinary tracheostomy tube. If a tube has been inserted, an extra sterile set the same size as the one inserted should be available at the bedside for emergency use if the first tube should come out.

The most important function of the nurse is to keep the airway clear. The nurse must be available to wipe or suction secretions when the patient coughs, or he may aspirate them. In the beginning, suctioning may be necessary as often as every 5 minutes. The suction catheter should not be inserted more than the length of the tube, and if secretions cannot be removed, the physician should be notified. Efforts should be made the prevent wound infection through maintaining aseptic technique. Oxygen is administered for a day or two to make breathing easier.

The character of respirations must be observed for any increase in rate, wheezing, or crowing sounds. Secretions may be tinged with blood for the first day or two, but any continued bleeding may be from internal hemorrhage and should be reported. Meticulous mouth care with an antiseptic mouthwash should be given frequently. If intravenous fluids are given, they should not be placed in the arm that the patient uses for writing, if possible. The patient may not be allowed anything by mouth for about a week. Feedings are given by means of a gastric tube passed through the patient's nose by the physician. When the patient is allowed food by mouth, it should be soft until healing is complete. Some surgeons do not order tube feedings but allow the patient to eat soft food and drink liquids if he feels well enough. A patient with a laryngectomy is usually most comfortable in a 45-degree Fowler's position, which makes breathing easier (Fig. 11-8). The lips should be kept

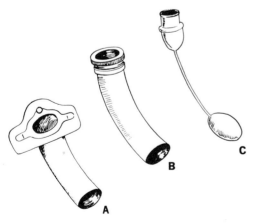

Fig. 11-21. Laryngectomy tube. **A,** Outer cannula. **B,** Inner cannula. **C,** Obturator.

moist with cold cream, and crusts should not be allowed to form about the nares.

As the patient improves, he should be taught how to care for his own tracheostomy, and if he will be unable to do so, some member of the family should be taught. When a tube is used, it may be left in place for approximately 6 weeks. As soon as the neck wounds have healed, the therapist may begin speech training. Esophageal speech has proved to be the most successful means of communication after a laryngectomy. This is taught at special speech clinics in larger cities. If esophageal speech cannot be learned, a vibrator or an electronic artificial larynx can be used. Much assistance can be obtained from local chapters of the American Cancer Society, Inc., including information on a Lost Cord Club or a New Voice Club. There is little reason today why the patient with total laryngectomy should not return to his normal role in life. However, he should be advised against occupational hazards such as dust and fumes and should seek to protect himself against respiratory infections.

Cancer of the lungs

The incidence of malignant tumors (carcinoma) of the lung has been increasing and is more common in men than in women. Tumors may result from metastasis from somewhere else in the body or may appear as primary tumors. Depending on the location and size of the tumor, the patient may or may not experience symptoms. A cough and dyspnea are usually the only signs, and the tumor may have been present for some time when they occur. Immediate treatment is essential, and surgical removal of the part is usually indicated. The removal of one or more lobes of the affected lung or the entire lung depends on the location and extent of tumor growth. X-ray therapy and chemotherapy are also used.

Chest surgery

Surgery on the chest is performed to cure or relieve disease conditions such as bronchiectasis, lung abscess, lung cancer, cysts, and benign tumors. Open heart surgery also involves opening the chest. The kind of operative procedure used depends on the purpose for which it is to be done. An exploratory thoracotomy is done to confirm a diagnosis of lung or chest disease. Often a biopsy is taken and the chest is closed, with the possibility of future operations to treat the disease process. In some conditions only a small portion of lung tissue may be removed, and this procedure is called segmental resection of the lung. Removal of an entire lobe of one lung is lobectomy, and the removal of an entire lung is pneumonectomy (Fig. 11-22). The latter is done most frequently for treatment of bronchogenic carcinoma. After surgery many patients will be cared for in intensive care units or in cardiopulmonary units during the most critical postoperative period.

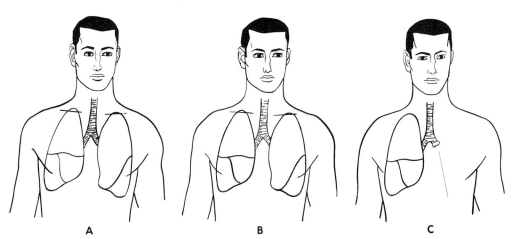

Fig. 11-22. Lobectomy and pneumonectomy. **A,** Normal lung. **B,** Lobectomy with lower lobe of left lung removed. **C,** Pneumonectomy with entire left lung removed.

Patients being considered for lobectomy or pneumonectomy are carefully screened by the surgeon, since not all patients are eligible for this kind of surgery. Many patients will be seen in the surgeon's office, and tests and examinations will be performed on an outpatient basis. Some patients will be admitted to the hospital for their preoperative preparation, which is both psychologic and physical. The patient may have been chronically ill for a long time, leaving his physicial condition at low ebb. His emotional reaction to the proposed surgery may be affected by his general physical condition. While efforts are being directed toward improving his general physical condition, efforts should be made to remove the patient's fears and to reassure him. The nurse should encourage the patient to communicate his feelings and should report any special problems to the physician. During this period efforts are made toward correcting any condition that might affect the outcome of surgery.

The patient should know that he will have several examinations and tests performed, and he should be carefully prepared for each one. He may have a bronchoscopic examination, electrocardiogram, gastric washings, x-ray examination of the chest, and sputum examination. Tests of pulmonary function and a number of blood tests may be done. Most patients receive blood transfusions preoperatively, and antibiotic or sulfonamide drugs are administered. Drugs by nebulization may also be ordered. Mouth hygiene is extremely important, and the nurse should ascertain that the teeth are brushed after each meal, in the morning, and at bedtime. Postural drainage is done several times daily, first when the patient is awakened in the morning and the last time at bedtime. The patient should be encouraged to cough deeply and to expectorate as much mucus as possible during postural drainage. The diet should be nourishing, and the patient should be weighed daily. Unless his condition contraindicates it, the patient should be ambulatory during the preoperative preparation to maintain muscle tone. An explanation concerning the nursing procedures that will be carried out postoperatively should be given to the patient. He should be told that he will have pain because the nerves

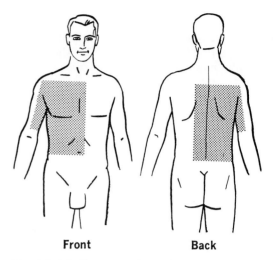

Fig. 11-23. The area of the skin to be prepared for thoracic surgery.

between the ribs have been cut, that he will receive blood and other fluids, that he will receive oxygen, and that vital signs will be checked frequently for several hours. If a chest catheter will be used postoperatively, the patient should be told that it will drain the fluid and air that normally accumulate after chest surgery. He should be taught how to cough and how to do arm and shoulder exercises (Fig. 11-23).

The immediate preparation before going to surgery includes postural drainage and mouth care. Patients are not given a narcotic as a rule, but they may be given a larger dose of atropine or barbiturate than that ordinarily administered to surgical patients.

The room should be prepared for the patient's return from surgery and should include equipment for any emergency that might arise. The patient will be more comfortable if he is placed on a firm bed with hinged bed boards beneath the mattress. Oxygen should be brought to the room as well as a thoracentesis tray and a tracheotomy tray. If the patient is having a lobectomy, there will be drainage tubes; sterile equipment for closed drainage with a pleural pump should be secured if it is ordered. A suction machine with catheters for oral and nasal suction and additional supplies may also be needed. If the patient is having a pneumonectomy, there usually are no drainage tubes. It is the responsibility of the nurse to understand the operation of all equipment and to be sure that it is in working order.

Postoperatively the blood pressure, pulse, and respiration rates are checked every 15 minutes for 3 hours, and then every 30 minutes until ordered otherwise by the surgeon. Oxygen is administered by tent, mask, or oropharyngeal method, and it is continued as long as necessary. When he returns to his room, the patient may be receiving blood intravenously, to be followed by intravenous fluids. The nurse must realize that the reduction in lung capacity requires a period of physiologic adjustment so that fluids must not be allowed to drip at a faster rate than 50 or 60 drops per minute, unless ordered by the surgeon, to avoid overloading the circulation and thus precipitating pulmonary edema. This is especially important in older patients. Fluids by mouth are allowed early in the postoperative period.

When the patient is conscious and the vital signs have stabilized, the head of the bed may be elevated to an angle of approximately 30 to 45 degrees. The nurse must understand the surgeon's orders concerning the positioning of the patient. The patient with a pneumonectomy is usually turned every hour from the back to the affected side and should never be completely turned to the unoperated side. This allows the fluid left in the space to consolidate and prevent the remaining lung and the heart from shifting toward the operative side (mediastinal shift). The patient with a lobectomy may be turned to either side, and the patient with a segmental resection is usually not turned onto the affected side unless this position is ordered by the surgeon.

Medication for the pain will be needed for several days and must be planned for the individual patient. Coughing will be painful, and better cooperation will be secured from the patient if pain-relieving medication is administered before he is instructed to cough. Coughing must be deep enough to bring up secretions, and the nurse should splint the chest when the patient coughs. There are several ways in which this may be done, but both the anterior and posterior chest must be splinted. The nurse's forearms or palms of the hands, or a towel placed around the

chest and held tightly may be employed. If the mucus is thick and the patient has difficulty bringing it up, steam inhalations or aerosol therapy may be ordered to thin secretions. If efforts to cough and bring up the mucus fail, the surgeon should be notified.

Exercises are begun early in the postoperative period to facilitate lung ventilation and to maintain normal muscle tension in the shoulder and the trunk. At first the exercises are performed passively by the nurse, but as soon as the patient is ambulatory or able to sit on the side of the bed and stand, they are performed actively by the patient. The physical therapist will assist with exercises, but in the absence of the physical therapist the nurse must be able to teach and to help the patient with exercises.[10]

The nurse must be constantly on the alert for signs indicating serious complications. Cyanosis, dyspnea, and acute chest pain may foretell atelectasis and should be reported immediately. The nurse must be able to check the apex beat of the heart and note its location; if any change is noted in its location, it should be reported. Pallor, increase in the pulse rate, and any significant drop in blood pressure may indicate internal hemorrhage. Dressings should be checked frequently for the presence of bright red blood, which may indicate external hemorrhage.

Early ambulation of the patient with lobectomy may begin as early as the first or second postoperative day. The patient is allowed first to sit on the side of the bed or to stand beside the bed. Patients having a pneumonectomy are usually not allowed out of bed before the fifth postoperative day. Ambulation depends on the individual patient and his progress.

Chest wounds

Injuries to the chest are serious surgical emergencies and may involve the thoracic cage, pleura, lungs, heart, diaphragm, and abdominal organs. The care of the patient will be largely determined by the extent of the injury. Patients with chest wounds are often apprehensive, and the nurse should explain procedures done to or with the patient. Patients with fractured ribs usually have considerable pain, and the administration of a sedative before turning or moving the patient is advisable. With only simple rib fractures the chest may be strapped from the side of injury to the unaffected side. Adhesive tape, elastic bandage, or foam rubber bandage may be used. The patient should be encouraged to cough and breathe deeply and should be ambulatory as soon as his condition permits.

Penetrating wounds may be caused by any foreign object. Knife and bullet wounds may penetrate the lungs, resulting in an air leak. When this occurs, the air may compress the lung, causing pneumothorax, or bleeding into the pleural cavity may occur, causing the lung to collapse. Both are serious because they may lead to cardiac or respiratory arrest unless immediate emergency treatment is given. The patient should be observed for dyspnea, and the blood pressure, pulse, and respiratory rates should be checked at frequent intervals. Oxygen may be administered, and a thoracentesis may be done with a catheter inserted and connected to closed drainage to remove air and blood. If the injury is such that surgical repair is necessary, a thoracotomy is performed at a later time. An antibiotic and tetanus toxoid injection is generally administered. In cases in which respiration is severely compromised a tracheotomy may be required to provide for adequate ventilation. (See p. 574 for emergency care of other types of chest wounds.)

HEALTH, SOCIAL ASPECTS, AND REHABILITATION

Through public health education and the use of chemotherapeutic agents the incidence of many infectious respiratory diseases has been reduced and serious complications avoided. However, much remains to be done, and nurses can set an example by isolating themselves when they have an acute respiratory infection. When caring for patients with infection, nurses should realize the importance of self-protection and protecting other patients and workers. Nurses should use every opportunity to emphasize to patients with respiratory disease the importance of avoiding acute infections.

Many patients are handicapped socially, vocationally, and emotionally because of respiratory diseases. When severe dyspnea is present, it interferes with work capacity, and the individual may be totally unemployable. Persons with copious bronchial secretions and sputum may become self-conscious, and they may be isolated socially because others may fear that these individuals have a communicable disease. The individual then becomes insecure and tends to withdraw from society, sometimes becoming preoccupied with his health problems and often magnifying them beyond reason. Prolonged unemployment and chronic illness bring financial responsibilities and worries to the patient and his family. Providing emotional support and encouragement and being a good listener may go far in helping the patient adjust to his illness.

Persons with certain types of respiratory conditions, such as the patient with laryngectomy, lobectomy, or pneumonectomy, may need special rehabilitation services. Speech training may be needed to enable the individual to assume his normal position in society. Rehabilitation of this type usually includes reeducation and training for occupations requiring less expenditure of energy for persons with reduced vital capacity. The necessity to provide leisure-time activities and recreational pursuits for persons who will not be able to work is another aspect of rehabilitation. The nurse should be familiar with the community agencies offering services that will assist the individual in becoming an independent, useful member of society.

Summary outline

1. Structure and function of respiratory system
    A. Components of respiratory system: nasal cavities, trachea, larynx, bronchi, lungs
    B. Alveoli are functional units of lungs
    C. Thoracic cage, pleura, diaphragm, and muscles are closely related to respiratory system
    D. Function of respiratory system: exchange of oxygen and carbon dioxide between blood and air
        1. External respiration—inhalation and exhalation
        2. Internal respiration—oxygen transfer from blood to body cells and utilization of oxygen within cell
2. Abnormal types of respiration
    A. Dyspnea—labored breathing
    B. Hypoxia—lack of oxygen in tissues

C. Apnea—temporary cessation of breathing
D. Cheyne-Stokes respiration—irregular breathing with periods of apnea
E. Asphyxia or suffocation—increase of carbon dioxide and decrease in oxygen
F. Cyanosis—caused by incomplete ventilation and decreasing oxygen in bloodstream, resulting in blueness of skin and mucous membranes
G. Hyperventilation—oxygen entering alveoli greater than physiologic needs
H. Hypoventilation—oxygen entering alveoli less than physiologic needs
3. Diagnostic tests and procedures
   A. Routine blood examinations
   B. Blood gas studies
   C. Sputum examination and culture
   D. Pulmonary function tests
      1. Total capacity of lungs
      2. Vital capacity of lungs
      3. Inspiratory capacity of lungs
      4. Residual capacity of lungs
   E. Gastric washings—aspiration of gastric contents for examination
   F. X-ray examination and fluoroscopic studies—permit diagnosis and follow course of a disease
   G. Bronchography—x-ray examination of lungs after injection of radiopaque material
   H. Bronchoscopy—visual examination of lungs
   I. Thoracentesis—removal of air or fluid from pleural cavity for diagnosis or treatment
   J. Thoracotomy—surgical opening into chest cavity to drain blood or pus or to remove air and to explore cavity for evidence of disease
      1. Closed chest gravity water-seal drainage; one or two bottles
      2. Closed chest suction water-seal drainage; two or three bottles or Pleur-evac
   K. Tracheotomy—surgical incision into trachea to provide temporary airway; when tracheotomy is to be permanent, it is called *tracheostomy*
   L. Endotracheal intubation—usually emergency procedure
4. Specific aspects of nursing care
   A. Nurse must be able to recognize signs of oxygen deficiency
      1. Symptoms include increased pulse and respiratory rates, headache, yawning, sighing, nausea and vomiting, anorexia, restlessness, and excitement, but all signs may not appear in patient
   B. Psychologic care—nurse must be able to control own emotions and to maintain calm approach to situation
   C. Methods for maintaining free airway
      1. Coughing—must be deep to be effective and should be accompanied by splinting chest for patient having surgery
         a. Cough medicines are classified as demulcents, expectorants, or sedatives; may be narcotic or nonnarcotic

   2. Suctioning with use of suction catheter and electric suction machine
      a. Use of Y tube will permit fingertip control
      b. Separate catheters must be available for nasal and for tracheobronchial suctioning
   3. Postural drainage—used to drain secretions from bronchi and lungs; oral care should be given after procedure
   4. Percussion—aids in drainage of secretions
   D. Procedures for providing relief of irritation in respiratory passages
      1. Throat irrigations with physiologic saline solutions heated to 120° F.
      2. Plain or medicated steam inhalations
      3. Medications by nebulization
   E. Mechanical ventilation—mechanical devices used to increase flow of air or oxygen through lungs
      1. Assisted ventilation—machine assists breathing when patient breathes spontaneously
      2. Controlled ventilation—machine is set to ventilate lungs without any stimulation from patient
      3. Pressure cycled—machine ventilates until a preset pressure is reached
      4. Volume cycled—machine ventilates until a preset volume is delivered
   F. Rotating tourniquets—to decrease venous pressure and venous return of blood to lungs; used in pulmonary edema
   G. Oxygen therapy—used as supportive therapy when pulmonary ventilation is poor
      1. Oropharyngeal insufflation—nasal catheter inserted through nose and taped to forehead
      2. Oxygen by mask—provides high concentration of oxygen if mask fits face tightly
      3. Oxygen by nasal cannula—provides low concentration of oxygen; care must be taken to avoid direct stream of oxygen against nasal membrane
      4. Oxygen by tent—several types of tents are available but use is limited
      5. Precautions important when oxygen is being used; supports combustion
      6. Hyperbaric oxygen—oxygen under pressure in special steel chamber; use limited at present
5. Nursing patient with diseases and disorders of respiratory system
   Diseases may result from infection, tumors, physical and chemical agents, allergy, senescence, and emotional factors
   A. Noninfectious respiratory conditions
      1. Epistaxis (nosebleed), which occurs in several conditions; may be controlled by a few simple nursing measures
      2. Chronic obstructive pulmonary diseases (COPD)—causes psychologic, physical, and social problems for patients
         a. Pulmonary emphysema

(1) Pathophysiology
   (a) Narrowing of lumen of airway passages
   (b) Loss of elasticity
   (c) Increased pressure in alveoli
   (d) Decrease in vital capacity
   (e) Increase in residual volume of air
   (f) Decreased supply of oxygen in arterial blood
   (g) Increase of carbon dioxide in blood—may lead to acidosis or carbon dioxide narcosis
b. Chronic bronchitis—often occurs with emphysema; changes functional
  (1) Pathophysiology
   (a) Increase in mucus-producing cells and glands
   (b) Thickening with fibrosis of bronchioles and infiltration of inflammatory cells
   (c) Sputum contains variety of pathogenic microorganisms
   (d) Mucous secretions may form plugs in small bronchi
   (e) Chronic persistent cough with large amounts of sputum
   (f) Vital capacity reduced
   (g) Dyspnea, cyanosis, and wheezing
c. Asthma
  (1) Extrinsic—from without body; usually hypersensitivity to allergen involved
  (2) Intrinsic—from within body; possibly from recurrent respiratory infections
  (3) May contribute to emphysema
  (4) Paroxysms of coughing, wheezing, shortness of breath, cyanosis
  (5) Factors in treatment—relief of attack, control causal factors, and general patient care
3. Bronchiectasis—permanent dilation of bronchi involving one or more lobes of lung; both lungs may be affected
 a. Occurs in young
 b. Characteristic symptom is cough
 c. Diagnosis is made by x-ray examination, bronchography, and bronchoscopic examination
 d. Treatment is palliative—only cure is surgery
4. Pulmonary embolism and infarction—blood clots or other foreign material originate in venous system and carried to lung
 a. Can cause death of lung tissue and infarction
5. Pulmonary edema—medical emergency, left ventricle cannot pump blood out as fast as it is being returned to right side of heart

 a. Cyanosis; dyspnea; weak, rapid pulse; respiration wheezy and moist, with gurgling sound; restlessness and apprehension
 b. Patient requires continuous care
6. Atelectasis and pneumothorax related to collapse of lung
 a. Atelectasis may result from accumulation of fluid or air in pleural cavity, tumors, enlarged heart, or obstruction of bronchus; thoracentesis may be done to relieve condition
 b. Pneumothorax or collapse of lung may occur spontaneously with no known cause
B. Infectious respiratory conditions
1. Pathophysiology
 a. Pathogenic microorganisms cause inflammation and edema of mucous membranes of upper respiratory tract
 b. Cervical lymph nodes enlarged and tender
 c. Impaired pulmonary ventilation
 d. Mucous membranes of throat become red, dry, and sore; voice is hoarse with painful cough
 e. Leukocytosis occurs to combat infection
2. Acute coryza (common cold)—of viral origin, but bacteria may take over
3. Acute pharyngitis—may be of viral or bacterial origin
4. Acute laryngitis—usually secondary to other upper respiratory infections and may occur in children at night as croup
5. Tonsillitis—may be caused by streptococcus or staphylococcus bacteria, and severe complications such as rheumatic fever or nephritis may occur
6. Sinusitis—bacteria may enter sinuses from respiratory tract and may lead to complications if infection is not treated
 a. May be acute or chronic
7. Treatment and nursing care of patients with infections of upper respiratory tract—directed toward preventing complications, preventing spread of infection, and relieving discomfort from symptoms
8. Influenza—caused by virus that has been identified as type A, B, C, or parainfluenza 1; strains of A are A_1, A_2, and A_2 Hong Kong–like virus
 a. Influenza vaccine not recommended for healthy adults and children
 b. Persons who should receive influenza vaccine
  (1) Rheumatic heart disease
  (2) Cardiovascular disorders
  (3) Chronic pulmonary disease
  (4) Diabetes
9. Acute bronchitis—caused by inflammatory condition of bronchial tree; often a complication of some communicable disease

10. Pneumonia—may be viral or bacterial in origin, usually caused by pneumococcus
    a. Pathophysiology
       (1) Infected secretions from upper respiratory tract drain into alveoli
       (2) Inflammatory process begins, and increased edema fluid is released into affected area
       (3) Serous fluid moves into alveoli and bronchioles
       (4) Leukocytes begin to accumulate and fill each alveolus, causing consolidation
       (5) Phagocytosis eventually clears consolidated area
    b. Symptoms of bacterial pneumonia occur suddenly; patient is acutely ill and in acute stage requires expert nursing care
    c. Viral type of pneumonia appears as patchy infection throughout lung; it is rarely fatal, but requires longer convalescence than for bacterial pneumonia
11. Pleurisy and empyema
    a. Pleurisy results from inflammation of pleura and may occur in several forms, including dry pleurisy, wet pleurisy, or pleurisy with effusion, and empyema, or pus in pleural cavity
    b. If fluid becomes purulent and empyema develops, temperature may reach 105° F.
6. Obstructions of respiratory system
   A. Deviations of nasal septum may result from injury
   B. Nasal polyps—small tumorlike projections on mucous membrane of nasal cavities, which may be result of chronic infection
   C. Submucous resection—surgical procedure for removal of polyps or correction of deviated septum
   D. Enlarged tonsils and adenoids
      1. Pharyngeal tonsil is located in back of nose in upper part of pharynx
      2. Palatine tonsils, located on each side of soft palate, may become sufficiently enlarged to obstruct breathing and affect hearing, usually making surgical removal necessary
         a. Tonsillectomy for adult usually performed while he is under local anesthesia
         b. If general anesthetic is given, position patient postoperatively on stomach with head hyperextended, check vital signs, and watch for bleeding
   E. Foreign bodies
      1. Obstruction by foreign bodies occurs more commonly in children
      2. Creates acute emergency, since aspirated objects are likely to lodge in right

main bronchus or continue into lung, making bronchoscopy necessary
7. Tumors of respiratory system
   A. Carcinoma of larynx most common in men 45 years of age and older who are heavy smokers
      1. Hoarseness of voice—if this symptom is neglected, carcinoma may metastasize to other structures
      2. Laryngectomy—surgical removal of larynx, may be partial or total
      3. Psychologic preparation for surgery very important
      4. Self-care as patient improves
      5. Speech training
   B. Cancer of lung—incidence is increasing in heavy smokers
      1. Difficult to diagnose; cough and dyspnea may be only symptoms
      2. Treatment by surgery, x-ray therapy, and chemotherapy
8. Chest surgery
   A. Types
      1. Exploratory thoracotomy
      2. Segmental resection
      3. Lobectomy
      4. Pneumonectomy
   B. Preoperatively patient needs extensive evaluation and preparation psychologically and physically
   C. Postoperative care
      1. Maintain closed drainage system
      2. Observe drainage
      3. Position according to type of surgery
      4. Encourage frequent coughing
      5. Observe for complications
      6. Postoperative exercises begun early
9. Chest wounds
   Represent serious medical or surgical emergencies
   A. Fractured ribs—may be extremely painful
      1. Administer sedation to relieve pain before moving patient
      2. Patient with simple fractures should be ambulatory as soon as possible
   B. Penetrating wounds—may involve lungs, pleura, heart; care depends on extent of injury
10. Health, social aspects, and rehabilitation
    A. Patient with respiratory disease should be instructed concerning general health, avoiding acute infections, and preventing spread of infection
    B. Nurse should be example through self-protection and protection of patients and others
    C. Respiratory diseases may handicap individual socially, vocationally, and emotionally
    D. Some respiratory conditions require specialized services in rehabilitation such as speech therapy, vocational counseling, and occupational adjustment

Review questions

1. Define the following types of abnormal respirations.

a. Hypoxia *not enough O₂ to tissues*
b. Dyspnea *difficult breathing*
c. Cheyne-Stokes *irreg. resp: near death*
d. Cyanosis *paleness due to lack of O₂ in blood*

2. What do blood gas studies measure?
   a. *how O₂ & CO₂ are being exchanged in lungs*

3. What are the three parts of a tracheostomy tube called?
   a. *inner cannula*
   b. *outer "*
   c. *obturator*

4. What is the major difference between a regular and a cuffed tracheostomy tube? What precaution must be taken in the care of a patient with a cuffed tracheostomy tube?
   a. *cuffed - air tight*
   b. *reduce pressure occasionally*

5. Name and describe the three classifications of cough medicines.
   a. *demulcents - soothe irritations*
   b. *expectorants - produce sputum*
   c. *sedatives - depress cough reflex*

6. Describe three important principles involved in the suctioning of a tracheostomy tube.
   a. *keep patent airway*
   b. *aseptic technique*
   c. *10 sec. limit on suctioning*

7. What are the two major types of mechanical ventilation?
   a. *pressure cycled*
   b. *volume "*

8. Name two characteristics of chronic obstructive pulmonary diseases.
   a. *chronic cough*
   b. *pain*

9. What emergency measure would be best for a child who is choking on a penny?
   a. *hold him upside down by the feet*

10. What is the major cause of cancer of the lung?
    a. *smoking*

11. Define the following types of chest surgery:
    a. Exploratory thoracotomy
    b. Lobectomy- *one lobe removed*
    c. Pneumonectomy *lung removed*

12. Explain the difference between two-bottle and three-bottle closed chest water-seal drainage.
    a.
    b.

Films

1. Chronic bronchitis and emphysema—W.S.U. (32 min., sound, color, 16 mm.), Audiovisual Utilization Center, Wayne State University, Detroit, Mich. 48202. Describes the relationship between chronic bronchitis and emphysema. Several patients representing different degrees of disability are presented and describe their own symptoms. Treatment is reviewed.

2. Chronic bronchitis and pulmonary emphysema —M-821 and M-822 (part 1—29 min., part 2—24 min., sound, color, 16 mm.), Media Resources Branch, National Medical Audiovisual Center (Annex), Station K, Atlanta, Ga. 30324. Part 1: physiology and pathology of chronic bronchitis and pulmonary emphysema; equipment, diagnostic techniques, and management demonstrated. Part 2: treatment and rehabilitation; postural drainage, breathing exercises, and other clinical methods to help meet demand of daily activities demonstrated.

3. Intensive respiratory care—M-693 (30 min., sound, color, 16 mm.), Media Resources Branch, National Medical Audiovisual Center (Annex), Station K, Atlanta, Ga. 30324. Presents overview of intensive respiratory care unit with emphasis on role of each member of team in diagnosis and treatment. Actual patients shown.

4. The cough: diagnosis and management—research (26½ min., sound, color, 16 mm.), Eli Lilly & Co., Audiovisual Library, Indianapolis, Ind. 46206. Describes anatomy and physiology of cough, conditions that can cause cough, and methods of diagnosis.

5. Spirometry—early detection of chronic obstructive pulmonary disease (25 min., sound, color, 16 mm.), National Tuberculosis Association, 1740 Broadway, New York, N. Y. 10019. Film introduces two men, one with chronic bronchitis, other with emphysema. Normal respiratory physiology, ventilation, diffusion, and perfusion is reviewed, and the changes are portrayed.

6. A breath of air (22 min., sound, color, 16 mm., 8 mm.), American Cancer Society, 219 East 42nd St., New York, N. Y. 10017. Presents medical and scientific evidence on health hazards of smoking.

7. Fair warning (28 min., sound, color, 16 mm.), Media Resources Branch, National Medical Audiovisual Center (Annex), Station K, Atlanta, Ga. 30324. Presents motivations for smoking and information for health professionals that will assist in dealing with smoking problems.

8. The Mark Waters story (25½ min., sound, color, 16 mm.), Modern Talking Picture Service, 2323 New Hyde Park Rd., New Hyde Park, N. Y. 11040. Presents a true story of a man who wrote his own obituary while dying of lung cancer. Stars Richard Boone. Free loan.

9. Chronic obstructive pulmonary disease: breathing patterns—M-1569 (10 min., sound, color, 16 mm.) Media Resources Branch, National Medical Audiovisual Center (Annex), Station K, Atlanta, Ga. 30324. Presents methods used to teach patterns of breathing to the COPD patient.

10. Chronic obstructive pulmonary disease: the use of oxygen in physical therapy management—M-1572 (10 min., sound, color, 16 mm.), Media Resources Branch, National Medical Audiovisual Center (Annex), Station K, Atlanta, Ga. 30324. Shows various machines being used to supply oxygen to COPD patients.

11. Management of the emphysematous patient —M-1216 (6 min., sound, color, 16 mm.),

Media Resources Branch, National Medical Audiovisual Center (Annex), Station K, Atlanta, Ga. 30324. Presents rehabilitation measures for the emphysematous patient.
12. Postural drainage—M-1217 (6 min., sound, color, 16 mm.), Media Resources Branch, National Medical Audiovisual Center (Annex), Station K, Atlanta, Ga. 30324. Shows the effects of postural drainage with the emphysematous patient.

References

1. Adler, Sol: Speech after laryngectomy, American Journal of Nursing 69:2138-2141, Oct., 1969.
2. Beeson, Paul B., and McDermott, Walsh, editors: Cecil-Loeb textbook of medicine, Philadelphia, 1971, W. B. Saunders Co.
3. Belinkoff, Stanton: Introduction to inhalation therapy, Boston, 1969, Little, Brown & Co.
4. Bergersen, Betty S.: Pharmacology in nursing, ed. 13, St. Louis, 1976, The C. V. Mosby Co.
5. Brunner, Lillian S., and Suddarth, Doris S.: Textbook of medical-surgical nursing, ed. 3, Philadelphia, 1975, J. B. Lippincott Co.
6. Conn, Howard F., editor: Current therapy 1976, Philadelphia, 1976, W. B. Saunders Co.
7. Daley, Billee: Hyperbaric nursing, Nursing Times 69:203, Feb. 15, 1973.
8. Egan, Donald F.: Fundamentals of respiratory therapy, ed. 2, St. Louis, 1973, The C. V. Mosby Co.
9. Foss, Georgia: Postural drainage, American Journal of Nursing 73:666-669, April, 1973.
10. Kearns, Barbara: Tracheotomy suctioning technique, The Canadian Nurse 66:44-48, Feb., 1970.
11. MacVicar, Jean: Exercises before and after thoracic surgery, American Journal of Nursing 62:61-63, Jan., 1962.
12. Marks, Anna E.: Hyperbaric medicine, The Journal of Practical Nursing 19:24-26, Oct., 1969.
13. Morbidity and mortality weekly report, week ending June, 15, Atlanta, 1974, Center for Disease Control.
14. Neyland, Margaret P.: Anxiety, American Journal of Nursing 62:110-111, May, 1962.
15. Scott, Betty H.: Tensions linked with emphysema, American Journal of Nursing 69:538-540, March, 1969.
16. Secor, Jane: Patient care in respiratory problems, Philadelphia, 1969, W. B. Saunders Co.
17. Shafer, Kathleen N., Sawyer, Janet R., McCluskey, Audrey M., Beck, Edna L., and Phipps, Wilma J.: Medical-surgical nursing, ed. 6, St. Louis, 1975, The C. V. Mosby Co.
18. Smith, Dorothy W., Germain, Carol P. Hanley, and Gips, Claudia D.: Care of the adult patient, ed. 3, Philadelphia, 1971, J. B. Lippincott Co.
19. Sweetwood, Hannelore: Emphysema, Nursing 72 2:8-12, Nov., 1972.
20. The health consequences of smoking, a report of the Surgeon General, pub. no. 72-7516, Washington, D. C., 1972, Government Printing Office.
21. von Hippel, Arndt: Chest tubes and chest bottles, Springfield, Ill., 1970, Charles C Thomas, Publisher.
22. Zilm, Glennis: Hyperbaric oxygen units—high-pressure nursing, The Canadian Nurse 65:37-40, Feb., 1969.

CHAPTER 12

Nursing the patient with diseases and disorders of the blood and blood-forming organs

KEY WORDS

[handwritten: decrease in rbc, iron or hbg]

anemia *[handwritten: decrease or ↓]*
agranulocytes *[handwritten: disease or disorder of blood]*
blood dyscrasias
corpuscles
cryoprecipitate *[handwritten: ↑ amt. bleeding into tissues]*
ecchymosis *[handwritten: lg. amt. bleeding rbc's into tissues]*
erythrocytes
erythropoiesis
extracellular *[handwritten: outside the cells]*
granulocytes
hematogenic shock *[handwritten: blood loss]*
homeostasis
hemoglobin
  electrophoresis
hemophilia
Hodgkin's disease
hypochromia

immunoglobulins (Ig)
leukemia
leukocytosis *[handwritten: increase in wbc]*
leukopenia *[handwritten: decrease in wbc]*
lymph nodes
molecules
osmotic pressure *[handwritten: normal function, physiology is ↑ poet]*
pathophysiology
petechias *[handwritten: pinpoint hemorrhages, cut into vein to remove blood, returning, to donor, plasma is removed]*
phlebotomy
plasmapheresis
purpura *[handwritten: bleeding into the skin, rbc-mal-formed cells]*
sickle cell disease
splenomegaly *[handwritten: enlargement of the spleen]*
viscosity *[handwritten: thickness of fluid]*

THE BLOOD—ITS FUNCTION AND STRUCTURE

Function

The blood is the transportation system of the body. Through its vast network of vessels it carries oxygen to the cells and returns carbon dioxide to be eliminated. It transports food to nourish the cells so that they may carry on their normal functions. Water, electrolytes, hormones, and enzymes, all of which have important functions in helping to keep the body in a state of equilibrium (homeostasis), are transported by the blood. Heat is carried by the blood and helps to regulate body temperature. Blood carries immune bodies and antibodies that help to prevent disease and infection. Through a complex system that is not completely understood the blood functions to provide clotting and prevent serious loss of fluids in case of injury. It also functions to prevent clot formation in blood vessels, which would seriously interfere with oxygen reaching the cells of the body. Any disease or condition that affects the blood or its transport system may pose a serious threat to the individual.

Structure

The blood is slightly sticky and has a characteristic odor and a faint salty taste. It is bright red in the arteries because it is carrying oxygen, and it is dark red in the veins because the cells have taken up the oxygen and it is carrying carbon dioxide to be eliminated by the respiratory system. The blood is composed of two parts: the liquid part called plasma, which constitutes

[handwritten: ½ plasma, ½ cells]

slightly more than half of the total volume, and the formed elements, or cells. Blood volume remains fairly constant in one person, but there are variations among individuals. Factors such as age, sex, and the amount of adipose tissue may affect the volume of circulating blood.

Plasma 55% of blood

Plasma contains no cells and is estimated to be about 90% water. It is a clear straw-colored fluid with a large number of substances dissolved in it. Among the most important of these substances are the plasma proteins, which include serum albumin, serum globulin, and fibrinogen. The serum albumin and fibrinogen are synthesized in the liver, whereas the serum globulins are part of the immunity system related to the circulating antibodies. These proteins have several important functions essential to the regulation of blood volume, providing nutrition to body cells, blood clotting, and circulating the antibodies. Approximately 2% to 4% of the other substances dissolved in plasma include urea, uric acid, glucose, respiratory gases, hormones, and electrolytes. Minute amounts of other substances essential to meet the body's needs are also found in plasma. Plasma can be separated from the formed elements, and because it contains the proteins that assist in the clotting of blood, it is administered for several bleeding disorders.

Formed elements 45%

The formed elements, or corpuscles, have been divided into several groups: (1) erythrocytes, or red blood cells, (2) leukocytes, or white blood cells, and (3) platelets, or thrombocytes.

Erythrocytes. The erythrocytes are formed in the red marrow, which is found near the distal ends of certain long bones and in some flat bones. The formation of erythrocytes in the bone marrow does not begin until after birth. Prior to birth the production is carried on by the liver and the spleen. The production of erythrocytes, *erythropoiesis,* is a continuous process, and in the absence of disease the number remains relatively constant. Every hour of the day millions of erythrocytes are being destroyed and replaced by millions of new ones. The exact way in which homeostasis

is maintained is not clearly understood. However, it is known that the red marrow must remain in a healthy condition for normal production to take place.

The main ingredient of the erythrocytes is hemoglobin. Within each red blood cell there are millions of molecules of hemoglobin, each one of which contains iron and a pigment that gives color to the blood. Hemoglobin is measured in grams per 100 ml. of blood, whereas red blood cells are measured in millions per cubic millimeter of blood. Hemoglobin carries oxygen to the cells of the body, thus the amount of oxygen available to the cells will depend on the amount of hemoglobin in the blood. The number of erythrocytes in men is usually slightly higher than that in women. In the newborn infant the number may be increased, but gradually it decreases to the adult level by 15 years of age. Loss of blood through hemorrhage will cause a decrease in circulating fluid and in hemoglobin, and in turn the amount of iron will be decreased. Since the oxygen-carrying power of the blood has been decreased, the heart will have to work harder to supply the cells with oxygen. Thus a person suffering from loss of blood may be expected to have an increase in the pulse rate and may also develop anemia, since the iron content of the blood is reduced. Certain diseases of the blood and the blood-forming organs may affect the production of erythrocytes so that the number is decreased or their structure is immature, whereas in some diseases there may be an overproduction of erythrocytes. In some genetic diseases the erythrocytes may have an abnormal shape.

Leukocytes. Leukocytes, or white blood cells, are not as numerous as the erythrocytes, or red blood cells. The number of white blood cells in 1 mm.³ of blood varies between 5000 and 10,000. The number is essentially the same for men and women. When there is an increase of more than 10,000 white blood cells, it may indicate the presence of some pathologic condition. Such an increase is called *leukocytosis* (p. 31). Under some conditions there may be a decrease in the number of leukocytes, which is called *leukopenia.* Leukocytes are classified as granular or nongranular, depending on the color of their cytoplasm and the shape of their nuclei. Granular leukocytes are called *granulocytes,* and approximately 50% to 75% of the leukocytes are granulocytes. The nongranular leukocytes, or *agranulocytes,* comprise less than one third of the cells and include the lymphocytes and monocytes. There are several varieties of granulocytes, and they are formed in the red marrow along with monocytes. The lymphocytes are formed in certain tissues of the lymph nodes and the spleen. The leukocytes have many functions in the body, and their ability to move about helps to protect the body from infection and to repair damaged tissue (Fig. 2-2). A count of white blood cells is often an important aid to the physician in establishing a diagnosis; for example, in suspected acute appendicitis an increase in the number of white blood cells together with clinical symptoms may indicate to the physician the need for an appendectomy.[1]

Differential count. A differential count is a count of several kinds of white blood cells. Only one drop of blood is needed. After placement on a slide and staining the slide is placed under the microscope, and each kind of leukocyte is counted and identified. The various cells are reported as a percentage of 100 of all kinds of white blood cells. In various diseases certain kinds of cells may be increased; for example, in some bacterial infections the number of lymphocytes may be increased.

PLATELETS

Platelets, or thrombocytes, are tiny fragile elements in the blood. They are formed in the red marrow and are thought to be minute fragments of large cells called *megakaryocytes.* The exact number of platelets is unknown, but various estimates have placed the number from 150,000 to 500,000/mm.³ of blood. The primary function of platelets is to control bleeding. When an injury to a blood vessel occurs, the platelets concentrate at the site of the injury and control bleeding by forming thrombotic plugs and by releasing a substance, factor 3, that is necessary for coagulation and the formation of fibrin. They continue their activity in helping to shrink the clot and bring together the margins of the damaged vessel. In certain

hemorrhagic disorders there may be a decrease in the number of platelets, which may cause serious bleeding, whereas in other diseases there may be an abnormal number of platelets, called *thrombocytosis.*

Average normal blood values are as follows:

Erythrocytes
  Men   4.5 to 6.0 million/mm.³ blood
  Women   4.3 to 5.5 million/mm.³ blood
  Newborn   5.0 to 7.0 million/mm.³ blood
Leukocytes
  Men   5000 to 10,000/mm.³ blood
  Women   5000 to 10,000/mm.³ blood
  Newborn   15,000 to 45,000/mm.³ blood
Platelets   150,000 to 500,000
Hemoglobin
  Men   14 to 18 grams/100 ml. blood
  Women   12 to 16 grams/100 ml. blood
  Newborn   15 to 20 grams/100 ml. blood

BLOOD FRACTIONS

Blood may be broken down into its component parts so that patients with certain conditions may be given specific blood fractions to meet their individual needs.

Blood plasma. Plasma may be separated from whole blood that has been stored, or it may be separated from fresh blood taken from a donor and immediately frozen. The primary use of plasma is for defective clotting of the blood. When fresh blood plasma is used, it contains all of the factors essential for clotting, including the antihemophilic factor. The use of plasma for some conditions has decreased as other more effective fractions have become available.

Platelets. Platelets may be separated from whole blood and administered to patients with severe hematologic disorders, open heart surgery, and postoperative bleeding. The demand for platelets has increased, and it is now believed that patients with active bleeding from any site, internal or external, whose platelet count is below 20,000/mm.³ of blood should receive platelets. The administration of platelets has been a life-saving measure for many patients receiving chemotherapy for malignant disorders. Platelets may be administered in fresh whole blood, in plasma that is rich in platelets, or as a platelet concentrate. The advantage of the platelet concentrate is that it involves only 5 to 10 ml. of fluid. When long-term administration is required, it avoids overloading the circulatory system. With the exception of hemolytic reactions the patient receiving platelets may have similar reactions as from whole blood transfusions. Therefore close observation of the patient is essential.

Globulins

The globulins have several important functions in the body. They may be classified as follows:

    Serum globulins
       Immunoglobulin Ig (gamma globulin)
       Albumin
       Fibrinogen
    Hyperimmune human gamma globulin
    Immune serum globulin

The globulins are serum proteins and include several groups of gamma globulins, now called immunoglobulins (Ig).[12] The primary use of the immunoglobulins is in the prevention or modification of infectious disease. Immune serum globulin is used in the prevention of hepatitis A but is not effective in hepatitis B. The hyperimmune human gamma globulins are fractions of human blood of persons with circulating antibodies. Such persons may have antibodies as a result of having had the disease or having been immunized against it. Hyperimmune human gamma globulin is given to nonimmune persons to prevent infectious disease or its complications in diseases such as tetanus, mumps, or pertussis. The Center for Disease Control has recently released a zoster immune globulin (ZIG). It is recommended for nonimmune children exposed to chickenpox and for whom the disease might be serious. Human rabies immune globulin (HRIG) has been available since September, 1974.

Purified human serum globulin may be administered to assist in maintaining osmotic pressure of the plasma. It is useful in any condition in which the albumin globulin ratio has been lowered. It may be administered to burned patients, for hypovolemic shock, and in liver disease.

Fibrinogen is an essential factor for the clotting of blood. A deficiency may be a congenital disorder or an acquired condition resulting from massive hemorrhage, prolonged active bleeding, or other hematologic conditions dependent on the clotting mechanism. Purified fibrinogen concentrate is prepared from human plasma. Because it is made from pooled blood and its preparation does not ensure the destruction of the hepatitis virus, there is some attendant risk of hepatitis when it is administered.

Cryoprecipitate is a fraction prepared from fresh frozen plasma and contains the antihemophilic factor essential to control bleeding in hemophilia. Administration of cryoprecipitate is considered the treatment of choice, but if it is not available purified antihemophilic globulin or plasma is administered.[5]

Packed red blood cells are red blood cells without the plasma. By centrifuging whole blood, the cells and the plasma are separated. In conditions where the blood volume is normal but the number of red blood cells and hemoglobin is decreased, packed red blood cells may be given. Since packed red blood cells are placed in only a small amount of fluid, the danger of overloading the circulatory system is avoided. In some types of anemia packed red blood cells may be administered in place of whole blood.

HEMATOGENIC (HYPOVOLEMIC) SHOCK

Shock is a condition that may occur in several conditions and is classified as to type. In each case the volume of circulating fluid, the vascular system, and the heart are involved. The loss of blood, internal or external, sufficient to reduce the volume of circulating fluid may lead to a type of shock classified as hematogenic volemia.

Pathophysiology. Pathophysiology means that normal physiologic function has been upset. In hematogenic shock the normal function of the cardiovascular system is affected.

When the output of blood from the heart is decreased, there is a corresponding decrease in the return of venous blood to the heart. With less blood returning to the heart there is less blood to be pumped out from the heart into the vascular system. Since the red blood cells with their hemoglobin carry oxygen to the tissues of the body, the cells are being deprived of their essential supply of oxygen. During the early stages when blood has been or is being lost, the body attempts to compensate for the loss by initiating several actions. The sympathetic nervous system causes norepinephrine to be produced, resulting in constriction of small peripheral blood vessels. This action increases the amount of venous blood being returned to the heart. The red bone marrow increases the production of red blood cells and releases them to supply more oxygen-carrying power. However, with the increased production many cells will be immature and will be unable to transport the normal amount of oxygen. The kidneys release substances to increase the tone of the arterioles, increasing their ability to constrict. The kidneys also begin to retain sodium that is normally excreted with water. Since the body is in need of fluids, the retention of the sodium keeps fluid in the blood and results in a decreased urinary output. Several other compensatory activities are initiated to help overcome the loss of circulating fluid. During the early stages of bleeding the body will be able to compensate for the loss, but if bleeding continues the body will be unable to maintain the volume of circulating fluid. The blood pressure will begin to fall. As the heart works harder, the pulse rate will increase and gradually become weaker. The increasing amount of carbon dioxide in the body stimulates the respiratory center in the brain, causing an increase in the respiratory rate. The decrease in oxygen supply to the brain may cause loss of consciousness. Because of the vasoconstriction of the peripheral blood vessels, the skin becomes pale, cool, and moist. The temperature becomes subnormal. Because of inadequate oxygenation of the blood, cyanosis may be observed around the mouth, lips, fingers, and toes. The diastolic blood pressure becomes imperceptible, and the systolic pressure continues to drop. The pulse and respiratory rates continue to increase, and oliguria occurs. At this stage the condition is irreversible and the patient lapses into coma and death.

Nursing care. The nurse should observe the patient who is bleeding for the following: (1) restlessness, (2) anxiety and apprehension, (3) blood pressure, (4) pulse rate and volume, (5) respiration rate and depth, (6) color, (7) urinary output, (8) thirst, and (9) state of consciousness. The nurse is responsible for the prompt and accurate observation, reporting, and recording for any patient who is bleeding internally or externally. Early treatment may save the patient's life by preventing shock from reaching the stage when it is irreversible.[4, 9]

COLLECTION OF BLOOD

The collection and storage of blood began in 1937 during World War II. Because of the progress of medical science, the need for whole blood, plasma, and blood fractions has become essential in the practice of modern medicine. Along with the increased demand, improved methods of collection storage and distribution have taken place. At the present time there are three main collection systems: the American Red Cross, hospitals, and commercial centers. The American Red Cross maintains regional centers for the collection of blood and mobile units that may be taken to communities, industrial plants, or college campuses. The arrival of the mobile unit is usually the culmination of drives for donors sponsored by local citizens. Most hospitals collect blood to meet their individual needs. Frequently donors are members of the patient's family, friends of the patient, or other persons interested in the patient. In an emergency, when large amounts of blood may be needed, the hospital may call on citizens of the community or the American Red Cross to help meet its needs. In most instances donors to hospitals and the American Red Cross do not receive payment for their blood. In recent years commercial centers have been opened and a small fee is paid to the donor. These centers have come under attack and are being scrutinized by state governments. Donors are often derelicts of the street from whom little or no information can be obtained concerning infectious diseases such as malaria, hepatitis, and syphilis. In meeting the individual needs of patients, centers have been opened for the collection of plasma. The plasma and red blood cells are separated at the time of collection, and the red blood cells are returned to the donor. This process is known as *plasmapheresis.*

BODY FLUIDS AND ELECTROLYTES

A large part of a person's body weight is composed of fluid. It has been estimated that in the average person from 60% to

70% of the fluid is water. Approximately one half of the fluid is found within the cells as *intracellular* fluid. A lesser amount is outside the cells as *extracellular* fluid. A portion of the extracellular fluid is in the blood vessels as plasma or *intravascular* fluid, whereas some is located between tissues as *interstitial* fluid. In general, body fluids are found in cells, outside cells, and in the vascular system. In the absence of disease these fluids remain in a state of equilibrium. A proper balance is maintained by the intake and output of fluid. The intake of fluid is through the ingestion of water, other fluids, or food, and some fluid is derived from conversion of substances by the cells into simple compounds. The output is carried on mainly by the kidneys, skin, lungs, and intestines. When output exceeds intake, dehydration may occur, whereas when intake exceeds output, edema may result. To maintain the proper balance of fluid in their respective compartments the semipermeable membranes permit water to pass from the cell or into the cell from the extracellular fluids.

Substances that are dissolved in body fluids are called *electrolytes*. The term *electrolyte* is derived from the fact that when electrolytes are placed in water, they develop an electric charge. The principal electrolytes are sodium, calcium, potassium, and magnesium. Some of these are found in the extracellular fluids and others in the intracellular fluids. Electrolytes can be measured by chemical analysis of the blood plasma. In a healthy person electrolytes remain in balance, but any condition that alters the fluid balance in the body will cause a decrease or an increase of some or all of the electrolytes. As with water, electrolytes are acquired through the ingestion of food and water. They are lost from the body in many different ways. Especially important is the loss through vomiting, diarrhea, ostomies, gastric suction, increased respiration when there is a high temperature, draining wounds, and burns. In almost all illnesses there will be some disturbance of electrolyte metabolism caused by inadequate intake of water. In many situations throughout this book the nurse has been told to encourage patients to drink water. In some conditions serious deficiencies in electrolyte balance may occur, leading to major metabolic changes.

In such conditions the physician may order electrolytes to be administered by infusion[11] (p. 152).

Normal values of principal electrolytes* are as follows:

Sodium	313 to 334 mg./100 ml. blood serum
Calcium	9 to 11 mg./100 ml. blood serum
Potassium	14 to 20 mg./100 ml. blood serum
Magnesium	1.8 to 3.0 mg./100 ml. blood serum

DIAGNOSTIC TESTS AND PROCEDURES

A large number of tests performed on the blood are done for diagnostic purposes, but some are useful in guiding the physician in the course and treatment of disease. Some tests are performed on capillary blood and require only a few drops, which is usually secured by pricking the finger or the ear lobe. Blood for other tests requiring a larger amount of blood is secured from a vein with a needle and syringe. Some of the more common tests will be reviewed here, and others will be found in different sections of this book according to their relation to specific diseases.

Complete blood count (CBC). The complete blood count is the most common of all tests made on the blood. It consists of a count of the erythrocytes and leukocytes, measurement of hemoglobin, and a differential count, which includes a count of a large number of other cells. The physician orders the examination, which is made by persons trained in laboratory methods. However, it is often the responsibility of the nurse to execute the proper forms and notify the laboratory of the physician's request. Many hospitals require that routine blood counts be completed for all patients on admission, and some hospitals route the patient from the admission office to the laboratory for the examination before the patient is admitted to the clinical unit.

Blood gas analysis. A blood gas analysis is used to measure the oxygen and carbon dioxide content of the blood and to determine the functional ability of the lungs to maintain adequate gas levels in the blood. Blood is secured from the brachial or femoral artery. The test is used primarily in respiratory diseases and disorders and guides the physician in the administration of oxygen and/or medications.[18]

---

*Values may vary, depending on the laboratory method used.

Hemoglobin electrophoresis. Hemoglobin electrophoresis is used to identify various abnormal hemoglobins in the blood. Abnormal hemoglobins can produce genetic disorders transmitted from parent to child. The most common abnormal hemoglobin causes sickle cell anemia.

Paul-Bunnell (heterophil antibody) test. The Paul-Bunnell test is used to determine the presence or absence of infectious mononucleosis in an individual.

Coagulation time. The test for coagulation time measures the ability of the blood to clot, which may be affected by many factors. Since there are so many variables related to the results of the test, it is usually considered significant only if the time necessary for the blood to clot is prolonged. Hemophilia is one disease in which there is a prolonged clotting time.

Hematocrit. The test for hematocrit measures the relative volume of cells and plasma in the blood. In anemia and after hemorrhage the hematocrit is lowered, and in dehydration it is increased. A microhematocrit test may be done using capillary blood secured by pricking the finger.

Icterus index. The icterus index is a test of liver function and measures the amount of yellowness of the blood serum. The test is useful in discovering early jaundice. Patients with severe jaundice may have as high as 100 units.

Prothrombin time. Prothrombin is related to the process of clot formation. With a decrease of prothrombin in the blood it is generally believed that there is also a decrease in the clotting tendency of the blood in the blood vessels. The time may increase in the presence of some diseases or when the patient is receiving anticoagulant therapy. The test should be performed daily on all patients who are receiving an anticoagulant drug.

Phlebotomy. See p. 243.

Sedimentation rate. The test for sedimentation rate measures the time required for the red blood cells to settle to the bottom of a test tube, usually based on duration of 1 hour. The test is used for diagnostic purposes and to follow the course of some diseases such as rheumatic fever and arthritis.

Bone marrow aspiration. Aspiration of bone marrow is done to obtain a specimen of cells for biopsy. Examination of the cells may indicate their reproductive ability and is useful in the diagnosis of certain blood dyscrasias in which defective production occurs. In adults the puncture may be made into the sternum, and in children the iliac crest or the tibia is recommended as a puncture site.

Normal hematologic values are as follows:

Bleeding time	1 to 4 minutes
Coagulation time	6 to 17 minutes with test tube method
Hematocrit	
Male	40% to 54%
Female	37% to 47%
Icterus index	4 to 7 units
Prothrombin time	11.0 to 12.5 seconds
Sedimentation rate	
Male	0 to 6.5 mm./hr.
Female	0 to 20 mm./hr.

Values will vary with the particular method of analysis used.

Blood chemistry. The chemical analysis of blood involves a large number of tests, some of which are carried out on whole blood, a few on plasma, and others on blood serum. A chemical analysis of the electrolytes previously referred to in this chapter are frequently ordered by the physician. Some of these tests will be discussed in various sections of this book as they relate to specific diseases.

Blood serology. Blood is secured by a venipuncture and sent to the serology laboratory for a serologic test for syphilis. The procedure is routine in most hospitals and may be done on admission of the patient or at the same time that blood is secured for the CBC.

Blood typing and cross matching. In administering blood it is important for the blood of the donor and the blood of the patient to be compatible. If it is not, the patient may suffer a severe or fatal reaction. To date there are fifteen different systems for matching blood and more than 100 different blood factors known. However, the most familiar system classifies blood types as A, B, AB, and O. The AB type contains agglutinogens of both the A type and B type and cannot be administered to persons with either the A or B type. It is always best to transfuse the patient with blood of his own type when possible; however, if the same type cannot

Universal donor - O type - me!

be secured or if there is a delay in typing and cross matching, the O type may be used in an emergency, but the patient must be watched carefully for indications of a reaction. The type O blood contains tiny amounts of both A and B agglutinins, but since the small amount in the donor's blood is mixed with the larger amount of the recipient's blood, the A and B factors are not likely to produce symptoms.[8] Thus type O blood is often referred to as *universal donor* blood, since it can be administered to anyone with type A, B, or AB blood. Usually 500 ml. of whole blood administered to a patient will elevate the number of red blood cells and the amount of hemoglobin 15% in 24 hours. Plasma may be administered to anyone, but since reactions may occur from plasma, the same precautions should be taken as for administering whole blood.

Rh factor. In addition to the kinds of protein substances found in the four types of blood, some persons have an extra protein substance called the *Rh factor.* Approximately 85% of all persons have this protein and are said to be Rh positive; the remaining 15% are said to be Rh negative. Since they do not have this extra protein, it is just as important to determine the Rh factor in cross matching blood for transfusion as it is to determine the blood type. If an Rh-negative person is transfused with Rh-positive blood, he may develop antibodies against the Rh-positive factor. If given further transfusions with Rh-positive blood, he may develop severe reactions. An Rh-positive fetus in utero may precipitate the formation of antibodies in an Rh-negative mother. If any of these antibodies reaches the fetal circulation, it may cause the baby to be still-

born or result in the disease called *erythroblastosis fetalis.*   *Rh baby*

Blood transfusion. The nurse will encounter many situations in which physicians will order the patient to be transfused with whole blood. There are three primary reasons for administering blood: (1) to replace or maintain blood volume, (2) to preserve the oxygen-carrying function of the blood, and (3) to increase or maintain the coagulation abilities of the blood.

SPECIFIC NURSING FUNCTIONS

Blood transfusion therapy. When the physician writes the order for the patient to be transfused, it may be the responsibility of the nurse to transmit the request to the laboratory so that typing and cross matching may be done and the number of pints (units) ordered will be prepared. The nurse may not begin administering blood but may assemble the necessary equipment and may assist in observation of the patient. Blood brought to the unit must be used immediately or refrigerated. The nurse should recheck the physician's order and should check the patient's blood type against the label on the blood sent to the clinical unit. The information is frequently recorded on the patient's chart to facilitate checking should it be necessary.

A fatal reaction from a blood transfusion may be caused by air that is allowed to enter the circulation. This is most likely to occur when blood is being given under pressure. As has been stated previously, elderly patients do not tolerate infusions of blood or fluids as well as younger persons and patients with cardiac disease and must be watched carefully during such

non white Rh + 99%
Rh - 1%

Table 12-1. Blood transfusion reactions

Type of reaction	Cause	Symptoms
Allergic reaction	Hypersensitivity to antibodies in donor's blood	Urticaria, pruritus, fever, anaphylactic shock *edema*
Hemolytic reaction	Incompatibility *chills fever oliguria*	Nausea, vomiting, pain in lower back, *dyspnea* hypotension, increase in pulse rate, decrease in urinary output, hematuria, *chest pain* death *renal damage*
Pyogenic reaction	Contamination of blood	Fever, chills, nausea, blood in vomitus, headache *"bld shock" - flushed*

procedures. Overloading the circulatory system may cause left ventricular failure.

In addition to transfusion reactions, several diseases may be transmitted by means of blood transfusions. These include hepatitis, malaria, and syphilis. Blood from donors with a history of these diseases is not used; however, often it is not possible to secure an accurate history. The nurse should be thoroughly familiar with the symptoms of blood reactions and at the slightest indication should stop the blood transfusion and call the physician. The nurse should remain calm, reassure the patient, cover him with a blanket, and remain with him. A 1:1000 solution of epinephrine with a sterile syringe and needle should be readily available (Table 12-1).

When blood has been discontinued because of a reaction, it should not be destroyed but should be saved for checking in an effort to determine the cause of reaction.

Blood chemistry. Blood for chemical analysis is usually collected early in the morning while the patient is in a fasting state. The requests are filed with the laboratory the evening before. The nurse should be familiar with the policies of the laboratory concerning food and fluids. Breakfast is usually withheld, and in some instances the patient is allowed nothing by mouth after midnight, although in other situations he may be permitted to have water. The patient's room or bed should be marked to avoid any error, and it is advisable to instruct the patient concerning the examination and the need to withhold food. If the blood specimen is not secured before breakfast is served, the patient's tray should be kept warm for him, or the meal may be reordered from the dietary service.

NURSING THE PATIENT WITH DISEASES AND DISORDERS OF THE BLOOD AND BLOOD-FORMING ORGANS

Diseases and disorders of the blood and the blood-forming organs are called blood dyscrasias. They cover a wide range of diseases and disorders, some of which respond to treatment and others in which treatment is only palliative. Some diseases may be controlled, but the patient must live with the disease the rest of his life. Some diseases are hereditary, and some individuals may be predisposed to some disorders because of their life style.

Following is a partial classification of diseases and disorders of the blood and the blood-forming organs[9]:

Anemia
    Hemorrhagic anemia
    Iron-deficiency or nutritional anemia
    Pernicious anemia
    Sickle cell anemia
Polycythemia
Disorders of white blood cells
Hodgkin's disease
Leukemia
    Myelogenous leukemia
    Lymphocytic or myelocytic leukemia
    Granulocytic (chronic) leukemia
Hemophilia
Purpura

Anemia

Anemia is not a disease but a condition resulting from one or a combination of causes. It accompanies several diseases, and its development may be so insidious that an individual is unaware of the condition until symptoms appear. It may develop slowly when there is a slow bleeding from the intestinal tract, or it may develop quickly if there is a massive hemorrhage. Anemia is usually present in diseases in which there is destruction of red blood cells or when there is immature development of the red blood cells. Any condition that causes a decrease in red blood cells, in hemoglobin, and in iron will cause varying degrees of anemia.

Hemorrhagic anemia

Anemia due to loss of blood may be acute or chronic. Acute anemia occurs when there has been a sudden loss of a large amount of blood. This may be caused by traumatic injury, hemoptysis, hemorrhage at childbirth, ulcerative lesions, and disorders of coagulation. Loss of as much as one third of the blood may be fatal. Anemia may result from lesser degrees of hemorrhage or slow bleeding such as that from a bleeding gastric ulcer or bleeding hemorrhoids.

Pathophysiology. The loss of blood decreases the amount of circulating fluid and hemoglobin, lowers the hematocrit value, and decreases the amount of oxygen carried to the tissues of the body. The tissues of the body must have oxygen to survive. Severe blood loss may be caused by trauma if large blood vessels are ruptured or severed. Massive uterine hemorrhage may accompany childbirth, or it may result from cancer. A ruptured tubal pregnancy may release large amounts of blood into the peritoneal cavity. Less severe blood loss occurs in many conditions including prolonged or frequent menstrual periods, bleeding gastric ulcer, or bleeding hemorrhoids. When blood loss is severe, the patient may experience hematogenic shock. There is prostration, thirst, rapid pulse rate, pallor, hypotension, clammy skin, or mental confusion because of decreased oxygen supply to the brain. When anemia is caused by slow bleeding, symptoms are less dramatic. Fatigue is a primary symptom. The volume and rate of the pulse is normal. On exertion the blood pressure may drop, and tachycardia may occur. There is a tendency toward fainting and dizziness. If bleeding continues for a prolonged period, pallor will develop and shortness of breath on exertion, headache, drowsiness, and menstrual disturbances may occur.

Emergency care. In a case of massive hemorrhage, measures are taken to control the bleeding, treat for shock, and replace the volume of circulating fluid. If the bleeding is external, external pressure should be applied to control the bleeding if possible. If it is necessary to apply a tourniquet, a tag should be attached to the patient to alert the physician or emergency clinic of its presence and time of application. After a tourniquet has been applied it should not be removed except by the physician or clinic. The most satisfactory method of treatment is to transfuse the person with whole blood of the correct type. Plasma expander such as dextran, isotonic saline solution, and 5% glucose in saline may also be administered.

Follow-up care. After the immediate emergency it may or may not be necessary to administer iron in some form. The immediate concern in chronic bleeding is to locate and remove the cause. This requires a carefully taken history and physical examination. Laboratory examina-

tions and x-ray studies may be required. Depending on the degree of anemia, blood transfusions may be given and iron therapy instituted.

Nursing care. The nurse who may assist with the care of patients who have suffered loss of blood, whether of large or small amounts, should observe the patient for evidence of any further bleeding. Observation of the patient during transfusion has been emphasized earlier in this chapter. The patient should be kept lying down; the foot of the bed may be elevated for patients with uterine hemorrhage. The patient should be kept warm with lightweight covering, but excessive perspiration should be avoided. Hot-water bottles should not be used because of the danger of burning the patient. Blood pressure, pulse, and respiration rates should be taken at frequent intervals until well stabilized. Care should be taken to prevent injury to a restless patient by tying a pillow at the head of the bed and padding side rails. If the patient complains of thirst, water may be given unless hemorrhage is internal or the physician has directed that nothing be given by mouth. Temperature is extremely important and should be taken every 4 hours.

For lesser bleeding the patient may or may not be hospitalized. While the cause of the bleeding is being determined through tests and examinations, he may be cared for on an outpatient basis. If the patient is hospitalized, he needs physical rest, relaxation, and relief from emotional strain. Physical exercise should be limited to the amount the individual can tolerate without fatigue. Personal hygiene should include a daily warm bath and good oral care.

The patient may or may not be given iron preparations. If the patient is receiving iron, his teeth should be brushed several times a day. If liquid preparations are administered, they should be given through a straw or drinking tube and the teeth and mouth cleansed after each administration. If there is any disorder of the intestinal tract that makes the oral administration of iron undesirable, it may be given intramuscularly in the form of iron dextran (Imferon). It is given in the gluteal muscle in 1 to 5 ml. injections daily or less frequently and may be con-

Imferon—
Iron prep.—gluteal muscle

tinued until the hemoglobin returns to normal.

A patient receiving oral iron therapy should be observed for gastrointestinal symptoms such as nausea, vomiting, and pain. These should be reported to the physician, since the dose may have to be reduced temporarily. Iron given with or directly after meals is less likely to cause gastric irritation than that given before meals.

Best Time

Many patients, particularly elderly persons, suffer from some degree of constipation; since iron is an irritant to the gastrointestinal tract, it may relieve constipation without employing other means. If necessary, a small low enema is preferred to a drastic cathartic. Some patients may become alarmed when they observe tarry stools, and the nurse will do well to prepare the patient in advance for the color change.

The nurse can contribute much to the patient's progress by exhibiting a sympathetic attitude, being familiar with the dietary needs of the patient, and being able to explain them and assist the patient in planning for adequate nutritional requirements.

Iron-deficiency anemia

Anemia caused by iron deficiency is the most common type of anemia. It is estimated that 90% of the iron-deficiency anemia in adults is found in women. It is the most common cause of anemia in infancy and childhood. The newborn infant stored iron in utero, but these stores are depleted during the first 6 months of life. Iron deficiency after 6 months is usually due to inadequate iron in the diet.

About 50% of all iron in the body is in the hemoglobin of the blood. For the most part this iron is used over and over, with essentially no excretion, and small reserves are available if needed. Since iron is not lost through normal excretion, anemia due to loss of iron has to result from some other cause. In the adult, diet is a factor only if another cause exists. These causes include excessive menstrual bleeding in the adolescent girl and the adult woman, repeated pregnancies with blood loss and transfer of iron to the fetus in utero, and blood loss from the gastrointestinal tract, as might occur from carcinoma. In some cases the body fails to assimilate and utilize the iron.

Pathophysiology. Iron-deficiency anemia is caused by an abnormal decrease in hemoglobin in the red blood cells. Although the red blood cell count may be within a normal range, the cells are small and poorly shaped and therefore are unable to carry their normal amount of hemoglobin. The body gradually exhausts its supply of stored iron, and the blood develops an abnormally low color index (hypochromia). Iron is an essential constituent of enzymes within the cells, and without it the metabolism of the cell is affected and eventually the entire body suffers. Except for pregnancy and infancy, blood loss is the most frequent cause of iron-deficiency anemia. The condition develops gradually, and the individual may consult a physician because of fatigue and weakness. Sometimes during the early stages the anemia may be found on a routine physical examination. Symptoms include pallor, dyspnea, palpitation, and loss of appetite. The nails become brittle and poorly shaped, the tongue is sore, and in some instances there may be difficulty in swallowing. The hemoglobin level will be found to be as low as 10 mg./100 ml. of blood, and if the condition is severe it may be lower.

Treatment. In the absence of observed bleeding a thorough examination should be made to locate any internal source of bleeding. Treatment for iron-deficiency anemia is the administration of iron, which may be given by the oral or the intramuscular route and occasionally intravenously. Iron is absorbed much more slowly when administered orally than it is when injected, and administration may have to be continued for several months. For varying reasons some patients cannot be given iron orally and they usually receive it intramuscularly. When iron is injected, the results are faster and the duration of therapy is shortened; however, it does carry some risk, since fatal reactions have been reported.

Nursing care. Most patients with iron-deficiency anemia will be cared for in the physician's office or the outpatient clinic. If the patient is hospitalized, nursing care is the same as that outlined for hemorrhagic anemia.

Average normal daily iron requirements are as follows:

Men and postmenopausal women	10 mg.
Women during childbearing period	18 mg.
During pregnancy	15 to 35 mg.
Infants	1.5 mg./kg. body weight or about 5 to 15 mg.
Children	10 to 18 mg.
Adolescent boys	10 to 15 mg.
Adolescent girls	12 to 25 mg.

Commonly used iron preparations and their dosages are as follows:

Oral administration	Average daily dose*
Ferrous sulfate (Feosol)	300 mg.
Ferrous gluconate (Fergon)	900 mg.
Ferrous fumarate (Ircon)	600 to 800 mg.
Ferrocholinate (Chel-Iron, Ferrolip)	1 to 2 Gm.
Intramuscular injection	
Iron dextran complex	50 to 250 mg.
Iron sorbitex (Jectofer)	2 to 4 ml.
Intravenous injection	
Dextriferron (Astrafer)	1.5 ml. in 5% solution

Pernicious anemia (primary anemia)

Until 1928, pernicious anemia was considered incurable, and the patient was subject to remissions, relapses, and ultimately death. Although the disease remains incurable, modern treatment has made it possible for the patient to have a normal life-span. At the present time patients with pernicious anemia who die do so from some other cause. The disease primarily affects older persons. Individuals who have had a total gastrectomy will inevitably develop the disease because the source of the intrinsic factor has been removed. Pernicious anemia is not the same as iron-deficiency anemia; however, it is believed that iron-deficiency anemia of long duration may predispose to pernicious anemia.

Pathophysiology. Pernicious anemia is caused by a deficiency of vitamin B_{12}. An intrinsic factor secreted by the fundus of the stomach is necessary for the absorption of vitamin B_{12} by the intestinal mucosa. A person with this type of anemia

does not have the intrinsic factor. In pernicious anemia the red blood cells in the bone marrow fail to mature, and their rate of destruction exceeds their rate of production. The erythrocytes that do reach the bloodstream may be few in number and abnormally large. The red blood cell count may be low, and the hemoglobin will be decreased. The skin may appear a pale lemon yellow because of the excessive death rate of the red blood cells, which cause the bile pigments to be increased in the blood serum. There is little or no secretion of hydrochloric acid in the stomach.

The onset of pernicious anemia is usually insidious with symptoms of a slowly developing anemia. Pallor develops gradually with the yellowish tint to the skin. There may be palpitation, nausea, vomiting, flatulence, indigestion, constipation, and often diarrhea. There is soreness and burning of the tongue, which appears smooth and red with infection about the teeth and gums. Fever, weakness, anorexia, and difficulty in swallowing may also occur. Neurologic symptoms may develop, including tingling of the hands and feet and loss of sense of body position. Cerebral symptoms include loss of memory, mental confusion, and depression. There may be partial or complete paralysis with loss of sphincter control. Death is usually from complications arising from confinement to bed.

Treatment. Once the diagnosis has been established, the treatment consists of injections of hydroxocobalamin (vitamin B_{12}), 1000 μg administered in the gluteal or deltoid muscle every 2 or 3 days until six injections have been given. If the anemia is severe, the patient may be transfused with packed red blood cells. The patient may also require treatment for coexisting conditions such as cardiovascular disorders. Injections of vitamin B_{12} must be continued during the person's lifetime. Treatment is individualized, and one injection bimonthly or every 2 or 3 months may keep the patient free of symptoms.[6]

Nursing care. The nursing care of the patient will depend to some extent on the stage the disease had reached when it was discovered. The nursing care may include complete bed rest, but as the

---

*Dosage must be planned for the individual patient based on the extent of his anemic disorder.

patient responds to therapy, some ambulation is desirable unless severe neurologic changes have occurred. As the patient improves and when he returns home, he may be encouraged to have several short rest periods during the day. While he is confined to the hospital, the vital signs should be checked daily and recorded. An increase in pulse and respiration is to be expected from the body's adjustment to get oxygen to the cells, but any great change should be reported immediately. Special mouth care should be given several times a day, using cotton applicators and a cleansing solution that is nonirritating to the mucous membrane of the mouth. Some patients have found that rinsing the mouth with one of the carbonated beverages is refreshing and helpful. Petroleum jelly or cold cream may be applied to the lips. Mineral oil should not be used, since there is danger that the oil will run down into the lungs and cause pneumonitis.

Meals should be carefully planned to provide a diet high in protein, vitamins, and minerals. It is better to use complete proteins of a high order. Since the patient may have a poor appetite, he may need considerable encouragement to eat. The attractive preparation and serving of food will often stimulate the appetite. Unusually hot, acid, salty, and spicy foods should be avoided because of the soreness of the mouth.

Urinary output should be watched carefully because the loss of sphincter control may cause urinary retention. Constipation may be treated with mild laxatives prescribed by the physician.

Patients with pernicious anemia are especially sensitive to cold, and extra lightweight warm blankets may be needed. Cotton flannel nightclothing, a warm bed jacket, and bed socks will make the patient more comfortable. Hot-water bottles and electric heating pads should be used with caution, particularly with older patients, because of the danger of burning the patient.

If neurologic symptoms such as paralysis have occurred, more intensive care will be needed. The patient will have to be turned at regular intervals, and deep breathing must be encouraged. Special skin care should be given, using an emollient lotion after bathing. Every precaution should be taken to prevent the development of decubiti. (See Chapter 6.) The use of a bed cradle to support covers, a footboard to prevent foot drop, and good body alignment will help to make the patient more comfortable and contribute to rehabilitation. If the patient is mentally confused or restless, side rails should be used.

Passive exercise may be given by the nurse and will help to maintain muscle tone and improve circulation. The patient with limb paralysis may be taught to walk again, but much will depend on his desire to walk and his willingness to make a real effort.

Most patients with pernicious anemia are past 40 years of age, and lifetime patterns have been established. It may cause considerable emotional shock for the patient to learn that he has an incurable disease. The patient may reject the diagnosis and lose valuable time needed for therapy. The nurse may help the patient by stressing how regular treatment will help the patient feel well, be well, and live a happy normal life. Persons who are economically depressed may need assistance from a community social agency, and elderly persons may be provided for through the social security Medicare or Medicaid program.

Sickle cell anemia

Until recently little attention was given to sickle cell anemia. The disease is found almost exclusively in blacks, and its distribution is world wide. Various estimates have placed the number of persons with the disease to be from 50,000 to 75,000. The disease is a genetic blood disorder affecting both men and women, and approximately one of every ten black persons carries the trait. The disease is transmitted to the offspring by the parent who has the defective gene. The disease is seen most frequently in children, rarely in infancy, and the mortality rate is high. The high death rate during childhood accounts for the small number of cases among adults. Screening clinics have been established in many areas of the United States to identify persons with the trait. Although there is no preventive treatment or cure for the disease, counseling helps the person to avoid the factors that may predispose to a serious exacerbation.

Pathophysiology. Sickle cell anemia is caused by an abnormal hemoglobin molecule. When the molecule is present in the red blood cell, it causes the cell to acquire a sickle or crescent shape. The sickle-shaped cell cannot move normally through the blood vessels and tends to block or clog small vessels. The cells are fragile and may break apart, causing blood clots to form. The life of the sickled cell is short, and the production of new cells is not fast enough to keep oxygen supplied to the tissues of the body. As a result, the person may experience attacks of severe pain in various organs and in the bones. There may be fever, anemia, thrombi in the lungs and the spleen, and the spleen may be enlarged. The hemoglobin level is low, but the patient does not appear to be affected by it. Leg ulcers may occur. These persons are especially susceptible to salmonella infections and pneumonia caused by the pneumococcus bacteria. The rate of maternal complications such as hemorrhage and eclamptic conditions is reported to be high.

Treatment. Treatment is preventive and supportive. Children should be immunized against preventable diseases. Any activity that causes stress or requires strenuous exercise and that would limit oxygen supply should be avoided. Good health habits including rest, proper diet, avoiding respiratory infections, and regular medical supervision should be encouraged. Although most persons may remain asymptomatic, an acute exacerbation (crisis) may occur. The patient is admitted to the hospital and placed on a regimen of bed rest. There may be fever, severe pain in the arms, legs, and abdomen, and leukocytosis. Treatment may include small doses of a mild analgesic such as codeine to relieve pain and oral fluids; if dehydration is present, intravenous infusion of electrolyte solutions is prepared to combat acidosis. The patient with sickle cell disease needs a great deal of encouragement and emotional support. This is especially true of the parent who has a child with the disease and who knows that the child may not live to reach his tenth birthday.[7, 16]

Polycythemia

Polycythemia is a chronic disease usually found in white males of middle age, and people of Jewish ancestry are often affected. The disease is caused by a proliferation of erythrocytes in the bone marrow. The red blood cell count may range from 7000 to 10 million/mm.[3] of blood. The disease occurs in two forms, primary and secondary. The cause of primary polycythemia is unknown. In the absence of cardiorespiratory disease the oxygen content of the blood is normal, but the rate of flow is decreased and the viscosity is increased. The decreased rate of flow and increased viscosity may lead to thrombosis in small blood vessels. The leukocyte count is increased and may reach 25,000 to 50,000/mm.[3] A defective platelet factor increases coagulation time and predisposes to intravascular thrombosis. The spleen and liver are enlarged, and bleeding in the form of ecchymosis occurs in mucous membranes and skin. The patient appears cyanotic with a look of fullness and may complain of headache, fatigue, and dizziness. These persons appear to be predisposed to gout and peptic ulcer. The secondary form of the disease accompanies several other chronic disorders, including cardiac and pulmonary disease. This form has been associated with benign and malignant tumors, particularly malignant tumors of the kidney. In the absence of infection the leukocyte count is near normal. The primary factor in secondary polycythemia is decreased oxygen in the blood.

Treatment. The objective of treatment of polycythemia is to suppress the bone marrow, reduce the blood cell mass, maintain the hematocrit value at or below 50%, and reduce the leukocyte and platelet count. Phlebotomy and the removal of up to 500 ml. of blood at intervals may accomplish the objectives for some patients. Chemotherapeutic drugs may also be used, including melphalan (Alkeran), chlorambucil (Leukeran), and busulfan (Myleran). Radioactive phosphorus (³²P) may be administered intravenously. Combinations of phlebotomy with chemotherapy and radioactive phosphorus are also used.

Survival time is long, and patients will be required to continue receiving medication. Persons who survive 10 years or longer frequently develop leukemia. The role of the nurse is supportive. The patient should be encouraged to maintain good health habits and regular medical supervision.[6, 9]

Disorders of white blood cells
Leukocytosis

Leukocytosis is an increase in the number of white blood cells. It is both a protective and a destructive mechanism. On p. 28 the role of the leukocytes in defending the body against infectious agents was discussed. In many diseases that are potentially dangerous, leukocytes are increased and play an important role in helping the body to overcome an infection. In some forms of leukemia large numbers of immature leukocytes are produced, causing changes in the spleen, liver, and lymph nodes.

Leukopenia

Leukopenia is a condition in which the number of leukocytes are greatly reduced. When the granulocytes (granulocytosis, p. 232) are reduced, serious bacterial infection may occur. There are numerous conditions causing leukopenia, including chemical agents known to be toxic to the body. Among these agents are the analgesic and antipyretic drug aminopyrine (amidopyrine), sulfapyridine, radioactive phosphorus (previously mentioned), and nitrogen mustard preparations. Whenever leukopenia occurs, the patient should be isolated and protected from infection. The nurse should recall that the protective mechanism afforded by the leukocytes no longer exists, and the patient's life could be in danger if infection should develop.

Infectious mononucleosis

Infectious mononucleosis is an acute infectious disease involving the white blood cells. The number of leukocytes may be increased from 10,000 to 25,000/mm.[3] The lymphocytes (agranulocytes) are also increased, some of which will be immature although most will be mature. The clinical manifestations of the disease involve the lymphoid tissues of the body, particularly the lymph nodes and the spleen. (See Chapter 23.)

Agranulocytosis

Agranulocytosis is an acute disease that is more common in women than in men. The white blood cells decrease to an extremely low level with the neutrophil leukocytes greatly decreased. The cause of the disease is believed to result from sensitization to drugs and/or chemicals. With the great reduction of leukocytes, infection develops with high temperature, chills, ulceration of the skin, mouth, and mucous membranes, septicemia, and acute prostration. Before the development of antibiotics the mortality rate for this disease was high. Treatment includes withdrawal of the drug responsible for the condition and controlling the infection with broad-spectrum antimicrobial agents. Fortunately, the disease is uncommon, but if it should occur, most patients will recover with proper treatment.[6]

Hodgkin's disease

Hodgkin's disease, generally considered to be a malignant condition, involves the lymph nodes and lymphatic tissues. The disease was thought to be fatal, but now many persons can be cured and the lives of others may be prolonged. Hodgkin's disease represents only a small percent of all malignant disorders; however, the American Cancer Society, Inc., predicted that 4800 new cases would be diagnosed during 1973. The disease occurs in a ratio of about 10:7, more frequently in men than in women, and rarely occurs in those under 20 years of age,[14] although it may occur at any age. The cause of Hodgkin's disease is unknown. The first sign of the disease may be an asymptomatic enlargement of a lymph node in the neck. As the disease progresses, the deep lymph nodes in the mediastinum and the retroperitoneal cavity with the adjacent tissues are involved. The spleen and liver become enlarged, and in about one fifth the cases the bone marrow is affected. Symptoms include pruritus, which begins early in the disease, and dyspnea because of pressure from lymph node enlargement. Fever varies with the extent of involvement. There is a loss of weight, difficulty in swallowing, edema of the extremities, and jaundice.

Treatment and nursing care. Hodgkin's disease is classified into groups according to pathologic findings and the probable prognosis. Based on these findings, the disease is further classified into stages. From stage one each subsequent stage represents increased activity and progression of the disease. Depending on the stage, treatment may be curative or only palliative. In the early stages treatment consists of radiotherapy of the involved lymph nodes and the contiguous tissues with a view toward cure. In later stages a combination of radiotherapy and chemotherapy is used. When the disease becomes widespread, radiotherapy has little benefit and chemotherapeutic drugs and steroids are administered in cycles. All of these drugs are toxic, and the patient must be carefully observed. Although cure may not be achieved in the late stage of the disease, remission extending over several years may occur.[5, 6]

The nursing care of the patient is the same as that for leukemia. Special attention must be given to the care of the mouth and lips, which become dry and fissured because of the elevated temperature. These patients often suffer from severe itching of the skin (pruritus), and the physician may order a cooling soothing lotion to be applied several times a day. The patient is especially susceptible to infection and should be protected against respiratory infections and skin infections, which may result from scratching.

Leukemias

Leukemia and Hodgkin's disease are now classified together as "neoplasms of lymphatic and hematopoietic tissue." Mortality rate from leukemia in children in the United States has shown some small progress. Variations in survival rates depend on the type of leukemia and the age group affected. In 1968, the last year when statistics became available, the highest death rate was for children 0 to 4 years of age. In adults 55 to 64 years of age the death rate began to rise sharply and continued to rise for all age groups after 64 years of age.[14]

Leukemia may be acute or chronic and is usually classified according to the type of cells involved. Acute leukemia is the form most common in children, but chronic forms may also occur. Chronic leukemia is most common in persons past 45 years of age,[3] but acute leukemia may occur in adult persons of any age. Approximately 50% to 60% of all leukemia in the United States is classified as acute leukemia.

Acute leukemia

Acute leukemia is most common in children under 10 years of age; most deaths occur in children under 4 years of age. In children the disease develops suddenly, whereas in adults it is more insidious. In children leukemia usually occurs as acute lymphocytic or myelogenous leukemia and in adults as acute lymphocytic or myelocytic leukemia (referring to the type of cells involved). Regardless of the type of cells involved, whether in children or adults, the characteristics and progress of the disease are essentially the same.

Pathophysiology. Early in the course of acute leukemia, lymphatic tissues are involved, including lymph nodes and the spleen. The enlarged lymph nodes may be the first signs of the disease in some persons. The leukemic cells (lymphocytes, nongranular leukocytes) multiply in the bone marrow. Their proliferation causes a decrease in the production of red blood cells and shortens their life. The platelets are also reduced. With the reduction of erythrocytes, anemia may develop, and the decreased platelets interfere with the blood clotting mechanism, which results in bleeding. During the course of the disease almost all organs of the body become involved. With treatment, remissions may occur during which erythrocyte production may return to nearly normal.

The onset of the disease often begins with a slight cold or tonsillitis. The temperature may range from low grade to high. The child may complain of headache and abdominal pain; in the very young child, pain may be evidenced by crying, restlessness, and reluctance to move or be moved. In the adult the onset of the disease may be traced to a cold from which recovery was slow. This is followed by prostration, weakness, anemia, and anorexia. If the anemia is severe, there may be pallor. Ulcerations occur about the mouth, skin, and rectum. Bleeding varies from ecchymosis and petechiae to purpura, which may become necrotic and ulcerative.

Symptoms will vary widely as various organs or parts of the body are involved.[10]

Treatment. Tremendous progress in the treatment of leukemia has been made during the last decade. In 1968 the survival rate for acute lymphocytic leukemia was from 1 to 1½ years, but it has now been increased to 3 years for 90% of the patients treated. Acute myelogenous leukemia has shown less response to treatment. Until the present time little could be done for acute leukemia in adults. The National Cancer Institute reports that there is the possibility that some patients are being cured. In acute myelocytic leukemia more than half the patients treated have achieved complete remissions during which all evidence of the disease disappeared. Treatment with a combination of drugs administered for 5-day periods with rest intervals of 5 to 10 days and continued over a long time has provided significant results. Drugs currently being used in this type of treatment are vincristine, prednisolone, methotrexate, and 6-mercaptopurine. Several new drugs have been found effective in the treatment of the disease. These include cytosine arabinoside, daunomycin, and L-asparaginase. In acute lymphocytic leukemia, cytosine arabinoside has been found increasingly useful.[13] A number of other drugs are under investigation.

Nursing care. The nurse who is caring for the patient with acute leukemia should remember that all the drugs being used produce toxic symptoms. Many of the symptoms concurrent with the disease are the result of the treatment rather than the disease. If the person receives blood transfusions, packed red blood cells, or platelets, he must be observed for transfusion reaction. When numerous transfusions are given, the danger of reaction is increased. The nurse must also help to protect the vein used for administration of medications. It is well to remember that hematomas or hemorrhage may occur from any puncture of the skin. Since infections and hemorrhage account for many of the deaths from leukemia, the nurse must be constantly alert to protect the patient from infection and to report immediately any severe bleeding or indication of infection.

The child with acute leukemia may come into the hospital several times during the course of the disease. The care of this child offers a real challenge to the nurse. Examinations and treatment may be painful experiences for him, and he may be fearful. The nurse should do everything possible to relieve the anxiety of both child and parent. Many times the child will be ambulatory. If he is of school age, he may work on lessons, or a visiting teacher may visit him in the hospital. He may enjoy television or radio. His room should be attractive, and the toys that he has learned to love and care for should be nearby. Everything possible should be done to help the child lead as normal a life as possible.

Although the parents may have known for weeks that the child cannot live, they continue to hope that the diagnosis will prove to be wrong or that some new drug will be discovered that will save the child's life. Parents need tender loving care at this time as much as the child, and perhaps more. Nurses should be sympathetic and understanding and above all must identify and clarify their own feelings concerning death before giving supportive help to parents who are facing the loss of their child.[15] The hospital chaplain or family religious counselor may give comfort and support to the parents and family of the child.

When the child enters the hospital for the last time, the nurse will provide the care of the child. The child suffers from bone pain, and gentleness and tenderness must be exercised when moving or handling him. He will be irritable, and the nurse must have unlimited patience and attend to his needs promptly. The administration of medications and treatments should be done on time. The child may be unable to use a toothbrush because of ulcers in the mouth and soft bleeding gums, and there may be a foul odor from the oral condition. Soft cotton applicators with a cleansing solution should be used. One teaspoonful of sodium bicarbonate in a glass of warm water with a little peppermint as flavoring or a solution of hydrogen peroxide that can be tolerated may be used. The most meticulous care must be given to the mouth to prevent infection, but care must be taken not to cause bleeding. Care of the nose is of equal importance, and cotton applicators should be used to clean the nares, with care exercised to prevent epistaxis. A mild lubricant such as cold cream should be applied to the nose and lips. The external genitalia need special care, since ulcerations may occur about the area. There may be bleeding about the rectum, and the membrane may be sore and tender. Rectal temperatures should be taken carefully to avoid undue discomfort and pain for the child. All urinary output and feces should be carefully checked for evidence of bleeding from the gastrointestinal and urinary tracts. If the child is receiving cortisone, he may be receiving a sodium-restricted diet. Because of anorexia and soreness of the mouth, he may refuse food. Permitting parents to eat their meal with the child may encourage him to eat. Food should be attractive and should be of a consistency that will not require a large amount of effort on the part of the child. Avoid encouraging the child in play activities at this stage because the exhaustion may be overwhelming. As the child lapses into coma, it is important for the nurse to remain with the child and the parents. All nursing care should be continued as long as the child lives.

Chronic lymphocytic, granulocytic, and myelocytic leukemia

Chronic leukemia is confined almost entirely to adults, and about 90% of chronic leukemia consists of the lymphocytic and myelocytic types. Chronic lymphocytic leukemia develops slowly, and the individual may be completely asymptomatic when the disorder is discovered on a routine physical examination. In chronic myelocytic leukemia the spleen becomes enlarged to the extent that the patient can palpate it, and he becomes aware of a heavy feeling in his upper left abdomen. In granulocytic leukemia there is increased production of granulocytes with splenomegaly. Chronic lymphocytic leukemia may progress slowly, or it may progress rapidly to a fatal termination. The leukocyte count is increased, and lymph nodes throughout the body are enlarged but are not painful; lymph node enlargement occurs less frequently in the myelocytic form of the disease, but when it does occur, the lymph nodes are painful. All forms of the disease are characterized by similar symptoms, including weakness,

fever, loss of appetite, loss of weight, anemia, enlargement of body organs, and hemorrhage.

The desired objectives of treatment in chronic leukemia partially depend on the kind of cells that are involved. In chronic myelocytic leukemia the purpose of treatment is to bring about a reduction in the number of leukocytes. When the white blood cell count is kept at or near normal, other symptoms are modified. In chronic lymphocytic leukemia the primary consideration is directed toward relief of the conditions that arise from the increased production of lymphocytes, such as the enlarged and painful lymph nodes and spleen, anemia, and decrease in the number of platelets. In granulocytic leukemia treatment is directed toward controlling the proliferation of granulocytes. Drugs commonly used in chronic leukemia include chlorambucil (Leukeran), corticosteroids, and cyclophosphamide (Cytoxan), all of which are administered orally. Irradiation of lymph nodes is often used, and blood transfusions may be given if the anemia is severe. In granulocytic leukemia, busulfan administered orally is generally considered to be the drug of choice. The drug produces toxic symptoms, including nausea, vomiting, loss of appetite, weakness, and loss of weight; therefore the physician determines the smallest dose possible to maintain the patient. Patients who cannot tolerate busulfan may be given 6-mercaptopurine (6MP) or hydroxyurea, which is administered in oral doses.[6] Although these drugs are not curative, they help to prolong life expectancy for patients with chronic leukemia. Life expectancy for patients with chronic leukemia is longer than for those with acute leukemia, and with the work being done with some of the newer drugs it is possible that life expectancy may be further increased.

The patient with chronic leukemia should be on a regimen of bed rest until the temperature is normal and should be confined to bed if hemorrhage or severe anemia occurs. The nursing care during severe relapses is the same as that for patients with acute leukemia. When the patient is ambulatory in the hospital or in the home, regular daily planned rest periods should be observed to minimize fatigue and weakness. The public health nurse may visit the patient in the home to encourage him to live within his limitations and to remain under medical supervision.

The patient may be having blood transfusions and must be observed carefully each time for early signs of reaction. The nurse should review Chapter 5 for the care of the patient receiving x-ray therapy. If nausea and vomiting should occur, the patient may feel better if he is given less solid food. Concentrated types of soluble carbohydrates found in sugars are readily absorbed; therefore they may be better tolerated.

Hemorrhagic disorders
Hemophilia

Hemophilia is a general term that is applied to a group of diseases that have certain things in common. They are all hereditary bleeding diseases that have a prolonged bleeding time. They all exhibit a deficiency in one or more of the factors essential for coagulation of the blood. The most common form of the disease is *classic hemophilia A.* This form appears only in males and is transmitted by the female. *Christmas disease* (hemophilia B) occurs most commonly in males; however, the female carrier may have a deficiency of an essential factor that may cause mild bleeding. Such episodes of bleeding are usually not of a serious nature. A third form of the disease is *von Willebrand's disease* (hemophilia C, vascular hemophilia), which occurs in both males and females.[9]

Symptoms. Severe bleeding may occur in any part of the body. Repeated hemorrhages into joints such as ankles, knees, and elbows may damage them to the extent that mobility is difficult. Hemorrhage into muscles may lead to contractures. Bleeding occurs into soft tissues and throughout the gastrointestinal tract, and minor injuries such as cuts, lacerations, or bruises may lead to fatal bleeding. There may be hematomas, and hematuria, and anemia is often present.

Treatment and nursing care. Treatment is first preventive. The individual with hemophilia in any form must be guarded against injuries. Athletic activities are usually advised against. Parents should receive instruction concerning activities for young children and should know when an injury is serious enough to call the physician. Genetic counseling should be available to the family. If there has been a severe hemorrhage, fresh whole blood may be given. At the present time cryoprecipitate is the treatment of choice for persons with hemophilia A. In hemophilia B, plasma concentrates containing the deficient factors may be administerd. In hemophilia C, fresh frozen plasma or cryoprecipitate is given. Patients having pain from joint or muscle complications may need analgesics to relieve pain. Analgesics containing aspirin or narcotics are usually avoided.

When giving injections, the nurse should use a small needle and apply firm pressure to the injection site for some time after the injection. The patient should be kept quiet by the use of the recommended sedation if necessary. Diet should be high in iron, vitamin C, and protein, with high-protein drinks between meals. The application of cold compresses and pressure sometimes lessens the amount of bleeding into the tissues.

Vascular purpuras petechiae & ecchymoses

Purpura is a condition in which there are small, spontaneous hemorrhages into the skin or mucous membrane. Tiny hemorrhages appearing as pinpoint purplish spots are called *petechiae;* larger hemorrhages are called *ecchymoses.* Purpura may be divided into two categories: those associated with the destruction of platelets and those caused by failure of the bone marrow to produce platelets. *Idiopathic thrombocytopenic purpura* is caused by the destruction of the platelets in the blood. The destruction results in a greatly reduced number of platelets and leads to bleeding. The disorder occurs in an acute form in children and may progress to a chronic disorder. It also occurs as a chronic disorder most commonly in young adult females. Destruction of the platelets is caused by an antiplatelet factor in the plasma. In the chronic form it may occur as a complication of a primary disease or after the ingestion of certain drugs. The platelets may collect in blood vessels, blocking and damaging them. In some forms the platelets are deposited in large numbers in

enlargement
of the spleen

the spleen, causing splenomegaly, and a splenectomy may be performed. The second form of the disease, _thrombocytopenic purpura_, is caused by a failure in production of platelets, which may be the result of damage to the bone marrow (p. 232). Drugs and chemicals or conditions that require massive blood transfusions may result in purpura.[9]

Treatment and nursing care. Treatment and care are dependent on discovering and eliminating the cause. If purpura is caused by the destruction of platelets, both the acute and the chronic stages of the disorder are treated with steroids. In some situations removal of the spleen may be indicated.[6] If purpura is caused by a drug, withdrawing the drug will usually correct the condition. Senile purpura is frequently seen in elderly persons, often occurring on the back of the hands, and is caused by a loss of elasticity of the subcutaneous tissue. A diet high in iron and protein is usually ordered, and iron therapy may be instituted.[15]

Splenomegaly

The spleen is located in the upper part of the abdominal cavity under the lower part of the rib cage. In blood dyscrasias in which blood cell production in the marrow is compromised, the spleen may assume the function of producing all the blood cells. It is also the organ that produces antibodies. Not all of the functions of the spleen are understood. Enlargement of the spleen occurs in several diseases and is called _splenomegaly_.

Splenectomy

Chronic congestive splenomegaly is frequently associated with certain blood dyscrasias in which removal of the spleen (splenectomy) may be indicated. Various disorders affecting the spleen may also require its removal. Injury to the organ, especially a crushing type, is always a surgical emergency.

Postoperative nursing care. The nursing care of the patient after a splenectomy is essentially the same as that for other patients after abdominal surgery. (See Chapter 9.) Since the spleen has a rich blood supply and the patient may have a blood dyscrasia, it is important that the patient be carefully observed for postoperative hemorrhage. An elevation of temperature may exist for 7 to 10 days after surgery.

Summary outline

1. The blood—its function and structure
   A. Function—transportation of oxygen, carbon dioxide, water, electrolytes, hormones, and enzymes
      1. Heat to help regulate body temperature
      2. Immune bodies and antibodies to help prevent disease and infection
      3. To provide clotting of blood in case of injury
      4. To prevent clot formation in blood vessels
   B. Structure
      1. Plasma—liquid part of blood; contains no cells; about 90% water, remaining 10% carries large number of substances dissolved in it
         a. Plasma proteins—serum albumin, serum globulin, and fibrinogen
            (1) Regulation of blood volume
            (2) Provide nutrition to body cells
            (3) Functions in clotting of blood
            (4) In circulating antibodies
      2. Cells—formed elements
         a. Erythrocytes—red blood cells
            (1) Erythropoiesis—production of erythrocytes
            (2) Main ingredient is hemoglobin; each molecule of hemoglobin contains iron and a pigment
            (3) Carries oxygen to tissues and returns carbon dioxide
         b. Leukocytes—white blood cells; increase is called leukocytosis; decrease is called leukopenia
            (1) Granular leukocytes called granulocytes
            (2) Nongranular leukocytes called agranulocytes; include lymphocytes and monocytes
         c. Differential count—several different kinds of white blood cells
         d. Platelets, or thrombocytes; may be fragments of large cells, megakaryocytes
            (1) Function to control hemorrhage
            (2) Abnormal increase called thrombocytosis
2. Blood fractions
   Blood may be broken down into its component parts
   A. Blood plasma—contains all factors necessary for blood clotting
   B. Platelets—increased demand for platelets; may be administered in fresh whole blood, in plasma, or as platelet concentrate
   C. Globulins—serum proteins
      1. Immunoglobulin (Ig), gamma globulin
      2. Albumin
      3. Fibrinogen
      4. Hyperimmune gamma globulin
      5. Immune serum globulin

D. Cryoprecipitate—contains antihemophilic factor to control bleeding
E. Packed red blood cells—contain no plasma; used when blood volume is normal but red blood cells and hemoglobin are decreased

3. Hematogenic (hypovolemic) shock
   A. Pathophysiology
      1. Volume of circulating fluid decreased
      2. Venous return to heart decreased
      3. Less blood being pumped out, depriving cells of oxygen
      4. Body tries to compensate during early stages
      5. Blood pressure begins to fall, increase in pulse and respiratory rates, loss of consciousness, skin cool, pale, moist, temperature subnormal, cyanosis, coma, death
   B. Nursing care and observations

4. Collection of blood
   A. American Red Cross maintains regional centers and mobile units
   B. Hospitals collect blood for their own use and emergency needs
   C. Commercial centers pay fee to donors
   D. Centers to separate plasma from red blood cells and return red blood cells to donor; process is called plasmapheresis

5. Body fluids and electrolytes
   Estimated that 60% to 70% of body fluid is water
   A. Intracellular fluid—within the cells
   B. Extracellular fluid—outside the cells
      1. Intravascular fluid within blood vessels as plasma
      2. Interstitial fluid between tissues
   C. Balance is maintained by intake and output
   D. Electrolytes—substances dissolved in body fluids
      1. Principal electrolytes are sodium, calcium, potassium, and magnesium
         a. Measured by chemical analysis of blood plasma
         b. Acquired by ingestion of fluids and water, lost by loss of fluids from body

6. Diagnostic tests and procedures
   Large number of tests are performed on blood, some for diagnostic purposes and others for following course of disease
   A. Complete blood count—most common test performed on blood and includes count of red blood cells, white blood cells, hemoglobin, and other cells (differential)
   B. Blood gas analysis—measures oxygen and carbon dioxide content of blood; used in respiratory diseases to measure functional ability of lungs
   C. Hemoglobin electrophoresis—identifies abnormal hemoglobins
   D. Paul-Bunnell test—determines presence or absence of infectious mononucleosis
   E. Coagulation time—not always reliable because many factors may affect it, and test may be significant only if time is prolonged
   F. Hematocrit—measures volume of cells and plasma in blood
   G. Icterus index—measures amount of yellowness in blood
   H. Prothrombin time—indicates clotting ability of blood, usually performed daily on patients receiving anticoagulant therapy
   I. Sedimentation rate—measures time necessary for red blood cells to settle to bottom of test tube
   J. Bone marrow aspiration—to obtain specimen for biopsy
   K. Blood chemistry—is chemical analysis of blood and may be performed on whole blood, plasma, or blood serum
   L. Blood serology—serologic examination of blood for syphilis
   M. Blood typing and cross matching—essential for purposes of blood transfusion
      1. Types A, B, AB, and O
      2. Patient should be transfused with same type of blood as his own
      3. Administration of 500 ml. of whole blood will usually elevate number of red blood cells and hemoglobin 15% in 24 hours
   N. Rh factor—extra protein substance found in blood of some persons
      1. Rh-positive persons who have this protein comprise 85% of population
      2. Rh-negative persons who do not have this protein comprise remaining 15%
      3. Rh factor must be determined when cross matching is done for transfusion purposes
   O. Blood transfusion—may be administered for following reasons:
      1. To replace or maintain blood volume
      2. To preserve oxygen-carrying power of blood
      3. To increase or maintain coagulation ability of blood

7. Specific nursing functions
   A. Blood transfusion therapy
      1. Transmit request to laboratory
      2. Assemble equipment
      3. Check and identify information on label of blood from laboratory with patient's blood type
   B. Causes for reaction to blood
      1. Incompatibility of patient's blood and donor's blood
      2. Allergy in donor
      3. Contamination of blood or equipment
      4. Air in circulation
   C. Elderly patients and patients with cardiac disease must be observed carefully during transfusion
   D. Diseases transmitted by blood transfusions
      1. Hepatitis
      2. Malaria
      3. Syphilis
   E. Blood chemistry
      1. Transmit request to laboratory
      2. Identify bed and room
      3. Give nothing by mouth after midnight
      4. Hold breakfast until blood specimen has been taken

8. Nursing patient with diseases and disorders of blood and blood-forming organs
   Diseases and disorders of blood and blood-forming organs are called *blood dyscrasias*

A. Causes—cover wide range of diseases and disorders
  1. Some may be controlled
  2. Some are hereditary
  3. Predisposition to some because of life style
B. Anemia—not disease, but condition in which there is reduction of red blood cells, hemoglobin, and iron
  1. Hemorrhagic anemia—may be acute or chronic; result of sudden loss of large amount of blood or slow bleeding over long period of time
    a. Traumatic injury
    b. Hemoptysis
    c. Childbirth
    d. Ulcerative lesions
    e. Disorders of coagulation
    f. Gastric ulcer
    g. Hemorrhoids
    h. Pathophysiology
      (1) Loss of blood decreases circulating fluid, decreases hemoglobin and lower hematocrit, decreases amount of oxygen to tissues
      (2) In severe blood loss hematogenic shock may occur
      (3) Symptoms—fatigue, drop in blood pressure, tachycardia; if bleeding prolonged, pallor, fainting, dizziness, shortness of breath, headache, drowsiness
    i. Emergency care
    j. Follow-up care
    k. Nursing care
  2. Iron-deficiency anemia—most common type
    a. Hemoglobin of blood contains 50% of iron in body
    b. Causes
      (1) Excessive menstrual bleeding
      (2) Repeated pregnancies
      (3) Blood loss as in gastrointestinal malignancy
    c. Pathophysiology
      (1) Blood loss causing abnormal decrease in hemoglobin
      (2) Red blood cells are small and poorly shaped; unable to carry normal amount of hemoglobin
      (3) Body exhausts stored supply of iron
      (4) Hypochromia develops, caused by decreased pigment
      (5) Symptoms—fatigue, weakness, pallor, dyspnea, nails become brittle, tongue sore, difficulty in swallowing
    d. Treatment—administration of iron
    e. Patient usually treated on outpatient basis
  3. Pernicious anemia
    a. Pathophysiology
      (1) Caused by deficiency of vitamin B_{12}; intrinsic factor in stomach is absent

      (2) Intrinsic factor is necessary for absorption and utilization of vitamin B_{12}
      (3) Decrease in hemoglobin
      (4) Bile pigments increase in blood, causing pale yellow color of skin
      (5) Little or no hydrochloric acid in stomach
      (6) Symptoms
    b. Treatment
    c. Nursing care
  4. Sickle cell anemia—found almost exclusively among blacks
    a. Disease is hereditary and has no known treatment
    b. Pathophysiology
      (1) Red blood cells are sickle shaped because of abnormal hemoglobin molecule in blood
      (2) Cells do not move freely through bloodstream; may break apart causing clots
      (3) Production of new cells not fast enough to supply oxygen to tissues
      (4) Symptoms
    c. Treatment
C. Polycythemia
  1. Chronic disease found in white males, often affecting Jewish people
  2. Two forms of disease
    a. Primary and secondary
  3. Cause—proliferation of erythrocytes in bone marrow, cause unknown
  4. Decreased rate of blood flow and increased viscosity
  5. Increase in leukocytes
  6. Defective platelet factor causing increased coagulation time
  7. Spleen and liver enlarged
  8. Bleeding into mucous membranes and skin
  9. Treatment
D. Disorders of white blood cells
  1. Leukocytosis—increase in number of white blood cells
  2. Leukopenia—reduction in number of white blood cells
  3. Infectious mononucleosis—infectious disease with increased leukocytes and lymphocytes
  4. Agranulocytosis—acute disease with white blood cells greatly decreased
E. Hodgkin's disease—involves lymph nodes and lymphatic tissues
  1. Some persons cured, others have life prolonged
  2. Cause unknown
  3. Nursing care—same as for leukemia, with special attention to mouth and lip care
    a. Pruritus a common symptom; may be relieved by application of soothing lotion to skin
F. Leukemias—malignant disease classified with cancer; may be acute or chronic; type depends on type of cell involved

1. Acute leukemia—most common in children
   a. Pathophysiology
      (1) Onset usually sudden in children
      (2) In adults onset is insidious
      (3) Enlarged lymph nodes and spleen
      (4) Leukemic cells multiply in bone marrow
      (5) Decrease in production of red blood cells
      (6) Reduction in platelets
      (7) Anemia
      (8) Symptoms
   b. Treatment
   c. Nursing care
2. Chronic leukemia—confined almost entirely to adults
   a. Chronic lymphocytic or myelocytic leukemia
   b. Chronic granulocytic leukemia
   c. Treatment based on clinical findings and planned for individual patient
   d. Life expectancy for chronic leukemia patient longer than that for acute leukemia patient

G. Hemorrhagic disorders
   1. Hemophilia—includes group of diseases
      a. All are hereditary bleeding diseases
      b. All are deficient in factors essential for coagulation of blood
      c. Forms of the disease
         (1) Classic hemophilia A
         (2) Christmas disease or hemophilia B
         (3) von Willebrand's disease, or hemophilia C
      d. Symptoms
      e. Treatment and nursing care
   2. Vascular purpuras—from many causes, including drugs, chemicals, and disease
      a. Petechiae are pinpoint purplish spots on skin
      b. Ecchymoses are larger hemorrhages into skin
      c. Categories
         (1) Idiopathic thrombocytopenic purpura—caused by destruction of platelets in blood
         (2) Thrombocytopenic purpura—caused by failure to produce platelets
      d. Treatment—steroid therapy

H. Splenomegaly—enlargement of spleen, which occurs in certain blood diseases
   1. Splenectomy (surgical removal of spleen) because of injury, or certain blood dyscrasias may be necessary
      a. Preoperative and postoperative care—same as that for other abdominal surgery
         (1) Postoperatively patient must be carefully observed for hemorrhage
         (2) Elevation of temperature for 7 to 10 days

Review questions

1. What three substances would you expect to find in hemoglobin?
   a. *O₂ Serum globulins*
   b. ~~Hyper~~immune serum globulins
   c. *Hyperimmune gamma globulins*
2. If a patient is receiving an anticoagulant drug, would you expect the prothrombin time to be decreased, increased, or unchanged?
   a. ~~decres~~ *increased*
3. List four important electrolytes found in body fluids.
   a. *sodium*
   b. *calcium*
   c. *magnesium*
   d. *potassium*
4. What term is applied to the production of erythrocytes?
   a. *erythropoiesis*
5. What three types of reactions may occur during a blood transfusion?
   a. *allergic (hypersensitivity)*
   b. *hemolytic (incompatibility)*
   c. *pyogenic (contamination)*
6. What specific treatment is given to a person who has pernicious anemia?
   a. *Vit. B₁₂*
7. At what ages would you expect to find the highest death rate from acute leukemia?
   a. *0-4*
8. What conditions may cause loss of electrolytes from body fluids?
   a. *vomiting*
   b. *diarrhea*
   c. *gastric suction*
   d. *ostomies*
   e. *inc. respiration*
   f.
   g.
9. What is the basic factor involved in hematogenic shock?
   a. *loss of blood*
10. What is the name of the process of separating plasma from the red blood cells and returning the red blood cells to the donor?
    a. *plasmapheresis*

Films

1. Fresh blood, whole blood, packed red cells—T2017 (32 min., sound, black and write, 16 mm.), Media Resources Branch, National Medical Audiovisual Center (Annex), Station K, Atlanta, Ga. 30324. Discusses the advantages and disadvantages of usage of whole blood and packed red blood cells in medical situations, during surgery, and after traumatic hemorrhage.
2. Nutritional anemia. Part 1, Hypochromic anemia—M2089 X (22 min., sound, color, 16 mm.), Media Resources Branch, National Medical Audiovisual Center (Annex), Station K, Atlanta, Ga. 30324. Describes hypochromic anemia and compares the normal color indexes with anemia deficiencies. Discusses the treatment program.

3. Pathogenesis of anemia—T1504 (30 min., sound, black and white, 16 mm.), Media Resources Branch, National Medical Audiovisual Center (Annex), Station K, Atlanta, Ga. 30324. Shows normal and abnormal red blood cell mass in different types of anemia.
4. Platelets and leukocytes—T2018 (20 min., sound, black and white, 16 mm.), Media Resources Branch, National Medical Audiovisual Center (Annex), Station K, Atlanta, Ga. 30324. Shows how cryoprecipitate can be prepared for the treatment of hemophilia. The film discusses other blood fractions.

References

1. Anthony, Catherine P.: Textbook of anatomy and physiology, ed. 9, St. Louis, 1975, The C. V. Mosby Co.
2. Barber, Janet M., Stokes, Lillian G., and Billings, Diane M.: Adult and child care, St. Louis, 1973, The C. V. Mosby Co.
3. Beeson, Paul B., and McDermott, Walsh, editors: Cecil-Loeb textbook of medicine, ed. 13, Philadelphia, 1973, W. B. Saunders Co.
4. Bordicks, Katherine J.: Patterns of shock, New York, 1965, The Macmillan Co.
5. Bruner, Lillian, and Suddarth, Doris: Textbook of medical-surgical nursing, ed. 3, New York, 1975, J. B. Lippincott Co.
6. Conn, Howard F., editor: Current therapy 1976, Philadelphia, 1976, W. B. Saunders Co.
7. Davis, Ruth W.: The patient with sickle cell anemia, Bedside Nurse 5:22-24, Sept., 1972.
8. Foster, Mary Ann: Teaching blood groups and reactions, Nursing Outlook 14:49-50, Feb., 1966.
9. Gardner, Alvin F.: Paramedical pathology, Springfield, Ill., 1971, Charles C Thomas, Publisher.
10. Leukemia—in children and adults, The Journal of Practical Nursing 22:22-23, June, 1972.
11. Metheny, Norma M., and Snively, William D.: Nurses' handbook of fluid balance, ed. 2, Philadelphia, 1974, J. B. Lippincott Co.
12. Morbidity and mortality weekly report, week ending Jan. 5, Atlanta, 1974, Center for Disease Control.
13. Progress against cancer 1969, a report of the National Advisory Council, Washington, D. C., 1969, Government Printing Office.
14. Recent mortality from Hodgkin's disease and leukemia, Statistical Bulletin 48:6-8, March, 1973, Metropolitan Life Insurance Co.
15. Shafer, Kathleen N., Sawyer, Janet R., McCluskey, Audrey M., Beck, Edna L., and Phipps, Wilma J.: Medical-surgical nursing, ed. 6, St. Louis, 1975, The C. V. Mosby Co.
16. Simpson, Elizabeth: Understanding sickle cell anemia, The Journal of Practical Nursing 23:16-17, Feb., 1973.
17. Smith, Alice L.: Microbiology and pathology, ed. 11, St. Louis, 1976, The C. V. Mosby Co.
18. Sweetwood, Hannelore: Nursing in the intensive respiratory unit, New York, 1971, Springer Publishing Co., Inc.
19. Young, Clara G., and Barger, James D.: Introduction to medical science, ed. 2, St. Louis, 1973, The C. V. Mosby Co.

Nursing the patient with diseases and disorders of the cardiovascular system

KEY WORDS

aneurysm *dilated bulge on bl. vessel*
angina pectoris *pain - due ... to dec O₂ to myocard*
arrhythmia *deviation from normal heart rhythm*
arteriosclerosis *arterial hardening*
atherosclerosis *fat depo... on bl. vessels*
atrial fibrillation
ascites *peritoneal fluid*
bacterial endocarditis *valve & heart lining infection*
cardiogenic shock *heart pumping action interference*
central venous pressure *rt side of heart ability*
cholesterol *natural body substance*
defibrillation *current to stop ventricular fib.*
diuretic *inc. urinary output*
electrocardiogram *recording of heart ele. activity*
embolectomy *removal of a blood clot from vein*
hypertension *↑ BP*
ischemic heart disease
lumen *opening c̄ in a tube*

lymphangitis *inflam. of lymph vessels*
myocardial infarction *obstruction of a coronary artery*
occlusion *blockage*
oscilloscope *visual wave on a screen*
pacemaker *ele. stimulator in heart block*
paroxysmal atrial tachycardia *very rapid heart beat*
plaques *fatty deposits*
Purkinje fibers *part of bundle of His*
sinoatrial node *heart's natural pacemaker*
sinus bradycardia *under 60 heartbeat*
sinus tachycardia *heart rate ↑ 100*
stenosis *constriction of a passageway*
thrombophlebitis *vein inflammation*
varicosities *dilated veins*
ventricular fibrillation *disorganized heartbeat*
ventricular tachycardia *rapid contraction of ventricle - reduced cardiac output*

STRUCTURE AND FUNCTION OF THE CARDIOVASCULAR SYSTEM

The heart is a hollow muscular organ located at the back of the sternum in the lower part of the mediastinum, between the lungs and above the diaphragm. It is divided into four chambers, with a septum that divides the right from the left side. The right upper chamber (atrium) receives venous blood returning from the body, whereas the left atrium receives oxygenated blood from the lungs. The lower right chamber (ventricle) pumps the venous blood through the pulmonary artery to the lungs, where it receives a new supply of oxygen and discharges its carbon dioxide. The left ventricle pumps the oxygenated blood through the aorta, from which it goes to all parts of the body. The lower part of the heart is called the *apex,* which is slightly to the left and downward. The upper part, or base, is located slightly below the second rib. There are four sets of valves in the heart. The tricuspid valve guards the opening between the right atrium and the right ventricle, and the bicuspid (mitral) valve is between the left atrium and the left ventricle. Located between the right ventricle and the pulmonary artery is the pulmonary valve, and the aortic valve is between the left ventricle and the aorta. The pulmonary valve and the aortic valve are also called the *semilunar valves.* These valves normally allow the flow of blood in only one direction; however, if they are diseased, blood may seep in the opposite direction. After birth there is no communication between the right and the left sides of the heart. The muscular substance of the heart is called *myocardium,* and the entire organ is covered with a membranous sac called *pericardium.* The inner structure of the heart is lined with a serous membrane called *endocardium.* The heart has its own electrical conduction sysetm, which is responsible for the contraction of the ventricles. This activity is the result of specialized cardiac muscle fibers. Located in the upper wall of the right atrium near the opening of the superior vena cava is the sinoatrial (SA) node, which has been called the pacemaker of the heart. The cells of the sinoatrial node have an internal rhythm causing them to contract at a constant rate. The rhythmic contractions cause impulses to spread throughout the heart muscle and set the pace or the rate at which the heart will beat. However, under certain conditions the human pacemaker may not perform its normal function adequately. Then it is necessary to use an artificial pacemaker to take over the task of establishing and maintaining the heart rate.

Below the sinoatrial node in the right atrial wall is the atrioventricular (AV) node. Impulses reaching the atrioventricular node are transmitted through fibers called the *bundle of His.* There are two branches of the bundle of His. One branch extends down the right side of the interventricular septum and the other branch down the left side until they reach the apex of the heart. The bundle of His is for transmitting impulses rather than for contraction. When the bundle branches reach the heart apex, the fibers begin to divide and subdivide extending out into the walls of the right and left ventricles as *Purkinje fibers.* Stimulation from the Purkinje fibers causes the ventricles to contract. During contraction small electrical currents are generated that extend to the surface of the body. The electrocardiogram is a record of these electrical currents and will indicate variation of the cardiac activity. (See Fig. 13-1.) The heart muscle receives its blood supply from two coronary arteries[3], [36] (Fig. 13-12).

The primary function of the right side of the heart is to pump blood into the capillary system of the lungs, where carbon dioxide can be released and oxygen absorbed into the blood. The primary function of the left side of the heart is to pump oxygenated blood to the body tissues, where oxygen can be released and the waste products of metabolism received.

The blood vessels are a network of tubes, arteries, veins, and capillaries that carry

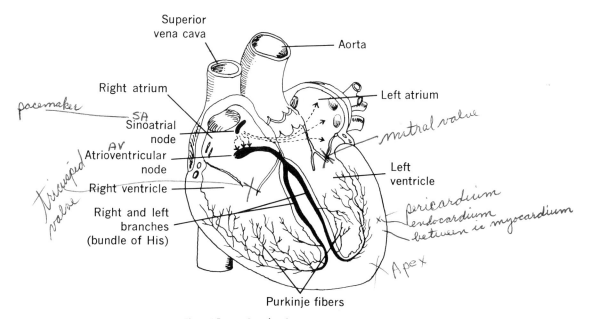

Fig. 13-1. Conduction system.

the blood to and from the heart. The blood leaves the heart by way of the aorta, which sends off branches that divide and subdivide and finally terminate in minute capillary vessels. By a similar but reverse process the smallest arteries (arterioles,) connect with the smallest veins (venules), which unite to form larger veins that finally empty into the superior and inferior vena cava, which in turn empty into the right atrium of the heart.

The blood vessels represent a vast transportation system by which essential substances are carried to the tissues and their waste products are returned to be eliminated. In the final analysis it is the tiny capillary vessels in which the exchange takes place.

LYMPH-VASCULAR SYSTEM

In addition to the tubes carrying blood, another system of tubes carries lymph. The lymphatic system is similar to the blood-vascular system without the heart and arteries. It is a system through which excess tissue fluid accumulating between the cells may be drained off. The level of tissue fluid must be kept constant, but it is continuously being added to; however, by means of the lymph-vascular system it is possible to maintain tissue fluid in a state of equilibrium. The lymphatic vessels begin in tiny lymphatic capillaries similar to blood capillaries. These unite to form larger vessels, which finally empty into veins. Distributed along the lymphatic vessels are small, round bodies of varying size called *lymph nodes*, which act as filters to remove certain solid materials that have been picked up by the lymph. Lymph node cells play a primary role in the immune system of the body. The nodes are more numerous in some areas of the body than in others. The lymph nodes in the neck, axilla, and groin are relatively superficial, whereas those in the abdomen are deep, Some diseases are characterized by an enlargement of the lymph nodes, which become inflamed and tender.

For a better understanding of the patient with diseases and disorders of the cardiovascular system, it is suggested that the nurse review in detail the structure and function of the cardiovascular system.

DISORDERS OF RATE AND RHYTHM OF THE HEART

The pulse is one of the most sensitive indices for determining how well the heart is functioning. Nurses should develop a trained sensitivity to what they feel when taking a pulse. When the heart is functioning normally, the pulse is felt as smooth, regular, equally spaced beats of equal strength and volume, which will occur from 72 to 80 times per minute. Under certain conditions, some of which are not well understood, changes occur in the pulse rate, its rhythm, and volume. Some of these conditions are called *cardiac arrhythmias*.

Cardiac arrhythmias

Cardiac arrhythmias occur in well persons and in some patients with heart disease. The nurse may be the first person to detect changes in the patient's pulse and should always report them to the physician. In patients with some disorders the pulse rate may exceed 150 beats per minute, and the volume will be weak, since the ventricle empties before it has time to fill completely. Arrhythmias resulting in an extremely rapid pulse rate are called *tachycardias*. In well persons they usually are not serious unless the increased rate continues over a considerable period of time. Persons with severe tachycardia may need to be hospitalized for treatment. Prolonged tachycardia occurring in a person with heart disease may lead to heart failure.

A slow pulse rate of 60 beats per minute or less is called *bradycardia* and occurs normally in many persons. Bradycardia may exist in some persons with conditions such as cerebral disorders in which intracranial pressure is increasing.

Extrasystole (premature beats). Some disorders result in a premature contraction of the heart chamber, which is characterized by premature beats, or *extrasystoles*, and are the most common of the arrhythmias. A premature contraction occurs when either an atrial or ventricular beat occurs earlier than anticipated in the normal rhythm of the heartbeat. Extrasystoles are uncommon in children but become more frequent with increasing age, and they occur in almost all persons over 70 years of age. The premature beat can be detected immediately after the regular beat; then there is a pause and the next regular beat. If the premature beat occurs too early, it may not give rise to a pulse wave and only the pause will be noted, appearing as a missed beat. Sometimes several premature beats will occur in a regular pattern, as in every third beat, or they may occur at irregular intervals. When a series of two premature beats occur in rapid succession separated by a longer interval, it is called *bigeminy,* or *bigeminal pulse.* An individual may experience this disturbance occasionally, or it may occur frequently and may feel like a little "flutter." Other symptoms may include faintness, apprehension, and diaphoresis. Some persons become apprehensive and believe they are suffering from heart disease. If the disorder causes the individual too much anxiety, it may be necessary to administer medications to relieve it.

Cardiac arrhythmias cause the heart to beat ineffectively, resulting in a decreased cardiac output, decreased blood flow through the coronary arteries, and cardiac ischemia. It has become evident that the "sudden" cardiac arrest is often preceded by various arrhythmias. If these forewarning symptoms can be identified early and treatment begun, the incidence of cardiac arrests can be decreased.

Atrial fibrillation

Atrial fibrillation is a serious disorder of the heartbeat in which the heart rate is greater than the pulse rate. The atrium may receive as many as 400 to 600 stimuli per minute, but the ventricle usually does not contract more than 150 times per minute. The sinoatrial node no longer controls the heart rhythm, and various parts of the atrium are being stimulated to contract at the same time, resulting in a quiver. Many stimuli also reach the ventricle, which responds irregularly to as many impulses as possible. Many of the contractions of the ventricle are too weak to open the valve and force the blood out so that a radial pulse wave may be felt. As a result the pulse is felt to be irregular in both volume and rhythm, and weak rapid beats may be difficult to count. The physician may request that both the radial and apical pulse be taken and recorded. When this is done, one nurse counts the radial pulse, and another

nurse, using a stethoscope placed over the apex of the heart, counts the heartbeats. One nurse should give the signal to begin so that each will be counting for the same period of time. The difference between the radial pulse and the apical pulse is called the *pulse deficit.*

Atrial fibrillation occurs largely in patients with heart disease such as rheumatic heart disease and arteriosclerotic and hypertensive heart disease. It may occur occasionally in persons who do not have heart disease. The disorder requires medical treatment, and digitalis and quinidine sulfate are usually ordered by the physician. The pulse for rate and rhythm should be checked before giving digitalis or quinidine; if it is unusually slow, the drug is not given, and a report is made to the physician. The patient should be observed for increased pulse rate, nausea, dizziness, and visual disturbances, which may indicate toxic manifestations. If the patient's condition still deteriorates, an attempt may be made to return the heartbeat to normal by cardioversion, which is the administration of a brief electrical shock. Paddles are placed on the external chest, and the electrical current must be delivered during the QRS complex of the heartbeat. This procedure is normally performed by the physician, who also can prepare the patient and receive his consent. The patient's heart rate is observed on a monitor during the procedure.

Ventricular fibrillation

Ventricular fibrillation is a rapid twitching of the ventricles, producing a decreased cardiac output, cardiogenic shock, and death. It is commonly called a cardiac arrest and requires emergency treatment. No pulse rate or blood pressure can be obtained, and there are no drugs to control the disorder. Cardiopulmonary resuscitation and electrical defibrillation are necessary. Defibrillation is similar to cardioversion, and the electrical shock is administered by a physician or adequately prepared nurse.

Sinus tachycardia

Sinus tachycardia is the most common disturbance of the rhythm of the heart. Impulses are initiated by the sinoatrial node, and the rate is regular but above 100 beats per minute. It is a normal physiologic response to exertion, fever, and emotional states in the normal person. It is also present in abnormal states, such as anemia, rheumatic fever, hemorrhage, hyperthyroidism, myocardial infarctions, congestive heart failure, and shock. The underlying cause must be found and treated, since if the condition persists, heart failure may occur.

Paroxysmal atrial tachycardia occurs when the heart suddenly begins to beat rapidly, at two or three times its normal rate. It is seen more frequently in young people and may be present in people with or without other heart diseases. It is believed that paroxysmal atrial tachycardia in otherwise normal persons could be due to a spot in the atrium which is hyperirritable from birth.[6] The majority of patients have few or no symptoms; however, shortness of breath, exhaustion, and a fluttering sensation may occur. Tachycardia may be treated with sedatives or tranquilizers, and patients should stop smoking and ingesting stimulants such as coffee.

Sinus bradycardia   *Slow rate*

Sinus bradycardia occurs when the heart rate falls to 60 beats per minute or below. It commonly occurs at night and in young athletes and laborers. It can sometimes be seen in patients with brain lesions and in patients receiving digitalis preparations for other heart disorders. There is no treatment other than removing the underlying cause.

Paroxysmal ventricular tachycardia is a sudden onset of rapid ventricular beats, which unpredictably will return to normal. It is more common in older patients and can be induced by excessive alcohol intake, smoking, and acute infections. Treatment is bed rest and the administration of an antiarrhythmia drug such as procaine amide hydrochloride (Pronestyl), either orally or intravenously.

Ventricular tachycardia

In ventricular tachycardia the atrial rate is normal but the ventricular rate may reach 150 to 200 beats per minute. Usually it indicates a badly damaged myocardium and may lead to ventricular fibrillation. If the process is not treated, it will lead to an inadequate cardiac output and cardiogenic shock. Cardioversion and medications that reduce the irritability of the heart are used to treat the condition. Lidocaine (Xylocaine) has recently become one of the most frequently used drugs in the treatment of patients with ventricular arrhythmias. It is effective in the treatment of patients with premature ventricular contractions (PVCs) and in controlling other ventricular arrhythmias. It is administered intravenously, and its effects are almost immediate. While the medication is being administered, it is essential that the blood pressure be checked for possible hypotension.

Heart block

Heart block is a disturbance in the atrioventricular bundle in which the mechanism responsible for transmitting impulses from the atrium to the ventricle is interrupted. It is usually the result of some disease of the heart, but it may result from other causes. Impulses to the ventricle may be blocked at any point along the conduction route. When impulses to the ventricle are delayed but eventually reach the ventricle, it is considered as partial block. Ordinarily an electrocardiogram is necessary to determine the disorder. When conduction to the ventricle is completely interrupted, a complete heart block has occurred. Depending on the level of the block, the bundle of His and its fibers may take over the pacemaker function, which normally belongs to the sinoatrial node. In this situation the ventricles establish their own rhythm for the heartbeat without assistance from the atrium. If the nurse counts the pulse, a pulse rate of approximately 30 to 40 beats per minute will be observed. The irregular heart rhythm produces sudden reductions in the cardiac output, which can produce hypoxia of the sensitive cerebral tissue, which can result in the Stokes-Adams syndrome. Convulsions may occur, the patient may feel dizzy and weak, and he may lose consciousness because of decreased cardiac output. If the ventricles do not recover, the patient dies. Heart block may be treated with drugs. For immediate treatment, epinephrine or isoproterenol hydrochloride (Isuprel) is given intravenously, and ephedrine may be used for long-range treatment. When these drugs are administered, the patient should be observed for side effects, including irregular heartbeat, tachycardia and palpitation.[40] A pacemaker is considered essential.

Pacemaker. The pacemaker is an electrically operated mechanical device that enables the ventricle to contract normally. It may be used in a number of cardiac disorders, including Adams-Stokes syndrome. It may be used in an emergency or for a temporary period, or it can be implanted permanently in the patient's chest. Several approaches are possible in initiating the use of the pacemaker. If it is to be temporary, a catheter may be inserted through a vein, often the jugular vein, and it is attached to an external pacemaker. Patients with an occasional blockage of the electrical impulses in the heart, such as after heart surgery or a myocardial infarction, may need this type of pacemaker. Usually it is inserted in the operating room or in a special laboratory, such as the cardiac catheterization laboratory, and the catheter is passed directly into the right ventricle under fluoroscopy. Permanent pacemakers are necessary if the patient has irreversible cardiac damage to the conductive nerve pathways of the heart. It is also inserted through a vein, but the battery box is permanently implanted within the subcutaneous tissue of the patient's chest or abdomen. Occasionally the patient's chest is opened and the electrodes are sutured into the ventricle. This procedure involves a major operation, a thoracotomy, and therefore is less desirable. The procedure chosen is determined by the patient's need for temporary or permanent assistance. Internal pacemakers may be powered by a mercury battery which lasts 1½ to 2 years, by lithium which lasts 7 to 10 years, or by nuclear energy which lasts 10 to 20 years.[9]

The nursing care of the patient is determined by the procedure used. In any case the patient will have a wound that must be protected from infection. If a catheter is inserted into a vein, care must be taken to prevent its displacement. When a temporary pacemaker is in use, all electrical equipment in the room must be grounded, and only one machine may be connected to any electric outlet. Any exposed electrodes should be insulated. The nurse should remember that the implanted pacemaker is a foreign object, and the patient should be observed for any elevation of temperature that might indicate trouble. The nurse should also be certain that an infusion set and a defibrillator are at the bedside for emergency use.[22] Patients with implanted pacemakers are apprehensive and fearful. The primary responsibilities of nurses include assisting the patient in accepting the instrument and relieving fear and apprehension. The patient must be taught the importance of counting his pulse twice a day and remaining under medical supervision. The patient needs to understand that the heart defect still exists and that if anything happens to the pacemaker, his symptoms will return.[31]

CARDIOPULMONARY RESUSCITATION

The sudden cessation of cardiac output and respirations is called cardiac arrest. Cardiopulmonary resuscitation is the technique of maintaining these vital functions until further treatment can be given. Currently, all nurses are expected to be trained in this technique, and many institutions are requiring that all persons involved either directly or indirectly with patient care be capable of initiating resuscitation. The general public is becoming more knowledgeable, and many nonmedical businesses are instructing their employees in this lifesaving measure. Recently, two Chicago businessmen saved the life of a fallen 70-year-old man by administering mouth-to-mouth resuscitation and cardiac massage.

When a patient suddenly loses consciousness and appears to stop breathing, the nurse should immediately check the carotid pulse in the neck or the femoral pulse in the groin. If they cannot be felt, circulation is inadequate. The pupils of the eye begin to dilate within 45 seconds after circulation becomes ineffective. If both signs are present, help should be summoned and cardiopulmonary resuscitation should be initiated at once.

The most satisfactory method of breathing for the patient is by mouth-to-mouth resuscitation. First, an open airway must be established. Any obstruction should be removed at once, and the head should be tilted backward as far as possible by lifting the back of the neck with one hand and pushing on the forehead with the other. The tongue must be kept forward to prevent its obstructing the airway. If the victim is a small child, the nurse's mouth should be placed over his mouth and nose, followed by gentle blowing. An adult's nose should be pinched and the nurse's mouth should be placed over his mouth. The nurse should blow forcefully and watch to see if the patient's chest rises. The nurse's mouth is then removed, and the nurse should listen for the return rush of air. About twelve breaths of air per minute should be given. If the chest does not rise, it indicates that the airway is still obstructed.

The best method of performing cardiopulmonary resuscitation is to have one person breathe for the patient and another administer external cardiac massage. The patient should be placed on a hard surface, such as the floor. The sternum should be palpated, the heel of one hand placed on the lower half of the sternum, and the heel of the opposite hand placed on top of the first. Fingers should be spread and raised. Firm even pressure should be applied, depressing the chest 1½ to 2 inches. This requires effort, and the best position may be on one's knees beside the patient. Sixty to eighty compressions per minute should be done. The breathing and cardiac massage should be coordinated so that one breath is given for every five compressions without interruption of rhythm. Unless oxygen is in the lungs, the massage is useless. Care must be taken to avoid extreme compression of the chest, since ribs may fracture and puncture lung tissue or the heart. (See Fig. 13-2.) The pupils should be checked for dilation or constriction. Constriction indicates that cerebral tissue is receiving enough oxygen for tissue function. Other signs of improvement include body movement, improved color, and spontaneous respirations.[13, 14, 35]

Many hospitals have an emergency team who can be called when an emergency occurs, and all units have cardiac arrest equipment nearby. An electrocardiograph, a defibrillator, endotracheal tubes, intravenous materials, laryngoscope, tracheostomy set, oxygen, and a suction machine should be available. Epinephrine may be injected directly into the heart, sodium bicarbonate given to combat acidosis, and calcium chloride given to stimulate cardiac contraction.

CORONARY CARE UNIT (CCU)

The coronary care unit or the cardiopulmonary unit is a specially designed unit of the hospital. The unit is equipped with all supplies and equipment, including emergency drugs to meet the needs of each patient admitted to the unit. It provides for continuous monitoring of the cardiac function.

The overall objective of the coronary care unit is to save life. During the early development of these units emphasis was placed on the prompt treatment of patients with cardiac arrest. With increased knowledge and understanding about coronary

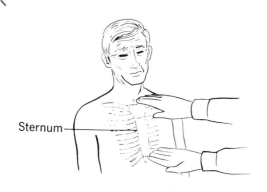

Sternum

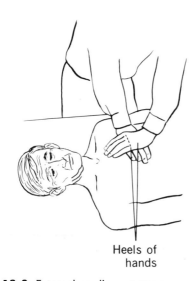

Heels of hands

Fig. 13-2. External cardiac massage.

heart disease the emphasis is now placed on preventing cardiac arrest. If not identified, treated, and/or controlled, minor disorders of rhythm and arrhythmias may lead to serious arrhythmias, heart failure, and death. It cannot be expected that all patients admitted to the unit will survive.[5]

Large medical centers have specially designed separate coronary care units; however, most community hospitals care for coronary disease patients in intensive care units along with other seriously ill patients. There are definite disadvantages to this system, especially when the intensive care unit (ICU) is a ward type of arrangement. However, the environmental location of the patient is not always what is most important, but the quality of nursing care. "In fact, the number of lives saved in a coronary care unit and the excellence of care rendered are directly related to the competence of the nurse."[*] Nurses are with the patient 24 hours a day and are in a position to detect the first sign of trouble. Their immediate assessment of the problem and appropriate emergency action may be life saving.[31] The coronary care unit with its effective monitoring system and trained personnel has effectively reduced in-hospital death from heart attacks by about 30%.[21]

Cardiac monitoring

Cardiac monitoring is increasingly becoming a part of the nursing care of the cardiac patient. A bedside monitor records a continuous electrocardiogram on an oscilloscope or screen, and it is simultaneously channeled to a console at the nurse's station. In this way the patient's cardiac activity can be observed at all times. Electrodes are placed on the patient's chest so that the best tracing appears on the oscilloscope. The electrodes may be stainless steel needles that are inserted into the subcutaneous tissue or one of the many varieties of paste-on skin electrodes. High and low rate limits are set on the monitor, and if the patient's pulse rate falls below or above the limits, a blinking light and alarm system is activated. Depending on the equipment used, the alarm may trigger the console monitor to produce an electrocardio-

*From Pinneo, Rose: Nursing in a coronary care unit, Cardiovascular Nursing **3:**1, Jan.-Feb., 1967.

gram tracing. The highly trained nursing personnel in the unit can then observe the patient and the tracing and begin immediate treatment if necessary. Loosening of an electrode or excessive muscular activity can result in false alarms and irregular patterns on the electrocardiogram.[30] Paste-on electrodes should be removed and the area washed frequently. Needle electrode sites are checked for inflammation daily.

Patients in a coronary care unit often are under extreme emotional as well as physical stress. They are anxious about loss of function, helplessness, finances, family, and the possibility of death. The environment itself is foreign and frightening. Coronary care nurses have achieved a high level of technical proficiency, but unfortunately they tend to neglect the psychologic care of the patient. In a recent survey 95% of the nurses responded that they did nothing when an interpersonal situation arose except to refer the problem to the physician or clergyman.[23] Much can be done to reassure the patient by supplying information that will relieve anxiety, by listening carefully to the patient, and by treating him honestly as an adult. The caring and empathy on which nursing was founded should be demonstrated in perhaps the most serious crisis the patient has faced.

Nurses in the coronary care unit are often responsible for taking electrocardiograms, observing and recording cardiac monitor readings, maintaining oxygen therapy, and observing and regulating intravenous fluids. They should also be prepared to provide external cardiopulmonary resuscitation and defibrillation, to rotate tourniquets, to insert pacemakers, and to perform other duties.

DIAGNOSTIC TESTS AND PROCEDURES
Physical examination

One of the initial steps taken by the physician in examination of the cardiovascular system is to estimate the size, shape, and position of the heart, to estimate the character of the heartbeat, and to detect any abnormal sounds. The examination is carried out by five routine methods: inspection, percussion, palpation, auscultation, and blood pressure.

Inspection. By locating the apical beat, the physician can estimate the approximate

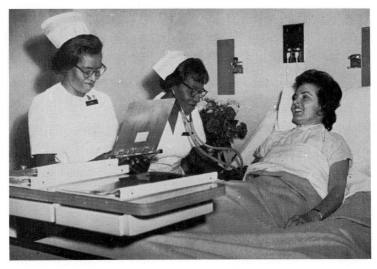

Fig. 13-3. Nurses take blood pressure and maintain the patient's chart. (Courtesy Medical Center, Columbus, Ga.)

location of the heart. If the apex beat is located too far to the right or too far to the left of its normal position, the physician knows that there is displacement of the organ.

Percussion. Since the heart is a fairly solid organ, when it is gently tapped with the fingertips it will give a dull sound in contrast to the lungs, which will give a resonant sound. Thus the physician will gain some idea of the size and the shape of the heart.

Palpation. By placing the hand over the apex beat, the physician is able to estimate the force with which the heart muscle contracts.

Auscultation. Using the stethoscope, the physician listens to the heart sounds. In addition to the rate and rhythm, he may detect abnormal sounds that are present in diseases of the heart. Some of these sounds, called *murmurs,* indicate disease of the valves of the heart.

Blood pressure. The measurement of arterial blood pressure is important in the examination of the patient and often supplies vital information concerning cardiac function and the condition of the peripheral blood vessels (Fig. 13-3). Other observations include rate and character of the pulse, quality of the respirations, and presence of pain, color, and edema.

Laboratory examination

Several laboratory studies are usually important in establishing accurate diagnosis or in following the course of the disease.

Complete blood count. The routine laboratory examination comprises a count of red and white blood cells, an estimate of hemoglobin, a serologic test for syphilis, and a differential count, which includes many different cells that are usually few in number (p. 235). An increase in the number of white blood cells indicates that an inflammatory condition or tissue destruction is present. The determination of red blood cell count and hemoglobin level helps physicians to determine how well the blood is being oxygenated.

Sedimentation rate. The sedimentation rate is used to determine the extent of inflammation and infection that is present in the patient. It is usually increased in rheumatic fever and in myocardial infarction. It is useful both in diagnosing rheumatic fever and in following the course of the disease (p. 236).

Blood cultures. When evidence of endocarditis of bacterial origin is found, diagnosis may be established by finding the causative organism in the blood. Often several blood cultures may be necessary before a positive diagnosis can be made.

Cholesterol. The exact relationship between atherosclerosis and cholesterol has not been specifically determined; however, many believe that it may have some part in producing myocardial infarction, since deposits (plaques) of fatty material are often found to be blocking coronary arteries. It has been estimated that cholesterol above 250 mg./100 ml. increases the risk of coronary heart disease approximately four times. The normal cholesterol value is 150 to 260 mg./100 ml. of serum. However, at the present time a reduction of cholesterol in the blood serum does not indicate a reduction of the risk factor.[11]

Circulation time. The purpose of the test for circulation time is to determine the speed with which the blood flows. Either of two methods can be used. One is the arm-to-tongue time, in which a substance is injected into a vein in the arm and the time observed until the patient indicates that he notices the taste in his mouth, which may be bitter or sweet, depending on the substance used. The second is the arm-to-lung time, in which ether or dehydrocholic acid (Decholin) is injected into a vein in the arm and the time observed until the patient coughs or smells the substance. In patients with congestive heart failure the circulation time is prolonged. The normal circulation time is 10 to 16 seconds (arm-to-tongue method).

Venous pressure. The test for venous pressure measures the pressure of the circulating blood against the walls of the veins. The pressure is measured in centimeters of water rather than blood to avoid clotting of blood in the equipment. The procedure is carried out at the bedside by the physician. A small three-way stopcock is attached to the hub of a syringe with a needle, and a manometer is attached to the stopcock. Physiologic saline solution is placed into the manometer. After the physician does a venipuncture the stopcock is adjusted to allow the saline solution to flow into the patient's vein. The manometer is read at the level at which the saline solution ceases to flow into the vein. The normal venous pressure is 60 to 100 ml. of water. The nurse who may assist the physician should be sure that all equipment is sterile, including the physiologic saline solution. The patient should be positioned so that the arm is at the level with the

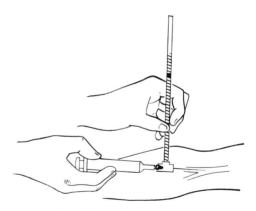

Fig. 13-4. Venous pressure.

heart. The patient may lie flat in bed or may sit up, in which case the arm may be supported on pillows[40] (Fig. 13-4). The nurse can observe changes in venous pressure by carefully noting changes in the patient's neck veins. Normally a person's neck veins are not visible when his head is elevated 30 to 45 degrees. When increased venous pressure is present, neck veins will bulge and look distended in this position. Hand veins can also give the nurse an indication that increased pressure is present. Normally hand veins are collapsed when they are held above the level of the heart and distended when held below the level of the heart. Veins of the hand will stay distended at shoulder level if increased venous pressure is present.

Central venous pressure. Determination of central venous pressure, which differs from that of venous pressure, is an important method of learning the circulatory state in relation to blood volume, the ability of the heart to pump blood, and the capacity of the blood vessels. The physician introduces a polyethylene catheter into a vein through a cutdown and guides it into the right atrium or vena cava. The pressure is measured in centimeters of water as in venous pressure. The procedure for determining central venous pressure is similar to that for determining venous pressure. The catheter is attached to a three-way stopcock and then to an intravenous infusion, usually 5% glucose in water. This is allowed to drip slowly to keep the vein open. When a reading is to be taken, the stopcock is opened to the manometer and it is filled with the intravenous solution. The stopcock is then

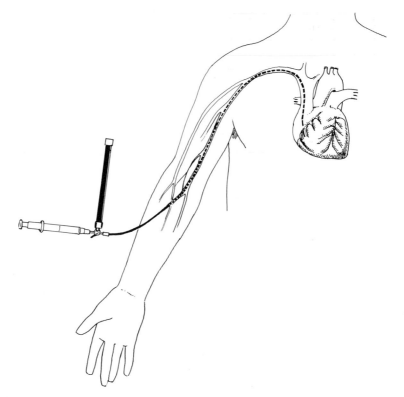

Fig. 13-5. Central venous pressure.

turned to the venous opening, and the level of the fluid in the manometer should vary with each respiration. The highest level of fluid within the column is read, and the stopcock is turned to resume the intravenous infusion.[26] The normal range for central venous pressure is 4 to 10 cm., or 40 to 100 ml. of water. The patient should be kept in the same position for each reading, and the infusion site should be covered with sterile dressings. When the pressure continues to rise, it may indicate that the pumping action of the heart is becoming weak, and cardiac failure may occur. If the pressure is low or continues to fall, it may indicate a need for an increase in circulating fluid. Depending on the patient's condition, he may be given whole blood or intravenous fluid[2, 4] (Fig. 13-5).

Electrocardiography. The electrocardiogram is a graphic tracing of the electrical currents resulting from the activity of the heart. However, only the electrical potential reaches the skin surface. When possible, the patient is advised to avoid smoking

and having cold drinks or a heavy meal just prior to the examination. The patient is placed in the supine position and should be relaxed and comfortable. When the examination is done in the outpatient clinic or the physician's office, it is desirable for the patient to rest for 30 minutes before the examination. Electrodes are attached to the extremities and placed at various positions on the chest after the application of a special jelly. Wires from the electrodes are attached to the electrocardiograph, which traces the pattern on heavy paper. To read and record these tracings each wave has been lettered: P, Q, R, S, and T. The P wave represents the spread of impulses from the sinoatrial node throughout the atria. The P-R interval is the period of time it takes for the impulse to reach the ventricle and start the contraction. The QRS complex represents the time that is necessary for the impulse to spread through the bundle of His and Purkinje fibers and cause ventricular contraction. The S-T segment indicates the re-

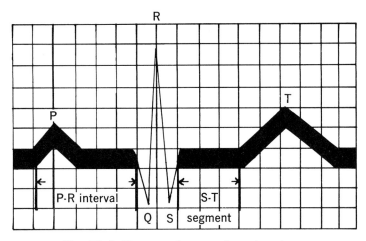

Fig. 13-6. Electrocardiogram of one heartbeat.

covery stage of the ventricular muscles (Fig. 13-6). Pathologic processes in the heart invariably are indicated by a change in one of these areas.[7] The patient should be assured that he will feel nothing and will not receive a shock. The examination is of value in recording changes in the normal rhythm of the heart, in diagnosing myocardial damage, and in detecting conduction defects such as those occurring in heart block. When the electrocardiogram is made in the hospital at the bedside and the patient is receiving oxygen, the nurse should remember to turn the oxygen off during the examination. EKG

X-ray examination and fluoroscopy

X-ray films. The use of x-ray examination is one of the physician's most valuable tools in the diagnosis of heart disease and appraisal of the size and shape of the heart. The heart is opaque to x rays, but the contour may be readily outlined, and the thoracic aorta may be seen. Fluoroscopic examination allows the physician to see the heart in motion. The outline of the heart may be traced on the fluoroscope screen and copied on paper for further study, a procedure called *orthodiagraphy*. The physician will evaluate the lungs at the same time, since congestion of the lungs occurs early in heart failure and may be detected before other signs of heart failure occur. Many new techniques and devices have been developed in recent years that have increased the value of the x-ray film in the examination of the heart and blood vessels.

Angiocardiography (angiography). Examination of the chambers of the heart, valves, and blood vessels is made by injecting a contrast medium into a vein or artery. X-ray films called *angiograms* are then taken. Selective angiography uses a smaller amount of the contrast medium and injects it in or near the area to be studied. This method has proved more satisfactory than injecting the contrast medium into the vein. Selective angiography makes it possible to study any part of the vascular system.[16] Patients undergoing this procedure should be questioned carefully concerning allergies, since some persons are sensitive to the dye. Food is usually withheld from the patient preceding the examination to avoid nausea and vomiting, and a mild sedative may be given. These patients are usually fearful and apprehensive and need a great deal of reassurance. After the procedure the patient should be observed for bleeding from the site of the injection, and blood pressure readings should be taken for 2 hours.[35]

Cardiac catheterization. Cardiac catheterization requires a staff of well-trained physicians and nurses and is usually done only in medical centers where facilities exist for open heart surgery. The purposes of cardiac catheterization are to measure the pressure in the heart chambers and pulmonary arteries, to obtain blood samples from the heart and vessels for determination of the amount of oxygen and carbon dioxide present, and to detect congenital or acquired defects. The catheterization may be done on either the right side or the left side of the heart. A cutdown is usually made over a vein in the arm, and a small catheter similar to a ureteral catheter is introduced into the vein. It is gradually passed through the vein to the heart with the aid of the fluoroscope, and x-ray films are then taken or may be taken at any point along the route. The examination enables the physician to make a more precise diagnosis. The left side of the heart may be catheterized in a similar way by inserting a catheter into the femoral artery and passing it up the aorta and into the heart. If atrial stenosis is present, a needle can be passed into the heart by means of a special bronchoscope, or the heart may be entered directly through the chest wall.[35]

The nurse should not attempt to discuss the procedure with the patient or his family but should refer the patient's questions to the physician. The nurse may reassure the patient. If he is to be given an anesthetic, the nurse should be sure that his breakfast is held. When he returns to his room, his pulse should be taken at 15-minute intervals for 1 hour and then frequently for several hours. Any change in the rate and rhythm should be reported immediately. The wound at the site of the cutdown should be observed for any signs of inflammation, since thrombophlebitis may occasionally occur.

NURSING THE PATIENT WITH DISEASES AND DISORDERS OF THE CARDIOVASCULAR SYSTEM

Heart disease continues to be the leading cause of death in the United States, and the majority of deaths are caused by coronary artery disease. The probability of eventually dying from arteriosclerotic heart disease gradually increases from birth to 65 years of age and older. The way in which morbidity and mortality from heart disease may be reduced is the primary concern of physicians and researchers. Many factors in the personal habits of individuals increase the risk of heart disease. Research has provided reasonable evidence of the risk factor associated with smoking cigarettes. Studies have shown that an increase in blood pressure and serum cholesterol and atherosclerosis of the coronary arteries have a direct relationship to smoking and to the number of cigarettes smoked.[42] Persons with diabetes and gout have a two to four times greater risk of heart disease than other persons. Other factors that may predispose an individual to heart disease include hypertension, obesity, physical inactivity, diet, and menopause, at which time estrogens are lost and serum cholesterol rises. Frequently a combination of these risk factors exists in an individual so that in the presence of any one of them others should be looked for. The nurse should be aware of the risk factors and in contacts with patients should encourage them to modify habits that may predispose to heart disease.[11] The nurse must be an example: If the nurse smokes or is obese, encouraging the patient to stop smoking or to consult his physician about weight reduction may be difficult. The present approach to preventing morbidity and mortality from heart disease is prevention, and the risk factors are receiving more attention in the preventive program.

Diseases and disorders of the heart
Congenital heart disease

Congenital heart disease includes a wide variety of conditions representing developmental errors that occur during intrauterine life or at the time of birth (Figs. 13-7 to 13-11). These conditions may involve the heart itself, its valves, or both and may include blood vessels. Many babies born with heart defects die soon after birth, some die within the first year, and a few reach adult life. Some persons may reach adult life without knowing that the defect exists, whereas others may be severely handicapped. Some defects are severe enough to produce symptoms, and the overburdened heart fails.

Treatment and nursing care. With the development of open heart surgery, new diagnostic aids, and improved techniques, it has become possible to correct some kinds of congenital defects. However, limitations still exist, and not all individuals are suitable candidates for heart surgery. Patients with some conditions can be helped through surgery but not cured, and some risk is involved in all heart surgery. Nurses who come in contact with parents

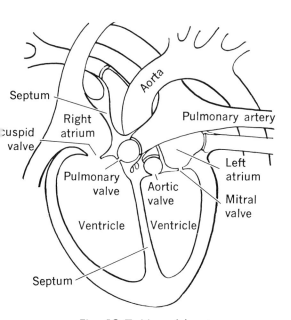

Fig. 13-7. Normal heart.

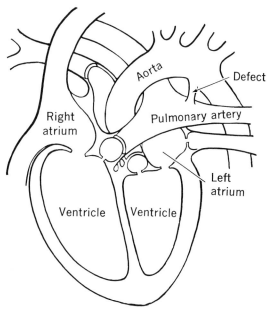

Fig. 13-8. Congenital heart defect—patent ductus arteriosus. The tube called the *ductus* should close during the first 2 weeks of life.

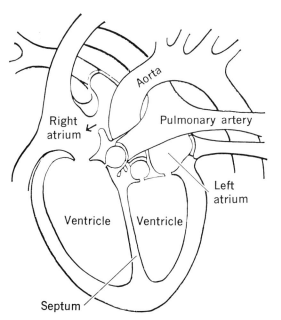

Fig. 13-9. Septal defect allows blood to flow from the left atrium into the right atrium of the heart. Note the arrow indicating the defect in the septum.

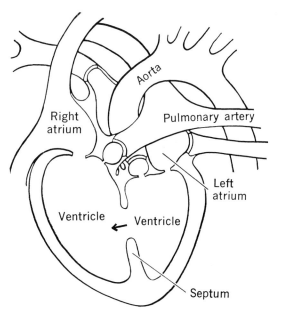

Fig. 13-10. Septal defect allows blood to flow from the left ventricle into the right ventricle. The arrow indicates the defect in the septum between the two ventricles.

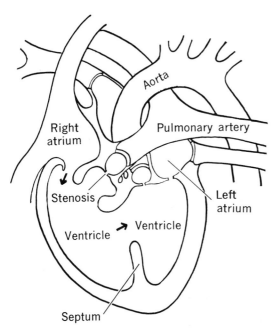

Fig. 13-11. Tetralogy of Fallot. There is a septal defect between the right and left ventricles and a stenosis of the pulmonary valve, which allows a mixing of the venous and the arterial blood and results in cyanosis (blue baby).

of children with congenital defects should encourage them to seek competent medical advice.

Arteriosclerosis and atherosclerosis

Arteriosclerosis is a process of degeneration and hardening of the walls of arteries due to chronic inflammation and scarring. This process tends to weaken the walls of the vessels and predispose to hemorrhage, thrombosis, and hypertension, and it appears to be related to the aging process. Atherosclerosis is a type of arteriosclerosis that affects large arteries that are normally flexible and elastic, such as the aorta and its major branches, the coronary arteries, and the large arteries of the brain. It has been called *the* most important disease in the United States because it is the underlying cause of most infarcts, or death of tissue, in the heart and brain.

The disease is characterized by deposits of fat (usually cholesterol) within the inner lining of the arteries. This deposit initiates a low-grade inflammatory reaction and healing process, which eventually re-

sults in hard, irregular, multicolored plaques, which fibrose and calcify within the inner lining of the arteries. This process weakens and narrows the walls of the major arteries, and partial or complete obstruction can occur. Whenever obstruction occurs, the tissue beyond the obstruction is deprived of its blood supply, and death of the tissue may result. The deprivation of blood to the heart is referred to as ischemic heart disease, and the pathology involves the coronary arteries.

Treatment and nursing care. There is no effective treatment or cure for arteriosclerosis and atherosclerosis. The process probably begins early in life and develops gradually over the years. Surgical procedures have been developed that will remove plaques from certain areas and increase the circulation beyond. Earlier in this chapter several factors that increase the risk of heart disease were reviewed. To decrease the risk factors that may lead to ischemic heart disease the individual must establish good health habits during his early years. It is generally believed that the destructive process can be slowed, even if it cannot be cured, by modification in daily living. A reduction of dietary cholesterol will usually cause a decrease of the serum cholesterol. Most cholesterol in the diet comes from animal fats. Foods that should be eliminated from the diet include whole milk, butter, eggs, organ meats, and other animal fats. The use of polyunsaturated oils, skim milk, and cheese should be considered. The nurse should encourage young persons to establish good dietary patterns and not to smoke or to stop smoking if they have already begun.

Hypertension and hypertensive heart disease

Hypertension refers to an elevation of blood pressure, that is, a blood pressure higher than would normally be expected for the individual's age, weight, and sex. When an abnormally high blood pressure occurs without any known cause, it is called essential hypertension,[24] which comprises 80% to 90% of hypertension.

Prior to this decade, little scientific information was available, and little research was done on hypertension, although many theories existed. Since 1971, intensive programs to gather, study, evaluate, and make recommendations concerning hypertension have been under way. Agencies and organizations now working include the Department of Health, Education, and Welfare, the National Heart and Lung Institute, the American Heart Association, Inc., and the American Medical Association. Community programs have been organized to locate and identify persons with hypertension who are not under treatment or whose hypertension is not controlled. Through the mass media of radio and television persons have been encouraged to secure a blood pressure check. Results so far indicate that there are thousands of persons with hypertension who are unaware of the condition.[28]

Recent studies have shown that arteriosclerotic changes leading to eventual hypertension are present at birth and that they progress through childhood and adolescence. This is followed by a period of latency, during which a person is asymptomatic. Finally, there is a period during which clinical signs begin to make their appearance.[27]

When symptoms do occur, the first sign may be headache, followed by fatigue, dyspnea on exertion, deteriorating vision, and kidney disorders. As the flow of blood from arteries into capillary vessels and veins meets resistance, blood from the heart must be pumped at an increased pressure to compensate for this resistance and to maintain the circulatory flow. Gradually the walls of the left ventricle and the arterioles become thickened, and as the left ventricle works harder and harder to force the blood out, it becomes enlarged. Eventually it will no longer be able to function, and congestive heart failure occurs.[35]

Treatment and nursing care. All authorities do not agree on methods of treating essential hypertension. However, most do agree that a number of factors need to be considered, including age, sex, family history, living habits, and whether vascular changes have occurred. It is recognized that the height of the diastolic blood pressure is more important than the height of the systolic pressure. It is also believed that a single blood pressure is not diagnostic but that several readings should be made at weekly intervals. There is evidence among some physicians that no specific blood pressure should be sought for the patient but that a pressure with which the patient is comfortable should be maintained.

Hypertension may be classified as early mild uncomplicated, moderate, and severe. Treatment may be based in part on this classification. If the patient has hypertension and is taking medication, it usually means that he will continue taking medication for the rest of his life. Many physicians believe that the least amount of medication that is consistent with the patient's hypertensive state is the preferred treatment. "A pill a day" is a statement often used by physicians.

Many patients with essential hypertension are given a diuretic, alone or in combination with another drug. Several diuretic drugs are in current use, all with the same or similar effect but different in cost. The physiologic effect of diuretics in reducing blood pressure is that they reduce the volume of extracellular fluid and the sodium in the fluid. Some of the diuretics in common use include ethacrynic acid (Edecrin), furosemide (Lasix), chlorthalidone (Hygroton), and chlorothiazide (Diuril). Patients receiving diuretics lose potassium along with the water and sodium, and their diet should contain foods that are rich in potassium and include two glasses of orange juice daily. Complications that may occur from the long-time use of the chlorothiazides include an increase in serum uric acid and the development of gout (p. 516). Several other drugs may be given with or without the diuretic, including spironolactone (Aldactone) and reserpine (Serpasil, Sandril, and others). Side effects of Aldactone include sleepiness, whereas reserpine causes nasal congestion. Other hypotensive drugs in current use include hydralazine (Apresoline), methyldopa (Aldomet), and guanethidine (Ismelin), which is a highly potent hypotensive drug usually given to patients with severe hypertension. Drugs known as adrenergic blocking agents that act on the autonomic nervous system may be given to some patients. All drugs and their dosage are planned for each individual patient, based on his hypertensive condition, symptoms, and complications.

It is important that the patient with essential hypertension modify his life style to delay the serious effects of his hypertension. Cigarette smoking increases the chances of complications and should be avoided. Weight reduction is desirable, but many physicians believe that long-time weight reducing programs are often unsuccessful. There should be a program of regular exercise that is within the limits of the patient's capability based on his symptoms. Patients who are extremely anxious and apprehensive may be given a tranquilizer. However, there is a growing belief that because of cost and the economic status of many persons with hypertension, medications should be kept at the minimum necessary to control the blood pressure.[32]

Malignant hypertension differs from essential hypertension. It occurs principally in younger persons and runs a rapid course, with the blood pressure remaining extremely high. The condition affects the kidneys and eyes, and death often results from uremia.

Patients who are hospitalized because of hypertension should be provided with a quiet environment and optimum conditions for maximum rest. Procedures designed for relaxation such as warm baths, rubs, and warm drinks should be provided. Other nursing care is directed toward observing and reporting symptoms and planning care to relieve them.

Foods rich in potassium

Buttermilk	All citrus fruits and juices
Brussels sprouts	Prunes
Mustard greens	Raw carrots
Turnip greens	Asparagus
Bran flakes	Raw cabbage
Puffed wheat	Bananas
Cauliflower	Broccoli
Corn bread	Okra
Seafood	Sweet corn
Chicken	Soybeans

(margin note: Potassium rich foods)

Rheumatic fever and rheumatic heart disease

Rheumatic fever is primarily a disease of children and young persons, occurring between 5 and 15 years of age. Rheumatic fever usually begins with hemolytic streptococcus sore throat, which develops rapidly. The throat appears very red, and swallowing is difficult. The glands under the jaw are enlarged and tender, and the temperature may be elevated as high as 104° F. Throat cultures may be taken and the causa-

(margin note: hemolytic streptococcus)

tive organism isolated. Two or three weeks after recovery from the throat infection, indications of rheumatic fever appear. It is not the streptococcus organism that is thought to be the causative agent, but rather the toxins released by the organism. The body forms antibodies against these toxins that can react with many tissues of the body, producing a wide variety of symptoms.[20] Rheumatic fever, however, is a preventable disease.[19] Through the use of antibiotic therapy for patients with streptococcal infections almost all primary attacks of rheumatic fever could be eliminated. Once it has occurred, however, the patient is susceptible to future attacks.

Rheumatic fever has no specific set of symptoms, since the signs will vary with the age of the individual. The diagnosis is established through careful laboratory examinations and observation of the patient. The leukocyte count and the sedimentation rate usually increase. Fever may occur, including a pulse rate consistent with the fever. Any increase in the pulse rate should be viewed as serious, since it may be the first indication of heart damage. Some degree of anemia may be present because of dietary deficiencies. The younger the child the less likely it is that the joints will be involved. When the joints are involved, they are swollen and tender, and a characteristic of the disease is that the joint pain moves from joint to joint. Nodules may appear on the joints and subcutaneously, developing in crops. As one crop disappears, another appears. More than half of the patients with rheumatic fever develop inflammation of the heart (carditis). This may be followed by a systolic murmur that is heard at the apex of the heart, and endocarditis is always a possibility. Rheumatic fever may be recurring, and each new attack further damages the heart. The formation of scar tissue in the heart may cause the valves to leak, resulting in insufficiency, or a narrowing of the valve may occur, resulting in stenosis. The mitral and aortic valves are the ones most often affected, but the other valves may be involved. Extensive damage to the heart muscle at the time of a severe attack of rheumatic fever may result in heart failure and death. However, the disease is likely to become chronic, resulting in death years later. Some individuals recover with no heart damage, but careful medical supervision over a long period of time is necessary to eliminate the possibility of heart involvement.

Treatment and nursing care. Emphasis is placed on prevention, through extensive and immediate treatment of patients with throat infections with chemotherapeutic drugs to eradicate the hemolytic streptococcus bacteria. Physicians may advise that antibiotic therapy be continued at regular intervals for as long as 5 years after an attack of rheumatic fever. The care and treatment of a child with rheumatic fever and heart involvement is largely symptomatic. The very ill child with an acute attack is rarely seen today, largely because of improved social conditions and the availability of antibiotics. The use of a drug such as aspirin is generally ordered for the relief of painful joints and should be administered after meals with milk. When several joints are involved, any movement or jarring of the bed causes the patient severe pain. The parts involved should be supported with pillows with the joint slightly flexed. The patient will be more comfortable if bed boards are placed under the mattress. A footboard should be placed at the foot of the bed to keep weight from affected ankle joints. A bed cradle may be used to keep weight from other joints. Mild heat such as that provided by an electric heating pad set on low may be used, and oil of wintergreen (methyl salicylate) may be applied locally (do not rub or massage) to the joints, which may be wrapped in flannel or cotton. The antipyretic action of aspirin may cause profuse sweating; warm baths should be given and flannel garments used. In many instances cotton flannel sheets are preferred to cotton sheets, which become damp and cold. Great care should be taken in moving and turning the patient. The patient should be observed for dyspnea and any increase in pulse rate or temperature; observation of any such change should be reported.

Since diet may have been deficient over a period of time, a well-balanced diet high in calories, vitamin B, and vitamin C should be given. The appetite may be poor, and the patient may need considerable encouragement in taking food. Small meals at frequent intervals are often preferable to three

meals a day. Fluid intake should be from 2500 to 3000 ml. in a 24-hour period, and accurate records should be maintained. Since rest is of prime importance, nursing care should be planned to provide for undisturbed periods. Cooperation and coordination with other hospital departments may be needed to assure the patient of desired rest. The physician will determine how long the patient is to remain in bed and when exercise may be permitted. Complete bed rest may be required for complicated acute rheumatic fever, and the nursing care as just outlined should be given. In the absence of complications and during convalescence a more liberal regimen may be planned. The patient may have a modified program of bed rest, be taken to the bathroom, be allowed to feed himself, and engage in handicrafts with the assistance of the occupational therapist.

The child with rheumatic fever and rheumatic heart disease will often be cared for by his mother in his own home. To keep an active child quiet and in bed often poses a real problem. It will require all the ingenuity that everyone has to keep quiet an adolescent boy who wants to be out playing football or basketball. The public health nurse can give valuable assistance to the mother in supervising and teaching simple procedures and suggesting activities to keep a child interested. The American Heart Association, Inc., will provide free educational material giving guidance in caring for the child and in providing activities for teen-agers.

After the acute attack has subsided children who have rheumatic heart disease are usually advised to lead relatively normal lives but to restrain from vigorous competitive sports.

Complications of rheumatic fever

Mitral and aortic stenosis. Mitral stenosis and aortic stenosis are the most serious complications of repeated attacks of rheumatic fever. In these two conditions the respective valves become thickened and fused together, causing heart failure. Symptoms include dyspnea on exertion and pulmonary edema, a direct result of failure of the left side of the heart.

Treatment varies with the severity of the condition. Conservative treatment involves limitation of activity, reduction of sodium intake, and administration of digitalis and diuretics. If the patient becomes increasingly incapacitated when undergoing this therapy, surgery may be necessary. Mitral stenosis can be treated surgically by performing a mitral commissurotomy. The surgeon makes an incision into the left atrium and inserts the finger, a knife, or a dilator through the valve and breaks apart the stenosed tissue. Aortic stenosis is treated with open heart surgery using a heart-lung machine, as is mitral stenosis if a commissurotomy is unsuccessful.[35]

Bacterial endocarditis *heart lining*

The endocardium is the serous membrane that lines the inside of the heart and covers the flaps of the valves. Bacterial endocarditis is an inflammation of this lining caused by bacteria, and it may be acute or subacute.

Subacute bacterial endocarditis. Subacute bacterial endocarditis may occur in persons who have had rheumatic fever and whose heart valves have been damaged or in persons with congenital defects of the valves. It is believed to result from hospital-acquired infection after various types of surgery, including open heart surgery. It may also occur after dental extraction or tonsillectomy. Usually the causative organism belongs to the viridans group of streptococci.

The organism is present in the bloodstream and directly invades the heart. The valves are usually involved and become inflamed and covered with bacterial growth. The healing process may result in scarring, which will gradually reduce the effectiveness of the heart. The onset is generally insidious over a period of several weeks, and the symptoms, which may be numerous, gradually become worse and more serious. Anemia is usually present and there may be fever, loss of weight, cough, headache, and joint pains. One of the most characteristic symptoms is the appearance of petechiae, small hemorrhages from capillaries. These frequently occur in the conjunctiva, mouth, and legs. Small nodes, called Osler nodes, occur on the tips of the fingers and toes, and clubbing of the fingers is frequent. The hemorrhagic tendency gives rise to menstrual disorders, and hematuria may

occur. Emboli from the vegetative lesions on the heart valves may be carried to the lungs, spleen, or kidneys. Confirmed diagnosis is usually made on finding the organism in the blood culture.

Treatment and nursing care. Prior to the use of antibiotics patients with subacute bacterial endocarditis could be expected to live about a year. Prompt treatment with intensive antibiotic therapy will now cure about 90% of the patients with the disease. Bed rest is indicated for all patients, and transfusions of blood or packed red blood cells may be given. The diet is high in calories, vitamins, and protein; the patient may need encouragement to eat because of loss of appetite. The nursing care is based largely on the symptoms; however, observation of the patient for petechiae, location of pain, vomiting, speech difficulty, paralysis, and visual disturbances is important, and the occurrence of any of these signs should be reported at once.

Coronary artery and heart disease

The two coronary arteries, right and left, arise from the aorta just above the aortic semilunar valves, or the point where the ascending aorta begins. They are the first blood vessels to branch off from the aorta. Each coronary artery fans out over the heart muscle (myocardium) and subdivides into smaller branches that supply the myocardium with oxygen and nutrients (Fig. 13-12).

Pathophysiology. The primary cause of coronary artery disease is atherosclerosis. The development of atherosclerosis is closely related to a person's way of life (p. 268). The major factor in coronary artery disease is the gradual buildup of deposits consisting of cholesterol, other fatty substances, macrophages, and various cellular debris within the inner lining of the arteries. The walls of the vessels become inflamed, and eventually calcification of the deposits takes place, forming *plaques* that obstruct the flow of blood. Obstruction of the vessels is a slow, insidious process that develops over the years with few or no symptoms. Symptoms do not occur until obstruction of one of the coronary arteries or its branches becomes severe enough to deprive the heart of its oxygen supply. When the oxygen supply is cut off from any part of the heart

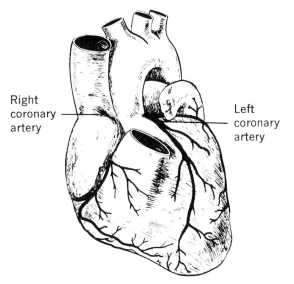

Fig. 13-12. Coronary arteries arise from the aorta just above the heart, one on the left side and one on the right side of the aorta.

muscle, the part affected will die. The most common diseases resulting from the obstruction of the coronary arteries or their branches are angina pectoris and myocardial infarction.

Angina pectoris (anginal syndrome)

The cause of angina pectoris is a decreased flow of blood from the coronary arteries and oxygen deficiency to the myocardium. The disease is usually the result of atherosclerosis; however, conditions such as hypertension, diabetes mellitus, syphilis, or rheumatic heart disease can predispose a patient to the disorder.

The characteristic symptom of the disease is a sudden, agonizing pain in the substernal region of the chest; the pain may be sufficiently severe to completely immobilize the person. The pain may radiate to the left shoulder and down the inner side of the arm into one or more fingers (Fig. 13-13). The pain is inconsistent, and frequently the patient is unable to describe it because of its many variations. At times it may appear only as a digestive upset. During an acute episode the face may have an ashen appearance, the patient may be covered with cold, clammy perspiration, and he may be unable to speak. The pulse rate remains normal, pulse volume does not change, and the blood pressure shows little or no

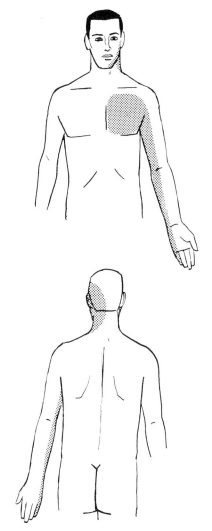

Fig. 13-13. Area to which pain radiates in angina pectoris.

change. The patient is extremely apprehensive, and the great physical and mental pain cause him to believe that he will die.

Any one of several factors may precipitate an attack of angina, including exposure to cold, emotional upsets, an unusually heavy meal, particularly at night, or any activity that will increase the work of the heart or cause a decreased supply of blood to the heart muscle.

Treatment and nursing care. The treatment of angina pectoris requires the treatment of the individual as a whole rather than treatment of the disease only. The individual needs to understand the nature of the pain and the factors that cause it. He needs help to regulate his daily plan of living to eliminate the attacks of pain. The individual should protect himself from cold by wearing warm clothing in cold weather. The use of tea, coffee, and tobacco should be discouraged, and meals should be regular and of moderate proportion. If the patient is overweight, plans should be made for a gradual reduction to a nearly normal range for age and height. Rest and relaxation are essential elements of treatment. Adjustments should be made when necessary to relieve the individual of tension and emotional strain. Treatment of angina is directed toward relieving the attack and decreasing the frequency and severity of attacks. The sublingual administration of nitroglycerin, 0.32 to 0.65 mg., or isosorbide dinitrate (Isordil), 5 mg., to relieve the immediate attack may be ordered. These medications dilate the capillary system and increase the blood flow to the heart muscle. Amyl nitrite is sometimes preferred because of its immediate action. This medication is dispensed in a small capsule, which can be crushed and then the contents inhaled. A longer acting medication, pentaerythritol tetranitrate (Peritrate), 10 mg., is administered three times daily, or erythrityl tetranitrate (Cardilate), 10 to 30 mg., is administered daily. All nitrate preparations will cause flushing of the skin and an increase in pulse and respirations, and a headache may occur. Patients with angina pectoris should always carry a nitrite preparation with them and may use it freely. Occasionally, theophylline ethylenediamine (aminophylline) will be given several times a day to produce a prolonged vasodilatation.[35]

A major aspect of nursing care is to relieve the patient's fear. This is particularly important if attacks occur at night. The nurse must rely on the patient for information concerning the quality, intensity, and duration of pain. Medication should not be withheld but should be given promptly. The patient may be raised to a sitting position and made comfortable. He needs support and reassurance, and these can best be provided if the nurse is calm, has a well-modulated voice, is firm, yet provides care with gentleness, understanding, sympathy, and efficiency. The nurse must be able to differentiate between dyspnea as a subjective complaint and dyspnea resulting from congestive failure, when the respiration is wheezy and the patient is cyanotic.[18]

Myocardial infarction

Myocardial infarction occurs when one of the coronary arteries or its branches (Fig. 13-12) suddenly becomes occluded. The cause may be a coronary thrombosis in which a blood clot forms and interrupts the blood supply. Blockage from other causes, such as vasoconstriction of the arteries or sudden atherosclerotic changes, is referred to as a coronary occlusion. The part of the heart supplied by the vessel is deprived of its blood supply and as a result dies. The area becomes soft and necrotic (infarct), it is gradually replaced by fibrous tissue, and a collateral circulation is established.

Men in middle life who generally consider themselves to be in robust health are often the persons who have a myocardial infarction. They usually have some degree of atherosclerosis and may or may not have hypertension. In some cases the condition may develop slowly, and often the individual has what he believes to be a mild indigestion. Diagnosis may be difficult to establish at this stage. For example, Mr. H., a 66-year-old retired businessman, had complained of indigestion for several days. The pain in the upper gastric region was slight, and he did not think he needed medical attention. Finally a member of the family persuaded him to see his physician, which he did. The physician examined his heart and told him that his heart was all right. The following morning Mr. H. got out of bed and started to the kitchen to begin breakfast, which was his usual custom. As he reached the kitchen door, he fell and was later pronounced dead.

The typical symptoms of acute myocardial infarction include a severe pain in the area of the lower sternum and upper abdomen, which may continue to increase in severity and radiate to the shoulders and down the arms. The left shoulder and the left arm are more frequently affected. The pulse becomes rapid, weak, and irregular. Vomiting occurs, and the patient is covered with cold, clammy perspiration. The blood pressure may fall, and all the signs of cardiogenic shock are present.

Cardiogenic shock occurs when the heart

fails to pump an adequate amount of blood to the vital organs. Whenever a portion of the heart muscle dies, that area can no longer contract and do its share of the work required to pump the blood through the circulatory system. Therefore the cardiac output will decrease and less blood will be available to supply oxygen and nutrients to the body tissues. Symptoms of the resulting cardiogenic shock include cold, clammy, and moist skin, pallor, apathy, decreasing blood pressure, a weak, thready, irregular, and rapid pulse, shallow and rapid respirations, and as the condition progresses, cyanosis of the lips and nailbeds, and dilated pupils. Approximately 10% of all patients with myocardial infarctions die of this shock syndrome. Most patients are acutely aware of their condition and are extremely apprehensive. In a few hours the temperature rises, but the elevation does not exceed 101° F. Both the leukocyte count and the sedimentation rate are increased. An electrocardiogram may be made on the patient's admission to the hospital and will be repeated at intervals to follow the patient's progress. An x-ray examination of the chest is made as soon as the patient's condition permits.

Three laboratory tests have proved to be beneficial in assessing the damage that occurs to the heart. The death of cardiac muscle results in the release of intracellular enzymes into the bloodstream. These enzymes are also located in tissue other than heart muscle; however, their presence indicates that damage of tissue has occurred. This plus electrocardiogram changes and the presence of typical symptoms leads to a rather firm diagnosis. The serum glutamic oxaloacetic transaminase (SGOT) level may rise as early as 4 to 6 hours after the infarct. It peaks in 1 or 2 days and returns to normal in about 4 days. The lactic dehydrogenase (LDH) level becomes elevated within a day after cardiac damage, peaks in 3 days, and returns to normal within 1 or 2 weeks. The creatine phosphokinase (CPK) level is often elevated within 3 to 5 hours after the initial symptoms, peaks in about 1½ days, and returns to normal in 3 days if no further damage has occurred.[38]

Treatment and nursing care. Most patients are placed in the coronary care unit or intensive care unit. The relief of pain is of primary importance, and morphine or meperidine hydrochloride (Demerol) is usually administered. When the patient is in shock or when cyanosis or dyspnea is present, oxygen may be administered by mask or nasal catheter. Theophylline ethylenediamine (aminophylline) or papaverine hydrochloride may be ordered to relax smooth muscle and dilate the coronary vessels. If the fall in blood pressure is severe and does not respond to conservative treatment, levarterenol (Levophed) or other vasopressor drugs may be ordered and administered by slow intravenous drip. The rate of drip is regulated by the blood pressure, which is taken with the pulse every 3 to 5 minutes. The nurse who is caring for a patient receiving vasopressor drugs should remember that they are dangerous drugs, and extreme caution must be used while they are being administered. The temperature is taken every 4 to 6 hours. An anticoagulant drug such as heparin sodium or bishydroxycoumarin (Dicumarol) is usually given to prevent venous thrombosis or pulmonary embolism. A daily test of prothrombin time must be made as long as the patient is receiving an anticoagulant drug. It is generally believed that if laboratory facilities are not available for testing prothrombin time, the anticoagulant drug should not be given to the patient. The prothrombin time is maintained at approximately 10% of normal, or 30 seconds. The patient should be observed for signs of bleeding while he is receiving anticoagulant therapy. Bleeding may occur from gums or from sites of injections. All emesis, urine, and stools should be inspected for any evidence of blood. Any sudden signs of dyspnea and changes in rate, rhythm, or volume of the pulse should be reported at once.

The patient with myocardial infarction must be assured of maximum rest from the moment of the attack. Nursing procedures should be planned to allow for long periods of undisturbed rest. It is often desirable to plan with other hospital departments so that a minimum of persons enter and leave the room. During the acute stage only close members of the patient's family are allowed in the room, and visits should be spaced so that they do not interfere with rest. Complete bed rest is the usual way of providing maximum rest; however, studies appear to indicate that the work demanded of the heart may be lessened if the patient is in an upright position. Therefore some physicians will permit the patient to be lifted into an armchair for short periods of time several times a day. The patient should be watched carefully for changes in his condition while in the sitting position. The physician will order increasing amounts of activity and generally uses electrocardiograph readings and serum enzyme levels as a guide. Intravenous infusions will be started immediately if a myocardial infarction is suspected. Cardiovascular shock and consequent collapse of the vessels are a constant threat, and a vein should be kept open for the administration of emergency drugs. The diet should be suited to the patient's condition and may be liquid, soft, or regular. No iced or very hot drinks should be given because they may precipitate cardiac arrhythmias, and foods known to be gas producing should be avoided. The urinal and bedpan may be offered at regular intervals to spare the patient the effort of having to ask for them. Bowel elimination may be regulated by mild laxatives or a low enema on medical order, and the patient should not be permitted to strain at defecation.

As the heart starts to heal, collateral circulation develops and the necrotic tissue in the myocardium begins to be repaired with fibrotic scar formation. The first 2 weeks after a myocardial infarction are considered the most dangerous, and the patient's condition must be watched closely for 4 weeks. Healing usually occurs in 6 weeks, although convalescence generally takes 2 to 3 months. Gradually the patient will be able to return to a normal or nearly normal life.

The management and care of the patient with myocardial infarction must be individualized, depending on the severity of the attack, complications, and progress. The use of modern monitoring equipment has made it possible to detect cardiac disturbances that otherwise would have been missed. Several new methods of treating patients with myocardial infarction, including the use of hyperbaric oxygen, are in the experimental stage. Nurses should realize that machines can contribute much to the care of the patient but may also increase the patient's fear, anxiety, and apprehension unless he understands their contribution to his care. Above all, it should be remembered that machines cannot provide emotional support and intelligent, sympathetic understanding essential to the patient's progress.

Several surgical techniques have been attempted to remove the atherosclerotic deposits that obstruct the coronary arteries. One surgical approach opens the coronary artery and removes the plaque in the diseased vessel. This procedure is called an *endarterectomy*. The diseased plaques can also be excised and replaced with a vein graft or artificial materials. In gas endarterectomy, carbon dioxide jets loosen the plaques, which then can be removed surgically.

However, the coronary artery bypass is rapidly becoming one of the most frequently performed heart operations in the United States. The operation involves the use of the heart-lung machine and a highly trained operating room staff (p. 283). To create the bypass the surgeon removes a vein from the patient's leg and sutures one end to a new hole in the aorta near the junction of the coronary arteries. The other end is connected to a part of the coronary artery past the diseased area. This procedure "bypasses" the obstruction to blood flow and increases the oxygen supply to the heart muscles immediately. The patient is able to lead a nearly normal life after the operation; however, the long-term effects of the surgery have yet to be determined.[24, 29]

Aneurysm

When the wall of an artery becomes weakened from disease or from injury, it may become distended at the weakened place. The distended part is called an *aneurysm*. The most frequent causes are syphilis and arteriosclerosis. Almost all aneurysms involve the aorta, with most of them occurring in the arch of the aorta. However, they may occur in arteries located elsewhere in the body. A fusiform aneurysm affects the entire circumference of the artery, similar to a partially blown-up long balloon (Fig. 13-14). A saccular aneurysm involves only a portion of the artery wall and forms an outpouching on the side of an otherwise normal artery (Fig. 13-15).

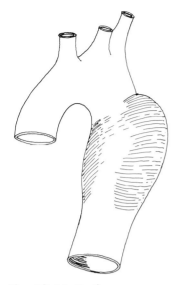

Fig. 13-14. Fusiform aneurysm.

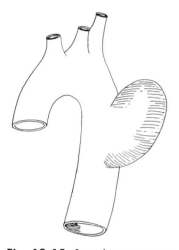

Fig. 13-15. Saccular aneurysm.

The distended part fills with blood and gradually becomes larger and larger, until it may appear as a pulsating tumor. The symptoms are related to the structures, bones, or nerves against which the aneurysm presses. A pulsating aneurysm pressing against the ribs may erode through the bone to the chest wall and then protrude through under the skin. The patient may have severe pain in the chest, and there may be dyspnea and cyanosis. Sometimes the pupils are of unequal size, and the radial pulse may vary in the two arms. Aneurysms are usually diagnosed by fluoroscopic examination and a reactive serology test for syphilis.[6]

Treatment consists of decreased physical activity to reduce the work of the heart and to decrease the arterial pressure. Many aneurysms may be corrected or improved through surgical techniques, since there is no other cure. A fusiform aneurysm can be removed and replaced with a graph of a synthetic fiber such as Dacron or Teflon or with a vessel taken from another region of the patient's body. Saccular aneurysms can be removed and the vessel sutured, or a patch graph can be used to replace the deformity. For patients who are not suitable candidates for surgery, treatment and nursing care are based on their symptoms, and the prognosis is poor.

Congestive heart failure

Congestive heart failure occurs when the cardiac output can no longer meet the needs of the body tissues. It may be the result of bacterial endocarditis, damage from rheumatic fever, syphilitic heart disease, arteriosclerosis, hypertension, or myocardial infarction. It may also occur from other disorders including blood transfusions or infusions. It may affect the right or the left side of the heart, but ultimately both sides are affected.

Pathophysiology. When the heart fails to pump blood sufficient to meet the needs of the body, all body organs and tissues are affected. The pulmonary vascular system becomes congested, since it is no longer emptied sufficiently by the left atrium and ventricle. As the pressure in these chambers increases, the blood begins to back up in the atria and the large veins. Blood returning to the heart cannot be pumped rapidly enough into the congested pulmonary vessels, and the venous system becomes engorged. As the pressure in the venous system rises, other organs of the body become congested. The decreased cardiac output causes a diminished flow of blood to the kidneys and reduces the glomerular filtration rate. With reduced renal blood flow, sodium and water are retained in the body and contribute to generalized edema. Because of increased venous pressure and stasis, fluid is pushed out of the capillaries and venules. The liver and other organs become congested, and fluid escapes into the abdominal cavity (ascites).

The early symptoms of congestive heart

failure are (1) shortness of breath, usually apparent on exertion such as climbing stairs or walking rapidly, (2) a slight cough, more of a hacking type, (3) a tendency to become easily fatigued, (4) slight abdominal discomfort, and (5) swelling of the feet and ankles. The edema of the feet and ankles subsides at night when the person is in a supine position. As the disease becomes advanced, the dyspnea may be of a panting type and may be so severe that the person must remain in an upright position (orthopnea). The cough is dry, and hemoptysis may occur. The edema may extend to the face, neck, sacrum, and extremities and is a pitting type (dependent edema). There may be cyanosis, enlargement and tenderness of the liver, and decreased urinary output. Abnormalities of the pulse may be found, and the patient may or may not complain of pain in the chest and abdomen. When there is left ventricular failure, acute pulmonary edema may occur. Dyspnea is increased, cyanosis occurs, and productive cough is present. This is always a serious emergency, and immediate treatment is necessary. When right ventricular failure occurs, there may be excessive weight gain. As the venous pressure increases, the patient complains of more pain in the upper abdomen. The patient is weak with loss of appetite, excessive perspiration, and nocturnal diuresis. Pitting edema, particularly noticeable in the lower extremities, occurs, which is related to the abnormal weight gain. The central venous pressure is elevated but will gradually decrease with effective treatment.

Treatment and nursing care. In the treatment of congestive heart failure there are three primary objectives: to reduce oxygen requirements, decrease the edema, and increase the cardiac output. To accomplish these objectives three approaches are usually taken: rest to reduce the oxygen requirements, drugs to reduce the edema, and digitalis to improve the cardiac output.[39]

Rest. The patient with congestive heart failure must be treated on an individual basis, and many patients with mild or moderate failure will avoid serious complications such as venous stasis or pulmonary embolism if they are up and leading a relatively normal life. Because of this, many physicians do not confine such persons to long periods of bed rest. If the condition is severe, bed rest is usually necessary, and the length of rest is determined for the individual patient. When the patient is hospitalized, he should be placed in a quiet, restful environment. The nurse needs to understand that emotional exertion, like physical exertion, increases the metabolic activity and increases oxygen needs. The patient may fear immediate danger and prolonged helplessness. The nurse should be alert to signs that indicate anxiety, frustration, and fear. The patient may express these feelings verbally or may show them by uncooperativeness and hostility. The patient may feel safe only when someone is with him, and arrangements may have to be made for a member of the family to stay with him. Reassuring the patient may often be accomplished best by a calm, cheerful attitude and efficient, confident administration of care.

Drugs. Diuretics are drugs administered for the purpose of removing the excess water that has been retained by the body. In the presence of the diuretic, urinary output is increased, edema and ascites are relieved, and breathing is made easier. Mercurial diuretics include meralluride (Mercuhydrin), chlormerodrin (Neohydrin), mercumatilin (Cumertilin), and mercaptomerin (Thiomerin), which are administered intramuscularly. The patient should be observed for toxic symptoms such as drowsiness, numbness, dizziness, and digestive disturbances. Mercurial diuretics may be given with ammonium chloride, a diuretic that enhances the effects of the mercurial drugs, or they may be alternated every other day with acetazolamide (Diamox). The most widely used oral agent is chlorothiazide (Diuril), a synthetic thiazide compound. At the present time several similar agents are available under various trade names, including Hygroton, Esidrix, Enduron, Renese, Saluron, Naturetin, and others. Furosemide (Lasix) is a rapid-acting oral diuretic that has come into popular use. It is more powerful than the thiazides and is highly effective in congestive heart failure. All produce similar effects—excretion of sodium chloride and water. Since potassium is also lost, the patient must be given a glass of orange juice each morning unless he is receiving potassium chloride.

When severe ascites is present, the physician may perform an abdominal paracentesis, or if fluid has accumulated in the chest cavity, a thoracentesis may be done.

The physician usually orders digitalis in some form to slow the heart rate and increase the force of the beat, thereby improving cardiac output. The physician may wish the maximum effect to be obtained as quickly as possible and may order several doses large enough to accomplish this; this treatment is called *digitalization*. During this time the patient must be carefully observed for toxic symptoms such as nausea, vomiting, irregular pulse, diarrhea, anorexia, and visual disturbances. If any of these symptoms occur, the drug should be withheld and the physician notified. As soon as the maximum effect has been obtained, the patient is placed on a maintenance dose. The nurse should remember to count the pulse before administering digitalis. If the rate is below 60 or over 100 beats per minute, the drug is not given and the physician is notified. Digitalis is marketed under several different trade names, among which are Digalen, Lanoxin, Cedilanid, and others.

A mild sedative may be needed for sleep and rest at night. Chloral hydrate or one of the slow-acting barbiturates may be ordered. Meperidine hydrochloride (Demerol) may be ordered to relieve pain; however, simple nursing measures such as changing the patient's position, rearranging the pillows and bedding, letting the patient empty his bladder, and rubbing his back may be soothing and relieve the need for sedation. A mild cathartic or a stool softener may be given to avoid straining while defecating. When dyspnea or cyanosis is present, oxygen may be administered by tent, mask, or nasal catheter. In some cases intermittent positive-pressure breathing may be ordered.

Diet. Patients with congestive heart failure, as well as patients with some other heart diseases, are often placed on a sodium-restricted diet. The body requires a certain amount of sodium, and any excess is excreted by the kidneys. In patients with congestive heart failure, when water is being retained in the tissues, the sodium is being retained also. The sodium contributes to water retention, but when the sodium is absent, the water will be excreted. The physician will prescribe the diet and the amount of sodium that may be permitted. The sodium-restricted diet is difficult for the patient to accept, and he will need a great deal of encouragement. The nurse should review basic nutrition to give the patient as much help as possible. The sodium-restricted diet is often misunderstood and interpreted by the patient to mean no consumption of salt. The selection of foods that are low in natural sodium is perhaps more important. In some instances when the patient is receiving a diuretic, he is not placed on a sodium-restricted diet. The diuretic promotes excretion of the sodium and the water. Meals for the patient should be small to keep the diaphragm low, providing for expansion of the lungs. Most physicians allow the patient a liberal amount of fluids to provide for adequate diuresis, which will result from the sodium restriction and the administration of the diuretic. The nurse must understand the physician's orders for the amount of fluid permitted.

Nursing care. The patient should be placed in the position affording him the greatest amount of comfort and rest. Most patients are made comfortable in a high Fowler's position with the back, arms, and knees supported with pillows. A small pillow may be placed at the back of the head and one in the small of the back. Pillows should be secured to prevent their slipping. This position gives the patient more room for adequate ventilation and slows the return of venous blood to the heart. A footboard should be placed at the foot of the bed to keep the weight of bedding from edematous extremities and to help keep the patient from slipping down. Side rails should be placed on the bed. The patient may rest his head on pillows placed on an overbed table while the bed is being changed. The head of the bed may then be lowered and the bed made from the top to the bottom.

It should be remembered that the patient on a regimen of complete bed rest is predisposed to venous stasis. If the patient is unable to move his legs, the nurse should give passive exercise every 1 or 2 hours, flexing the extremities; however, the patient should not be disturbed when he is asleep.

Some patients are not allowed to participate in any part of their care or feed themselves during the acute stage of heart failure. Complete bed baths may be too fatiguing for the patient, and partial baths, with special care of the skin and all bony prominences, may be adequate. Because of poor circulation, the patient is predisposed to decubitus ulcers, and frequent inspection and massage are required for their prevention. (See Chapter 6.) Sponge rubber bra cups with twill tape ties will fit over elbows and heels to prevent friction. Accurate intake and output records must be maintained, and the patient should be weighed daily when possible. The patient should be weighed at the same time each day and under the same conditions. Loss of fluid will cause a marked decrease in weight. Since dyspnea may be present, the temperature should be taken rectally. The patient should be lifted on and off the bedpan, or if his condition permits, less energy is expended by both patient and nurse if the patient is gently rolled onto the bedpan. A child's bedpan or an orthopedic pan may facilitate the procedure with less strain on the patient. Some patients may be permitted to use a bedside commode. The automatic bed used in many hospitals may be lowered to the height of the commode, or in some instances the commode may be elevated to the height of the bed. The patient must not be permitted to strain while defecating.

The patient should be observed for any change in the rate, rhythm, or volume of the pulse, color, dyspnea, increase or decrease of edema, and any evidence of mental confusion or psychoses. During the acute stage of the illness, visitors should be limited to immediate members of the family, who should not tire the patient with lengthy conversations or disturbing affairs. As the patient improves, activity is permitted, but the process should be gradual. The nurse should understand the physician's orders and the amount of exercise the patient is permitted.

Heart disease complicated by pregnancy

It is estimated that 2% to 4% of pregnant women have heart disease, which is a cause of maternal mortality and may contribute to premature and perinatal deaths.

The largest number of cases of heart disease in pregnant women result from rheumatic fever, with a small number from congenital defects and about the same number from hypertensive heart disease. Frequently the woman may be unaware that she has heart disease until she visits an obstetrician for antepartum care. Every young woman anticipating marriage should visit her physician for examination prior to marriage. Many cardiac defects could be corrected before marriage, which would assure safe pregnancies through the childbearing years.

Treatment. Treatment is designed to prevent congestive heart failure. The obstetrician may secure a cardiologist to assist with the management of the patient. The medical history should include any history of rheumatic fever, chorea, congenital heart disease, and heart murmur. A careful evaluation of the cardiac condition is made, and the patient's activity is planned according to the cardiac findings. Activities requiring the greatest amount of energy output should be reduced or eliminated. Some of these activities include climbing stairs, polishing floors, sweeping rugs, and making beds. The patient is advised to spend 10 hours in bed at night and to have several rest periods during the day. She is cautioned against exposure to respiratory infections such as colds and sore throats. Beginning at the third trimester of pregnancy, the greatest burden is placed on the heart. At this time the patient should be carefully observed for increased dyspnea, cough, hemoptysis, peripheral edema, anemia, or increased pulse rate. The patient may be hospitalized, with fluids restricted, undergo digitalization, and placed on a sodium-restricted diet.

Nursing care. Most patients will be seen in the physician's office or in a clinic during their antepartum period. The nurse in the physician's office or clinic may be the first person to see the patient. The nurse should observe the patient carefully on each visit and report any noticeable symptom to the physician. The nurse should be familiar with the physician's orders to the patient and be able to help the patient understand them. The patient will usually be required to visit the physician every 2 weeks. The nurse may assist in encouraging the patient and in helping to prevent and relieve anxiety.

When the patient enters the hospital for delivery, the nurse should not leave the patient alone during labor. Dyspnea may be relieved by placing the patient in a semirecumbent position, and not permitting her to bear down during contractions, since this places more strain on the heart. The pulse and respiratory rates should be taken frequently, and any increase in the pulse rate above 110 beats per minute should be reported. The patient should be observed for increased dyspnea or cyanosis, which should be reported immediately. Emergency equipment and supplies should be available for any emergency. During the postpartum period the patient should not be permitted to become fatigued. In most instances there should be help in the home when the patient returns from the hospital. Rest periods and moderation in activities should be continued, and the patient should remain under the care of the physician.[12, 17]

Diseases and disorders of the veins and lymphatics
Thrombophlebitis

Simple phlebitis is the inflammation of the wall of a vein, whereas thrombophlebitis is inflammation with the presence of a blood clot in the vein. Many factors predispose a person to this condition, including age, occupation, obesity, prolonged abdominal or pelvic surgery, injury to the extremities, dehydration, and any condition that requires the individual to be on a regimen of bed rest over an extended period of time. Thrombophlebitis may occur easily in older persons with sclerotic changes in the veins that cause the blood to flow slowly.

The nurse can contribute much toward the prevention of thrombophlebitis by understanding and carrying out simple nursing procedures. Active exercise while the patient is in bed, including dorsiflexion (bending backward) and plantarflexion (bending forward) of the toes, should be done several times each hour or for 3 minutes each hour while the patient is awake. This simple exercise will do more to stimulate circulation than will massage or telling the patient to move his legs. Fluid intake should be encouraged to prevent dehydration, and accurate intake and output records should be maintained. When patients have Levin tubes connected to suction, the nurse should be sure they are working properly. Elevating the knees by changing the position of the Gatch bed and placing pillows under the knees should be avoided, since these procedures will compress the undersurface of the knee, causing a pooling of blood and increased pressure in the veins of the calf of the leg. The same situation occurs when the patient is sitting in a chair, which permits the calf of the leg and the knee to be compressed. Placing the patient's feet on a stool will avoid pressure on veins under the knee. Tight abdominal binders and dressings and the use of drugs that depress respiration should be avoided postoperatively.

The veins of the lower extremities are the ones usually affected. The patient may complain of pain or cramps in the calf of the leg, and these pains may follow the course of the vein. Tenderness and abnormal distention of the vein may be noted. There is usually an elevation of temperature, and the sedimentation rate is also elevated. The most serious complication of thrombophlebitis is pulmonary embolism with a possible pulmonary infarct (p. 210).

Treatment and nursing care. Treatment of the patient with thrombophlebitis depends on whether only superficial veins or deep vessels are involved and the extent of involvement. Physicians differ concerning elevation of the extremity, and the nurse should understand the physician's order. If the phlebitis involves only the superficial veins, anticoagulant therapy may not be ordered. Bed rest with continuous hot moist packs is generally ordered, and as soon as the acute condition has subsided, the patient may be allowed out of bed with an elastic stocking on the extremity. If the phlebitis involves the deep veins, anticoagulant therapy with heparin sodium is usually ordered. An x-ray film (phlebogram) may be made to determine the exact site and extent of the involvement. A surgical procedure known as thrombectomy (removal of a thrombus from the vein) may be done.[15]

For hot compresses Turkish towels are dipped in warm water, wrung fairly dry, and then wrapped loosely about the extremity and covered with plastic. An electric heating pad on a low setting may be used to keep the dressing warm, or the Aquamatic K pad may be used (Fig. 18-6). When elastic stockings or bandages are used, they should be put on before the patient gets out of bed, and they should be removed several times during the day and the leg inspected. Elastic stockings should not be rolled at the top.

Varicose veins

Varicose veins are greatly and permanently dilated veins in the lower extremities, in which the blood flow becomes stagnant. Other forms of venous varicosities are hemorrhoids and varicocele. Several factors contribute to the cause of varicose veins. The underlying cause may be a congenital weakness in the walls of the vein, an abnormal placement of the valves in the vein, or a defect of the valves. The immediate causes include severe physical strain such as that produced by long standing and lifting heavy objects. Pressure on pelvic veins during pregnancy from the enlarging uterus, pelvic tumors that may press on veins, obesity, and wearing tight round garters also contribute to the development of varicose veins.

About 50% of all women and 25% of men 40 years of age or older have varicose veins. They develop insidiously, beginning in young adults and gradually increasing in severity with increasing age. At first there may be no symptoms, but eventually the patient may complain of pain in the feet and ankles, with a tired, heavy feeling in the legs.[15] Swelling may occur in the feet, which usually subsides during the night and reappears as soon as the patient is up on his feet again. Pigmented areas may appear on the skin above the ankles with eczema-like lesions; these lesions ultimately may break down, and ulcers may occur. The rupture of a varicose vein through an ulcer may cause the loss of a considerable amount of blood, since such a vein will bleed from both ends.

Treatment and nursing care. The treatment of patients with varicose veins includes bed rest and elevation of the extremity, the use of an elastic stocking or an elastic bandage, or the surgical removal of the vein (vein stripping). Sometimes when small veins are involved, the physi-

cian may inject a solution into the vein that will cause its sclerosing without providing a permanent cure.

Vein ligation and stripping. Ligation and stripping is one of the most common types of surgery performed on the veins. Prior to surgery the physician will determine that the deep veins of the extremity are open. Not all patients with varicose veins will need to have them surgically removed, but when edema and pigmentation (which may lead to ulceration) occur, surgery is usually advised. Sometimes veins are so distended that they become unsightly, and surgery may be done for cosmetic reasons.

The physician usually visits the patient on the evening before surgery and marks the route of the veins that are to be removed. The long saphenous vein, which branches from the groin and extends to the ankle, is often the one removed. One or both extremities may be involved. The entire leg and pubis are shaved, with special care being given to the groin, which will be the site of ligation. Other preparation is the same as that for other surgical patients. Although the surgical procedure may be performed while the patient is under local anesthesia, it is long and painful, and the patient is usually given a general anesthetic.

Postoperative nursing care. When the patient returns from surgery, the extremity will be wrapped with elastic bandages. Small sterile dressings will cover the areas in which veins were ligated. These dressings should be checked frequently for evidence of bleeding. Bandages should be removed only on the physician's order. The knee section of the Gatch bed should not be raised, but the foot of the bed may be elevated about 8 inches to facilitate the return of venous blood. The foot and toes should be observed for color and edema, and the patient should be encouraged to move them about as soon as possible. The patient may have some pain for 2 or 3 days, and meperidine hydrochloride may be ordered for relief of the pain. Most physicians order the patient to be ambulatory by the first day after surgery or as soon as she has recovered from anesthesia. The patient should not sit or stand, but should walk. Patients are usually discharged after 2 or 3 days, and an elastic stocking is worn for several weeks. Patients should be advised against the use of depilatory cream on the legs, especially where the skin may be thin. They should avoid scratching and bruising of the legs. They should not sit with the legs crossed and are advised to avoid the use of panty girdles that may compress veins in the groin and thighs.[33]

Lymphangitis

Lymphangitis is an acute inflammation of the lymph vessels caused by the invasion of bacteria such as the streptococcus organism. It is characterized by red streaks that follow the course of the vessel involved. The patient may have an elevation of temperature and chills. In some patients the lymph nodes along the course of the vessel may be involved and become swollen and tender. Usually, however, the inflammatory condition will terminate at the first lymph node. The condition may be serious if the causative organism reaches the bloodstream, since septicemia may occur.

Treatment and nursing care. Treatment of lymphangitis is based on controlling the underlying cause. Warm moist dressings may be ordered for application over the affected vessels, and scrupulous skin care and immediate attention to all abrasions should be given. The affected part is elevated, and sulfonamide or antibiotic therapy is ordered. The condition generally responds quickly to therapy. In some cases, abscess formation may occur, and incision and drainage may be necessary.

NURSING THE PATIENT WITH OPERATIVE CONDITIONS OF THE CARDIOVASCULAR SYSTEM

Surgery of the cardiovascular system is one of the most significant accomplishments of medical science in this century. Today it is saving lives and providing lifetimes of health free from crippling cardiac conditions. There is every indication that an increasing number of persons will be helped in the future.

Modern heart surgery requires a vast array of equipment and a staff of highly trained, efficient professional persons. In no other aspect of medical-surgical care is the team concept of greater importance than in operative procedures involving the heart. Judgment, technical competency, and skill in observation are demanded of the nurse, and an ability to understand the feeling and emotional response of the patient is of equal importance. Whether the patient is an adult or a child, the nurse's responsibility may begin in the physician's office and continue until long after the surgery has been completed and convalescence and rehabilitation have returned the patient to his optimum capacity.

Since almost all cardiac surgery is performed only in large medical centers, most patients will be away from their families and friends. They will be in a strange environment among strange people and will be fearful of what is happening to them. The warm, friendly attitude of the nurse may contribute greatly to the patient's feeling of security and may lead him to verbalize fears, anxiety, and problems.

Cardiovascular surgery may be performed to correct congenital or acquired conditions. It may be performed inside the heart (open heart surgery), or it may be done to relieve or correct some condition outside the heart (closed heart surgery). It may involve the valves of the heart, the heart muscle or its covering, or the great blood vessels of the body.

Open heart surgery can be performed only through the use of a heart-lung machine. Although there are many models, all machines are similar in that they provide for gas exchange (oxygen and carbon dioxide), which normally occurs in the lungs, and they pump the oxygenated blood to the body tissues, duplicating the action of the heart. This process is called a cardiopulmonary bypass. In addition, the patient's body temperature may be lowered during surgery to reduce the metabolic processes.

Cardiac surgery may be performed on very young infants, middle-aged persons, and selected older persons; however, most people undergoing cardiac surgery are young adults. Not all persons needing help are suitable candidates for cardiac surgery, and not all those having surgery will be completely cured. Sometimes damage already done cannot be corrected, but further damage can be prevented. The physician may recommend surgery to the patient, but the final decision is always left to the patient. In the case of a young child the parent must make the decision, which is not always easy because there is some risk involved and sometimes, even though the child may be helped, there is no possibility of complete cure.

Cardiac surgery

Preoperative care. The patient is admitted to the hospital several days before surgery, and most patients are very apprehensive. During this time he receives detailed examination, including laboratory studies and special tests and examinations outlined earlier in this chapter. The physician will plan for a conference with the patient and give him as much information as advisable. The nurse should accompany the physician in order to know what the patient has been told.

Preoperatively the blood pressure and apical-radial pulse are taken every 4 hours, and the patient is weighed daily to establish a basis for determining what is normal for the patient and to estimate the amount of blood that will be needed for the heart-lung machine if open heart surgery is to be done. If the patient has been on a sodium-restricted diet or has been receiving a diuretic or digitalis, these may be continued. If permitted, the patient should be up and walking about to maintain strength and muscle tone. If the patient is a child, the nurse may utilize the opportunity to learn the child's interests, habits, likes, and dislikes and to establish a friendly mutual acceptance. This will be extremely important in the postoperative care of a child. The child's room should be attractive and cheerful and provided with some of his most cherished toys.

The surgeon and nurse will prepare the patient for some of the details of his postoperative nursing care. He should be taught how to breathe deeply, slowly, and noiselessly and how to tighten the muscles of the abdomen, which will stimulate coughing on exhalation. The patient should practice this procedure under supervision many times, since it will be essential postoperatively. He should know that he will have chest tubes, that he will be receiving oxygen, that intravenous fluids will be given, and that he may have a Levin tube in his nose. The patient should also know that vital signs will be checked frequently for a considerable time. He should be told that

he will have pain, but that his pain will be relieved and the nurse will be at his bedside and will not leave him alone.

The physical preparation is similar to that for most surgical patients. The skin preparation usually covers a wide area, and the wrists and ankles are shaved in anticipation of a venous cutdown. An enema and a sedative for sleep and rest may be given the evening before with fluids restricted after midnight.

Operative day. Although the fear is not always verbalized, the patient probably expects to die and may have made necessary material preparation. On the day of surgery members of his family and his religious counselor should be permitted to visit him. The physician will come to the room and do a venous cutdown and start an infusion. Usually a vein in one of the ankles is used. The patient may be given a mild sedative, but narcotics are not usually ordered preoperatively because of the danger of depressing the respiration. A small dose of atropine may be given to decrease secretions. Other preparation is the same as that for other surgical patients. (See Chapter 9.)

While the patient is in surgery, all equipment that will be needed for postoperative care is brought to the room and checked for working order. Supplies to meet any emergency must be in the room, including emergency drugs. Open heart surgery may be performed under hypothermia, and equipment for warming the patient should be available. The cardiac care unit brings together all the necessary equipment, including emergency needs. A check should always be made to be sure that everything is working properly and that nothing has been omitted.

Postoperative care. The first 48 hours after heart surgery are the most critical for the patient. The patient may be kept in the recovery room during this period or may be transferred to an intensive care unit, to the cardiac care unit, or to his own room on medical order. Cardiac monitors are generally used continuously for the first few days.

Vital signs. The apical-radial pulse, blood pressure, and respiration are checked and recorded every 15 minutes for not less than 8 hours and sometimes for as long as 24 hours. The rhythm, rate, and strength of the pulse should be observed, and the nurse should constantly observe for arrhythmias. The central venous pressure will be monitored frequently. The physician should indicate the lowest level of systolic pressure that the patient can tolerate without harmful effects. If the surgery has involved coronary arteries, systolic pressure must be watched more closely. Any elevation of temperature of more than 102° F. should be reported, since temperature elevation increases the work of the heart.

Oxygen. For the first few hours postoperatively the patient is usually given assisted ventilation and oxygen. This procedure decreases the possibility of hypoxia and resulting arrhythmias. Oxygen may continue for several days. Intermittent positive pressure breathing may be used to facilitate deep breathing and coughing when continuous assisted ventilation is discontinued.

Closed drainage system. Chest catheters may be used for both the right and the left pleural cavities or for one side only. They are attached to a closed drainage system (underwater drainage) and must be kept free of clots by milking or stripping. They must not be allowed to become kinked. (See Chapter 11.) Drainage should be observed for excessive amounts of blood. The amount of drainage in 24 hours will depend on the type of surgery and may vary from 400 to 1200 ml. in some patients. Absence of drainage must be promptly reported, since fluid may be accumulating in the chest cavity and will result in cardiac embarrassment. When turning the patient, the nurse should provide for adequate slack in the tubing to prevent disconnection or displacement of the chest catheters.

Levin tube. When patients have undergone surgery of the coronary arteries, a Levin tube is inserted and connected to suction to keep the stomach empty. Food and fluids by mouth are withheld until the patient begins to expel flatus. The patient is usually maintained on a regimen of intravenous fluids for 2 or 3 days. Blood samples may be taken daily for several days to be examined for serum electrolyte content, and electrolytes may be administered. The nurse should understand the physician's orders concerning the rate of administration of infusions; unless they drip slowly, the

circulation may be overloaded, causing serious complications.

Exercise. The patient is encouraged to cough and breathe deeply every 2 hours. There must be specific physician's orders for positioning the patient. Some patients may be placed in a semi-Fowler's position and turned from side to side every 2 hours; others may be turned to one side only; and patients undergoing some types of surgery must remain flat and may not be turned. When the patient is first elevated from a supine position, the blood pressure should be taken in 5 minutes, and if it has dropped since the previous reading, the head is lowered for 30 minutes before elevating it again. Passive exercises of the extremities are started after 24 hours, with special attention to the left arm. As soon as the patient is able, exercises should become active rather than passive. The patient should be encouraged from the beginning to use the left arm and to put it through a complete range of motion.

Urinary output. When open heart surgery has been done, a retention catheter may be placed in the urinary bladder. Output is checked and recorded hourly and should be from 15 to 30 ml. Specimens are collected hourly, and the specific gravity is checked and recorded. Urine should be observed for evidence of blood, and any decrease in output should be reported because a kidney shutdown may be occurring.

Relief of pain. The patient will have considerable pain for the first 48 hours, largely because of rib retraction. Drugs for relief will be administered, but care must be exercised not to sedate the patient to the extent that he will be unable to breathe deeply and cough. Meperidine hydrochloride is usually ordered in amounts from 25 to 100 mg., depending on the age and condition of the patient.

Airway. One of the purposes of coughing is to bring up deep secretions and maintain a free airway. The nurse may assist the patient by splinting the chest and upper abdomen. Deep coughing often becomes a problem because the patient fears the pain; however, if it is not successful, endotracheal suctioning will have to be used to maintain a free airway.

Diet. Most patients are allowed fluids by mouth as soon as nausea and vomiting have ceased; however, intravenous infusions are maintained for a few days. Occasionally fluid intake is restricted, and an accurate measurement must be maintained. Very hot or very cold fluids should be avoided because they may cause an irregularity of the heartbeat. Some physicians omit fruit juices during the early postoperative days. Diet is usually given to the patient as tolerated, and if the patient has been receiving a sodium-restricted diet, it may be continued.

Antibiotics are routinely given to all patients to prevent infection. An x-ray examination of the chest and an electrocardiogram are usually made after the first 24 hours following surgery. Dressings should be checked frequently during the first 48 hours for evidence of any unusual bleeding. The patient is observed for cyanosis, and if he should complain of numbness, tingling, or pain in the extremities or if there is any loss of motion, it should be reported. Observations for possible shock, hemorrhage, pneumothorax, pulmonary edema, and congestive heart failure must be made. Disorientation is common after heart surgery but should always be noted and reported.[6] The patient may have profuse sweating. The bed should be kept dry and the patient protected from drafts.

Ambulation. The type of surgery and the condition and progress of the patient will determine when he may become ambulatory. The process should be a gradual one and should proceed from sitting on the side of the bed once or twice a day to standing beside the bed, sitting in a chair for short periods, and finally walking. Walking may consists of only a few steps in the beginning. Most patients are dismissed to their homes in approximately 2 weeks. Close medical supervision and convalescence continue for several weeks.

• • •

In some large medical centers the surgical removal of a patient's diseased heart and its replacement with a normal heart (heart transplant) has been accomplished. However, such surgical procedures are limited at this time and are considered experimental.

Embolectomy

The surgical removal of an embolus from an artery or a vein is called *embolectomy.* Throughout this book stress is placed on the prevention of venous stasis and clot formation. Arterial embolism occurs most frequently in persons with heart disease or in persons who have recently experienced an acute coronary episode. An embolus may lodge in an artery and completely shut off blood flow to the part. If it lodges at the distal end of the aorta or in its branches to the extremities, death of the extremity will occur and amputation of the part will be necessary.

Postoperative nursing care. When embolectomy has been performed, the extremity must be protected from injury. No external heat or cold should be applied. Anticoagulant drugs are administered to prevent clot formation, and antibiotics are given to prevent infection. Vital signs are observed, as in all surgical procedures. (See Chapter 21 for a discussion of nursing care in amputation.)

REHABILITATION—SOCIAL, PSYCHOLOGIC, AND ECONOMIC FACTORS

The rehabilitation of the cardiac patient is closely related to his emotional response to his illness. One of the primary functions of rehabilitation is helping the patient develop a healthy mental attitude toward his disease and toward the future. To most patients a heart attack means "dropping dead" or a life of semi-invalidism. Nothing could be more wrongly conceived. The American Heart Association, Inc., has established criteria for classifying the patient according to his limitations.

Social and psychologic factors that affect a patient's return to normal living may include how he views his symptoms, how he regards his medical care, and what happens to him during recovery. Social status is closely related to these factors. A person of lower social and economic status may view his symptoms more seriously than will a person of higher social and economic status. A person with limited economic reserve may view his illness as a threat to his security and that of his family. He is likely to discuss his illness and work potential with his physician. The failure of the physician to discuss prognosis and help the patient make plans for work may create emotional anxiety and tensions that affect his progress toward recovery.[10]

Patients have reported that while in the coronary care unit their greatest source of assurance was the constant attendance of the nurse. When the patient was unable to see the nurse, his level of anxiety rose. The patient in the coronary care unit should have information about the monitor and alarms. He should understand that false alarms occur and what causes them. In medical centers where several physicians make rounds together the patient should understand that this is routine, or he may believe that his condition is worse. The fears and anxieties that arise in the coronary care unit are usually from lack of information and communication.[8, 41]

Children, like adults, respond to illness in different ways. Some are angered by the restrictions placed on them and strike back by sudden outbursts of temper. Some children hold their feelings in and appear depressed and refuse to eat or to talk. Parents may have overprotected the child and find it difficult after surgery to realize that the child should do things for himself. Older children may withdraw, feeling they are different from other children. Many children find it difficult to give up their privileged position and to begin to make independent decisions. Some children will understand the importance of trying to live a normal life to the extent that they are able. For many children nursing care will be a matter of keeping them interested and providing them with things to do. Visiting teachers and educational television are available in many places to assist the child. The wide range of do-it-yourself activities for all age groups may fill many hours of leisure time.

The population of the United States is increasing, and every year more people are reaching the age when heart disease manifests itself and when it takes its greatest toll. Rusk[34] has stated that heart disease is costing the country more than $4 million annually. The intangible results are deprivation of the family, physical and mental suffering, and loss to society when the in-dividual is unable to function as a social being. Research has provided guideposts to the prevention of some kinds of heart disease. Through adequate medical care and evaluation, followed by sound programs of rehabilitation, many persons can become contributing members of society.

Summary outline

1. Structure and function of cardiovascular system
   A. Heart consists of four chambers, right and left atria and right and left ventricles
      1. Lower part of heart is apex, upper part is base
      2. There are four valves—tricuspid, bicuspid, pulmonary, and aortic
      3. Heart muscle is called myocardium; inner serous membrane is endocardium
      4. Electrical conduction system is responsible for contraction of ventricles
         a. Sinoatrial (SA) node called the pacemaker
         b. Atrioventricular (AV) node
         c. Bundle of His arises from AV node
         d. Purkinje fibers extend from bundle into walls of ventricles
   B. Blood vessels consist of arteries, veins, and capillaries
   C. Function of cardiovascular system is to pump blood from heart to be carried to body tissues and to return it to heart, where it discharges carbon dioxide and receives new supply of oxygen
2. Lymph-vascular system
   Similar to the blood-vascular system without heart and arteries
   A. Lymph nodes are distributed along vessels and act as filters; they are more numerous in some areas than in others
3. Disorders of rate and rhythm
   A. Cardiac arrhythmias—occur in well persons and in those with heart disease
      1. Pulse may be abnormally rapid or slow
      2. Tachycardia—very rapid pulse
      3. Bradycardia—pulse rate of 60 or less
      4. Extrasystole or premature beat—heartbeat that occurs too soon
      5. Atrial fibrillation—heart rate greater than pulse rate
      6. Pulse deficit—difference between apical pulse rate and radial pulse rate
      7. Sinus tachycardia—most common disturbance of rhythm of heart
      8. Paroxysmal atrial tachycardia—heart beats rapidly two to three times normal rate; begins and ends suddenly
      9. Sinus bradycardia—heartbeat falls to 60 or below; normal in some persons; abnormal in digitalis toxicity or in patients with brain lesions
      10. Paroxysmal ventricular tachycardia—sudden onset of rapid ventricular beats, which may suddenly return to normal

11. Ventricular tachycardia—atrial rate normal, ventricular rate up to 200 beats per minute; indicates damaged myocardium and may lead to ventricular fibrillation
12. Ventricular fibrillation—rapid twitching of ventricles, causing decreased cardiac output, cardiogenic shock, and death
13. Heart block—caused by disturbance of electrical conduction system; may be partial or complete
    a. Adams-Stokes syndrome may accompany complete heart block and extremely serious
    b. Electronic heart or pacemaker is electrical device that stimulates ventricle to contract normally
4. Cardiopulmonary resuscitation
   Technique of maintaining vital functions until further care can be given
   A. Mouth-to-mouth resuscitation
   B. External cardiac massage
5. Coronary care unit (CCU)—cardiopulmonary unit
   A. Objective is to save life
   B. Continuous cardiac monitoring
   C. Need to reassure patient and relieve anxiety
6. Diagnostic tests and procedures
   A. Physical examination
      1. Inspection, percussion, palpation, auscultation, and blood pressure
   B. Laboratory examinations
      1. Complete blood count, sedimentation rate, blood cultures, and cholesterol
   C. Circulation time—determines speed with which blood flows
   D. Venous pressure—pressure of circulating blood against walls of veins
   E. Central venous pressure—to determine blood volume, ability of heart to pump blood, and capacity of blood vessels
   F. Electrocardiogram—graphic recording of electrical currents resulting from activity of heart
   G. X-ray examination and fluoroscopy—used to evaluate lungs and outline shape of heart
      1. Orthodiagram—tracing on paper of outline of heart
      2. Angiocardiogram—examination of heart by injecting iodine substance into vein and making x-ray films; selective angiography—medium injected in or near area to be studied
   H. Cardiac catheterization
      1. Measures pressures in heart chamber and pulmonary arteries
      2. Obtains blood samples to determine amounts of carbon dioxide and oxygen
7. Diseases of the cardiovascular system
   A. Heart disease leading cause of death
      1. Majority of these deaths due to coronary artery disease
   B. Risk factors
      1. Cigarette smoking

2. Hypertension
3. Increased serum cholesterol
4. Diabetes and gout
5. Obesity
6. Physical inactivity
7. Menopause
C. Congenital heart disease—caused by developmental errors during intrauterine life or at birth
   1. Disease may involve heart, its valves, or blood vessels
   2. Patients with some conditions may be helped by surgery
D. Arteriosclerosis and atherosclerosis (hardening of arteries) are pathologic conditions
   1. Atherosclerosis—formation of fatty deposits in inner lining of blood vessels (plaques)
   2. Arteriosclerosis—hardening of blood vessels from fibrous tissue formation
E. Hypertension and hypertensive heart disease
   1. Elevation of blood pressure above what is normal for individual
   2. Essential hypertension—without known cause; 80% to 90%
   3. Extensive program to locate persons with hypertension not under treatment or whose hypertension is not controlled
   4. Classification
      a. Early, mild, uncomplicated
      b. Moderate
      c. Severe
   5. Develops gradually over years
   6. Treatment and nursing care
      a. Newer concepts in treatment and control
      b. Diuretics to reduce volume of extracellular fluid and sodium
      c. Hypotensive agents with or without diuretics
      d. Adrenergic blocking agents act on autonomic nervous system
      e. Patient must modify his life style to delay serious effects of hypertension
   7. Malignant hypertension—occurs in younger persons and usually terminates fatally
F. Rheumatic fever and rheumatic heart disease
   1. Rheumatic fever—disease of children and young adults; usually begins as hemolytic streptococcus sore throat; joints may or may not be swollen and tender
      a. Toxins released by streptococcus organism thought to be cause
      b. Stenosis—narrowing of valve
   2. Treatment and nursing care—emphasis on prevention
      a. Treatment symptomatic
      b. Bed rest during acute phase, aspirin for pain, antibiotic therapy, support of painful joints, bed boards, footboard, bed cradle, mild heat, and warm baths

c. Diet high in calories and vitamins B and C
d. Fluid intake of 2500 to 3000 ml. in 24 hours
e. Child may be cared for at home, and assistance may be given by public health nurse
3. Complications
   a. Mitral stenosis requires surgery or mitral commissurotomy
   b. Aortic stenosis requires open heart surgery

G. Bacterial endocarditis—inflammation of lining of heart (endocardium)
   1. Causative organism usually viridans group of streptococci and may be found in bloodstream
   2. Often occurs in persons who have had rheumatic fever or may follow tonsillectomy and tooth extraction; may result from hospital-acquired infection
   3. Treatment and nursing care
      a. Prompt and intensive antibiotic therapy
      b. Bed rest, blood transfusions, high-calorie high-vitamin diet, care largely based on symptoms
   4. Prompt treatment will cure 90% of patients

H. Coronary artery and heart disease
   1. Two coronary arteries, right and left, supply myocardium with oxygen and nutrients
   2. Pathophysiology
      a. Primary cause is atherosclerosis
      b. Plaques in lumen of vessels obstruct flow of blood to myocardium
      c. When flow of blood and oxygen is cut off, part will die
      d. Most common diseases are angina pectoris and myocardial infarction
   3. Angina pectoris (anginal syndrome)
      a. Cause is decreased flow of blood to myocardium
      b. Predisposing factors—atherosclerosis, hypertension, diabetes mellitus, syphilis, and rheumatic fever
      c. Symptoms include sudden symptoms severe pain in substernal area radiating to left shoulder and inner left arm, ashen color, cold clammy perspiration; pulse rate remains normal with little or no change in blood pressure
      d. Precipitating factors are exposure to cold, emotional upset, heavy or irregular meals
      e. Treatment and nursing care involve whole individual and include protection from cold, avoidance of tea, coffee, tobacco, reduction in weight if obese, rest, relaxation, and relief of tension
      f. Drugs such as nitroglycerin (0.32 to 0.65 mg.) sublingually for relief of pain or prophylactically and iso-

sorbide dinitrate (Isordil), 5 mg., administered orally; pentaerythritol tetranitrate (Peritrate) or erythrityl tetranitrate (Cardilate)
   4. Myocardial infarction—occlusion of one of coronary arteries or its branches by clot or sclerotic condition
      a. Symptoms—severe pain in area of lower sternum and upper abdomen, elevation of temperature, nausea, vomiting, increased leukocyte count and sedimentation rate
         (1) Cardiogenic shock—symptoms include cold, clammy, moist skin, pallor, apathy, decreasing blood pressure, weak, thready, irregular, and rapid pulse, and shallow, increased respiration; about 10% of all patients die of this syndrome
      b. Electrocardiogram and chest x-ray film are done as soon as condition permits
      c. Laboratory tests used in diagnosis
         (1) Serum glutamic oxaloacetic transaminase (SGOT)
         (2) Lactic dehydrogenase (LDH)
         (3) Creatine phosphokinase (CPK)
      d. Treatment and nursing care
         (1) Relief of pain; meperidine may be ordered
         (2) Theophylline ethylenediamine (aminophylline) or papaverine hydrochloride to relax smooth muscle and dilate coronary vessels
         (3) Oxygen by tent, mask, or nasal catheter
         (4) Vital signs checked frequently
         (5) Anticoagulant therapy and daily test of prothrombin time
         (6) Care individualized—if possible place patient in coronary care unit
         (7) Surgery may be done for some patients
            (a) Endarterectomy — surgical removal of plaques
            (b) Coronary artery bypass

I. Aneurysm—distention of wall of artery from disease or injury
   1. Most frequent cause—syphilis or arteriosclerosis
   2. Types
      a. Fusiform—affects entire circumference of artery
      b. Saccular—affects only one side of artery
   3. Most aneurysms occur in arch of aorta, which may become pulsating tumor
   4. Symptoms are related to structures such as bones and nerves against which aneurysm may press
   5. Treatment and nursing care consists in decreasing work of heart, with some patients improved through surgery; nursing

care based on symptoms for those who are not suitable candidates for surgery
  J. Congestive heart failure—occurs when heart can no longer do its work and is caused by underlying heart disease
    1. Pathophysiology
      a. When heart fails to pump blood, all organs and tissues are affected
      b. Pulmonary vascular system becomes congested
      c. Pressure in left atrium and ventricle increases, and blood backs up in large veins
      d. Systemic venous system becomes engorged with blood
      e. Pressure in venous system rises, affecting other organs
      f. Diminished blood supply to kidneys reduces filtration rate
      g. Retention of water and sodium contributes to generalized edema
      h. Fluid is pushed out of capillaries and venules, and liver and other organs become congested
      i. Fluid escapes into abdominal cavity causing ascites
    2. May be mild or advanced
    3. Central venous pressure elevated
    4. Symptoms—shortness of breath, fatigue, cough, abdominal discomfort, edema of feet and ankles; dyspnea and cyanosis may occur and patient may complain of pain in chest; hemoptysis may occur
    5. Objectives of treatment
      a. Reduce oxygen requirements
      b. Decrease edema
      c. Increase cardiac output
    6. Treatment and nursing care
      a. Physical and mental rest to reduce oxygen requirements
      b. Drugs such as diuretics to reduce edema
      c. Digitalis to improve cardiac output—slows and increases force of heartbeat
    7. Sodium-restricted diet to prevent water retention and edema
    8. Nursing care—includes positioning patient for comfortable rest, prevention of decubitus ulcers, prevention of venous stasis, accurate record of intake and output, daily weighing, taking rectal temperature, lifting patient on and off bedpan or using bedside commode if permitted and observation for change in pulse rate, rhythm, or volume, color, dyspnea, increasing or diminishing edema, mental confusion or psychoses
  K. Heart disease complicated by pregnancy
    1. About 2% to 4% of pregnant women have heart disease
    2. Treatment designed to prevent congestive failure
    3. Activity dependent on severity of condition
    4. Observation during antepartum and

labor for increase in pulse rate, dyspnea, cyanosis, peripheral edema, or cough
  8. Diseases of veins and lymphatics
    A. Thrombophlebitis—inflammation of vein with clot formation
      1. Predisposing factors are age, obesity, prolonged abdominal or pelvic surgery, injury to extremities, dehydration, prolonged bed rest
      2. Preventive measures are active exercise postoperatively, adequate hydration, avoidance of pressure on popliteal space, and avoidance of tight abdominal dressings or binders and drugs that depress respiration
      3. Treatment depends on location of thrombus; continuous hot packs, may or may not be elevated or given anticoagulant drugs; surgical removal of clot may be done
    B. Varicose veins—greatly and permanently distended veins, usually in lower extremity
      1. Underlying causes—congenital weakness in vein or defect in placement of valves in vein
      2. Immediate causes—severe physical strain, pressure on pelvic veins due to pregnancy or tumor, obesity, and tight round garters
      3. Symptoms—pain, edema in feet and ankles, pigmented areas above ankles, eczema-like lesions, and ulcers
      4. Treatment and nursing care—bed rest, elastic stocking or elastic bandage, and surgical removal of vein
      5. Vein stripping and ligation is common surgery
        a. Indications for surgery include edema and pigmentation, which may lead to ulceration, and cosmetic reasons
        b. Preoperative care includes shaving entire extremity from groin and pubis downward and same care as that given other surgical patients
        c. Postoperative care
          (1) Check dressings over incisions for bleeding
          (2) Routine blood pressure, pulse, and respiration; observe foot for cyanosis and edema
          (3) Early ambulation—walking
          (4) Elevation of foot of bed first 24 to 48 hours
          (5) Elastic bandages should not be removed without physician's order
          (6) Elastic stockings may be worn several weeks after surgery
    C. Lymphangitis is disease of peripheral lymphatic vessels
      1. Caused by invasion by bacteria
      2. Symptoms—red streak along route of affected vessel, elevation of temperature, chills, and possibly tender and swollen lymph node

9. Operative conditions of cardiovascular system
   A. Cardiac surgery—requires highly trained professional persons who work closely as team
      1. Surgery may be done to correct congenital or acquired conditions and may be open heart or closed heart surgery
      2. Preoperative care
         a. Physical examination, including laboratory tests and special tests and examinations
         b. Planned conference by physician with patients
         c. Blood pressure, apical-radial pulse taken every 4 hours, and patient weighed daily
         d. Diet may be sodium restricted; drugs as ordered by physician
         e. Patient should be ambulatory to maintain strength and muscle tone
         f. Learn child's likes, dislikes, and habits and establish friendly relationship
         g. Preparation of patient for postoperative nursing procedures
      3. Operative day
         a. Venous cutdown and infusion started by physician
         b. Mild sedation—narcotics seldom given
         c. Secure all equipment needed for postoperative care
      4. Postoperative treatment and nursing care; first 48 hours are most critical; patient may be placed in intensive care unit or cardiac care unit; continuous cardiac monitoring
         a. Vital signs checked and recorded every 15 minutes for 8 to 24 hours
         b. Central venous pressure monitored frequently
         c. Assisted ventilation for several hours, and oxygen continued for several days
         d. Closed drainage system with one or two chest catheters
         e. Levin tube connected to suction
         f. Patient placed in flat or semi-Fowler's position and may be turned from side to side, back to side, or kept flat and not turned; depending on type of surgery, passive exercises begun as soon as possible
         g. Urinary output should be from 15 to 30 ml. every hour; urine is checked hourly for specific gravity
         h. Patient will have considerable pain for 48 hours; oversedation must be avoided
         i. Intravenous fluids for a few days
         j. Fluids may be given by mouth when nausea and vomiting have ceased, and other foods given as tolerated depending on condition; diet may be restricted for several days until flatus is passed
         k. Secretions must be coughed up, or endotracheal suctioning must be done
         l. Antibiotics are administered routinely to prevent infection
         m. Dressings should be checked frequently for bleeding
         n. Observe for cyanosis, numbness, tingling, pain, loss of motion of extremities, and disorientation
         o. Ambulation is gradual process
   B. Heart transplants still in experimental stage
   C. Embolectomy—surgical removal of embolus from artery or vein
      1. Preoperative preparation same as for other surgical patients
      2. Postoperative care
         a. Protect extremity from injury and avoid extremes of heat and cold
         b. Anticoagulant drugs with daily test of prothrombin time
         c. Antibiotics
10. Rehabilitation—social and economic factors
    A. Healthy mental attitude must be developed
    B. Social and psychologic factors affect return to normal living
       1. How he views his symptoms
       2. How he regards his medical care
       3. What happens to him during recovery
    C. Social status closely related to psychologic factors
    D. Patients in cardiac care unit report greatest feeling of assurance is constant attendance of nurse
       1. Patient needs to be informed about monitor and false alarms
    E. Children respond to illness in different ways
       1. May devote part of day to schoolwork; visiting teacher and educational television may be available to child at home
       2. Do-it-yourself activities for all ages
    F. More people reaching age when heart disease takes greatest toll
    G. Cost to country annually $4 million
    H. Intangible results—deprivation of family, physical and mental suffering, social isolation
    I. Medical care, evaluation, and rehabilitation helps many persons

Review questions

1. What is the term for very rapid beating of the heart?
   a. *Tachycardia*
2. What is the term for an electrically operated device that causes the ventricles to contract?
   a. *pacemaker*
3. What is the average normal cholesterol per 100 ml. of serum?
   a. *150-260*
4. List five factors that may increase the risk of heart disease.
   a. *obesity*

b. *smoking*
c. *diabetes*
d. *gout*
e. *physical inactivity*

5. What is another name for hardening of the arteries?
   a. *arteriosclerosis*
6. If a patient has had heart surgery, why should intravenous fluids drip slowly?
   a. *to prevent overloading the heart.*
7. What are three objectives in the treatment of congestive heart failure?
   a. *relief of pain — reduction of edema*
   b. *rest*
   c. *slowing heartrate*
8. What three things should the nurse avoid in the prevention of thrombophlebitis?
   a. *no ... pree ele . on bed.*
   b. *tight binders*
   c.
9. What one thing provides the greatest feeling of assurance for the patient in the coronary care unit?
   a. *seeing a nurse*
10. Define the following cardiac arrhythmias:
    a. Sinus tachycardia
    b. Atrial fibrillation
    c. Heart block
    d. Extrasystole
11. What are the two primary techniques involved in cardiopulmonary resuscitation?
    a. *breathing (mouth to mouth)*
    b. *compression*

Films

1. Angina pectoris—W.S.U. (58 min., sound, color, 16 mm.), Audiovisual Utilization Center, Wayne State University, Detroit, Mich. 48202. Describes etiologic factors, variations in the clinical picture, and problems of diagnosis, treatment, and prognosis. Patients presented to demonstrate points covered.
2. An introduction to nursing in a coronary care unit—M-1461 (26 min., sound, color, 16 mm.), Media Resources Branch, National Audiovisual Center (Annex), Station K, Atlanta, Ga., 30324. Shows specially designed coronary care unit and electronic monitoring devices.
3. Blood pressure readings—M-1582 (18 min., sound, color, 16 mm.), Media Resources Branch, National Medical Audiovisual Center (Annex), Station K, Atlanta, Ga. 30324. Presents a variety of clinical blood pressure measurements. Each scene shows a column of mercury descending on a sphygmomanometer scale with accompanying stethoscopic sounds. Viewers record their observations during the pause between segments.
4. Congenital anomalies of the heart (48 min., sound, color, 16 mm.), Squibb, 909 Third Ave., New York, N. Y., 10022, or your local Squibb distributor. Describes nearly all congenital anomalies of the heart.
5. Coronary occlusion—W.S.U. (35 min., sound, color, 16 mm.), Audiovisual Utilization Center, Wayne State University, Detroit, Mich. 48202. Describes diagnosis, differential diagnosis, and discussion of treatment. Problems of bed rest, resumption of activity, and prognosis are discussed.
6. Cardiac conditioning after myocardial infarction—M-1625 (18 min., sound, black and white, 16 mm.), Media Resources Branch, National Medical Audiovisual Center (Annex), Station K, Atlanta, Ga. 30324. Demonstrates physical conditioning for patients having had a myocardial infarction.
7. The nurse in emergency cardiopulmonary resuscitation (15 min., sound, color, 16 mm.), Chicago Heart Association, 22 West Madison St., Chicago, Ill. 60612. Pictures a hospital patient in acute cardiopulmonary distress. Illustrates nurse's functions and the team approach. Related materials can be obtained.

References

1. Aagaard, George: Treatment of hypertension, American Journal of Nursing 73:621-623, April, 1973.
2. Andreoli, Kathleen G.: The cardiac monitor, American Journal of Nursing 69:1238-1243, June, 1969.
3. Anthony, Catherine P., and Kolthoff, Norma J.: Textbook of anatomy and physiology, ed. 9, St. Louis, 1975, The C. V. Mosby Co.
4. Betson, Carol, and Ude, Linda: Central venous pressure, American Journal of Nursing 69:1466-1468, July, 1969.
5. Braum, Harold A., Diellert, Gerald A., and Wills, Vera S.: Coronary care unit nursing, Missoula, Mont., 1969, Mountain View Publishers.
6. Brunner, Lillian S., and Suddarth, Doris S.: Textbook of medical-surgical nursing, ed. 3, Philadelphia, 1975, J. B. Lippincott Co.
7. Butler, Herbert H.: How to read an ECG, RN 36:36-45, Jan., 1973.
8. Cassem, N. H., Hackett, Thomas P., Bascom, Caroline, and Wishnie, Howard A.: Reactions of coronary patients to the CCU nurse, American Journal of Nursing 70:319-325, Feb., 1970.
9. Cortes, Tara S.: Pacemakers today, Nursing 74 4:22-27, Feb., 1974.
10. Croog, Sidney H., and Levine, Sol: Social status and subjective perceptions of 250 men after myocardial infarction, Public Health Reports 84:989-997, Nov., 1969.
11. Dauber, Thomas R., and Thomas, H. Emerson, Jr.: Risk factors in coronary heart disease, Cardiovascular Nursing 6:29-33, Jan.-Feb., 1970.
12. Davis, Morris E., and Rubin, Reva: DeLee's obstetrics for nurses, ed. 18, Philadelphia, 1966, W. B. Saunders Co.
13. Deal, Jacquelyn: CPR and the ABC's, Part 1, Bedside Nurse 4:17-21, Feb., 1971.
14. Deal, Jacquelyn: CPR and the ABC's, Part 2, Bedside Nurse 4:11-17, March, 1971.
15. Dionne, Phillippe: Varicose veins of the

lower limbs, The Canadian Nurse 63:39-42, Feb., 1967.

16. Fernandez, Virginia, Reppert, Patricia A., and Reppert, Edmond H.: Contrast visualization of the cardiovascular system, Cardiovascular Nursing 1:5-9, Spring, 1965.

17. Fogg, Marguerite F.: The maternity patient with heart disease, Cardiovascular Nursing 2:27-30, Summer, 1966.

18. Griep, Arthur H., and DePaul, Sister: Angina pectoris, American Journal of Nursing 65:72-75, June, 1965.

19. Grossman, Burton J.: Rheumatic fever: declining but still dreaded, The Journal of Practical Nursing 24:23+, Feb., 1974.

20. Guyton, Arthur C.: Textbook of medical physiology, ed. 4, Philadelphia, 1971, W. B. Saunders Co.

21. Heart facts 1973, New York, 1972, American Heart Association, Inc.

22. Hunn, Virginia K.: Cardiac pacemakers, American Journal of Nursing 69:749-754, April, 1969.

23. Hutchinson, Sally: Some psychological aspects of CCU nursing, RN 36:1+, June, 1973.

24. Hypertension-high blood pressure, National Institute of Health Publication no. 1714, Washington, D. C., 1969, Government Printing Office.

25. Long, Madeleine L., Scheuhing, Mary Ann, and Christian, Judith L.: Cardiopulmonary bypass, American Journal of Nursing 74:860-867, May, 1974.

26. Marchiondo, Kathleen: CVP, the whys and hows of central venous pressure monitoring, Nursing 74 4:21-24, Jan., 1974.

27. Neufeld, Henry N.: Precursors of coronary arteriosclerosis in the pediatric and young adult age group, Modern Concepts of Cardiovascular Disease 6:93-97, July, 1974.

28. Paul, Oglesby: A survey of the epidemiology of hypertension 1964-1975, Modern Concepts of Cardiovascular Disease 7:99-102, July, 1974.

29. Phibbs, Brendan: The human heart, ed. 3, St. Louis, 1975, The C. V. Mosby Co.

30. Pinneo, Rose: Essentials of cardiac monitoring, The Journal of Practical Nursing 23:26-29, Nov., 1973.

31. Pinneo, Rose: Nursing in a coronary care unit, Cardiovascular Nursing 3:1-4, Jan.-Feb., 1967.

32. Review of modern medicine—hypertension and the cardiovascular system, New York, 1972, New York Times Media Co., Inc.

33. Rodrique, Murielle: Nursing care in varicose vein surgery, The Canadian Nurse 63:43-44, Feb., 1967.

34. Rusk, Howard A.: Rehabilitation medicine, ed. 3, St. Louis, 1971, The C. V. Mosby Co.

35. Shafer, Kathleen N., Sawyer, Janet R., McCluskey, Audrey M., Beck, Edna L., and Phipps, Wilma J.: Medical-surgical nursing, ed. 6, St. Louis, 1975, The C. V. Mosby Co.

36. Shepro, David, Belamarich, Frank, and Levy, Charles: Human anatomy and physiology, New York, 1974, Holt, Rinehart & Winston, Inc.

37. Smalser, Lloyd C.: Preparation for coronary care nursing, The Journal of Practical Nursing 24:22+, Jan., 1974.

38. Smith, Anysley M., Theirer, Judith A., and Huang, Shelia H.: Serum enzymes in myocardial infarction, American Journal of Nursing 73:277-279, Feb., 1973.

39. Smith, Barbara C.: Congestive heart failure, American Journal of Nursing 69:278-282, 1969.

40. Smith, Dorothy W., Germain, Carol P. Hanley, and Gips, Claudia D.: Care of the adult patient, ed. 3, Philadelphia, 1971, J. B. Lippincott Co.

41. Sobel, David E.: Personalization on the coronary care unit, American Journal of Nursing 69:1439-1442, July, 1969.

42. The health consequences of smoking, 1969 Supplement Public Health Service Publication no. 1696-2, Washington, D. C., 1969, Government Printing Office.

Nursing the patient with diseases and disorders of the gastrointestinal system

KEY WORDS

anabolism *construction*
anastomosis
appendicitis
biliary
cardiospasm
catabolism *destruction*
cholangiography
cholecystectomy
cholecystography
cirrhosis
colectomy
colostomy
decomposition
dysphagia
esophagoscopy
gastrectomy
gastroscopy
hemorrhoids
hiatus hernia
hepatic coma
hepatitis
herniorrhaphy
hydrolysis
hyperalimentation
ileostomy
ileus
intussusception
laparotomy
pancreatitis
peptic ulcer
peristalsis
protoscopy
pyloric spasm
sigmoidoscopy
stoma
stomatitis

STRUCTURE AND FUNCTION OF THE GASTROINTESTINAL SYSTEM

The gastrointestinal (GI) system, or alimentary tract, is also called the digestive system because its function is the digestion and absorption of food. The system begins in the mouth and terminates at the anus. The mouth is also called the *buccal*, or oral, *cavity*. Three sets of salivary glands pour their secretions through ducts that open into the mouth. The teeth and tongue are considered accessory organs of digestion. The esophagus, which is about 10 inches long, leads from the mouth to the stomach. In its desecent it passes through the thoracic cavity back of the trachea and the heart. A sphincter muscle, the cardiac sphincter, guards the opening between the esophagus and the stomach. The muscle relaxes to permit the passage of food or fluids, after which it contracts to prevent backward flow. The stomach is a pouchlike structure located in the upper part of the abdominal cavity under the liver and the diaphragm. It is divided into three parts: the fundus, the part nearest the esophagus, the middle section, or body, and the pylorus, which is the lower part. Located between the stomach and the small intestine is the pyloric sphincter, which relaxes to permit passage from the stomach into the small intestine and contracts to prevent the contents of the intestine from returning to the stomach. Spasms of the cardiac and the pyloric sphincter sometimes occur and are considered functional disorders (p. 323).

The small intestine, about 20 feet long,

consists of three sections but has no break in its continuity. The section nearest the stomach is the duodenum, the middle section is the jejunum, and the lower section is known as the ileum. Most of the digestion and absorption of food takes place in the small intestine.

The large intestine is only about 6 feet long but is much larger in diameter than the small intestine. It is also divided into three sections. The cecum, which begins where the large intestine joins the small intestine, is only a few inches long. The ileocecal valve guards the passageway between the ileum and the large intestine. The vermiform appendix, located at the end of the cecum, is a small, wormlike tube. The colon from the cecum ascends upward on the right side of the abdomen, then crosses over the abdomen below the stomach and continues downward on the left side. Thus the colon has been separated into the *ascending, transverse,* and *descending* colon. As the colon descends, the final portion is shaped like an S and is called the *sigmoid colon.* The sigmoid then joins the rectum, which is about 7 or 8 inches long. The final inch makes up the anal canal. The opening from the anal canal to the exterior is guarded by two sets of muscles, the internal sphincter and the external sphincter. The final opening to the exterior is the anus. Peristalsis is the involuntary contraction of the muscles that line the alimentary canal to propel the food content along.

The accessory organs assist the process of digestion by contributing specific secretions and enzymes essential for normal digestion and utilization of nutrients: the liver, gallbladder, and pancreas. The liver, located on the right side of the body under the diaphragm, is the largest of the organs. It has many functions and is considered one of the most vital organs of the body. The gallbladder is shaped like a pear and lies under the liver. It stores and concentrates bile and releases it into the duodenum during the process of digestion. The pancreas is a slender organ, fishlike in shape, which is located at the back of the stomach with a portion extending into a C-shaped curve of the duodenum. Located within the pancreas are the cells called *islands of Langerhans* that secrete insulin.[2]

Since much of the care of the patient depends on the specific parts of the gastrointestinal system affected, the nurse is encouraged to review in greater detail the structure and function of the system.

PROCESS OF DIGESTION AND ABSORPTION

Digestion is the process by which food is prepared so that it may be absorbed and utilized by the body. Absorption is the process in which nutrients pass into the circulation so that they may be carried to the body tissues. Digestion is accomplished by two processes: (1) mechanical digestion and (2) chemical digestion.

During mechanical digestion, which begins in the mouth, food is cut and ground into small pieces *(mastication)*. Its passage from the mouth to the stomach is facilitated by mucus from the salivary glands and the mucus-secreting glands along the esophagus that lubricates and aids in easy passage. Food entering the stomach from the esophagus passes through the *cardiosphincter* (valve). The muscle relaxes to allow food to enter the stomach, then contracts to prevent its backward flow. When the semiliquid contents of the stomach *(chyme)* enter the small intestine (duodenum), their passage is controlled by the *pyloric sphincter* (valve), which relaxes and contracts much the same as the cardiac sphincter. Food is moved along the entire route by wavelike muscular contractions *(peristalsis)*. Mechanical digestion may be best described as a cutting, grinding, and churning process. As this action goes on, numerous enzymes are being secreted that act on the various food constituents.

Chemical digestion is the action of enzymes on the proteins, carbohydrates, and fats by breaking them into simple compounds in preparation for absorption. *Ptyalin* is secreted in the mouth and acts on starches; however, the action is limited and largely destroyed by the hydrochloric acid in the stomach. Several enzymes are secreted in the stomach, including the hormone *secretin,* which stimulates the pancreas to secrete its enzymes. The breakdown of proteins begins in the stomach. Hydrochloric acid is secreted in the stomach, and the acidity must remain at about pH 2.0 for enzyme action. There is little action on fats in the stomach. The major part of chemical digestion occurs in the small intestine, where all of the food constituents undergo enzymatic action. An enzyme from the pancreas aids the digestion of fats. Bile produced in the liver and stored in the gallbladder is released into the duodenum and is required for the final action on fats. Vitamins, minerals, and water that are present require no enzyme action.

When chemical action is complete, through several processes, absorption begins. Carbohydrates and proteins enter the circulation through the portal system, whereas fats enter the lymph vessels and eventually reach the portal system near the thoracic duct. The large intestine (colon) has several functions before the cycle is complete. There are no enzymes in the large intestine. The residue from the small intestine passes through the *ileocecal valve*. After entering the colon, water and sodium are absorbed into the blood. Most of the other electrolytes are eliminated in the feces. Bacteria in the colon synthesize vitamin K and a few of the vitamin B group. The end products for which the body has no used are eliminated as feces.[28]

There are numerous factors that affect the process of digestion and absorption. An elderly person who has lost his teeth and has no dentures or has poorly fitting dentures will have a problem of mastication. Thus the process of cutting and grinding will be compromised. The patient who must remain in recumbent position may have difficulty in swallowing, since food does not pass down the esophagus as easily as in a sitting position. Emotions affect the secretion of enzymes or may cause severe and painful contractions of the sphincter muscles. Pathologic disease may affect any part of the system; some may be treated medically, whereas others may require surgery. The lack of specific nutrients or sufficient calories may result in malnutrition or starvation.

CAUSES OF DIGESTIVE DISEASES AND DISORDERS

Numerous diseases of the gastrointestinal system are pathologic, such as cancer. Many complaints are symptomatic of some underlying condition, such as abdominal

pain in appendicitis. Some gastrointestinal symptoms are characteristic of specific diseases; for example, nausea and vomiting are associated with many infectious diseases, or diarrhea may be a sign of food infection. Many complaints have no pathologic basis but result from some emotional problem, such as the child who resorts to vomiting because of an unpleasant school experience. These are called *psychosomatic* disorders.

Other conditions may be the result of traumatic injury or congenital malformation. In some conditions the body may be unable to utilize certain nutrients, as is the case in diabetes. When the islands of Langerhans in the pancreas fail to produce insulin, the body cannot utilize carbohydrates. Changes occur in the system that are normal results of the aging process. Frequently elderly persons do not understand these degenerative changes and believe they have some disease.

In spite of the multiplicity of digestive disorders, few symptoms are directly related to the digestive system. These symptoms are clinically defined as nausea, vomiting, constipation, diarrhea, loss of appetite, difficulty in swallowing, abdominal pain, blood in stools, and vomiting of blood (hematemesis); these symptoms may represent the total list attributable to digestive disease.

DIAGNOSTIC TESTS AND PROCEDURES

Several diagnostic tests and procedures are performed on the gastrointestinal system. Some are to aid the physician in establishing a diagnosis when symptoms of a disease are present. Tests may be done to rule out the existence of a specific disease, and some may be done as a preventive measure to discover a disease before symptoms occur, when treatment may be most advantageous. There may be some variation in procedures among physicians and hospitals, and the nurse should understand the physician's orders.

Gastric analysis. The test for gastric analysis is performed to determine the degree of acidity of the stomach contents. Cells of the stomach secrete hydrochloric acid, which aids digestion. Too much acid may be present in persons with conditions such as peptic ulcer, and in persons with diseases such as pernicious anemia or gastric malignancies the acid may be absent. The patient receives nothing by mouth after supper the evening before the test, and in the morning a tube is passed through the nostril into the stomach. A large syringe is attached to the tube, and the contents of the stomach are aspirated. Usually several specimens are secured at intervals according to the physician's direction. Each specimen must be carefully labeled with the time it was taken and its numerical order. A clamp is placed on the tube between specimens and the tube taped to the patient's face. The physician may wish to stimulate the flow of gastric secretions and will order the subcutaneous injection of histamine or betazole hydrochloride (Histalog). The gastric secretions are then aspirated at 15-minute intervals for 1 hour or longer. Since some patients are sensitive to histamine and may have a reaction, a tray with a syringe containing a 1:1000 solution of epinephrine should be ready for emergency use.

The procedure should be explained to the patient, and he should be assured that although it may be uncomfortable, it is not painful. An emesis basin should be given the patient in case he becomes nauseated during the procedure. The test may be performed in the physician's office or in an outpatient clinic. The procedure may be carried out by the nurse under the physician's direction, or it may be done by a laboratory technician.

Tubeless gastric analysis. The tubeless method of determining the presence of hydrochloric acid in the stomach is more comfortable for the patient because it does not require the passage of a tube. Although the method is not suitable if an exact analysis is needed, it is often satisfactory in many cases as a screening method. Preparation of the patient may be the responsibility of the technician or nurse. All food is withheld after midnight until the test is completed. In the morning the patient voids, and the specimen is discarded. The patient is then given 250 mg. of caffeine sodium benzoate. After 1 hour the patient voids, and the entire specimen is saved, labeled, and sent to the laboratory. The patient is then given one packet of an exchange resin, azure A or azuresin (Diagnex blue), with half a

glass of water; 2 hours later the patient voids, and the specimen is sent to the laboratory.[10]

Approximate normal values of gastric analysis tests are as follows:

Total acidity-fasting	10° to 50°/100 ml.
Histamine	After 1 hour, free acid 30° to 85°
Diagnex blue	In 2 hours, greater than 0.3 mg.

Esophagoscopy and gastroscopy. Esophagoscopy and gastroscopy are examinations that permit the physician to visualize the esophagus and portions of the stomach and to secure tissue for a biopsy when it is indicated. After the throat has been sprayed with a surface anesthetic a special lighted instrument (esophagoscope) is passed through the mouth, down the esophagus, and into the stomach. The procedure may be done as an emergency measure to remove a foreign body from the esophagus or the stomach. When the patient is a child, it may be necessary to administer a general anesthetic; otherwise the child must be securely restrained to prevent injury. Food and fluids are withheld for 6 hours prior to the examination. All dentures and glasses are removed, and the patient is allowed to void before beginning the procedure. Morphine or meperidine hydrochloride is usually given, and atropine sulfate may be given to decrease secretions. When the patient returns to his room, nothing should be given by mouth until the gag reflex returns. Patients who complain of sore throat may be given aspirin, and throat irrigations with warm saline solution may help to relieve the discomfort.

Proctoscopy and sigmoidoscopy. Proctoscopy and sigmoidoscopy are examinations that enable the physician to visualize the lower 10 inches of the gastrointetsinal system. (See Chapter 5.)

Gastrointestinal series and barium enema. The purpose of the gastrointestinal series and the barium enema is to detect any abnormal condition of the tract, any tumors, or other ulcerative lesions. The gastrointestinal series is an examination of the upper gastrointestinal tract. As the patient drinks a radiopaque substance such as barium, the physician observes its passage through the esophagus into the stomach with the fluoroscope. X-ray films are then taken over a period of several hours. (See Chapter 5.)

Stool examination. Stools may be examined for bacteria, parasites, blood, or for chemical analysis. The process of digestion changes blood that might be coming from the stomach or the intestine so that it will not be observed on inspection. Chemical examination is then necessary to detect obscure occult blood. In some instances the patient may be placed on a meat-free diet for 3 days prior to the test, whereas in other situations any random stool may be sent to the laboratory. Stools may also be examined for other substances that may indicate disorders of the biliary tract, pancreas, or some problem of digestion of food.

Stool specimens may be examined for various kinds of parasitic infections. (See Chapter 1.) The specimen is secured and kept in various ways, depending on the type of parasite sought. Most stool specimens must be taken to the laboratory as soon as they are secured and must be kept warm.

Liver function tests. The primary functions of the liver are to secrete bile, assist in the digestion of proteins and fats, assist in the regulation of blood glucose, and synthesize proteins that function in blood clotting and water balance in the body. Therefore a number of different tests are done to determine liver disorders and liver function. Most tests are made on blood serum and a few on urine and feces. Some laboratories may require that tests be made while the patient is in a fasting state. Because of variations in procedure, the nurse should understand the orders. The liver function tests that may be performed include the bilirubin, cephalin flocculation, thymol turbidity, and galactose tolerance tests.

Bilirubin test. The bilirubin test may be performed on blood, urine, or feces. Bilirubin, a pigment resulting from a breakdown of hemoglobin, is excreted with bile into the small intestine, where it is converted to urobilinogen. Some of the urobilinogen is excreted, and some is returned to the liver where it is reconverted into bilirubin. Normally, little appears in the blood, but when obstructions of the liver ducts occur, bilirubin is picked up by the

blood, resulting in jaundice. Thus in jaundice there will be an increase of bilirubin in the blood.

Cephalin flocculation test. The cephalin flocculation test, performed on blood serum, is useful in determining damage to the liver cells. It may be used to follow the course of cirrhosis of the liver.

Thymol turbidity test. The thymol turbidity test is performed on blood serum. When liver cells have been damaged by hepatitis, the test is positive. Patients may be required to be in a fasting state for the test.

Bromsulphalein test. The bromsulphalein test is used to determine the ability of the liver to remove a dye. After injection of the dye a blood sample is taken from the opposite arm in 30 minutes and again in 1 hour. In the presence of liver disease the dye remains in the blood. Warnings have been issued against the use of this test because of serious and fatal reactions. For this reason the test has limited use.[10]

Galactose tolerance test. Galactose, a sugar, is converted to glycogen by the liver. When liver cells are damaged, this function of the liver is impaired. The test is frequently done when jaundice is present and also when diabetes is suspected. The patient is required to be in a fasting state. The test may be oral or intravenous. If the oral test is done, the patient is given galactose in water to drink, and urine specimens are collected each hour for 5 hours. In the intravenous test a solution of galactose is injected into a vein, after which one or more blood samples are collected.

Several other tests may be performed, including the *icterus index* and *serum cholesterol* tests discussed in Chapter 13. The *serum glutamic oxaloacetic transaminase* (SGOT), *serum glutamic pyruvic transaminase* (SGPT), and *lactic dehydrogenase* (LDH) tests are used in several diseases, including liver disease. The *alkaline phosphatase level* is elevated in obstructive disorders of the biliary tract.[24]

Approximate normal values of liver function tests are as follows:

Bilirubin	Direct, 0.1 to 0.4 mg./ 100 ml. serum
	Indirect, 0.2 to 0.7 mg./ 100 ml. serum
Cephalin flocculation	0 to 1 in 24 hours

little used (handwritten margin note)

Thymol turbidity	Less than 0 to 5 units
Bromsulphalein	Less than 5% after 1 hour
Galactose tolerance	Not more than 3.0 grams after 5 hours
SGOT	5 to 40 units/ml.
SGPT	5 to 35 units/ml.
Alkaline phosphatase	1.5 to 4 Bodansky units/ 100 ml. (several methods, with some variation according to method used)

Liver biopsy. The procedure of liver biopsy is used to assist in establishing diagnosis in various diseases affecting the liver. Several other examinations precede the biopsy, including tests of bleeding time, prothrombin level, and venous pressure. (See Chapter 12.) A biopsy needle is inserted through a small incision in the skin, and a small cylinder of liver tissue is removed. After the procedure the patient must be carefully observed for signs of hemorrhage and should also be positioned on the right side for several hours.

Liver scanning. Radioactive isotopes are administered to the patient and are readily picked up by the liver. Radiation from the isotopes is recorded by a scanning device. The procedure helps to differentiate normally functioning areas of the liver from nonfunctioning areas.

Cholecystography and cholangiography. Through the use of a radiopaque dye it is possible to visualize the gallbladder and the extrahepatic biliary system. This enables the physician to determine the size, shape, and position of the organ and to observe the presence of certain kinds of calculi (stones) in the gallbladder. After a low-fat evening meal the patient is given one of the synthetic radiopaque drugs, iopanoic acid (Telepaque), iodoalphionic acid (Priodax), or iodipamide methylglucamine (Chlografin methylglucamine), by the oral route. The dye is removed from the bloodstream by the liver and is excreted into the bile. Only black coffee, tea, or water is allowed in the morning. An enema is given to clear the intestinal tract of feces and gas. After x-ray films a high-fat diet is given, and additional x-ray films are taken. A normally functioning gallbladder will contain bile and the radiopaque dye and shows up as a dense shadow on the x-ray film. Absence of opaque material in the gallbladder indicates a nonfunctioning organ. The fatty meal stimulates the gallbladder to contract, expelling the dye and bile into the bile ducts. X-ray examination at this point enables visualization of the biliary system. The nurse should be sure that the examination has been completed before permitting the patient to have food. The patient should be observed for any toxic symptoms from the radiopaque drug.

Gastric lavage. Gastric lavage refers to the washing out of the stomach. The purpose may be to remove poisonous ingested substances or any other irritating substance, to relieve nausea and vomiting, or in some cases to prevent nausea and vomiting. A stomach tube and approximately 4000 ml. of a solution, which may be tap water, physiologic saline, 5% solution of sodium bicarbonate, or in case of poison the specific antidote, is used. Not more than 500 ml. of solution should be instilled into the stomach at one time. It is then siphoned back and the procedure repeated. In case of poison the siphoned solution may have to be saved for laboratory analysis.

Gastric gavage. Gastric gavage is used to provide nourishment for patients who are unable to eat from loss of appetite, unconsciousness, excessive weakness or debilitation, or obstruction of the esophagus. Patients with depression psychosis, premature infants, or infants with plastic repair of the mouth may be fed in this manner. The tube is introduced into the stomach in the same manner as a Levin tube.

Gastrointestinal decompression. Decompression of the gastrointestinal tract may be employed for several different reasons. It may be employed to remove air and fluids from the stomach. A nasogastric tube is generally used for this purpose. The tube is lubricated with a water-soluble jelly and passed through the nostril down the esophagus to the stomach. The tube is taped to the cheek to avoid pressure against the nostril and is connected to an electric suction machine such as the Thermotic drainage pump (Fig. 14-1). Gastric suction is frequently used to prevent postoperative distention and to relieve postoperative vomiting. When used for these purposes, the tube may be inserted before the patient goes to surgery. When surgery on the stomach is performed, the surgeon may insert

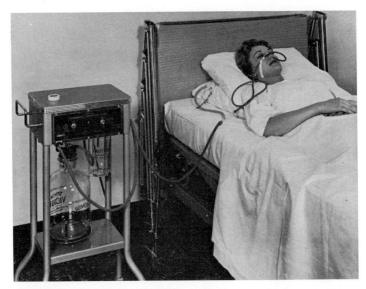

Fig. 14-1. The nasogastric tube is attached to suction, using the Thermotic drainage pump. (Courtesy Gomco Surgical Manufacturing Corp., Buffalo, N. Y.)

the tube after completing the surgery. The tube then protects the suture line from pressure postoperatively. The length of time that the tube remains in the stomach is determined by the physician; it may be approximately 48 hours or until peristalsis returns.

Intestinal decompression may be necessary when some obstruction along the intestinal route is suspected, or it may be used in case of paralytic ileus. Any of several types of tubes may be used for this purpose, including the Harris tube, Miller-Abbott tube, or Cantor tube (Fig. 14-2). These tubes are long, soft rubber tubes with a balloon at or near the end and eyes through which secretions may be drained. The Miller-Abbott tube has two lumens; one opens into the balloon into which mercury is placed, the other lumen is attached to suction. The tube is inserted through the nostril and is advanced along the intestine by peristaltic action or by the weight of the mercury. Secretions along the route are removed by gentle suction. The tube usually remains in the intestinal tract for several days, and when it is removed it is done gradually.

All decompression tubes are generally attached to some type of suction apparatus, and it is important that the equipment used be in working order. The tubing for gastric

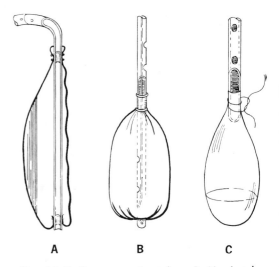

Fig. 14-2. Decompression tubes. **A,** Harris tube. **B,** Miller-Abbott tube. **C,** Cantor tube.

suction should be pinned or clipped to the sheet, allowing sufficient slack to permit the patient to turn without displacement of the tube. Care should be taken to prevent the tubing from becoming kinked or obstructed by the patient lying on it. Patients usually complain of considerable discomfort from the nasogastric tube. The nostrils become dry and crusted from increased mucous secretions. The throat is irritated, and the mouth and lips are dry. The patient is often receiving nothing by mouth but should be allowed to rinse the mouth frequently. Equal parts of glycerine and lemon juice may be applied to the mucous membrane of the mouth with an applicator. This preparation will form a protective coating that helps to prevent drying. Cold cream or petroleum jelly may be applied to the lips. The nares about the tube should be cleansed with applicators and warm tap water or a water-soluble jelly. Some physicians may allow the patient to have occasional chipped ice, sips of water, or hard fruit candy to relieve throat discomfort. Chewing of gum results in some swallowing of air, therefore some physicians disapprove of it.

Drainage tubes may become blocked with blood clots or mucus, which will obstruct the flow. The physician often orders irrigation of the tube with sterile physiologic saline solution every 2 hours or as necessary to keep it open and draining. Not more than 30 ml. of solution should be gently injected through the tube. Careful aspiration of the solution may be necessary to ensure patency of the tube, but any vigorous effort to aspirate the tube should be avoided. If the suction apparatus is working properly and the tube is open, the solution will return. Accurate records of irrigation solution used must be maintained, and the amount must be deducted from the total gastric drainage. The secretions in the drainage bottle are measured approximately every 8 to 24 hours and recorded. The appearance, odor, and presence of blood, bile, or mucus should be noted. If the nurse observes that the suction apparatus is not working properly, it should be reported immediately to the physician.

When intestinal decompression tubes are

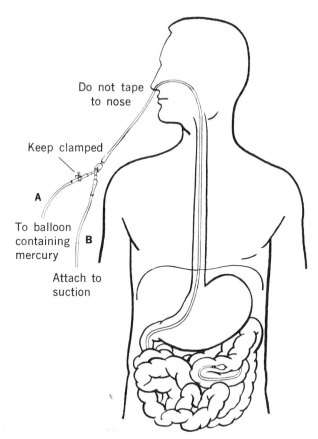

Fig. 14-3. Intestinal decompression tube in place. Note that the tube is not taped to the nose. **A,** Arm of Y tube leading to balloon containing mercury or air must be kept clamped. **B,** Arm of Y tube is attached to rubber tubing leading to suction.

used, they should not be taped to the nose because they are designed to move through the intestine by gravity and peristaltic action. Caution must be used in irrigating these tubes to be sure that the solution is injected into the opening that is attached to suction. The other opening is to the balloon containing air or mercury and is clamped off. To avoid error both outlets should be labeled. Measurement and observation of drainage are the same as that done with the gastric tube (Fig. 14-3).

Hyperalimentation. Hyperalimentation is the technique of administering large amounts of simple, basic nutrients by intravenous infusion. Although it is not a specific treatment for patients with gastrointestinal diseases, many patients suffering from these disorders may be possible candidates. Patients selected for this procedure are usually in an emaciated nutritional state and need basic foodstuffs readily available for tissue use. Generally protein hydrolysate in a concentrated dextrose and water solution is administered. It is a highly concentrated mixture and therefore must be given in a large vein such as the superior vena cava. The flow rate must be extremely slow and constant or complications will occur. Usually fractional urine measurements are done to watch for glucose appearance in the urine. Nausea and headache are often early signs of too rapid administration. Later symptoms may include severe dehydration and convulsions.[17]

NURSING THE PATIENT WITH DISEASES AND DISORDERS OF THE GASTROINTESTINAL SYSTEM
Abdominal surgery

The abdomen is opened for several surgical procedures, and the incision into the abdomen is called a *laparotomy.* Surgical procedures within the abdominal cavity may include surgery of the stomach, the small intestine, the large intestine, and the accessory organs of digestion. The upper part of the uterus, fallopian tubes, and ovaries are within the abdominal cavity. However, the abdomen may be opened for the surgical removal of all of the pelvic organs, or they may be removed by a vaginal hysterectomy (p. 376). Surgery may also involve certain other structures within the abdominal cavity such as lymph

nodes and blood vessels, or it may provide for drainage of blood or pus. An exploratory laparotomy may be performed when it is not possible to make an accurate diagnosis prior to surgery. Since the nursing care of the patient may involve procedures related to the particular type of surgery, the nurse should become familiar with the following terms and their meanings:

abdominoperineal resection Removal of the rectum and a portion of the colon, leaving a permanent colostomy.
appendectomy Removal of the appendix.
cholecystectomy Removal of the gallbladder.
colectomy Partial or complete removal of the colon.
gastrectomy Removal of all or part of the stomach.
gastrostomy A surgical opening into the stomach.
herniorrhaphy Surgical repair of a hernia.
hysterectomy Removal of the uterus.
oophorectomy Removal of the ovaries.
salpingectomy Surgical removal of the fallopian tubes.
splenectomy Surgical removal of the spleen.

Preoperative nursing care. The preoperative nursing care of the patient who is to undergo abdominal surgery is essentially the same for all the abdominal surgical procedures just defined (Fig. 14-4). The basic

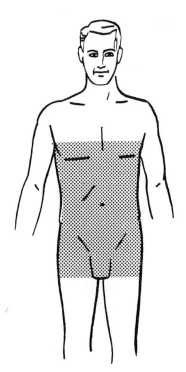

Fig. 14-4. Area of skin to be prepared for abdominal surgery.

postoperative care is also the same, with slight variations in specific nursing procedures. (See Chapter 9). The patient is usually admitted to the hospital 2 or 3 days prior to surgery, and during this time the nurse should try to get to know the patient and his family. The nurse should learn how the patient feels about the surgery and what he fears so that problems that may be encountered during the postoperative period may be identified. The nurse should seek to encourage the patient, relieve his anxiety, and reassure him that efforts will be made to meet his individual needs.

Nursing responsibilities for tests and procedures

When the physician writes the order for examinations and tests, the forms should be properly completed and the laboratory or x-ray departments should be notified without delay. Specimens to be collected by the nurse should be secured promptly, labeled properly, and sent to the laboratory. Proper identification of the patient's room or bed when food or fluids are to be withheld is a nursing responsibility. The patient should be readied and transported to the x-ray department or laboratory at the scheduled hour. If for any reason an appointment cannot be kept at the specified time, the department should be notified as early as possible. Medications ordered prior to and in preparation for tests and studies should be administered promptly and recorded. Any patient receiving intravenous dye should be carefully observed for reactions.

Most patients are completely unfamiliar with the various procedures and tests and will be nervous and apprehensive. They may be anxious and worried over what the examination will reveal. The nurse should be able to explain in simple words some of the things that the patient may expect. Through careful, thorough, and prompt preparation of the patient the nurse will be indicating an interest in his welfare and giving support and encouragement.

Observation

Earlier in this chapter reference was made to the limited number of symptoms characteristic of diseases and disorders of the digestive system. Similar symptoms may

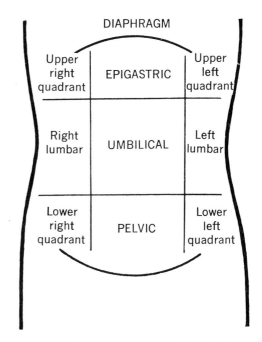

Fig. 14-5. Anatomic regions of the abdomen.

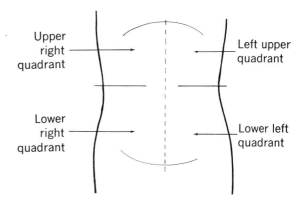

Fig. 14-6. Quadrants of the abdomen.

occur in several different diseases, and the nurse can assist the physician by making careful observation of the patient's complaints and reporting and recording them.

The nurse should be familiar with the correct anatomic location of abdominal pain so that it may be properly identified and reported as to location (Figs. 14-5 and 14-6). The pain should be described as throbbing, aching, stabbing, dull, intermittent, or constant. The abdomen should also be observed for distention.

Nausea and vomiting may be the result of organic disease or may occur from emotional disturbances. Nausea and vomiting frequently occur after the administration of a general anesthetic. The patient may complain of nausea but without any emesis. If vomiting occurs, the amount, character, relation to food or fluid intake, presence of bright red blood, and presence of fecal matter, which may be detected by appearance and odor, should be recorded and reported.

Stools should be observed for frequency, color, presence of mucus, bright red blood, coffee-ground appearance (indicating old blood), odor, and macroscopic parasites (worms).

Other observations that may be important to the physician include belching gas or expelling large amounts of flatus and the condition of the patient's appetite. The patient's mental state should also be observed with reference to depression, anxiety, apprehension, restlessness, or crying episodes. Vomiting, frequent liquid stools, excessive diaphoresis, and hemorrhage or oozing from wounds result in loss of electrolytes. Nursing procedures such as gastric suction siphonage and repeated enemas also cause loss of electrolytes. Since a serious imbalance of electrolytes may result, it is important for the nurse to observe patients carefully for any condition that may cause electrolyte loss and report it at once to the physician (p. 234).

Colostomy and ileostomy nursing care

Both colostomy and ileostomy provide an artificial anus through which fecal matter may be eliminated. A colostomy may be temporary or permanent, but an ileostomy is always permanent. Although both procedures are designed for the same purpose, the nursing care and the patient's problems are different. The basic nursing care of these patients is the same as that for any patient having abdominal surgery. The colostomy is usually performed on the left side of the colon (Fig. 14-7), and fluids and electrolytes have been absorbed, leaving a solid or semisolid fecal mass. The colostomy can be more easily managed because of the consistency of the stool and the absence of irritating chemicals and enzymes from the digestive juices. During the early postoperative period after a colostomy, considerable drainage may occur, which is increased after the return of peristalsis. If the

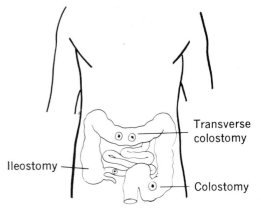

Fig. 14-7. The colostomy opening is usually on the left side of the abdomen, whereas the ileostomy is on the right side of the abdomen. A colostomy may be done on the transverse colon, with the proximal and distal ends of the colon brought out onto the abdomen.

colostomy is done on the transverse colon, the drainage is almost continuous and is in a semiliquid state.

A transverse colostomy is usually temporary and is performed to divert the feces from the affected portion of the bowel to allow healing. In a double-barreled colostomy the transverse colon is brought to the surface of the abdomen, and two openings (stomas) are present. One opening, generally the one on the patient's right, is the stoma through which stool will pass. The opening on the left will lead to the resting bowel. A similar procedure is the loop colostomy, in which the transverse colon is brought to the surface and a glass rod is inserted beneath the loop to prevent it from slipping back into the abdominal cavity. The bowel may not be opened to form the stomas for several days.[24] A permanent colostomy usually involves the sigmoid colon, and the proximal end is brought to the surface and sutured (Fig. 14-7).

The care of the patient is directed toward preventing contamination of the surgical wound and keeping the skin in a healthy state. Dressings that must be changed frequently are held in place with Montgomery straps, and dressings should be changed as necessary to keep the patient dry, clean, and free from offensive odors. The skin should be washed with mild soap and water after each dressing change. Various methods are used to protect the skin about the stoma, such as the application of petroleum gauze or a protective paste or ointment. Any protective preparation used should be ordered by the physician and must be removed at intervals to permit observation of the skin. The amount of drainage should be observed so that the colostomy does not become obstructed, since this might cause abdominal distention. After a few weeks it is often possible to regulate evacuation through the colostomy so that the fecal matter in the lower intestine, which is in a solid state, may remain so for varying periods of time. It may be necessary for the colostomy to be irrigated every day or two to stimulate the evacuation of the bowel. For some patients the regularity of emptying the bowel is such that only a small gauze dressing over the stoma is all that is required.

An ileostomy is an opening into the small intestine through which fecal material is eliminated (Fig. 14-7). The colon and rectum no longer function, and elimination occurs through an opening in the wall of the abdomen. Generally a loop of ileum is brought to the surface in the lower right quadrant and sutured to the skin. The procedure is usually permanent, and the colon and rectal tissue are removed (total proctocolectomy). Occasionally, the colon is re-

sected leaving a rectal stump (partial colectomy), and the ileum may be anastomosed to the rectum in a future operation. In this case the ileostomy is temporary, and there may be two openings (stomas) on the abdominal wall. Only one will excrete fecal material.

The contents of the small intestine are liquid and contain large quantities of digestive enzymes that are irritating and will cause excoriation and ulceration of the skin. The ileostomy drains freely and almost continuously day and night so that an appliance is necessary to collect the fluid. Regular bowel movements can never be achieved through the ileostomy. A temporary disposable ileostomy bag is applied at the time of surgery to prevent fecal drainage from coming in contact with the skin and the incision. The bag prevents ulceration of the skin and interference with wound healing. The temporary bag has an adhesive back, which is applied to the skin and will stay in place until it is pulled off or removed with a solvent such as ether or benzene. The bag will need to be changed frequently, depending on the particular type of bag used. The skin must be carefully cleansed and completely dried during the change, since moisture will result in failure of the appliance to adhere, allowing seepage onto the skin. The best

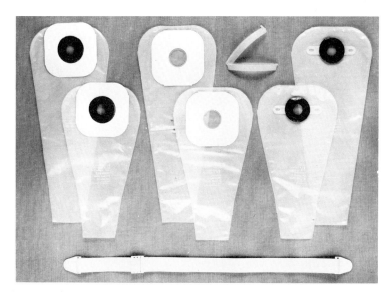

Fig. 14-8. Drainable stoma bags with karaya seal, adhesive or combination with clamp and belt. (Courtesy Hollister, Inc., Chicago, Ill.)

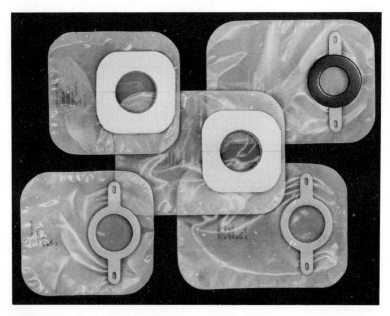

Fig. 14-9. Closed karaya seal adhesive and regular stoma bags for colostomies, abscesses, and draining fistulas. (Courtesy Hollister, Inc., Chicago, Ill.)

results will be obtained if the bag is changed several hours after the patient has eaten. Karaya gum powder or tincture of benzoin may be applied to protect the skin and promote healing if ulceration has occurred.

When the stoma has healed after approximately 6 weeks, a permanent appliance will be ordered for the patient (Figs. 14-8 and 14-9). They are made of plastic material and will last for a year or two. Disposable bags are available but normally are too expensive to use for a long period of time. The appliance is usually secured before the patient goes home so that he may be taught the steps in caring for the ileostomy and using the appliance. The patient's diet is restricted for several months. Fresh fruits and vegetables are avoided because of their tendency to cause diarrhea, and the diet is high in protein and low in residue. It may be months before the patient will be able to return to a normal diet. Gastrointestinal upsets are more serious for patients with an ileostomy. Fluid and electrolyte imbalances occur more readily, since the fluid reabsorption function of the colon no longer exists.

The necessity for good psychologic preparation for the patient cannot be over-emphasized. Usually the patient consents to the ileostomy so that he may once again become a contributing member of society. However, the creation of a new opening for the passage of fecal matter produces much emotional trauma. Preoperative preparation should begin in the physician's office and continue throughout the hospital stay. The nurse should explain the procedure, familiarize the patient with the equipment, and allow the patient to verbalize his feelings. Preoperative visits from other persons who have ileostomies can be extremely helpful. Volunteers from "ileostomy clubs" are usually available. Patients will need encouragement, instruction, reassurance, and praise when learning to care for the ileostomy. Dietary restrictions must be explained to the patient and family, and the patient must realize he will need continual medical supervision. Most of the patient's concerns will involve control of the odor and bowel excretions and the amount of time that must be devoted to care. Nursing personnel can assist the patient in planning schedules and referring the patient to helpful resources.[22]

The psychologic care of the patient with a colostomy or an ileostomy is more demanding than the physical care. No other type of surgery produces greater emotional trauma and requires greater understanding by all who care for the patient. The patient with a colostomy is usually of middle age or older, whereas the patient with an ileostomy is often a young adult or is in his teens with his whole life before him. The patient is often a frail, undernourished, debilitated person whose response to the shock may be so severe that he hopes to die. A colostomy may be only a palliative procedure to prolong the life of a patient with cancer.

In the weeks, months, or years ahead the patient must develop social confidence. This can be facilitated by careful teaching of the patient concerning care and control of his colostomy to avoid unpleasant incidents. During the early postoperative period the patient will be concerned and fearful about recurrence of the malignancy. An optimistic attitude and regular reexamination by his physician will do much to reassure the patient. If employed, the patient should return to his regular employment as soon as possible. If retraining is necessary, he should contact the Office of Social and Vocational Rehabilitation. Today a colostomy is no barrier to employment and social acceptance.

SPECIFIC DISEASES AND DISORDERS OF THE GASTROINTESTINAL SYSTEM
Inflammatory diseases
Stomatitis

Inflammation of the mouth results from several causes and may affect the entire mouth or only a small part of the mucous membrane. Among the causes of stomatitis are vitamin deficiency, infection by specific organisms such as fungi or bacteria, certain drugs, and some virus diseases. Symptoms may include a burning sensation, pain, formation of ulcers, presence of membrane as in diphtheria, tender bleeding gums, disagreeable odor to the breath, and sometimes fever. Treatment depends on identifying and treating the cause. Vincent's stomatitis, commonly called _trench mouth,_ often occurs in epidemics and is fairly common. The condition responds readily to penicillin and good mouth hygiene.

Thrush (moniliasis) is caused by a fungus organism, *Candida albicans*. The disease appears as small white patches on the mucous membrane of the mouth and tongue. The same organism is responsible for monilial vaginitis in the adult, and newborn infants may become infected as they pass through the birth canal. The infection may be spread in the nursery by carelessness of nursing personnel. Handwashing, care of feeding equipment, and cleanliness of the mother's nipples are important to prevent spread. There are several methods of treatment, including 1 to 4 ml. of nystatin (Mycostatin) dropped into the infant's mouth several times a day. Thrush may also occur in adults who are receiving broad-spectrum antibiotics, particularly chlortetracycline or tetracycline. Treatment for the adult is the same as for the infant.[7]

The possibility of transmission of some inflammatory diseases of the mouth has been questioned. However, when bacterial disease is known to exist, nurses should use every precaution to protect themselves and all patients, whether or not disease is present. Nursing care should consist of cleansing the mouth and teeth of any foreign material, rinsing the mouth, and lubricating the lips. The mouth should be inspected by using a flashlight and tongue blade. The frequency of oral care depends on the patient's condition, and whatever procedure is used should meet the needs of the patient and should be consistent and effective.[11, 24] The nurse should be alert in identifying patients who are in need of special mouth care and should encourage good oral hygiene in all patients.

Gastritis

Inflammation of the stomach is the most common stomach ailment and may result from substances that produce an irritation of the membrane. It may be caused by food infection, dietary indiscretion, excessive ingestion of alcohol, or excessive use of salicylates such as aspirin. If the condition is acute, fever, epigastric pain, nausea and vomiting, headache, coating of the tongue, and loss of appetite may occur. If the condition results from ingestion of contaminated food, the intestines are usually affected, and diarrhea may occur. Food is generally withheld as long as vomiting persists, and if vomiting is severe, intravenous infusions are administered. Drugs that relax smooth muscle, such as propantheline bromide (Pro-Banthine) and aropine derivatives, may be given. Chronic gastritis may indicate the presence of ulcers or malignancy, or it may accompany uremia and liver disease. The treatment consists of a bland diet, antacids, and avoidance of irritating foods and situations that might further the condition. The underlying cause must be treated.

Enteritis

Inflammation of the intestine accompanying gastritis is called *gastroenteritis.* Enteritis occurs in conjunction with some infectious diseases such as typhoid fever, dysentery, tuberculosis involving the intestines, and most cases of food infection. The severity of the condition depends on the virulence of the organism causing the condition. The primary symptoms are diarrhea and abdominal cramping. When the infection is from food, the symptoms occur within a few hours after the contaminated food has been eaten. Fever may or may not occur, but dehydration and weakness are usually present. Diarrhea is present in many types of infections and may be the forerunner of serious infections, especially in children.

Treatment is based on identifying the cause, which may be done by stool examination or cultures from suspected food. Precautions should always be taken until the cause of the diarrhea has been established. Patients with infectious enteritis should be isolated and medical asepsis carried out. Bed rest is indicated, and only liquids are given by mouth. When vomiting is present, oral fluids may be withheld, and the appropriate electrolyte solutions are administered parenterally to replace those lost through diarrhea and vomiting. Antibiotic or sulfonamide drugs may be ordered by the physician in treating some types of enteritis.

Ulcerative colitis

Ulcerative colitis involves the colon almost exclusively and is one of the most serious diseases of the gastrointestinal tract. Even though the disease has been reported since 1875, the specific cause is still unknown. There appears to be little evidence that the disease is caused by pathologic organisms. Possible causes include food allergies, emotional factors, and autoimmune reactions.[14] Many patients with ulcerative colitis are dependent people who are sensitive perfectionists and are easily frustrated.[24] Once the disease becomes established, it often becomes chronic. The disease may be acute, progressing rapidly to a fatal outcome, or it may remain low grade. No cure is known except by surgery. The disease usually attacks young adults and may be found in children and teen-age persons; it almost always occurs before 30 years of age. The disease is important because it may result in disability and dependence of the individual. The disease begins in the rectum and spreads upward in the colon, eventually involving the mucous membrane and all layers of the intestinal wall.

The symptoms begin rather insidiously, with increasing distress and frequency of stools until the individual may have as many as twenty to thirty stools a day. The presence of ulcers on the lining of the intestine results in blood loss and anemia and possibly in severe hemorrhage. The patient becomes debilitated, pale, weak, and thin, and electrolytes are constantly being depleted from the severe diarrhea. Because of the nutritional deficiency, symptoms of vitamin deficiency may occur. The diagnosis is made on the basis of the history and physical examination, including sigmoidoscopy, x-ray examination, and stool specimens. Some patients may be helped by medical treatment, and some may be cured by surgery.

Treatment and nursing care. Treatment includes complete bed rest. Bathroom privileges may be permitted in some cases. Rest must be both physical and emotional. Some physicians believe that psychotherapy should accompany medical treatment, since understanding the patient and his problems is a primary factor in his response to treatment. Sedation such as phenobarbital or a tranquilizer is given after meals and at bedtime, and a hypnotic such as pentobarbital sodium (Nembutal) or chloral hydrate may be ordered for sleep at night. Several drugs are designed to control diarrhea and abdominal discomfort, but unless dosage is large enough to produce side effects, they are ineffective. A hot-water bottle or electric heating pad to the abdomen and hot sitz baths may provide some relief. ACTH has given good results for some patients, but its effect may vary in the same patient at different times. Because of its side effects, it is seldom given unless other measures fail. The diet is high in proteins, calories, and vitamins.[7]

Patients with ulcerative colitis should have a quiet, pleasant environment and should be protected from chilling and secondary infection. Since diarrhea constitutes one of the major problems, bathroom facilities should be readily available; a bedside commode or, if the patient is not ambulatory, a padded bedpan should be within reach of the patient. After defecation the anal area should be carefully cleansed and a soothing ointment applied. The frequency, amount, and character of stools should be observed and recorded. Care must be taken if enemas are given, since perforation of the bowel may easily occur. Room deodorizers should be available to eliminate unpleasant room odors, and plans should be made for airing the room daily. Patients with ulcerative colitis are usually debilitated and thus are predisposed to decubitus ulcers.

Preventive measures should be taken early by using any of the procedures reviewed in Chapter 6. The skin is dry, and superfatted soap should be used, followed by lanolin. Special mouth care must be given several times a day with the application of cold cream or petroleum jelly to the lips. Since the appetite is poor, the patient will need much encouragement to eat, and consideration should be given to the patient's food desires because he will often know which foods cause him the most discomfort. Food intake should be carefully noted, since diet is important in treating patients with ulcerative colitis. During the acute stage of the disease the patient may be receiving intravenous infusions and blood transfusions. Perforation of intestinal ulcers may occur, resulting in hemorrhage and peritonitis. Any drop in blood pressure and increase in pulse rate or abdominal pain should be reported. The patient is usually given some mild sedative drug to relieve nervous tension and an antispasmodic drug to decrease peristalsis.

The psychologic care of the patient with ulcerative colitis requires the sympathetic understanding of everyone concerned with his care. The patient is often insecure, sensitive, and apprehensive. A carefully prepared nursing care plan will contribute to the continuity of care, which is important in meeting the patient's needs for a feeling of security. Since the patient's behavior may be characterized by periods of depression and changes in mood, the nurse must be prepared to accept such changes and continue to provide intelligent, personalized nursing care.

Appendicitis

One of the most common causes of an acute abdominal condition in children and young adults is appendicitis. The risk of fatal complications is increased when treatment is delayed. Factors that have helped reduce deaths from appendicitis during past years include early recognition of the disease, improvement of surgical techniques and anesthesia, use of antibiotics, and intensive nursing care.[3]

Pathophysiology. The vermiform appendix is a small tube in the right lower quadrant of the abdomen. The lumen of the proximal end is shared with that of the cecum, whereas the distal end is closed. The walls of the appendix contain lymphoid cells, and although the appendix has been generally considered to have no specific function, it is now believed to share with other lymphoid tissues of the body in preventing infection. The appendix fills and empties regularly in the same way as the cecum. However, the lumen is tiny and is easily obstructed. If it becomes obstructed, the blood supply is disrupted, it becomes distended, and inflammation occurs. Pathogenic bacteria present in the intestinal tract, often *Escherichia coli* (p. 68), begin to multiply in the appendix, and infection develops with the formation of pus. If distention and infection are severe enough, the appendix may rupture, releasing its contents into the abdomen. If this occurs, the infectious material may be walled off and the infection localized with an appendiceal abscess. If it is not localized, the infectious material spreads to the abdominal cavity and generalized peritonitis occurs.

The three symptoms most characteristic of acute appendicitis are pain, fever, and nausea and vomiting. In adults the pain may be felt in the lower right quadrant of the abdomen, halfway between the umbilicus and the crest of the ilium *(McBurney's point)*. In children pain may be experienced near the umbilicus. Mild leukocytosis and loss of appetite may also be present.

Treatment and nursing care. The surgical removal of the appendix (appendectomy) is often performed as an emergency operation; occasionally it may be performed as an elective procedure, and in most patients having any abdominal surgery the appendix is routinely removed. When appendicitis is suspected, surgery is usually done as soon as the diagnosis has been completed to avoid rupture and complications. If the appendix has ruptured, treatment will vary among physicians. Over the decades there has never been agreement among physicians as to the best method of treatment. Some physicians prefer a conservative approach and large doses of antibiotics are administered, whereas other physicians believe that the abdomen should always be opened and the appendix removed.

In clean appendectomy (without rupture) recovery is usually rapid, requiring 5 to 7 days. The postoperative care is directed toward preventing wound infection and pulmonary complications. The patient is ambulatory on the first postoperative day. When drainage is necessary because of an abscess, dressings must be changed as necessary and carefully disposed of. Re-covery is slower, and the patient must be watched for complications such as hemorrhage, intestinal obstruction, and increased elevation of temperature and pulse, which may indicate the formation of a secondary abscess.

Diverticulum and diverticulosis

A diverticulum is a protrusion of mucosa through the muscles of the intestinal wall (Fig. 14-10). Diverticulosis is an inflammation of the diverticulum. The disorder may occur in the duodenum, small intestine, or large intestine. It is estimated that 5% to 10% of persons 40 years of age and older will develop diverticula of the large intestine. Diagnosis is made by sigmoidoscopy, fluoroscopy, and x-ray examination. Any examination that would cause overdistention of the sigmoid is usually avoided.

Pathophysiology. The cause of diverticulum is unknown. Factors believed to contribute to the condition are weakness of the intestinal wall, pressure within the lumen of the intestine, or overdistention of the intestine. Pressure from outside or the existence of congenital factors may be contributing causes. About 20% of the patients with diverticula will develop diverticulosis. The disorder may be acute, or it may have existed over an extended period of time. When inflammation and infection are present, the colon becomes spastic, and perforation resulting in peritonitis may occur. With or without infection severe bleeding may occur. The continued presence of

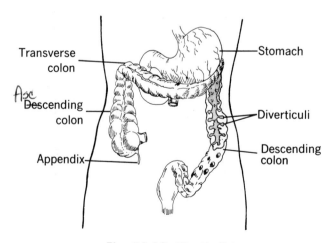

Fig. 14-10. Diverticuli.

diverticula in the intestine leads to scarring of the bowel, abscess formation, fistula, or intestinal obstruction.

Symptoms include a cramping type of pain in the lower left abdomen, diarrhea, or constipation. Blood may appear in the stools, flatulence, rectal pressure, and urinary urgency may be present.

Treatment and nursing care. Treatment is medical, and if conservative measures fail or if complications occur, surgery may be performed. A high-residue, low-roughage diet may be ordered. Antispasmodics such as propantheline bromide (Pro-Banthine), dicyclomine hydrochloride (Bentyl), or oxyphencyclimine (Daricon) may be ordered. They are administered orally before meals and at bedtime. Fecal softeners and wetting agents and retention enemas of warm oil are given if evacuation of the bowel fails to occur. Sedation in the form of phenobarbital and a tranquilizing agent such as diazepam (Valium) or chlordiazepoxide (Librium) are given to relieve tension and provide relaxation. If the symptoms are acute, the patient is hospitalized and placed on a regimen of bed rest. Intravenous fluids and electrolytes are administered, and antibiotics and analgesics may be required. Surgical intervention depends on the severity of the disorder; a colostomy, temporary or permanent, may be necessary. In some patients the involved part of the colon may be resected and the ends of the bowel anastomosed to each other.

The nurse should assist the patient in planning nutritional requirements consistent with the dietary plan. Stools should be observed for any evidence of bleeding. The patient should be encouraged to remain under medical supervision. When surgery has been done, the care of the patient is the same as that for other kinds of abdominal surgery discussed in this chapter.[26]

Intestinal obstruction

An obstruction of the small or large intestine may occur when any condition exists that prevents the free passage of bowel contents through the intestine. The obstruction may be partial or complete and is always regarded as serious. The relief of intestinal obstruction is ultimately a surgical procedure; however, the cause of the obstruction, its location, and the condition of the patient will be considered by the physician.

Pathophysiology. Intestinal obstruction has many causes, some of which include strangulated hernia, twisting of the bowel (volvulus), cancer, postoperative adhesions, paralytic ileus, and stricture. The most common causes are from postoperative adhesions and hernia. Obstruction may occur in the small or the large intestine. In the large intestine it is less dramatic than when it occurs in the small intestine. When an obstruction cuts off the blood supply, as in a strangulated hernia, the part will die and gangrene will develop. Most obstructions occur in the small intestine and affect the normal homeostasis of the body. The continuous vomiting causes loss of electrolytes and loss of hydrochloric acid from the stomach, leading to alkalosis. The loss of water and sodium from the body may cause acidosis and severe dehydration.

The symptoms will vary according to the location and the extent of the obstruction. When the obstruction is high in the small intestine, symptoms appear earlier and are more acute than when the large intestine is obstructed. The early symptoms are abdominal pain, vomiting, and constipation. The pain is often wavelike in severity, and vomiting may be projectile in type. The gastric contents are first vomited, but as peristalsis is reversed, bile and fecal matter from above the obstruction are vomited. When the obstruction is in the colon, vomiting may not occur. The patient may eliminate blood or pus from the bowel, but no fecal matter or flatus passes. Extreme thirst occurs, and the tongue and mucous membranes of the mouth and lips become parched. Abdominal distention occurs and is greater when the obstruction is in the colon. Signs of shock may appear, and without treatment the patient may die within a few hours.

Medical treatment and nursing care. An intestinal decompression tube such as the Miller-Abbott tube is inserted by the physician to remove gas and fluids from the stomach and intestine and to relieve the distention. Intravenous fluids are administered to correct the dehydration and replace the electrolytes lost through vomiting. All vomitus should be saved for the physician's inspection, and any fecal matter should be saved to be examined for occult blood. Temperature, pulse, and respiration rates are taken every 4 hours. The patient is placed in Fowler's position to prevent respiratory embarrassment, which might occur from the abdominal distention. Careful records of urinary output should be maintained, and if retention occurs, the patient should be catheterized. Often a retention catheter is inserted into the urinary bladder and connected to closed drainage. Measures designed for relief may include warm enemas or colonic irrigations and the application of heat to the abdomen. The patient should be assisted with frequent cleansing of the mouth and changing position. The environment should be kept well ventilated and free of odors by prompt care of vomitus and the use of a deodorizer if necessary.

Surgery. Surgery for intestinal obstruction depends partly on the cause of the obstruction, its location, and the condition of the patient. In some cases surgery may be relatively simple, whereas in other situations the cause may complicate the surgical procedure. In obstructions resulting from a strangulated hernia, the cutting off of the blood supply may have caused the bowel to become gangrenous, and resection of the affected bowel may be necessary. Preoperatively the patient is given a small enema under low pressure. Intravenous fluids are administered to replace electrolytes lost through vomiting and to provide nourishment. Postoperatively, if the bowel has been resected, oral feeding is withheld to give the anastomosis time to heal. A nasogastric tube attached to suction aids in keeping the stomach empty. Accurate intake and output records must be kept. Other postoperative care is the same as that for any abdominal surgery.

Peritonitis

Peritonitis is an inflammation of the peritoneum and the abdominal cavity and is often a complication of a bacterial infection. Infection may come from a perforated peptic ulcer or ruptured appendix. It may be caused by infection from the internal female organs. Although infrequent, it may occur from trauma to abdominal organs or be carried by infection in the bloodstream.

The inflammatory process may be localized, with abscess formation, or it may be generalized, with bacteria spreading throughout the entire abdominal cavity. Sometimes peritonitis occurs without any known cause.

Generalized peritonitis is an extremely serious condition characterized mainly by severe abdominal pain. The patient usually lies on his back with the knees flexed to relax the abdominal muscles, and any movement is painful. Nausea and vomiting occur. Constipation or diarrhea may occur early, but as the condition progresses, peristalsis ceases and constipation occurs with no passage of flatus. The abdomen becomes distended, tense, rigid, and very tender. The pulse is weak and rapid, and blood pressure falls. Leukocytosis and marked dehydration occur; the patient may collapse and die.

Treatment and nursing care. The patient is placed in semi-Fowler's position and is given meperidine hydrochloride or morphine sufficient to relieve pain. A nasogastric tube is inserted and connected to suction to keep the stomach empty. Intravenous fluids are administered to prevent dehydration and to maintain electrolyte balance, and appropriate antibiotic therapy is started. Further care or indications for surgery will depend on the cause of the peritonitis and the patient's condition. The patient receives nothing by mouth, and special mouth care is needed, including lubrication of the lips. All intake and output, including vomitus, must be accurately measured and recorded. The patient should be observed for pain and the type of pain and its location should be described, recorded, and reported. The patient often realizes the seriousness of his condition, and the nurse should reassure him and provide emotional support.

Tumors of the gastrointestinal system
Cancer of the mouth

Tumors of the lips, tongue, and mouth may be benign or malignant; cancer of the tongue is the most common type of tumor of the mouth. Although the cause of mouth cancer is unknown, it is believed that irritation resulting from smoking, consumption of alcohol, dental appliances, and rough, jagged teeth are predisposing factors. Malignant tumors of the mouth metastasize early to adjacent structures such as the lymph nodes in the neck and muscle tissue. Cancer of the mouth is often associated with leukoplakia, a condition characterized by the formation of white patches on the mucous membrane of the tongue or cheek. Cancer of the mouth is more common in men than in women and is responsible for 3% to 6% of deaths from cancer. Treatment is by x-ray and radium therapy or surgery. When the disease is discovered early, the prognosis is good.

Surgery of the mouth. Common surgical procedures of the mouth include operative treatment of carcinoma in or about the mouth. Malignant lesions may involve the lips, tongue, or mucous membrane lining the mouth, and surgery or radium or both may be used in the treatment. Any surgery of the mouth interferes with the normal functions of respiration, speech, and eating and will involve certain nursing problems. The mouth cannot be rendered completely free of pathogenic organisms but should be kept as clean as possible to prevent infection.

The preoperative care of the mouth for patients with malignant tumors requires meticulous attention. The teeth should be brushed before and after meals, and dental floss should be used to remove any particles between the teeth. Dentures and bridges should be cared for in the same manner. Warm mouthwashes or irrigations with an antiseptic solution may be ordered by the physician. If necrotic tissue is present, various preparations may be used to loosen the tissue and deodorize the mouth. A solution of 1 teaspoon of salt and 1 teaspoon of soda in 1 quart of warm water may be used for frequent mouthwashes. Also, 1.5% hydrogen peroxide may be used as a mouthwash with moderate pressure irrigation. All smoking and alcohol should be forbidden.[21] Depending on the site and the extent of the lesion, eating may be difficult. The diet should contain soft food and be free of acids and citrus foods, which may cause pain; frequent small feedings may be more desirable than large meals three times a day. The emotional factors involved in this kind of surgery require that the nurse have a sympathetic understanding of the patient's feelings. The patient may fear permanent disability or disfigurement and should be given as much information preoperatively as is desirable to help relieve his anxiety. If the malignancy involves the lymph nodes in the neck, a radical neck dissection may be done in an attempt to remove all affected tissue.

Postoperatively the patient's speech will be affected, and a pad and pencil should be at the bedside. The patient may have a tracheotomy or a tracheostomy, and nursing care will be the same as that outlined in Chapter 11. A nasogastric tube may be inserted through the nostril and connected to suction. The physician will order the position in which the patient should be placed. Depending on the suture line and the extent of surgery, suction of secretions and mucus may be gently done, or a wick of gauze may be placed in the mouth and allowed to drain into an emesis basin. The physician may order mouth irrigations done, using a prescribed solution and sterile equipment. Intravenous infusions may be given. If a radical neck dissection has been done, blood transfusions may be needed, and a large pressure dressing may be applied to help prevent edema and splint the part. Some physicians place a perforated catheter in the wound and attach it to a small portable suction apparatus (Hemovac). This removes secretions as soon as they accumulate and promotes healing. If this method is used, no dressings are applied and the area may be sprayed with a plastic material. The method of feeding will depend on the site and the extent of the surgery, and nasogastric tube feedings may be necessary in the beginning. When a portion of the tongue has been removed, a thread is often passed through the remaining portion of the tongue and fastened to the outside of the cheek with adhesive tape to keep it from obstructing the airway. The patient must be watched carefully for hemorrhage and respiratory difficulty, since edema may occur and obstruct the airway. A tracheostomy tray, a suction machine with a soft rubber catheter, and oxygen should always be available for emergency use.

Cancer of the mouth may be treated by external radiation or by implanting radium needles or radon seeds. (See Chapter 5.) When radium needles are used, they are attached to threads fastened to the outside of the cheek with adhesive tape, and the patient must be cautioned against any pulling on the threads. The threads must be checked and counted several times a day and recorded on the patient's chart. A pad and pencil or slate should be provided for the patient, since talking will be difficult. Mouth hygiene is important, and a spray may be ordered and used while the needles are in place. Any equipment used must be carefully inspected for radium that may have become dislodged. The physician will give directions concerning food and fluids. The patient should always be watched carefully for hemorrhage, edema, or choking.

Cancer of the esophagus

Malignant tumors of the esophagus occur in both men and women and account for a small number of cancer patients. The incidence in the nonwhite male is two times greater than in the white male, whereas the incidence in both nonwhite and white female is negligible. The only predisposing factor clearly established is the use of tobacco and alcohol.[5] The first symptoms that the patient may notice are difficulty in swallowing and hoarseness that becomes progressively worse. As the condition progresses, the individual is unable to swallow even liquids. Pain does not occur until the disease is well advanced, and since the swallowing difficulty is usually intermittent, in the beginning, the individual may delay medical care. The tumor metastasizes to the lymph nodes in the neck and chest and eventually to the liver and the bones. The patient becomes thinner and more malnourished as the disease progresses. The only hope for cure is early diagnosis and surgical removal of the lesion. The tumor may be removed and the esophagus anastomosed to the stomach (esophagogastrostomy), or a portion of the intestine may be anastomosed between the esophagus and the stomach after the tumor is removed. If the patient is not a candidate for major surgery, or if the tumor is inoperable, a gastrostomy may be performed.

Gastrostomy care. The patient with a gastrostomy has a permanent opening into the stomach through which a tube has been inserted for the purpose of feeding (Fig. 14-11). The stomach is sutured to the abdominal wall to prevent stomach contents

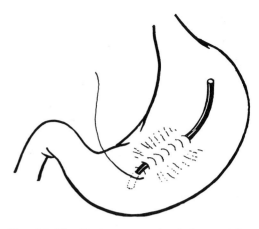

Fig. 14-11. Gastrostomy tube is inserted into the stomach and secured with sutures. The end of the tube or catheter is brought out through an opening in the abdomen so that feedings may be given.

from entering the abdominal cavity, and the catheter is secured into a small incision. The nurse should understand the physician's orders concerning the tube. If the tube inserted by the physician happens to come out, the physician should be notified immediately. Some physicians use the Barnes-Redo prosthesis, which is sutured into the gastrostomy opening. The appliance has a cap that may be removed for feeding and then replaced.[24] The nursing care of the patient includes care of the skin, maintaining patency of the tube, good oral care, and administering the prescribed feeding as ordered by the physician. Often there is a slight seepage of secretions about the tube, which will cause excoriation of the skin. Careful washing with mild soap and water, thorough drying, and the application of a bland ointment will usually keep the skin in a healthy condition. If the tube becomes blocked, it may be gently irrigated with a bulb syringe and warm tap water or physiologic saline solution. Force should not be used, and if the tube is not easily unplugged, the physician should be notified.[1] A second tube should be sterilized and available if a replacement is needed. When healing has occurred, the gastrostomy tube is removed and replaced only for feedings, and sterile technique is no longer needed.

The diet is prescribed by the physician,

and food should be warmed by placing it in a pan of warm water. The patient is placed in a semi-Fowler's position, and the feeding is allowed to flow by gravity. (Refer to a textbook on basic nursing.) The amount of food taken should be recorded so that the physician may determine if the amount of food that the patient is receiving provides sufficient calories. The preparation of gastrostomy feedings has been greatly simplified because of the commercial powdered feedings that are now available. These preparations contain all of the nutritional requirements of a normal diet. They liquefy easily in a blender and may be more acceptable to the patient.

The patient with a gastrostomy has an emotional adjustment to make that may be difficult for him. The realization that he will not be able to eat normally may be traumatic, and the patient will need a great deal of support and encouragement. The nurse can help the patient by providing privacy for the feeding, by preparing an attractive tray with the feeding in an opaque container such as an attractive pitcher or teapot, and by using a colorful tray cover. The patient is often allowed to chew some food but not swallow it, which stimulates the flow of the digestive juices and aids digestion. As the patient begins to accept this method of feeding, he should be encouraged to participate in administering the feeding and caring for the skin. It is usually important for a member of the family to be taught the preparation of the diet as well as the gastrostomy care and feeding of the patient. After the patient leaves the hospital the public health nurse may visit the patient in the home to supervise, instruct, and provide encouragement.

Cancer of the stomach

Cancer of the stomach is found primarily in men over 45 years of age and accounts for approximately 10% of all cancer deaths.[24] Cancer of the stomach occurs twice as often in the nonwhite male as in the white male, and the risk of the male having cancer of the stomach is 1.6 to 1 in the female. Although many deaths occur from cancer of the stomach, mortality from it has declined during the past few years.[5]

The early symptoms are so poorly defined that most individuals delay medical treatment until the malignancy is well established. Frequently symptoms related to the metastasis rather than the cancer prompt the patient to consult the physician. Symptoms include loss of appetite, a feeling of fullness after meals, epigastric distress, nausea and vomiting, weight loss, anemia, vomiting blood having a coffee-ground appearance, blood in the stools, which may have a dark, tarry appearance, and pain. Sometimes a palpable mass may be felt through the abdominal wall. The treatment is surgical, and early diagnosis is most important. The patient is admitted to the hospital, and a series of diagnostic tests are begun, including x-ray and fluoroscopic examination of the entire gastrointestinal tract. Cytologic examination using the Papanicolaou technique to determine the presence of cancer cells may be done. Emesis may be saved for examination, and stool specimens are examined for the presence of occult blood. When a palpable mass can be felt, the condition is often inoperable, and palliative treatment may be started. However, x-ray therapy has little benefit in gastric cancer. After completion of the examination the patient is prepared for surgery, and a gastrectomy is performed, the extent of which will depend on the surgeon's findings.

Cancer of the colon

Although cancer of the colon may occur in any part of the large intestine, approximately half the cases occur in the area of the sigmoid. Symptoms may partly depend on the portion of the colon involved. Obstruction is most likely to occur in the area of the sigmoid, since the fecal mass is more solid. Obstruction is least likely to occur if the tumor is on the right side or in the transverse colon, in which fecal contents are still fluid. One of the earliest signs is the alternating occurrence of constipation and diarrhea. There may be cramplike pains in the lower abdomen and abdominal distention. The individual may complain of weakness, loss of appetite, and loss of weight, and anemia may be present. Blood is frequently observed in the stools. Diagnosis is made on the basis of abdominal and rectal examination, which includes barium enema and a gastrointestinal series, proctoscopic and sigmoidoscopic examination, and examination of the stools for occult blood. A cystoscopy may be done. The treatment is always surgical and involves removal of part or all of the colon (colectomy) and the regional lymph nodes. Cancer of the colon may often be detected early through rectal examination, which should be included in all physical examinations. Any change in bowel habits from the normal pattern should always be viewed as suspicious.

Colon resection (colectomy). The partial or complete removal of the colon is usually done because of carcinoma of the colon, ulcerative colitis, and occasionally diverticulitis of the colon.

When a partial colectomy has been done, the affected area is removed and an end-to-end anastomosis of the bowel is done. In this way the normal continuity of the bowel is maintained. When the malignancy is in the sigmoid or the rectum, an abdominoperineal resection is done and the patient has a colostomy.

Preoperative preparation. Patients who are to have bowel surgery are usually admitted to the hospital several days before surgery to allow time for preparation. The patient is given a low-residue, high-caloric diet during this time. Sulfonamide agents and neomycin are administered orally to reduce the bacterial level in the colon. Enemas are given until the solution returns clear. The abdomen and perineal area is shaved, and a catheter is inserted for urinary drainage. An intestinal decompression tube is inserted to keep the stomach empty and prevent distention. The psychologic preparation of the patient is extremely important. If the physician anticipates that a colostomy will be necessary, the patient should be prepared for it. The patient needs to understand that he may expect to lead a normal life.[4]

Postoperative care includes the care of all tubes, such as a Miller-Abbott tube, a nasogastric tube, a urinary drainage catheter, or drains placed in the perineal wound. The character and appearance of all drainage must be observed and recorded. Considerable drainage may occur from the perineal wound for the first 24 hours, and dressings should be changed or reinforced frequently and observed closely for hemorrhage. Antibiotics are usually administered to prevent or control infection. The patient receives nothing by mouth, but intravenous fluids are given to maintain hydration and replace electrolytes. The perineal wound may have been packed, and the packing is removed gradually by the physician. When all packing has been removed, irrigation of the wound may be ordered once or twice a day. The physician should give specific directions regarding how the wound is to be irrigated and the solution to be used. Irrigation is a mechanical method of removing tissue and debris. Later the physician may order sitz baths.[13] When the patient returns from surgery, the colostomy will be clamped; depending on the type of procedure used, the physician will remove the clamp about the third day and may wish to do the first irrigation. The nurse should have the necessary supplies and equipment ready for the physician. Thereafter, routine care is given the colostomy. These patients usually require a longer time before ambulation is permitted, and the nursing procedures of encouraging deep breathing and coughing, turning the patient, and giving leg exercises are of special importance. The patient is usually very ill, and turning is difficult because of pain; the nurse should assist the patient and provide support with pillows (p. 304).

Cancer of the rectum

Malignant tumors of the rectum may be more easily diagnosed than those in other parts of the gastrointestinal tract, since symptoms appear earlier. Symptoms include constipation, often alternating with diarrhea, blood in the stools, and pain. The accessibility makes biopsy possible during a proctoscopic examination. The treatment is surgical, and an abdominoperineal operation is performed in which the rectum and anus are removed and the sigmoid colon is brought outside the abdomen and becomes a permanent colostomy (p. 304).

Benign tumors

Benign tumors may occur anywhere in the gastrointestinal tract and usually take the form of polyps, which occur most frequently in the stomach and the large intestine. Symptoms may resemble those of malignant growths, but surgical procedures are less radical. Diagnosis is made by proctoscopic examination and x-ray examination.

Peptic ulcer

It has been estimated that 14 million persons in the United States have peptic ulcer, with an estimated 10,000 deaths annually.[15] A peptic ulcer is an open lesion on the mucous membrane of the stomach or the intestine, where it is exposed to the acid present in the gastric juice. Peptic ulcers are most common in the duodenum (duodenal ulcers) just below the pylorus and in that location become chronic, whereas ulcers in the stomach (gastric ulcers) are more likely to produce acute symptoms.

Pathophysiology. The cause of peptic ulcer is unknown, but it is believed that hereditary predisposition may exist. Although pathologic disease elsewhere in the body or certain drugs such as steroids may be contributing factors, psychosomatic factors appear to play a major role by causing an increase in gastric secretions. The person with peptic ulcer has an increase of hydrochloric acid and pepsin in the stomach. When the flow of gastric secretions is stimulated by histamine (p. 297), about one half of the patients will demonstrate a marked increase in hydrochloric acid. Whether the increase in gastric secretion causes trauma to the mucosa depends partly on the normal protective substances in the stomach that neutralize the acid. The mucus-secreting cells may or may not secrete enough mucus to protect the mucosa, and if there is a deficiency, ulceration may occur. In the presence of increased hydrochloric acid and pepsin that has not been neutralized, an erosion may occur on the mucous membrane. The erosion may extend into the muscle layers and may even perforate, with subsequent peritonitis. If the ulcer erodes through into a blood vessel, bleeding or severe hemorrhage may result. In the case of hemorrhage, blood is vomited and large amounts may be lost. If slow bleeding is occurring, the blood generally passes through the intestinal tract, and stools are dark red and tarry in appearance.

Pain is the characteristic symptom and is described by the patient as dull, burning, gnawing, or boring; it is located in the right or left epigastric region. The pain occurs from 1 to 3 hours after eating and is relieved when food is eaten again. The pain is caused by the irritation of the ulcer by the gastric acid. Although pain is the typical symptom, many variations are found in its presence or absence, its character, and its duration. Nausea and vomiting may or may not be present and, when present, are often the result of obstruction. Many patients are anemic because of loss of blood but are usually well nourished because they eat to relieve the pain. Diagnosis is established through gastrointestinal series, gastroscopic examination, and examination of stool specimens for occult blood. Gastric washings may be done for cytologic examination to rule out cancer.

Medical treatment and nursing care. Treatment of the patient includes (1) rest and freedom from emotional tension, (2) proper diet, (3) drugs for sedation and relief of acidity and spasm, and (4) surgery. The nurse should become familiar with the purpose of the medical care plan and seek to understand the patient and his type of personality as well as the emotional factors that contribute to his condition. Although the patient may appear calm, inner tensions may cause him to be irritable and upset over the least irregularity or delay in his care. All treatments and examinations and the plan for care should be explained to him. Since the patient on a treatment regimen for peptic ulcer may need to follow it all his life, he will accept it more readily when he understands the reasons underlying the plan.

To ensure rest the environment should be controlled to prevent unnecessary noise and disturbance. The patient may be placed on a regimen of strict bed rest, but he may be allowed visitsors and should be permitted some diverisonal activity such as television to help keep his mind off himself. The nurse should be able to spend some time with the patient and in doing so may learn of problems that should be referred to the physician, the social worker, or the religious counselor.

The patient is given sedation, which may be in the form of tranquilizing drugs or mild barbiturates. If tablets are given, they must be crushed before they are administered. Since the drugs may make the patient drowsy, side rails should be placed on the bed for safety. The patient on a regimen of bed rest should be encouraged to breathe deeply and to turn from side to side frequently. Some physicians require patients to wear elastic bandages or elastic stockings while in bed to prevent thrombophlebitis. An antacid is ordered to neutralize the gastric acid. Several of these drugs are available, including aluminum hydroxide gel (Amphojel) and magnesium trisilicate. Antacids are usually administered every hour. Antispasmodic drugs are given to suppress gastric secretion and may include tincture of belladonna or atropine. Several synthetic drugs are also used including Banthine, Pro-Banthine, and Piptal. When belladonna or tropine is being given, the patient must be observed for toxic symptoms, which include dryness of the mouth and throat, thirst, difficulty in swallowing, flushed dry skin, rapid pulse and respiratory rates, dilation of pupils, and visual disturbance. Patients receiving antacids over a long period of time may develop alkalosis, characterized by loss of appetite, nausea and vomiting, weakness, headache, and visual disturbance.

During the acute stage of the symptoms the patient is given milk and cream hourly for 10 to 14 days. Depending on the patient's condition, the mixture may be given by continuous drip with the antacid added, or the feeding may be left at the bedside; if the patient is a responsible person, he may be permitted to administer the feeding and the antacid. The milk and cream may be given on the hour and the antacid on the half hour. Because of the possible association with the development of atherosclerosis, some physicians are prescribing skim milk or plain whole milk and eliminating the cream. As the patient improves and the pain subsides, he can receive a bland diet. Small feedings, attractively served, at frequent intervals are given. Foods that are chemically or mechanically irritating are avoided.[12] Constipation is frequently a problem, and care should be taken to prevent impaction. If impaction occurs, manual removal and small enemas may be necessary. No cathartics should be given unless ordered by the physician, since they increase peristaltic activity.

Complications. The major complications occurring in peptic ulcer include hemorrhage, perforation, and obstruction. When

a large hemorrhage occurs, measures are taken to control the bleeding and to restore the volume of circulating fluid. (See hypovolemic shock, p. 233.) The patient is transfused with whole blood or plasma, and intravenous fluids are administered to maintain urinary output and electrolyte balance. The patient may be given tranquilizing agents or barbiturates to relieve restlessness and apprehension. Any of several procedures may be used to help control the bleeding. Continuous gastric lavage using ice water or ice water and alcohol may be employed. A nasogastric tube may be inserted and milk and antacid allowed to drip into the stomach continuously. This prevents hunger contractions and keeps the gastric contents neutralized.

Gastric perforation occurs when an ulcer erodes through the wall of the stomach or the duodenum and the contents from the stomach are released into the peritoneal cavity. The result may be peritonitis (p. 312).

Another complication is obstruction of the pyloric sphincter, which is the result of scarring and fibrosis caused by the healing or breakdown of an ulcer. The muscle becomes spastic, edematous, and stenosed, gradually obstructing the passage from the stomach to the pylorus. Surgery is usually required to relieve the condition[4, 12] (p. 302).

Gastric resection (gastrectomy). Peptic ulcers that do not respond well to medical management and chronic peptic ulcers may be treated surgically by performing a gastric resection. A total or subtotal gastrectomy may be done, and several different types of surgical procedures may be used (Fig. 14-12). Usually the ulcer and a large amount of acid-secreting mucosa of the stomach are removed, and the remaining portion of the stomach is anastomosed to the small intestine (gastroenterostomy). A vagotomy may be done at the same time. This procedure includes resection of the vagus nerve, and stomach functions decrease as a result.

The patient who is about to have a gastrectomy has probably been ill for a long time and feels discouraged and worried, often fearing that the condition may be cancer. During this time an explanation of the various treatments and procedures and the

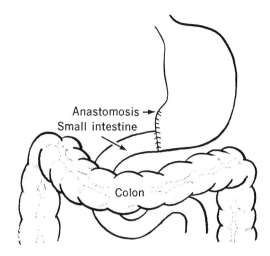

Anastomosis →
Small intestine

Colon

Fig. 14-12. Gastrectomy with a section of the stomach removed and the stomach anastomosed to the small intestine.

reasons for them will help to relieve his tension and apprehension. During the preoperative period the patient is encouraged not to smoke and is given an explanation of what to expect postoperatively.

Postoperatively the patient will have a nasogastric tube connected to suction siphonage and is given nothing by mouth for 24 to 48 hours. Drainage from the gastric tube should be watched carefully. Old blood with clots is expected at first, and some slight oozing from the suture line may occur, but any amount of bright red blood should be reported at once, since there is always the danger of hemorrhage. Dressings have to be watched also for any evidence of bleeding, which should be reported promptly if it occurs. The nurse should check the suction frequently to be sure it is working properly, since distention of the stomach will place strain on the suture line. Intravenous fluids are given to maintain fluid balance in the body. All intake, including fluids, output and gastric drainage must be measured and recorded. Mouth care and care of the nares about the tube must have frequent attention. When the tube is removed, the patient may be given small amounts of water, and diet may be resumed on the physician's order. Early feedings are small and are gradually increased as the patient can tolerate them. In approximately 1 week the patient will be receiving small meals and

should be observed for any feeling of fullness, nausea, or vomiting, which should be reported.

When a total gastrectomy is performed, the entire stomach is removed, and the small intestine (jejunum) is anastomosed to the esophagus. Patients having this procedure must be given injections of vitamin B_{12} for most of their life. The stomach mucosa secretes the intrinsic factor that is essential for the absorption of the vitamin from the intestinal tract. Without it no vitamin B_{12} will be absorbed. In addition, the patient must eat small frequent meals. A complication that occasionally occurs is the "dumping syndrome." After a meal the patient may complain of weakness, palpitations, diaphoresis, faintness, nausea, and a feeling of fullness in the epigastric area. These symptoms are thought to occur primarily as a result of food immediately entering the small intestine after eating.

On discharge from the hospital, the patient should be given instructions concerning diet and the importance of eliminating irritants such as coffee, alcohol, tobacco, and aspirin. Foods that contain many spices are usually advised against. The patient needs to follow a regimen that is relatively free from tension.

If the patient has a gastrostomy tube, the nurse must be careful when changing dressings to keep those around the tube separate from those around the wound. The tube must be handled carefully to avoid displacement (p. 314).

Hernia

A hernia, commonly referred to as a rupture, may be congenital or acquired; it is the projection of a loop of an organ, tissue, or structure through the abdominal wall. Most hernias have their origin in the abdomen (Fig. 14-13). The most common type of hernia is the umbilical hernia, which is frequently seen in infants as the result of a congenital weakness of the abdominal wall. A femoral hernia is more common in women, and an inguinal hernia is more common in men. Another type of hernia, *hiatus hernia*, is the projection of the stomach or the intestines through the diaphragm into the thoracic cavity. One of the most serious complications of hernia is the possibility that the intestine, which pro-

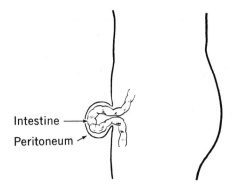

Fig. 14-13. A hernia in which the intestine pushes through a weakness in the abdominal wall.

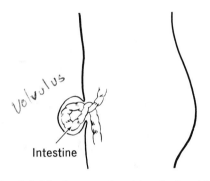

Fig. 14-14. A strangulated hernia in which the intestine becomes twisted, cutting off the blood supply and possibly resulting in gangrene.

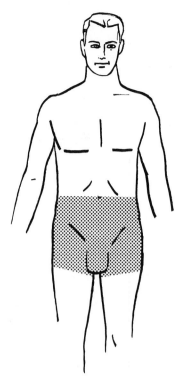

Fig. 14-15. Area of skin to be prepared for herniorrhaphy.

trudes through the abdominal wall, will become twisted (strangulated) (Fig. 14-14). If this occurs, the blood supply may be interfered with and gangrene may result, requiring immediate surgery. Some hernias may be pushed back into the abdominal cavity, but extremely large protrusions or those complicated by adhesions sometimes cannot be pushed back. These are said to be incarcerated hernias. In some cases incarcerated hernia may be reduced by elevating the foot of the bed and administering a narcotic to the patient to relieve pain. If the patient cannot reduce the hernia or if pain continues after reduction and the incarceration has existed for 6 hours, surgery is usually recommended.[7] The treatment of choice for all hernias is surgery; however, sometimes surgery is inadvisable because of the patient's poor condition or

some other reason. For such persons a mechanical appliance called a *truss* may provide some relief.

Surgery. The surgical procedure for repair of a hernia is called *herniorrhaphy* (Fig. 14-15). The preoperative care for the repair of a hernia is the same as that for any uncomplicated abdominal surgery. Postoperative care includes prevention of wound infection and avoidance of any strain on the wound for approximately 2 weeks. Early ambulation is encouraged to prevent abdominal distention. After repair of inguinal hernia, tenderness and swelling of the scrotum may be present. The use of a suspensory may provide some relief. The urinary output should be watched because retention sometimes occurs, and catheterization may be necessary. Food and fluids are usually permitted as soon as nausea ceases. If the operation is uncomplicated, progress is generally satisfactory, and the patient is dismissed in approximately a week but is not permitted to return to work for several weeks. Children and young adults are often ambulatory on the first postoperative day, and infants and young children are often sent home the first or second day, since they respond to recovery better in their home environment. If they remain in the hospital, they should be kept amused and prevented from crying, which might place strain on the sutures. Any evidence of abdominal distention or coughing after hernia repair should be reported to the physician immediately.[24] A few hospitals are attempting a type of outpatient, walk-in and walk-out surgery for simple hernia repairs and other types of uncomplicated surgery. The repair is completed in the morning, and the patient is resting at home in the evening.

Hiatus hernia

The hiatus hernia, hiatus meaning opening, is a common pathologic disorder of the upper gastrointestinal tract. It is most common in women 50 years of age or older. The disorder may be asymptomatic, or it may cause symptoms that are distressing to the patient. Diagnosis is made by esophagoscopy and barium and x-ray examination. Cytologic studies are usually made to eliminate a diagnosis of cancer.

Pathophysiology. Before entering the stomach, the esophagus passes through a small opening in the diaphragm. Under normal conditions the opening in the diaphragm encircles the esophagus securely. Thus the esophagus is held within the thoracic cavity, whereas the stomach remains in the abdominal cavity. For some reason, often congenital, the esophageal sphincter fails to remain tight, permitting the opening to become enlarged and relaxed. When this occurs, the upper portion of the stomach may protrude upward through the relaxed muscle into the thoracic cavity. Frequently this type of hernia may occur when the individual is in a prone position, and it will return to its normal position when the individual is in an upright position.

When symptomatic, a hiatus hernia may cause the person considerable distress. The primary symptom is heartburn caused by the gastric contents of the stomach being regurgitated into the esophagus. There may be substernal pain that may radiate, simulating angina pectoris. Vomiting and abdominal distention may occur.

suppresses gastric secretions

Treatment and nursing care. Treatment includes dietary measures with small meals consisting of bland foods. Antacids and anticholinergic agents may be given if symptoms are not relieved. The patient is advised not to smoke and to avoid wearing a tight girdle. Sleeping with several pillows at night may provide comfort. Straining for bowel elimination, coughing, and bending are discouraged. If the condition does not respond to conservative treatment, surgery may be performed. The surgical approach may be thoracic, and the patient will have a thoracotomy and chest drainage (p. 190). The surgery may be abdominal, and the nursing care is the same as that for other kinds of abdominal surgery.[12]

Hemorrhoids

Hemorrhoids (piles) are dilated veins similar to varicose veins. They may occur outside the anal sphincter as external hemorrhoids or inside the sphincter as internal hemorrhoids. The small bluish lumps characteristic of external hemorrhoids may disappear spontaneously, leaving a small skin tag. Occasionally, the hemorrhoid will become thrombosed, and a blood clot will develop within the vein. In addition to hemorrhoids, anal fissures (cracks in the mucous membrane) and anal fistula (duct extending from one tissue surface to another) may be present. Hemorrhoids result from numerous factors including (1) prolonged constipation, (2) heavy lifting, (3) straining in an effort to defecate, and (4) pregnancy or large pelvic tumors. Certain forms of liver disease and high blood pressure may also contribute to the disorder.

Symptoms may include an awareness of a mass in the rectum near the anus. Constipation is almost always present. Bleeding may occur and will appear as bright red blood that is not mixed with feces. The dilated veins may become thrombosed, causing severe pain. Since hemorrhoids may indicate disease further up the intestinal tract, a thorough examination of the colon is indicated, including sigmoidoscopy and barium enema with fluoroscopic and x-ray films. Hemorrhoids do not cure themselves, and medical or surgical care is necessary.[16]

The patient with rectal disorders has special problems in that "piles" have been a subject of jokes and laughter for decades.

Individuals have been reluctant to talk about the problem and even to seek medical care. When bleeding occurs, severe anemia may result unless medical care is obtained.

Treatment and nursing care. When the patient presents himself for examination, the nurse should be aware that this has been a difficult decision for him and should assure him of absolute privacy and protect his self-respect. Medical treatment of the patient with hemorrhoids consists of warm compresses to stimulate circulation and healing and analgesic ointments such as dibucaine (Nupercaine). Sitz baths help to reduce pain and edema, and mineral oil or stool softeners may be given to assist in the passage of fecal material. Steroid suppositories may be given to relieve inflammation. External hemorrhoids may be excised in the physician's office. Internal hemorrhoids occasionally are treated with an injection of a solution that will cause sclerosing or hardening of the dilated vein. This will cause the vein to shrink as it heals with fibrous tissue.[6] (See Fig. 14-16.)

Hemorrhoidectomy. If medical management fails to relieve the distressing symptoms, a hemorrhoidectomy is performed. Mineral oil and a laxative may be given preoperatively. Postoperatively, the patient is often positioned on his stomach, but he may lie on his back with a support under the buttocks. Although this surgery is not considered a major procedure, pain may be acute, and narcotics may be given and analgesic ointments applied. Sitz baths are given to relieve pain and promote healing.

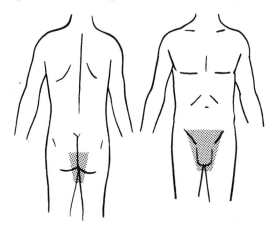

Fig. 14-16. Area of skin to be prepared for hemorrhoidectomy.

If a spontaneous bowel elimination does not occur within 3 days, an oil retention enema may be given followed by a cleansing enema. Dressings may or may not be used. Vital signs should be checked frequently for the first 24 hours to rule out internal bleeding, since hemorrhage is the most serious complication. Difficulty in voiding may occur, and the patient usually is allowed out of bed to urinate. Ambulation may be allowed on the night of the surgery or the next morning. A soft diet is permitted on the evening of the surgery day, and a full diet is given on the first postoperative day.

Functional disorders

Functional disorders are also called psychosomatic disorders and occur when no pathologic disease can be demonstrated. However, most functional conditions may also occur when there is pathology. Therefore they should not be considered lightly, but every effort should be made to determine the presence or absence of disease. The person whose complaints are psychosomatic may benefit from counseling and psychotherapy.

Indigestion

Indigestion may be the result of disease somewhere in the body, but as a functional disorder, it does not have a pathologic basis. Some hypersensitive persons who are tense and anxious may become aware of normal sensations present in the stomach, usually related to the digestive process. These individuals interpret such sensations as pain. They complain of pain in the upper abdomen, usually related to the eating of food. Such persons may describe the pain in a variety of ways and frequently attribute their discomfort to specific foods. Often these persons resort to the habitual use of sodium bicarbonate or some popularly advertised antacid, which may provide temporary relief. Treatment is based on examination to rule out the existence of disease and the encouragement of improved mental health.

Constipation

Constipation is the most common disorder of the gastrointestinal tract and is as old as the human race. Many people still believe that failure to have a daily bowel movement results in absorption of poisons, and they attribute several complaints to this "absorption of poison." There is no single cause for constipation; it may be the result of several factors, including nervous tension, faulty diet, inadequate fluid intake, lack of sufficient exercise, and inadequate toilet facilities. It must be kept in mind that constipation is a symptom of many organic diseases. During an acute illness constipation may occur because of reduced food intake and reduced intestinal motility. This type of constipation is usually relieved as soon as health returns. The patient in the hospital may repress the reflex of defecation because he does not want to ask for the bedpan or because he hates to use the bedpan. When there is delay in answering the patient's signal, the desire to defecate may also be repressed.

Constipation may occur during the latter part of pregnancy as a result of pressure on the lower bowel, or it may be a complication after delivery in the postpartum period. The patient may be able to relieve the disorder during the antepartum period by drinking more water, using fresh fruit and vegetables, and eating food containing roughage. Laxatives should be taken only on the physician's order.

Elderly people frequently suffer from constipation as a result of the slowing down of the digestive process and inadequate diet. Often they have a cabinet full of laxatives and fall prey to popular advertisements in an effort to have a daily bowel movement.

The treatment of constipation must be based on the type of constipation and the patient's individual needs, and the presence of possible organic disease must be ruled out. When mineral oil is administered for constipation, it should be given at bedtime to avoid interference with the absorption of the fat-soluble vitamins. Several laxatives, or stool softeners, are on the market under the trade names of Peri-Colace, Dialose, Sof-Cil, and Milkinol. Laxatives should be prescribed by the physician and should be discontinued as soon as possible.[27]

Cardiospasm and pylorospasm

Sphincter muscles are located between the esophagus and the stomach (cardiac valve) and between the stomach and its outlet into the duodenum (pyloric valve). Normally these muscles contract to prevent the backward flow of food material and gastric secretions and relax to allow food to enter the stomach from the esophagus and to permit the passage of food from the stomach into the duodenum. Under certain conditions these muscles fail to relax at the proper time and may contract vigorously. These severe contractions are called *spasms*. They give rise to symptoms of inability to swallow, regurgitation of food, epigastric pain, and vomiting. Spasms of the pyloric sphincter may be associated with peptic ulcer, but emotional factors are believed to be the primary cause of cardiospasm and pylorospasm. Treatment may include regulation of the diet, administration of antispasmodic and sedative drugs, and helping the individual to solve his emotional problems. If cardiospasm is severe, dilation of the constricted esophagus may be necessary.

Anal sphincter spasm

Sphincter muscles surrounding the anus and rectum relax to permit defecation. When the individual has severe hemorrhoids or fissures (cracks) in the anus or mucous membrane of the rectum, spasms of the sphincter muscles may occur. Difficult and painful defecation may then result. The treatment is correction of the cause or dilatation of the sphincter muscles.

Hyperacidity

Hyperacidity, commonly called *heartburn,* may occur as the result of a pylorospasm that contributes to reverse peristalsis. The gastric juice in the stomach is forced up through the cardiac valve into the esophagus, in which it gives the characteristic burning sensation.

Psychic vomiting

Psychic vomiting occurs in persons with emotional and psychologic problems. It may occur after every meal or infrequently, particularly when the individual is faced with a tense situation. Often the amount of food vomited is small and is regurgitated rather than vomited so that it does not interfere with the normal nutrition. However, if large quantities of food are regurgitated at frequent intervals, the individual may become malnourished. Psychologic vomiting is not uncommon in children and frequently occurs after breakfast. If the child expects to face an unpleasant situation at school, it may provide a means of escape.

Air swallowing

Air swallowing is a functional condition in which the person swallows air and then belches it up with a loud noise. Persons often master the technique so well that it is impossible to detect the individual swallowing the air.

Hyperemesis gravidarum (pernicious vomiting)

Nausea with or without vomiting during the first trimester of pregnancy (morning sickness) occurs in about 50% of pregnant women. It begins about the third or fourth week and lasts about 8 weeks. It is usually no more than a minor annoyance and is self-limiting. Nausea usually begins soon after the patient gets up in the morning and may be followed by vomiting, both of which are gone by the late morning. Occasionally it may continue until later in the day. The cause is not clearly known, but it is believed to be partly caused by normal physiologic changes that result from the pregnancy. Psychologic factors probably play some part in persons whose emotional patterns and adjustment may be somewhat unstable. Many remedies have been passed from mother to daughter or may have come from a helpful neighbor. Sometimes they help, and more often they offer limited relief. However, modern treatment is directed toward keeping the stomach from becoming completely empty by advising five or six small feedings a day. An antiemetic such as trimethobenzamide hydrochloride (Tigan), 250 mg. in the morning and at night, may be ordered by the physician.

Pernicious vomiting differs in that the nausea is continuous, with involuntary effort to vomit. The individual becomes exhausted and loses sleep, and as the condition continues, significant weight loss, serious dehydration, and starvation occur.

The temperature may rise to about 101° F., with an increase in pulse rate to 130 beats per minute or more. Abnormal constituents appear in the scanty urinary output. The condition is serious and, if not treated, may become fatal.

Treatment and nursing care. The patient should be hospitalized and placed on a regimen of bed rest in a quiet, well-ventilated room. Visitors should be limited, and in some cases it may be best to isolate the patient completely. Efforts are made to rule out any pathologic disease that may be the cause of the disorder. Then treatment is directed toward (1) hydration, (2) overcoming the starvation, and (3) psychotherapy and sedation. Intravenous infusion of 5% to 10% glucose is given, and physiologic saline solution may be given intravenously or subcutaneously. Thiamine hydrochloride (vitamin B_1) is given intravenously or intramuscularly, and when vomiting is controlled, 50 mg. may be given orally. After 24 hours small feedings of dry foods are offered every 2 to 3 hours, with about 100 ml. of fluids on alternating hours. Liquids such as cola drinks and tea may be better tolerated. If the vomiting has been relieved, other food is offered gradually. If vomiting continues, a nasogastric tube may be inserted and feedings given by continuous drip. Sedation such as phenobarbital sodium (Luminal sodium), 0.06 to 0.12 Gm. every 4 hours, may be given, or amobarbital sodium (Amytal sodium), 0.2 Gm. every 6 hours, may be administered by rectal installation.

Each patient is different and must have individualized nursing care. Frequently psychotherapy is available, and in its absence the patient's religious counselor may help the patient. The nurse caring for the patient should serve food attractively and in small amounts. It is equally important that hot food and drink be hot and cold food and drink be cold. Records must be maintained of all intake, including intravenous fluids, and all output, including vomitus. The nurse should be understanding, but firm in her expectation of recovery. The nurse should also remember that although the patient may have adjustment problems, she is also physically ill and needs sympathetic nursing care.[9]

DISEASES AND DISORDERS OF THE ACCESSORY ORGANS OF DIGESTION
Diseases and disorders of the liver
Hepatitis

Hepatitis is a viral disease that causes inflammation of the liver cells. The disease is recognized in two forms: infectious hepatitis, or hepatitis A, and serum hepatitis, or hepatitis B. Infectious hepatitis is the most prevalent form of the disease, and its incidence has been increasing. For the week ending September 7, 1974, the Center for Disease Control announced that 28,984 cases of infectious hepatitis had been reported since the first of the year,[19] whereas for 1973 a total of 50,749 cases were reported.[20] Virus A hepatitis is spread by the anal-oral route, with the virus present in the feces. Outbreaks resulting from contaminated food and water have been reported. Serum hepatitis is essentially the same, and the number of cases of serum hepatitis being reported is also increasing. The primary sources of transmission are blood transfusions and contaminated syringes and needles. Numerous outbreaks have occurred among drug addicts who use the same contaminated syringe and needle, thus introducing the virus directly into the bloodstream. The American Public Health Association reports that some research has been conducted that indicates the possibility that serum hepatitis may be transmitted by close personal contact, as well as by the parenteral route.[23] At the present time serum hepatitis is not believed to be transmitted through discharges from the bowel.

Pathophysiology. The incubation period for hepatitis may be as short as 15 days or as long as 50 days after exposure. Studies indicate that the virus may be found in feces from 2 to 3 weeks before symptoms develop and that the disease may be transmitted during this time. The virus continues to persist for from 8 to 18 days after jaundice (yellowing of the skin) develops and may be found in the blood during the febrile period. Recovery may take from 3 to 4 months. A diffuse inflammatory reaction occurs, and liver cells begin to degenerate and die. As the liver cells degenerate, the normal functions of the liver slow down.

Symptoms may be mild or severe and include loss of appetite, fatigue, nausea and vomiting, chills, headache, and temperature that may range from 100° to 104° F. Jaundice appears in from 1 to 10 days but may not occur before 30 days and may be absent in some patients. The jaundice is due to the inability of the liver to remove the waste products of red blood cell destruction (bilirubin) from the bloodstream satisfactorily. Bilirubin is a pigment that gives bile and consequently gives the stools their normal color. When an obstruction to the elimination of bilirubin occurs, the pigment accumulates in the bloodstream and is ultimately deposited in the body tissues. It can first be detected in the whites of the eyes. The urine becomes dark as the kidney attempts to remove the excess pigment from the bloodstream. Pruritus, abdominal pain with tenderness over the liver, and photophobia occur. Diagnosis is based on symptoms, liver function tests, and liver biopsy, with prothrombin and clotting time tests preceding the biopsy.

Treatment and nursing care. There is no specific treatment for hepatitis. Therapy is planned to strengthen the patient's resistance to the infection, and rest and a nourishing diet are primary considerations. Antibiotics may be administered to prevent secondary infection, and antihistamines may be given to relieve the itching. Fluid intake is encouraged during the acute stage, and if a sufficient amount is not taken, intravenous infusions may be given. Diet is of major importance and should provide all the necessary nutrients. Since the appetite is poor, the patient will need considerable encouragement to eat, and records of food intake should be kept. If the patient does not eat, tube feedings may be ordered.

All patients with infectious hepatitis should be isolated for at least 7 days and strict medical asepsis carried out. Patients with serum hepatitis do not have to be isolated, but if the form of the disease has not been clearly established, isolation should be instituted. The nurse caring for the patient has an important responsibility in preventing spread of the infection. As much disposable equipment as possible should be used, including paper dishes, disposable syringes and needles, and tissue wipes. Nondisposable dishes and utensils should be autoclaved. If boiling is necessary, it must be done for not less than 30 minutes after boiling begins. Gloves should be worn when handling bowel excretions, giving enemas, or taking rectal temperatures, and persons collecting blood samples or changing dressings are advised to wear gloves. Bowel excretions should be disinfected with full strength Wescodyne before disposal unless public sewage facilities are available.[8] However, exactly what it may take to destroy the hepatitis virus is not exactly known. It is known that ordinary chemical disinfection does not destroy the hepatitis virus. It is recommended that thermometers be destroyed when the patient leaves the hospital. Thorough handwashing is important for the patient after use of the bedpan, and nurses should wash their hands by the method previously discussed in this book. (See Chapter 3.)

The patient's environment should be made as pleasant as possible. Tepid baths, rubs, and oral care are important, and a soothing lotion may provide relief from skin pruritus. The patient may be disturbed over the long illness and the resulting financial problems. The nurse should attempt to encourage the patient and help to provide diversional activties to relieve the monotony of his convalescence. If the patient is a child, the problems of a long convalescence may be greater, and it will require the help of everyone to keep the child occupied and contented. Bed rest is indicated during the acute phase of the disease. When all symptoms have subsided, the patient may be allowed bathroom privileges. Physical activity is kept at a minimum throughout the convalescence.

Cirrhosis of the liver

Cirrhosis (scarring) of the liver is a disease in which the cells of the liver undergo degeneration and are replaced by fibrous tissue. The basic cause is not clearly understood but appears to be repeated injury to the liver cells. Although the liver cells have a great potential for regeneration, repeated scarring decreases their ability to be replaced. Cirrhosis is more common in men of middle and later life, but it may occur in younger persons. More than 20,000 persons in the United States die from the

disease each year. Several types of the disease have been identified, each with a different etiology, but the final result is the same for all types. The most common form of the disease in the United States is Laënnec's portal cirrhosis, which appears to be related to chronic malnutrition and alcoholism.

Pathophysiology. Cirrhosis is a disease that develops slowly and may progress gradually over a period of years. There is a slow destruction of the functional cells of the liver. As the cells degenerate, they become infiltrated with fat and the organ increases in size (fatty cirrhosis). The regenerated nodules are separated by bands of fibrous scar tissue. The process restricts the flow of blood to the organ and contributes to its destruction. As the blood supply continues to be diminished and the scar tissue increases, the organ becomes atrophied. The progressive damage causes obstruction of the portal vein as it enters the liver. This obstruction of the circulation results in portal hypertension. There is increased pressure in the veins that drain the gastrointestinal tract, and fluid accumulates in the abdominal cavity (ascites). Gradually veins in the upper part of the body become distended, including the esophageal veins, and esophageal varicosities develop that may rupture causing severe hemorrhage. Skin lesions appear on various parts of the body (spider angiomas), which appear to be small dilated blood vessels. Pressure on the center of the lesion will cause its temporary disappearance.

Early symptoms may include loss of appetite, nausea and vomiting, fever, and jaundice. When enough cells of the liver become involved to interfere with its function and obstruct its circulation, the gastrointestinal organs and the spleen become congested and cannot function properly and jaundice occurs. The patient loses weight and has diarrhea and constipation. Anemia occurs because of nutritional deficiency. There may be epistaxis, purpura, hematuria, and bleeding about the gums. The patient becomes extremely weak and depressed; he may lapse into a coma, and death may occur.

The most serious complication of cirrhosis is portal hypertension, which is responsible for the late symptoms including ascites, hematologic disorders, and splenic enlargement.

Treatment and nursing care. Treatment varies with the symptoms and their severity, but there is no specific treatment for the disease. Diet is the one important factor; when the patient has no appetite, it may take more than encouragement to persuade him to eat. Food should be served when the patient feels like eating. It should usually be high in protein, with little salt, and vitamin supplements may be given. Careful records of food intake should be maintained and recorded. All fluid intake and output are measured and recorded, and the patient is weighed daily. The patient may be given a diuretic such as chlorothiazide (Diuril) or chlorthalidone (Hygroton) to eliminate or decrease the edema and the accumulation of fluid.

When ascites is present, an abdominal paracentesis may sometimes be done. (Refer to a textbook on basic nursing.) Also, when ascites is present, the patient may be more comfortable if he is placed in a supine position, but his position should be adjusted to afford him the greatest amount of comfort and the least respiratory embarrassment. Special attention must be given to the skin, since the poor nutritional status and tissue edema may contribute to the development of decubiti. (See Chapter 6.) Oral care should be given frequently and regularly; a mouthwash before meals may make food a little more appetizing. If the patient is severely anemic or if hemorrhages should occur, transfusions with fresh whole blood may be given. The patient's environment should be quiet and conducive to rest, and precautions should be taken to protect him from exposure to secondary infections.

Several operative procedures can be used to reduce the flow of blood through the portal system. A portacaval shunt involves the anastomosis of the portal vein to the inferior vena cava so that the liver is bypassed, whereas the splenorenal shunt requires the removal of the spleen and the splenic vein is anasctomosed to the left renal vein. This is elective surgery that may be only palliative in nature.

Hepatic coma

Hepatic coma is a degenerative condition of the brain that follows liver failure. It is thought to be a result of increasing levels of ammonia in the bloodstream. Symptoms include changes in behavior, confusion, tremors and twitching of the extremities, stupor, and coma.

Treatment and nursing care. The underlying cause must be treated and the patient given supportive care that will prevent further damage to the liver. The patient should receive the supportive care necessary for any patient with liver disease or who is unconscious. However, special measures such as central venous monitoring and tracheostomy care may be necessary. Kidney output should be watched carefully, since renal failure may occur. Intravenous infusions and intermittent positve pressure breathing therapy may be given. Drugs that are normally detoxified by the liver are avoided, but medications that stimulate the removal of ammonia from the bloodstream through the kidney may be administered along with antibiotics to prevent infection. Hemodialysis may be used to remove the ammonia from the blood.

Diseases and disorders of the biliary system
Cholecystitis and cholelithiasis

Pathophysiology. Cholecystitis is an inflammatory disorder of the gallbladder and may result from infection by any one of a variety of pathogenic organisms. If stones are present in the gallbladder, it is called cholelithiasis. These two conditions constitute most of the diseases affecting the gallbladder and its ducts. The disease occurs with greatest frequency in women past middle life and often is found in obese persons. Cholecystitis may occur suddenly in an acute attack or may become chronic after several mild acute attacks. The inflammatory condition may involve only the mucous membrane lining the gallbladder, or it may invade the muscle layers. When the disease is severe enough to interfere with the blood supply, the walls may become gangrenous.

Pain is the chief symptom of gallbladder disease and is usually felt in the upper right quadrant of the abdomen. The patient may complain of heartburn, nausea, vomiting, and flatulence. Symptoms may first appear after ingestion of a heavy meal containing fatty foods. If the disease is severe, the pain and tenderness are increased, with elevation of temperature, increased pulse and respiratory rates, and increase in the number of leukocytes. Occasionally the patient may have an acute attack of pain in the upper right quadrant of the abdomen, caused by the obstruction of a duct with a stone. The pain is so severe that drugs must be administered for relief. The pain may be referred to the back and right shoulder and may last for several hours; it is usually accompanied by nausea and vomiting and profuse perspiration. Antispasmodic drugs may be given, a nasogastric tube is inserted and attached to suction, and intravenous fluids may be administered. The patient is usually scheduled for a gallbladder series (cholecystogram) of tests.

The direct cause of stones in the gallbladder or its ducts is not specifically known. The stones are found in a variety of shapes, and the number, size, and chemical composition vary. The amount of calcium or other solid deposits determines whether they can be seen on routine x-ray examination. Stones will sometimes cause an obstruction in the biliary tract, and the individual develops jaundice. In many instances stones may exist for years, and the individual will not have any symptoms. Although some mild attacks may be treated medically, the disease is primarily one that requires surgical intervention.

Cholecystectomy. Cholecystectomy, the surgical removal of the gallbladder, is usually indicated after the patient has had several acute attacks. However, careful evaluation and examination of the patient's general condition generally precede the surgery. The preoperative care is the same as that for any abdominal surgery. Since many patients are at an age at which degenerative changes may begin to make their appearance, the physician may order an electrocardiogram, chest x-ray examination, and if jaundice is present, tests of liver function and prothrombin time.

The postoperative care of the patient includes careful checking of vital signs and observation of dressings for drainage or hemorrhage. The patient may be placed in low Fowler's position but should be encouraged to turn and move about freely. Deep breathing and coughing are impor-

tant, and the patient will need considerable encouragement because of the location of the incision. The nurse can assist the patient by splinting the incision with a towel. The patient will need drugs for relief of pain for several days, and deep breathing and coughing may follow the administration of the medication. A nasogastric tube is usually inserted and connected to suction siphonage to prevent nausea, vomiting, and abdominal distention. The nurse should be sure the tube is draining properly, and if it becomes obstructed, it may be irrigated with physiologic saline solution. Usually 30 ml. of solution is sufficient to determine its patency. Sips of water or ice cubes may be allowed to keep the mouth moist, and the patient should be allowed to rinse the mouth frequently. Cold cream or petroleum jelly should be applied to the lips. Fluids and electrolytes may be administered by intravenous infusion. Tubes may be inserted in or near the wound, since drainage of bile is expected. The nurse should reinforce dressings as necessary until the physician gives an order for them to be changed. Dressings may have to be changed frequently to keep the patient dry and comfortable, and Montgomery straps should be used to prevent skin irritation from adhesive tape (Fig. 14-17). In some patients a T tube is inserted into the common bile duct, and the tubing is brought out through a stab wound near the surgical incision (Fig. 14-18). The tubing is attached to gravity drainage, and bile will drain out through the tubing. The drainage must be checked for color and amount at frequent intervals during the first 24 hours and recorded. After that it is measured and recorded daily. After a few days the tube is clamped before and after meals for approximately 1 hour. When the amount of drainage has decreased, the tube may be removed; however, some patients are discharged from the hospital with the tube, and drainage may continue for several weeks. The patient should be observed for yellowing of the skin, dark-colored urine, and lack of color in the stools, all of which should be reported to the physician.[24] As nausea and vomiting ceases and peristalsis returns, the nasogastric tube is removed, and the patient is given clear liquids, followed by diet as tolerated. The

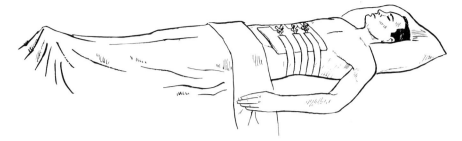

Fig. 14-17. Montgomery straps used to secure dressings when frequent changes are necessary.

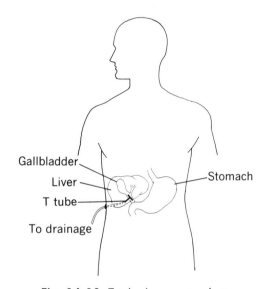

Fig. 14-18. T tube in common duct.

diet is usually kept low in fats. The patient is allowed out of bed on the first postoperative day, and ambulation is encouraged thereafter. When the patient is dismissed from the hospital, he should be encouraged to remain under medical supervision. His diet should maintain his nutritional requirements but should remain low in fats.

Diseases and disorders of the pancreas
Pancreatitis

Inflammation of the pancreas often occurs when chronic gallbladder disease is present. However, many persons who develop pancreatitis have no other illness, and the exact etiology is unknown. The condition may become chronic after several acute attacks. An acute attack may develop suddenly with intense pain in the epigastric region, vomiting, elevation of temperature,

and increased leukocyte count. In patients with a severe form of the disease the pancreas may be destroyed by its own enzymes, with hemorrhage into the pancreatic tissue and the abdominal cavity. Shock then occurs, and the patient dies.

In treating patients with simple pancreatitis, food and fluids are withheld to avoid stimulating pancreatic activity, and intravenous fluids are administered. The most common complaint is constant pain radiating to the back and both sides.[25] The pain is treated with morphine or meperidine hydrochloride. When the disease becomes chronic, the gland contains scar tissue so that its function is impaired. Mild to severe pain continues; weakness, jaundice, and diarrhea may occur, and the patient becomes weak and debilitated. Because of continued pain and the necessity for narcotic drugs, the patient may present problems of addiction. These patients need good nursing care and emotional support. The care is the same as that for other chronic diseases.

Pancreatectomy. There is no specific surgery to cure pancreatitis. An exploratory laparotomy may be done to confirm diagnosis and treat general peritonitis or perforation of the organ. In severe cases a partial or total pancreatectomy may be performed. If it is necessary to remove the entire pancreas, the secretion of insulin will be eliminated, and it will be necessary for the patient to take insulin for the rest of his life. The preoperative preparation of the patient is the same as that for other abdominal surgery. In addition to the routine postoperative care the patient should be observed for complications such as peritonitis, jaundice, and intestinal obstruction. Stools should be observed for a light-colored, frothy appearance and any evidence of undigested particles of fat.

Tumors of the accessory organs of digestion

Malignant or benign tumors may occur in any of the accessory organs of digestion. Tumors of the pancreas are usually malignant, and in some instances surgery may be done for their removal. Most malignant lesions of the liver are the result of metastasis from primary tumors elsewhere in the body. It was formerly believed that surgery of the liver could not be done; however, with the improved methods for determining liver function and blood replacement, improved methods of anesthesia, and antibiotics to prevent infection, it has become possible to remove entire lobes of the liver.[18] Liver transplants have been attempted but have not been successful.

Careful preoperative preparation and expert postoperative nursing care are necessary. Postoperatively the patient must be constantly observed for hemorrhage, since this is always a possibility. All vital signs are checked at frequent intervals. The patient will have chest tubes connected to underwater drainage and will have a nasogastric tube connected to suction siphonage. Food and fluids are withheld for several days, and mouth care is important. Ambulation is usually delayed for several days.[24] Cancer of the gallbladder and bile ducts is rare. When it occurs, it generally begins in one of the ducts and metastasizes to the liver. Patients with cancer of the accessory organs of digestion have loss of appetite, loss of weight, general weakness, secondary anemia, and a general feeling of discomfort. (See Chapter 5.)

Summary outline

1. Structure and function of gastrointestinal system (GI system, alimentary tract, or digestive system)
   A. Begins in mouth and ends with anus
      1. Mouth also called *buccal*, or oral, *cavity*
      2. Teeth and tongue accessory organs
   B. Organs consist of esophagus, stomach, small intestine, large intestine (colon), and rectum
   C. Colon divided into ascending, transverse, and descending
   D. Peristalsis—involuntary contraction of muscles that line alimentary tract
   E. Accessory organs of digestion—liver, gallbladder, and pancreas

2. Process of digestion and absorption
   A. Mechanical digestion
   B. Chemical digestion
3. Causes of digestive diseases and disorders
   A. Infection, emotional problems, diseases such as cancer, injury, congenital malformations, degenerative process, and faulty utilization of food
   B. Symptoms—nausea, vomiting, constipation, diarrhea, loss of appetite, difficulty in swallowing, abdominal pain, blood in stools, and vomiting blood
4. Diagnostic tests and procedures
   A. Gastric analysis—to determine degree of acidity of gastric contents
      1. Tubeless gastric analysis does not require passing of stomach tube
   B. Esophagoscopy and gastroscopy—to examine esophagus and portions of stomach
   C. Proctoscopy and sigmoidoscopy—to permit visualization of sigmoid and rectum
   D. Gastrointestinal series and barium enema
   E. Stool examination—to detect bacteria, parasites, blood, or for chemical analysis
   F. Liver function tests
      1. Bilirubin test
      2. Cephalin occulation test
      3. Thymol turbidity test
      4. Bromsulphalein
      5. Galactose tolerance test
      6. Icterus index
      7. Serum cholesterol level
      8. Serum glutamic oxaloacetic transaminase (SGOT) test
      9. Serum glutamic pyruvic transaminase (SGPT) test
      10. Alkaline phosphatase test
      11. Approximate normal values
   G. Liver biopsy—to establish diagnosis or determine extent of liver damage
   H. Liver scanning
   I. Cholecystography and cholangiography—using radiopaque dye to visualize gallbladder and extrahepatic biliary system
   J. Gastric lavage—to wash out stomach
   K. Gastric gavage—to provide nourishment for patients unable to eat
   L. Gastrointestinal decompression
      1. To remove air and fluids from stomach
      2. To prevent postoperative distention and vomiting
      3. To relieve intestinal obstruction or paralytic ileus
      4. To protect suture line
   M. Hyperalimentation—administration of nutrients by infusion
5. Nursing the patient with diseases and disorders of gastrointestinal system
   A. Abdominal surgery—includes surgery of esophagus, stomach, small intestine, large intestine, rectum, and accessory organs of digestion and may include other structures such as lymph nodes and blood vessels
   B. Nursing responsibilities for tests and procedures
      1. Completing laboratory forms
      2. Collecting specimens

3. Identifying room and bed
4. Preparing patient for examination
5. Administering any medications ordered
6. Reassuring patient
C. Observation—pain, nausea, vomiting, stools, flatus, appetite, mental state
D. Nursing care of colostomy and ileostomy
 1. Postoperative nursing care
  a. Care of nasogastric tube
  b. Coughing and deep breathing
  c. Administration of intravenous fluids
  d. Aseptic care of wound
  e. Observation for urinary retention
 2. Psychologic care
6. Specific diseases and disorders of gastrointestinal system
A. Inflammatory diseases
 1. Stomatitis—inflammation of mouth
  a. Vincent's stomatitis (trench mouth)
  b. Thrush (moniliasis)
 2. Gastritis—inflammation of stomach
  a. Caused by infection, dietary indiscretion, and excessive use of salicylates and alcohol
 3. Enteritis—inflammation of intestine that may occur with gastritis (gastroenteritis)
 4. Ulcerative colitis—severe disease involving colon; may be acute or chronic
  a. Treatment and nursing care
   (1) Quiet pleasant environment; protection from chilling and secondary infection
   (2) Psychologic care requires sympathetic understanding
B. Appendicitis—inflammatory condition of appendix most common cause of acute abdominal conditions
 1. Pathophysiology
 2. Appendectomy—surgical removal of appendix; generally performed as emergency surgery
 3. Treatment and nursing care
  a. With no complications, recovery after surgery is rapid
  b. If there is drainage, dressings must be changed frequently; watch for hemorrhage, intestinal obstruction, and increased elevation of temperature and pulse
C. Diverticulum and diverticulosis
 1. Diverticulum—protrusion of mucosa through muscle of intestinal wall
 2. Diverticulosis—inflammation of diverticulum
 3. Pathophysiology
 4. Treatment and nursing care
  a. Treatment is medical unless complications indicate surgery
  b. Dietary plan important
D. Intestinal obstruction—obstruction of small or large intestine may be partial or complete and is always serious
 1. Pathophysiology
 2. Medical treatment and nursing care
  a. Decompression tube
  b. Intravenous fluids
  c. Fowler's position

d. Urinary output—urinary retention and catheter may be inserted
 e. Warm enemas or colonic irrigation and application of heat to abdomen
 f. Oral care
 3. Surgery depends on cause, location of obstruction, and condition of patient
  a. May require resection of bowel
E. Peritonitis—inflammation of peritoneum, usually as complication of some other condition; if generalized, condition very serious
 1. Treatment and nursing care
  a. Fowler's position
  b. Relief of pain
  c. Nasogastric tube connected to suction
  d. Intravenous infusions
  e. Antibiotic therapy
  f. Surgery
F. Tumors of gastrointestinal system
 1. Mouth—may involve lip, tongue, or mucous membrane and are often malignant
  a. Surgery of mouth interferes with normal functions of eating, respiration, and speech
  b. Preoperative care
  c. Radical neck dissection may be necessary
  d. Tracheotomy or tracheostomy may be necessary
  e. Treatment may be with external radium or radon seeds
 2. Esophagus—malignant tumors usually have metastasized to lymph nodes of chest and neck before they are detected
  a. Gastrostomy care
   (1) Care of skin
   (2) Maintaining patency of tube
   (3) Good oral care
   (4) Administration of prescribed feeding
 3. Stomach—symptoms are often related to metastasis rather than tumor itself
  a. Gastrectomy is usually indicated
 4. Colon—cancer of colon may cause obstruction
  a. Treatment is always surgical, and colectomy (colon resection) may be done because of cancer, colitis, or diverticulitis
   (1) Colostomy done when there is abdominoperineal resection
   (2) Preoperative care
   (3) Postoperative care
 5. Rectum—malignancy may be diagnosed early
  a. Abdominoperineal resection with permanent colostomy is indicated
 6. Benign tumors—may occur anywhere in gastrointestinal system and usually are in form of polyps, which are more frequent in stomach and intestine
G. Peptic ulcer—open lesion on mucous membrane of stomach or duodenum, may be acute or chronic
 1. Pathophysiology
 2. May erode through wall and perforate, causing peritonitis

3. Severe hemorrhage may occur if erosion is into blood vessel
4. Medical treatment and nursing care
   a. Rest
   b. Diet
   c. Drugs for sedation and relief of acidity and spasm
5. Complications
   a. Hemorrhage
   b. Perforation
   c. Obstruction
6. Surgical treatment—gastric resection (gastrectomy)
   a. Procedures should be explained to patient to relieve apprehension and tension
   b. Nasogastric tube passed postoperatively, and nothing given by mouth for 24 to 48 hours
   c. Watch for hemorrhage
   d. Keep dressings around gastrostomy tube separate from those over wound

H. Hernia (rupture) may be congenital or acquired
   1. Umbilical, inguinal, or femoral
   2. Strangulation (bowel becoming twisted) may result in gangrene
   3. Incarcerated hernias cannot be reduced
   4. Treatment usually surgical
   5. Herniorrhaphy—requires same preparation and care as that for any uncomplicated abdominal surgery
      a. Postoperative care—avoid strain on surgical wound

I. Hiatus hernia
   1. Pathophysiology
   2. Treatment and nursing care
      a. Small meals of bland foods
      b. Antacids and anticholinergic agents
      c. Extra pillows under head at night
      d. Avoid coughing, straining for bowel elimination, and bending
      e. Surgery may be done
         (1) If procedure is into thoracic cavity, patient will have thoracotomy and drainage tubes
         (2) If abdominal route used, care is same as for other abdominal surgery

J. Hemorrhoids—dilated veins
   1. Causes
      a. Prolonged constipation
      b. Heavy lifting
      c. Straining to defecate
      d. Pregnancy and pelvic tumors
      e. Liver disease
   2. Surgery—hemorrhoidectomy
      a. Preoperative enemas
      b. Postoperative care—observe for unusual bleeding; warm sitz baths, oil retention enema, or stool softeners
      c. Analgesics as necessary for discomfort

K. Functional disorders—may be caused by disease or emotional problems; also called psychosomatic-disorders
   1. Indigestion—may be associated with disease

2. Constipation—symptom of many diseases
3. Cardiospasm and pylorospasm
4. Anal sphincter spasm
5. Hyperacidity—commonly called *heartburn*
6. Psychic vomiting
7. Air swallowing
8. Hyperemesis gravidarum (pernicious vomiting)
   a. Uncontrolled nausea and vomiting during first trimester of pregnancy
   b. May be result of normal physiologic changes of pregnancy
   c. Emotional factors play important part

7. Diseases and disorders of accessory organs of digestion
   A. Diseases and disorders of liver
      1. Hepatitis—inflammation of liver cells caused by virus
         a. Infectious hepatitis spread by oral-anal route
         b. Serum hepatitis spread by blood transfusions and contaminated syringes and needles; close personal contact may be possible means of transmission
         c. There is no specific treatment
         d. Isolate patient for 7 days
      2. Cirrhosis of liver—results in degeneration of liver cells
         a. Several types identified—Laennec's portal cirrhosis most common in United States
            (1) Related to malnutrition and alcoholism
         b. Pathophysiology
         c. Surgical procedures only palliative
            (1) Portacaval shunt
            (2) Splenorenal shunt
      3. Hepatic coma—may be caused by increased levels of ammonia in bloodstream
         a. Treatment and nursing care
            (1) Monitoring of central venous pressure
            (2) Tracheostomy care may be necessary
            (3) Observe for renal failure
            (4) Intravenous fluids
            (5) Intermittent positive pressure breathing therapy
            (6) Drugs to detoxify liver
            (7) Hemodialysis
   B. Diseases and disorders of biliary system
      1. Cholecystitis and cholelithiasis
         a. Pathophysiology
         b. Cholecystitis—inflammation of gallbladder
         c. Cholelithiasis—presence of stones in gallbladder
         d. Surgery—cholecystectomy requires that patient be observed for hemorrhage and jaundice
            (1) Observe drainage and change dressings to keep patient dry and comfortable
            (2) If gravity drainage is in place,

be sure tube is draining and not obstructed
- (3) Observe patient for jaundice, dark urine, and colorless stools
- (4) T tube may be placed in common bile duct and attached to gravity drainage

C. Diseases and disorders of pancreas
1. Pancreatitis—may be acute or chronic
   a. Pancreatectomy may be performed under certain conditions

D. Tumors of accessory organs of digestion
1. May be malignant or benign
2. May be result of metastasis

Review questions

1. What is the purpose of a gastric analyses?
   a.
2. Where would you expect to find occult blood?
   a. *stool*
3. What are two reasons for inserting a Levin tube after surgery of the abdomen?
   a. *keep stomach empty*
   b. *relieve vomiting*
4. Why should intestinal decompression tubes not be taped to the face?
   a. *they have to move forward along the intestine*
5. When a patient has an abdominoperineal resection, where would you expect to find the colostomy?
   a. *l. side*
6. What two processes are involved in digestion?
   a. *mechanical*
   b. *chemical*
7. List four nursing functions in the care of a patient with a colostomy
   a. *good skin care*
   b. *teaching*
   c. *prevent contamination of wound*
   d. *good post op care*
8. Why is an antacid ordered for a patient with peptic ulcer?
   a. *neutralize gastric acids*
9. How would you position a patient who has had a cholecystectomy?
   a. *Semi Fowlers*
10. What are two known ways in which hepatitis B may be transmitted?
    a. *blood transfusion*
    b. *contaminated needles*
11. When a patient has cancer of the mouth, what three normal functions are interfered with?
    a. *chewing (eating)*
    b. *talking (speech)*
    c. *respiration*

Films

1. Anorectal operations for hemorrhoids, abscesses, fissures, and fistulas—CS-990 (26 min., sound, color, 16 mm.), Davis & Geck Film Library, American Cyanamid Co., 1 Casper St., Danbury, Conn. 06810. Illustrates some of the diagnostic and technical surgical aspects in the management of hemorrhoids, abscesses, fissures, and fistulas. There is a small rental fee.

2. Clinical proctoscopy (20 min., sound, color, 16 mm.), Baxter Laboratories, Inc., 6301 Lincoln Avenue, Morton Grove, Ill. 60053. Features studies of the sigmoid colon, rectum, and anal canal. Common and uncommon problems in proctoscopy.

3. No. 9 Gastrointestinal problems: medicine or surgery? (90 min., sound, black and white, 16 mm.), Upjohn Professional Film Library, 7000 Portage Rd., Kalamazoo, Mich. 49001. Discusses the issues of whether to continue medical treatment in hiatus hernia, silent gallstones, ulcerative colitis, and chronic pancreatitis or to favor surgery. Also shown is a demonstration of gastric cooling in upper gastrointestinal bleeding and the psychologic approach in solving psychologic problems of postileostomy patients.

4. Postoperative management of colostomy—Mis-733 (22 min., sound, color, 16 mm.), Media Resources Branch, National Medical Audiovisual Center, (Annex) Station K, Atlanta, Ga. 30324. Role of the surgeon in the postoperative management and rehabilitation of the patient with colostomy. Shows irrigation by nurses and by the patient and demonstrates both the enema method and the bulb syringe method of irrigation.

5. Special problems in the management of peptic ulcer (16 mm., optical sound, color, 1 reel, 1,400 feet, 40 min.), Wyeth Film Library, P. O. Box 8299, Philadelphia, Pa. 19101. Presents therapeutic solutions to difficult ulcer conditions.

6. Intravenous hyperalimentation technique (30 min., sound, color, 16 mm. free loan), Abbott Laboratories, Abbott Park, North Chicago, Ill., 60064. Illustrates total intravenous feeding over long periods of time. Surgical and nursing procedures involving the care of the catheter are shown.

7. Nursing the cancer patient: diagnosis—cancer of the rectum (20 min., sound, color, 16 mm.), free from local chapter of the American Cancer Society. Shows the problems of a patient who has had surgery for cancer of the rectum and how the nurse can assist the patient and his family.

8. Caring for the patient with a colostomy (22 min., sound, color, 16 mm.), free from local chapter of the American Cancer Society. Depicts all aspects of caring for the colostomy patient, including emotional and social rehabilitation.

References

1. A cancer guide for practical nurses, New York, 1962, American Cancer Society.
2. Anthony, Catherine P., and Kolthoff, Norma J.: Textbook of anatomy and physiology, ed. 9, St. Louis, 1975, The C. V. Mosby Co.
3. Appendicitis in recent years, Statistical Bulletin **50:**5, Sept., 1969, Metropolitan Life Insurance Co.
4. Brunner, Lillian S., and Suddarth, Doris S.:

Textbook of medical-surgical nursing, ed. 3, Philadelphia, 1975, J. B. Lippincott Co.

5. Cancer rates and risks, United States Public Health Service Publication no. 1148, Washington, D. C., 1964, Government Printing Office.

6. Cantor, Alfred J.: Hemorrhoids: patient care essentials, The Journal of Practical Nursing **22**:20+, July, 1972.

7. Conn, Howard F., editor: Current therapy 1976, Philadelphia, 1976, W. B. Saunders Co.

8. Eisenmenger, William J., Uhl, Marilyn, and Lyndon, Jean: 1. Viral hepatitis. 2. From a nursing viewpoint, American Journal of Nursing **61**:56-59, Nov., 1961.

9. Fitzpatrick, Elise, Reeder, Sharon R., and Mastroianni, Luigi, Jr.: Maternity nursing, ed. 12, Philadelphia, 1971, J. B. Lippincott Co.

10. Garb, Solomon: Laboratory tests in common use, ed. 5, New York, 1971, Springer Publishing Co., Inc.

11. Ginsberg, Miriam: A study of oral hygiene nursing care, American Journal of Nursing **61**:67-69, Oct., 1961.

12. Given, Barbara A., and Simmons, Sandra J.: Gastroenterology in clinical nursing, ed. 2, St. Louis, 1975, The C. V. Mosby Co.

13. Halberg, Jeanne C.: The patient with surgery of the colon, American Journal of Nursing **61**:64-66, March, 1961.

14. Jackson, Bettie S.: Ulcerative colitis: from an etiological perspective, American Journal of Nursing **73**:258-261, Feb., 1973.

15. Kitzes, George: What the nurse should know about peptic ulcers, The Journal of Practical Nursing **20**:20-21, Jan., 1970.

16. Lehman, Geoffrey: Hemorrhoids, The Canadian Nurse **62**:36-37, March, 1966.

17. Metheny, Norma M., and Snively, William D., Jr.: Nurses' handbook of fluid balance, ed. 2, Philadelphia, 1974, J. B. Lippincott Co.

18. Molander, David W., and Brasfield, Richard D.: Liver surgery, American Journal of Nursing **61**:72-74, July, 1961.

19. Morbidity and Mortality Weekly Report, week ending Sept. 7, Atlanta, 1974, Center for Disease Control.

20. Morbidity and Mortality Weekly Report, year ending Dec. 29, Atlanta, 1973, Center for Disease Control.

21. Oral care for cancer patients, United States Public Health Service Publication no. 1958, Washington, D. C., Government Printing Office.

22. Reif, Laura: Managing a life with chronic disease, American Journal of Nursing **73**:261-264, Feb., 1973.

23. "Serum" hepatitis acquired by nonparenteral routes, Public Health Reports **85**:312, April, 1970.

24. Shafer, Kathleen N., Sawyer, Janet R., McCluskey, Audrey M., Beck, Edna L., and Phipps, Wilma J.: Medical-surgical nursing, ed. 6, St. Louis, 1975, The C. V. Mosby Co.

25. Simmons, Sandra, and Given, Barbara: Acute pancreatitis, American Journal of Nursing **71**:934-939, May, 1971.

26. Snively, William D., Jr., and Beshear, Donna R.: Textbook of pathophysiology, Philadelphia, 1972, J. B. Lippincott Co.

27. Steigman, Frederick: Are laxatives necessary? American Journal of Nursing **62**:90-93, Oct., 1962.

28. Williams, Sue R.: Nutrition and diet therapy, ed. 2, St. Louis, 1973, The C. V. Mosby Co.

Nursing the patient with diseases and disorders of the urinary system

KEY WORDS

anuria *no urine secreted by kidneys*
cystectomy *removal of bladder*
cystoscope *instrument to examine the bladder*
cystostomy *surgical opening into bladder*
dialysis *artificial kidney function*
diuresis *increase in urine output*
diuretic *drugs to ↑*
eclampsia *pregnancy complication*
enuresis *bed wetting*
glomerulonephritis *nephritis of R. glomerulus*
hematuria *blood in urine*
hemodialysis *kidney machine*
hydronephrosis *distension of R. pelvis*
ileal conduit *urinary diversion - ileostomy*
incontinence *can't hold urine*
lithiasis *formation of stones*
micturition *urination*
neobladder *urinary diversion (into colon)*
nephrectomy *R. removal*
nephron *unit of the R.*
nephrosclerosis *sclerosis of R. Bl. vessels of R.*
nephrosis *degeneration of renal tissue*
nephrostomy *opening into R. pelvis drainage*
oliguria *decreased urine*
pyuria *pus in urine*
uremia *toxic - urinary parts in blood*
ureterotomy
urinalysis *urine tests*

STRUCTURE AND FUNCTION OF THE URINARY SYSTEM

The organs of the urinary system consist of two kidneys located at the back of the abdominal cavity, one on each side of the vertebral column; two ureters, one from each kidney, which convey the urine from the kidney to the bladder; one urinary bladder located in the pelvis between the rectum and the pubis that stores urine; and one urethra to convey the urine from the bladder to the outside (Fig. 15-1).

The real work of the urinary system is done in the kidneys, in which more than a million tiny units called _nephrons_ are arranged in tiny coiled tubes called _tubules_. The top of each nephron is shaped like a cup and is called the _Bowman's capsule_. It surrounds a cluster of capillaries called a _glomerulus_. The serous portion of the blood filters out of the glomerulus and into the Bowman's capsule and then begins passing through the tubules. Here, substances that the body needs are reabsorbed into the bloodstream, and the waste products with some water continue to pass through a series of tubules until they reach the ureters and the bladder and are subsequently discharged from the body as urine. Approximately 1700 quarts of blood are filtered through this system each day.

The kidney is an extremely complex organ that has three main functions: (1) to filter materials from the blood that are no longer needed or that the body has an excess of and to return usable material to the blood, (2) to maintain water and electrolyte balance, and (3) to maintain acid-base balance. In other words the function of the kidneys is to maintain homeostasis.

Main function - to produce urine

Also regulates B/P

335

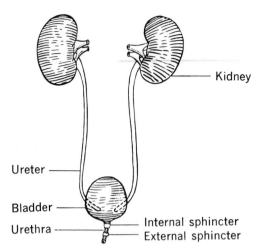

Fig. 15-1. Normal position of the organs of the urinary system.

They have the ability to regulate the amount of water and electrolytes that leave the body and the amount that remain in the body. These processes are vital to the normal functioning of the kidneys; if the kidneys become diseased so that they cannot perform their normal functions, death results unless another means of maintaining homeostasis is substituted. Each part of the urinary system has its own specialized function, but all parts must coordinate their functions for the system to work properly.

CAUSES OF URINARY DISEASES AND DISORDERS

Pathogenic organisms may gain entrance to the urinary tract by the bloodstream or from infections elsewhere in the body and result in an inflammatory process, or infection may spread from the urethra upward to other parts of the system. Obstructions may occur along the tract from stones, strictures, tumors, or a kinked ureter. Tumors, either benign or malignant, may involve any part of the system, and trauma may result in serious injury to the bladder, urethra, or kidneys. Injuries elsewhere in the body may also affect the kidney. Some diseases of the kidney may be the result of allergic factors, and others may be the result of degenerative changes.

URINARY OUTPUT

Life cannot continue for more than a few days when the kidneys fail to function. Under normal conditions they should filter, concentrate, and excrete from 1500 to 2000 ml. of urine in 24 hours. The first indication of serious disease may often be observed in the urine. The nurse can assist the physician in diagnosis and treatment by making and recording careful observations of the urinary output and its characteristics. A temporary decrease in urinary output may be caused by disease within the urinary system or elsewhere in the body, by restriction of fluids from surgery or disease, or by failure of the patient to drink an adequate amount of fluid.

Retention. Retention is a condition in which the patient is unable to void and may result from several factors, including surgery followed by delayed ambulation, obstruction, and traumatic injuries. It may follow childbirth, or in some persons it may be caused by emotional factors. The bladder becomes increasingly distended and may be felt above the pubis. Urinary retention may cause the patient considerable discomfort and anxiety, and nursing measures should be taken to relieve the condition. Drugs for discomfort should not be given when the discomfort is from urinary retention. The nurse should initiate measures to assist the patient to void, and if these measures fail, the physician should be notified and orders secured for catheterization. Retention with overflow results when the bladder becomes greatly distended and the patient voids small amounts, 25 to 35 ml., but is unable to empty the bladder.

Suppression. Suppression of urine (anuria) is an extremely serious condition indicating that the kidneys are failing to do their work. As a result the waste products are retained in the body and will give rise to generalized symptoms. The cause may be within the kidney as in acute nephritis, or it may be from causes such as shock, cardiac decompensation, or extreme dehydration. The nurse should observe the patient's failure to void and should be alert to signs of edema, nausea, vomiting, dizziness, drowsiness, and disturbance of vision. The physician will order the specific treatment indicated by the cause and the toxic symptoms.

Residual urine. Residual urine is the urine that is left in the bladder after the voiding patient has voided. If urine is allowed to remain in the bladder, it may give rise to infection and contribute to the formation of stones. Normally, little urine remains in the bladder after voiding. When the physician orders the patient to be catheterized for residual urine, the procedure should be explained to the patient. The patient is instructed to void, emptying the bladder as completely as possible. The nurse should have the catheterization tray ready, and the catheter is passed into the urethra immediately. There should be no delay, since urine is dripping into the bladder continuously, and delay will result in an inaccurate amount of residual urine. Both the voided urine and the catheterized residual urine are measured and recorded on the patient's chart as "voided" and "residual." If a sterile specimen is requested, the catheterized specimen may be saved and sent to the laboratory.

Incontinence. The inability to retain urine in the bladder through voluntary effort is called *incontinence.* Incontinence may result from any of several factors, including congenital defects of the urethra and bladder, causing true incontinence. Stress incontinence is caused by the displacement of pelvic organs or the presence of a cystocele, which tends to push or pull on the bladder so that leakage occurs in coughing, laughing, or sneezing. In patients in whom infection or urethral irritation is present, the urgency to urinate may cause incontinence. A constant dribbling of urine may be present when the bladder is full, but obstruction is present at the neck of the bladder or the urethra (paradoxical incontinence). Injury to the spinal cord and some neurologic diseases may result in relaxation of sphincter muscles of both the rectum and the urethra so that the patient has both urinary and fecal incontinence.

Some problems of incontinence may be corrected by surgery, and some are helped by the use of drugs. Many conditions can be helped by understanding the patient and his problems and planning a program to help him. The nurse should realize that incontinence in an adult is extremely embarrassing, and every effort should be made to keep the patient dry and to help him maintain his self-respect and dignity. In-

creasing emphasis is being placed on prevention and rehabilitation through a well-planned program of bladder control.[7, 13]

Enuresis (bed-wetting). Enuresis is the inability to retain urine in the bladder, frequently during sleep. Enuresis occurring during sleep is called *nocturnal enuresis.* The cause in an adult may be the same factors that cause incontinence in general, whereas enuresis in children may be symptomatic of emotional or behavior problems. The child may wet the bed while asleep or may wet the bed while wide awake. Enuresis should be thoroughly investigated to determine the cause. Punishing a child for wetting the bed rarely achieves results. If the cause is determined to be emotional, an investigation of home problems and psychotherapy for the child may be a more rational approach to the problem.[6]

DIURETICS

Diuretics are drugs that increase the urinary output. The excretion of large amounts of urine after the administration of a diuretic is called *diuresis.* The primary function of the kidneys is to control the composition and volume of body fluids to maintain the constancy of intracellular fluid. The excretion of urine is simply the result of the kidney function. Under normal conditions any excess of water and sodium is excreted along with the urine. In various kinds of heart disease, nephritis, and cirrhosis of the liver the kidneys are unable to perform their normal function; as a result, water and sodium are retained in the body, and edema and ascites occur. Diuretics do not cure the disease condition but help to restore kidney function by preventing the reabsorption of sodium and retention of water.

Diuretics have been found useful in other conditions, including premenstrual tension, hypertension, and edema of pregnancy.

The most commonly used diuretics are the mercurial diuretics and synthetic agents known as chlorothiazides, as well as several agents related to the chlorothiazides. The mercurial diuretics generally used are meralluride (Mercuhydrin), 1 to 2 ml., given parenterally, and mercaptomerin (Thiomerin sodium), 1 to 2 ml., administered parenterally. Use of the mercurial diuretics has decreased since the production of chlorothiazides. A primary advantage of the thiazides is that they are administered by the oral route. Chlorothiazide (Diuril) is widely used and may be administered in dosages from 0.5 to 1 Gm. daily. Since the development of Diuril, several related drugs having the same action have been produced. These include the trade names HydroDiuril, Esidrix, Hygroton, Saluron, Exna, Renese, and Naturetin. These may be administered in dosages of 50 to 200 mg. daily. The action of Hygroton may be as long as 72 hours, and it may be given twice a week.

Furosemide (Lasix) is a powerful oral diuretic that has recently come into widespread use. It acts quickly, and its effects last for approximately 8 hours. The normal dose is 40 to 80 mg. once a day. In addition, other types of drugs that may have a diuretic effect are classed as xanthine compounds and carbonic anhydrase inhibitors, such as acetazolamide (Diamox). The physician will order the drug or the combination of drugs that best suits the needs of the individual patient.

Nurses who may administer diuretics should observe patients for side effects, which include gastrointestinal disturbances, dizziness, weakness, fatigue, and skin rash. A common complication of continued diuretic therapy is a deficit of potassium in the body. Undue fatigue, weakness, loss of appetite, loss of muscle tone, and abdominal distention may be signs indicating that a potassium supplement is necessary. Patients receiving diuretics should be encouraged to eat bananas, oranges, dried fruits, fruit juices, nuts, and meats that are high in potassium. The physician may order a potassium supplement such as K-lyte, an effervescent tablet that is dissolved in water. Occasionally, potassium chloride is added to intravenous infusions. Diuretics should be administered early in the morning so that the patient's rest will not be disturbed at night. When patients are receiving diuretics, output and intake should be measured, and physicians usually request that patients be weighed daily.[10] Loss of weight indicates that the excess water is being excreted.

COMPOSITION OF URINE

Urine consists of excess water and substances considered waste products that result from body metabolism. Urine is approximately 95% water, and its physical characteristics vary, depending on several factors. Normal urine is slightly acid and clear, but it will become alkaline and cloudy on standing. Its color is pale yellow to amber, depending on the amount of pigment in it. The specific gravity varies with the amount of solids dissolved in the water. The kidneys are responsible for regulating the specific gravity, which may vary in the normal person from 1.003 to 1.030. When a large amount of urine is excreted, the specific gravity will be low; when the urine is concentrated, the specific gravity will be high. Many substances are dissolved in the urine, chief among which is urea, a waste product resulting from protein metabolism and accounting for half the solid material in urine. If the diet is high in protein, the urea will be increased; if the diet is low in protein, the urea will be decreased. Other waste products found in normal urine occur in lesser amounts, and the origin of some is unclear. In addition, normal urine contains several salts (electrolytes), of which sodium chloride accounts for more than half. Others are potassium, magnesium, and calcium. Earlier in this chapter it was stated that a function of the urinary system is to maintain a balance of electrolytes, and when an excess occurs above the body's needs, it is excreted.

In pathologic conditions the urine may contain certain substances, the presence of which is normal in the body but abnormal in the urine. The presence of albumin in blood plasma is normal, but its appearance in the urine is abnormal. Albumin may be present in the urine in some kidney disease, heart disease, and fevers. Glucose is normally found in the blood, but its presence in the urine is abnormal and may be an indication of diabetes; however, it may occur temporarily because of excess ingestion of sugar, which the body cannot immediately use. Other abnormal substances include acetone, found in diabetic acidosis, and casts of different kinds, which are formed in the kidney tubules. Stones may be formed in any part of the urinary tract and if small, may be washed out in the urine. The presence of pus, blood, or bile is abnormal and indicates some disease condition.[22]

DIAGNOSTIC TESTS AND PROCEDURES
Urinalysis—collection of specimens

The responsibility for the collection of urine specimens is often a nursing procedure. If the specimen is to be of value to the physician, certain factors should be kept in mind. All specimens will not keep for the same length of time. If bacteria are present, they will multiply rapidly and may alter other abnormal elements in the specimen. Therefore specimens should be taken to the laboratory immediately after their collection.

Routine collection. A carefully collected voided specimen is usually satisfactory for a routine examination. The specimen should contain the first urine voided in the morning and should be collected in a clean receptacle. To avoid the presence of unnecessary bacteria in the specimen the vulva or urinary meatus of the male patient should be bathed with warm water and a mild soap prior to collection of the specimen. Approximately 4 ounces should be placed in a specimen bottle, properly labeled, and sent to the laboratory. If the specimen is to be examined in the physician's office, the patient may be asked to void in the office or should void just before leaving home and take the specimen to the physician's office. (To collect a specimen from an infant, refer to a textbook on basic nursing.) The routine examination usually includes observing the urine's appearance, testing for acidity or alkalinity, specific gravity, albumin, and glucose, and microscopic examination for red blood cells, white blood cells, and epithelial cells.

Sterile specimens. Sterile specimens are collected by catheterizing the patient under aseptic conditions. (Refer to a textbook on basic nursing.) Some physicians require that catheterized specimens be secured from all female patients to avoid contamination. If vaginal bleeding is present, a voided specimen is generally unsatisfactory. If the patient is incontinent, catheterization may be necessary to secure a specimen. When a retention catheter is inserted into the urinary bladder, a sterile specimen may be secured at any time by sterilizing a spot on the catheter with an alcohol sponge and then using a sterile syringe and needle to puncture the catheter so that the specimen can be withdrawn.[20] A sterile, catheterized specimen may be required from a small child, and its collection often presents a nursing problem.[18] The nurse should recall previous discussion concerning the dangers of infection associated with catheterization. Many physicians are reluctant to order catheterization except in emergency situations.

"Clean-catch" specimen. Some hospitals use a procedure known as the *clean-catch* specimen to avoid catheterization. The patient is prepared as for catheterization and asked to void. The first urine voided is discarded, after which a sterile specimen container is held to catch the subsequent stream. The procedure should be explained to the patient and his cooperation secured. Specimens collected in this manner have been found to be as reliable as catheterized specimens, and the danger of introducing infection into the urinary system is avoided. The procedure is not suitable for all patients or for patients with urinary retention.

Commercial urine tests. There has been increased development of commercial urine tests designed to detect abnormal substances. Most of these tests consist of paper tapes or strips that are dipped into the urine and immediately compared with an accompanying color chart. These tests have been found useful in the physician's offices and hospitals because of their simplicity and the value of an immediate result. Some tests to detect sugar in urine may be taught to patients with diabetes and are suitable for home use.

Acetest Test used for detection of acetone, often in connection with the Clinitest.
Azostix Sixty-second test for blood urea nitrogen.
Bili-Labstix Dip and read test for pH, protein, glucose, ketones, bilirubin, and blood in urine.
Clinitest Most common test used in the home for detection of sugar in the urine.
Hema-Combistix Test for pH, glucose, protein, and occult blood.
Ketostix Test for ketones in the urine or serum plasma.
Phenistix Paper tape to detect the presence of ferric chloride in the urine; used in the diaper test to detect phenylketonuria.
Uristix Test for proteinuria and glycosuria.
Urobilistix Sixty-second colorimetric test for urine urobilinogen.

Fractional (two-glass) test. The fractional test is used for male patients when the urine contains blood or pus, and the test is diagnostic in determining whether the difficulty is in the upper or lower urinary tract. The patient is asked to void approximately 100 ml. into one container and, without interrupting the stream, to void the remaining urine into a second container. Each container must be properly identified.

Urine culture. When the patient appears to have a urinary tract infection, the physician may request that cultures be done. This involves a bacteriologic study of the urine for specific organisms. After the specific organism is isolated in the culture a sensitivity test is often done to determine which antibiotics can be used to eliminate the infection. Except in unusual circumstances, cultures are made only on sterile specimens. Sterile culture tubes with a sterile stopper are used, and the patient is catheterized, using aseptic technique. Before the specimen is collected a small amount of urine is allowed to flow out of the urethra. The urine is then collected directly into the tube. Care must be taken not to let the catheter or the hands come in contact with the rim or the inside of the culture tube. The stopper is placed in the tube, which is properly labeled and sent to the laboratory. When cotton plugs are used as stoppers, the tube must be kept in an upright position and the urine not allowed to touch the cotton. When properly carried out, the clean-catch specimen has been found satisfactory for cultures. Specimens for cultures may be obtained from the male patient without catheterization. The urinary meatus is thoroughly cleansed, and the patient voids a small amount to wash out the urethra. The subsequent stream is collected in a sterile container for transfer to the culture tube or may be collected directly into the culture tube.

Tests of kidney function

Tests to determine the functional capacity of the kidney may be divided into three groups: (1) tests to determine the ability of the kidney to filter materials from the blood, (2) tests to determine the ability of the tubules to reabsorb the usable substances and to concentrate and dilute urine, and (3) tests to determine the ability of the tubules to excrete waste materials as urine.

Nonprotein nitrogen (NPN) and blood urea nitrogen (BUN) tests. Nonprotein nitrogen and blood urea nitrogen tests are performed on the blood. Both tests give essentially the same information. In some kidney disorders the ability to remove urea from the blood is impaired, and the concentration of urea in the blood rises. When this occurs, the BUN and NPN levels will be elevated. When an increase or a continued rise occurs in the test results, the nurse should be alert for critical symptoms in the patient. Disorientation, mental confusion, convulsions, or coma may occur. Precautions that include side rails on the bed and a mouth gag should be available, and close observation of the patient should be provided.[26]

Concentration and dilution tests. The concentration test is done to determine the ability of the kidney tubules to concentrate urine. The fluid intake is restricted for approximately 12 hours, after which three urine specimens are secured at hourly intervals and the specific gravity determined on each. Normally the more concentrated the urine the higher will be the specific gravity; thus if the specific gravity is low, it may indicate renal damage.

Dilution tests measure the ability of the kidney tubules to dilute urine. Procedures vary according to the particular test used, but the principle is the same. Food and drink are restricted for approximately 12 hours. The patient then voids, and the specimen is discarded. He is then given approximately 1200 ml. of water to drink, after which specimens are collected at specified intervals. The patient with normal kidney function will excrete nearly the total amount of the 1200 ml. All specimens should be properly labeled, including the time of collection, and sent to the laboratory, where the specific gravity is determined for each specimen.

Phenolsulfonphthalein (PSP) test. The phenolsulfonphthalein test determines the excretory ability of the kidney tubules. The patient is instructed to drink several glasses of water, after which the phenolsulfonphthalein, a red dye, is injected intravenously. Specimens are then collected at intervals of 15, 30, 60, and 120 minutes. Each specimen is labeled with the time and sent to the laboratory. In patients with certain diseases or disorders such as chronic nephritis or obstruction, there is a decrease in the amount of dye excreted in the 2 hours, whereas normally all would be ex- *[more dependable than a BUN]* creted. *xxx*

Serum creatinine test. The serum creatinine test underlines measures kidney function and is being used more extensively because it appears to give a more accurate measure of renal function. With the patient in a fasting state a blood sample is taken. Normally creatinine is excreted in the urine and is relatively constant from day to day. When renal function is impaired, there will be an elevation of creatinine in the blood.

• • •

[handwritten: Renal Function Tests]

Approximate normal values of renal function tests may vary with the method used but are usually as follows:

Nonprotein nitrogen (NPN)	15 to 35 mg./100 ml. serum
Blood urea nitrogen (BUN)	10 to 20 mg./100 ml. blood
Phenolsulfonphthalein (PSP) IV	35% in 15 minutes 65% in 1 hour
Serum creatinine	0.7 to 1.5 mg./100 ml. serum
Creatinine clearance	
Male	110 to 150 ml./min.
Female	105 to 132 ml./min.
Concentration	
(after dry day)	Specific gravity 1.026
(after 1000 ml. water)	Specific gravity 1.003

Nursing responsibilities

The success of these tests depends to a large extent on the accuracy with which the nursing functions are carried out. These responsibilities include adequate explanation to the patient, withholding food and fluids for specified intervals, keeping the patient at rest when indicated, administering water and fluids as ordered, collecting specimens at exactly the specified intervals, and properly labeling and forwarding them to the laboratory. Since procedures vary among physicians and hospitals and since many different kinds of tests exist, the nurse must understand the directions for preparation of the patient for each particular test or examination.

Other tests and procedures

X-ray examination (KUB). A flat x-ray film is taken of the abdomen to visualize the kidneys, ureters, and bladder and serves as a screening prior to other procedures.

The preparation of the patient usually includes administration of a laxative on the day before the examination and a cleansing enema of tap water or physiologic saline solution 1 hour before the x-ray examination. Fluids are withheld after midnight, and breakfast is omitted. The nurse should be sure that the patient empties the bladder before reporting to the x-ray department. Since preparation may vary, the nurse should be familiar with the physician's orders.

Pyelography. *[IVP]* *[Pyelogram]* Two methods using a radiopaque dye are employed for securing x-ray films of the kidneys. In intravenous pyelography the dye is injected into a vein, and a series of x-ray films are taken at short intervals while the dye is being excreted. The physician will be able to determine the size, shape, and location of the kidneys and evaluate their exretory function. Careful preparation of the patient is necessary, and care must be taken to see that the patient receives no fluids for approximately 12 hours before the examination. *[cut liq. for 12 hrs]* Whenever an intravenous dye is to be given, the patient should be carefully questioned concerning any allergy, since some persons may be sensitive to the dye. Physicians will vary in some aspects of preparing the patient for the examination. Some physicians may order a laxative for the evening before, or enemas may be given in the morning. Fecal matter and gas in the intestinal tract will interfere with the visualization of the kidneys and the ureters on the x-ray film. The nurse should be certain of the effectiveness of whatever procedure is used, and failure to achieve satisfactory results should be reported. When the patient is returned to his room, fluids should be forced to help eliminate any dye that may be left in the body.

Retrograde pyelography, consists of injecting a radiopaque substance into the kidney pelvis through ureteral catheters passed into the ureters through the bladder and taking x-ray films. It is often done when an obstruction of the ureters is suspected. Urine specimens may be secured from each kidney prior to injecting the contrast medium; this procedure is called *ureteral catheterization.* The contrast medium may also be injected into the ureters and x-ray films taken. Retrograde pyelography is usually done in connection with cystoscopic examination of the bladder. Unlike intravenous pyelography, when the patient is to be examined by retrograde pyelography, he is encouraged to drink fluids prior to the examination. Otherwise, preparation of the patient is the same as that for intravenous pyelography.

Force Fluids (margin note)

Cystography. A catheter is introduced into the bladder, and the urine is removed, after which a radiopaque substance is injected into the bladder and x-ray films are taken. The examination assists the physician in detecting the presence of stones, tumors, or any other pathologic condition.

Bladder X-ray (margin note)

Cystoscopic examination. The cystoscopic examination allows the physician direct visualization of the inside of the urinary bladder. A cystoscope is a long, metal, lighted instrument that can be passed through the urethra and into the bladder to observe the bladder and ureteral openings for any abnormality. The examination may be done while the patient is under local anesthesia, or the patient may be given a general anesthetic. Unless a general anesthetic is to be given, fluids are forced, and the patient does not void prior to the examination. The cystoscopic examination is usually done as a part of a complete urinary study and is indicated for all patients who have blood in the urine (hematuria). A sedative such as phenobarbital or meperidine hydrochloride (Demerol) may be given 30 minutes before the procedure. The nurse should be sure that the patient knows what to expect prior to leaving the unit. After the procedure the urine may be blood tinged, or sometimes a blue or red dye may have been used to evaluate kidney function. The patient should understand that the discoloration is to be expected and that it will clear up. The patient may have some mild discomfort such as burning on urination or pain in the back. There may be chills, an elevation of temperature, and nausea and vomiting, and occasionally the patient may be unable to void after the procedure. Analgesic drugs, warm sitz baths, and external heat to the back and abdomen may be ordered. Occasionally the pain is severe enough to require the administration of a narcotic such as codeine or meperidine hydrochloride. Patients having a cystoscopic examination should al-

Bladder exam. (margin note)

Problems after cysto. (margin note)

ways be observed for possible hemorrhage after the procedure.

Radioisotope studies

Renography. A small amount of radioactive material usually [131]I Hippuran is administered intravenously to measure renal function. A graphic record (renogram) is made by spikes that trace the arrival of the material, its secretion, and drainage. When an obstruction is present in the renal artery, the arrival phase of the material will show very low spikes and those of the drainage phase will be prolonged.

Renoscan. The renoscan is a procedure that outlines the kidney by external scanning. A radioactive isotope such as [197]Hg (mercury) is tagged to the mercurial diuretic chlormerodrin (Neohydrin) and administered intravenously. A scanning device such as a scintillation counter is passed over each kidney on the patient's back over the areas of the kidneys. In the presence of tumors or nonfunctioning areas the radioactive material will not be detected by the scan.

Renovascular studies. Through the use of radioactive isotopes it is now possible to do a renal arteriogram, aortogram, venograph, and lymphangiogram. These studies may be made to examine the vascular supply. It is possible to detect the presence of thromboses, atherosclerotic plaques, and other obstructions in the flow of blood. Solid and cystic tumors, abdominal aneurysms, and other disorders may be detected that supply valuable information for the physician.[14]

SPECIFIC ASPECTS OF NURSING THE PATIENT WITH DISEASES AND DISORDERS OF THE URINARY SYSTEM
Intake and output

The fluid intake and urinary output must be accurately measured for all patients with urologic disease. Unless the patient's condition necessitates restriction of fluids, they should be given freely. Fluids should include a variety of juices, tea, coffee, and soups, as well as water. Adequate hydration keeps the urinary system irrigated and prevents urine from becoming concentrated. The fluid intake should not be less than 3000 ml. and for some patients may be as great as 5000 ml. a day. Unless fluids are being lost through excessive perspiration, vomiting, and diarrhea, the urinary output should be nearly equal to the fluid intake (Fig. 15-2). Many patients will be able to help maintain the record when they understand why it is important. However, the nurse will have to be responsible for many older patients whose condition prevents them from assuming the responsibility. If for any reason fluids cannot be given by the oral route, they often can be given intravenously.

Provision for urinary drainage

There are several types of drainage procedures. The most common method is to allow the urine to flow by gravity. It is recommended that a closed drainage system be used for all patients needing urinary drainage. Studies indicate that unless the patient is receiving antibiotic therapy, from 85% to 100% of patients will acquire a urinary tract infection within 2 to 4 days if an open system is used. Some studies show that the infection rate may be as high as 70% to 80%, even when the patient is receiving antibiotic therapy. In contrast, bacteria developed in only 21% of the patients with closed urinary drainage in one study of open and closed collection sets.[1] Closed systems have the drainage tube sealed to the container, whereas open systems are not sealed and allow air to enter the system freely.

Collection sets in widespread use contain sterile drainage tubing permanently connected to plastic containers. Most containers are flexible bags that have drains at the bottom of the bag to allow the urine to be emptied when the bag becomes full. The end of the drain is protected by a cap, and the tube is fastened to the container when it is not being used. Most containers have valves at the top of the container where the drainage tubing enters to prevent bacteria from entering the drainage tubing and traveling upward toward the urethra and bladder. Filter air vents are also located on the top of the containers that allow air to enter the system but prevent bacteria in the air from contaminating the urine. All collection containers have a bed hanger, which keeps the container in an upright position and off the floor[1] (Fig. 15-3).

The drainage tubing may be placed over the thigh, downward between the legs, or under the patient's leg near the popliteal space. Excess tubing should be coiled on the bed and not allowed to loop below the collection container. Many collection sets provide safety pins and rubber bands so that the tubing may be attached to the sheets in a proper manner. Care must be taken that the tubing does not become kinked or obstructed by the patient lying on it. Often the tubing is taped to the inner aspect of the patient's thigh. If the urine flow is blocked, stasis occurs and provides

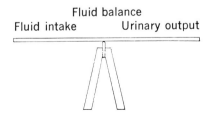
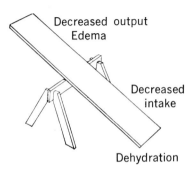

Fig. 15-2. Fluid balance. Output should equal intake.

Fluid balance
Fluid intake   Urinary output

Decreased output
Edema

Decreased intake

Dehydration

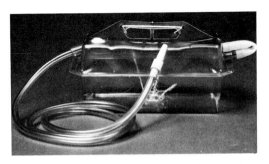

Fig. 15-3. Urinary collection set. Drain-box container. (Courtesy Abbott Laboratories, North Chicago, Ill.)

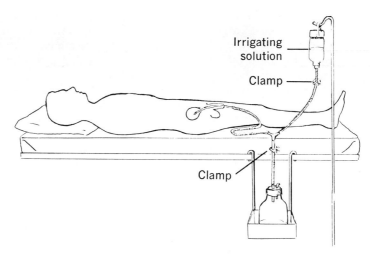

Irrigating
solution

Clamp

Clamp

Fig. 15-4. Retention catheter inserted for urinary drainage. Closed system with provision for catheter irrigation.

good media for bacteria to grow. The entire system should remain sterile and should not be disconnected. The collection set and tubing should not be lifted or elevated, since drainage may flow back into the bladder.

If bladder or catheter irrigation is ordered by the physician, a Y tube is attached with one arm connected to the catheter, one arm attached to the drainage tubing, and the third arm attached to tubing connected to a bottle of sterile irrigating solution that is hung on an irrigating stand beside the bed (Fig. 15-4). For irrigation to take place the drainage tube is clamped, the clamp on the irrigating solution is opened, and the specified amount of solution is allowed to run through the tubing into the bladder. The irrigating tubing is then clamped, the drainage tubing is unclamped, and the solution is allowed to drain out of the bladder. The physician will order the kind of solution, the amount, and the interval for irrigation. If continuous irrigation of the bladder is ordered, it may be accomplished by attaching a Murphy drip connector below the bottle of irrigating solution and regulating the rate of drip. For continuous irrigation the drainage tubing is left unclamped.

Several different types of apparatus are used for tidal drainage, and the nurse will need to understand the particular kind of apparatus to be used. However, the basic principle is the same regardless of the kind of equipment. It is an automatic system by which the bladder is filled and emptied through siphonage. The physician may set up the system and adjust it, but the nurse must observe it to be sure that sufficient solution is available and that it is filling and emptying properly. This type of drainage is often used for persons suffering from spinal cord damage with paralysis of the bladder and helps to maintain muscle tone and prevent infection.

Catheter care

Disposable catheterization trays, which are used once and then discarded, have reduced the threat of cross infection from one patient to another. The trays usually contain gloves, a protective pad, cotton balls, cleansing solution, lubricant, forceps, specimen bottle, and a catheter. Foley catheter trays often contain the collection set and a syringe of sterile water to inflate the Foley bag. Most catheters are made of plastic or are coated with Teflon or silicone, which does not irritate the mucosa of the urinary tract as much as a rubber catheter.

Patients whose condition necessitates the presence of indwelling catheters over an extended period of time often present nursing problems. This is especially true of chronically ill patients. Points that should be remembered are that the catheter should provide free flow of urinary drainage and should be comfortable for the patient. Having a catheter of the proper size is important. If the catheter is too small, leakage may occur around it, and if it is too large, it may be uncomfortable for the patient. The Foley retention catheter is available in various sizes with balloons of 30 and 5 ml. capacity. For most patients a size 16 Fr. catheter with a 5 ml. balloon is satisfactory and will be both comfortable and adequate for free drainage. Often, when a 30 ml. balloon is used, the tip of the catheter may bend on the balloon and obstruct the flow of urine.

Free drainage is facilitated when the patient receives adequate amounts of fluids. Adequate fluid intake helps to prevent accumulation of mucus, minerals, and exudate, which may adhere to the catheter and cause obstruction, and it also eliminates the necessity for irrigation.

Crusts and secretions about the vulva and around the catheter should be removed and the area cleansed twice daily. Povidone iodine (Betadine) ointment is often applied to the urethral opening and around the catheters and has been found to be effective against gram-positive and gram-negative bacteria. When it is necessary for patients to have retention catheters indefinitely, the catheter should be changed every 7 to 10 days, and the tubing should be changed weekly or more often if it becomes encrusted with organic deposits. Catheter care is a nursing responsibility, and every nurse entrusted with the care of patients having retention catheters must assume responsibility for good care in helping to prevent urinary tract infection.

Pyelostomy, nephrostomy, ureterostomy, and cystostomy catheters. Several surgical procedures are performed on the urinary system in which the patient will return from the operating room with a catheter placed in the kidney pelvis (pyelostomy) or in the kidney tissue (nephrostomy). The nephrostomy catheter is brought out through a stab wound or an incision in the flank and sutured to the skin. Catheters may be in one or both kidneys. Ureterostomy catheters may be passed through the ureters into the kidney pelvis and brought out through the abdomen. These catheters are attached to free drainage, and any catheter placed in the kidney pelvis is never clamped. Care must be taken to prevent any displacement of these catheters, since reinsertion may not be possible. The nurse should observe the catheters frequently to be sure they are open and draining, and any evidence of failure to drain must be reported to the physician immediately. All drainage is measured and recorded. Sometimes a catheter is placed in the bladder through an abdominal wound (cystostomy) and is attached to drainage at the bedside. All equipment used for pyelostomy, nephrostomy, ureterostomy, and cystostomy drainage must be kept sterile.

Catheter irrigation. A physician's order should be secured for catheter irrigation. If fluid intake is adequate and no blood clots occur, it should not be necessary to irrigate the urethral catheter unless the procedure is specifically ordered (p. 344). Thirty milliliters of physiologic saline solution is usually sufficient to determine patency of the catheter, or intermittent irrigation may be accomplished with the closed system referred to previously in this chapter. After irrigation the solution should return by gravity. If the irrigating fluid flows in well but does not return, a clot is usually present at the end of the catheter. If it cannot be dislodged by milking the tube, the physician should be notified. The nurse should remember that catheter irrigation is done to keep the catheter open and draining and not to irrigate the bladder.

If the patient has a bilateral pyelostomy and irrigations are ordered, separate equipment must be maintained for each catheter. The irrigating equipment and solution must be sterile, and only 8 to 10 ml., depending on the physician's order, is used for the irrigation. The solution must be injected extremely carefully and gently and its return by gravity observed. Failure of the solution to return must be reported, and additional solution should not be injected.

Patient care after catheter removal

The removal of the urethral catheter should be preceded by complete deflation of the balloon. After its removal the patient should be observed for retention or dribbling and often for residual urine. There may be a dribbling because of dilation of the sphincter muscles. Frequently the patient is unable to void normally, and sometimes catheterization and replacement of the retention catheter may be necessary. If the patient voids only small amounts, the bladder may not be completely emptying. Occasionally the capacity of the bladder may be temporarily decreased, and the patient will complain of discomfort soon after the removal of the catheter, while being unable to void. The patient should be instructed to assist in keeping a record of the time and the amount voided, and the appearance of the urine should be observed. If blood appears in the urine, the physician should be notified. Frequently it is necessary to maintain accurate output records for several days, especially if the patient has had urologic surgery.

Dressings

Many patients with disorders of the urinary system will have draining wounds. Although the patient may have understood this before surgery, when he is faced with the discomfort of wet dressings, the odor of urine, and the resulting skin irritation, he may become irritable and depressed and feel that adjustment is impossible. It may tax the ingenuity of the nurse to find ways to overcome these problems. Since dressings will need to be changed frequently, Montgomery straps or laced dressings should be used to avoid irritation from adhesive tape. Small dressings changed frequently will keep the patient more comfortable than large bulky ones that become saturated, heavy, and foul smelling. A ureterostomy cup may be applied and attached to free drainage, or the disposable plastic ileostomy bags may be used for some patients. Commercial suction cups are available that may be effective in some drainage problems. Any device used is only an adjunct to good nursing care, which includes cleansing the skin and protecting wounds from infection.

Follow-up care

Many patients are dismissed from the hospital to their homes with indwelling catheters, draining wounds, and permanent appliances. There should be a planned program teaching the patient self-care insofar as he is competent. This includes three steps: (1) observation, (2) participation, and (3) practice under supervision. The patient will observe the nurse in the various procedures; at the same time the nurse explains, step by step, what is being done and the reason for it. As the patient is able, he begins to assist the nurse or participate in the procedures, gradually assuming more and more of the care. Finally the nurse allows the patient to give all the care while observing him to correct any mistakes. When the patient leaves the hospital, he should feel secure because he knows what to do and how to do it. There may be catheters or dressings posteriorly that the patient cannot reach, and a member of the family should be instructed in the care. In addition, some hospitals provide written instructions with a list of the home equipment needed for the patient or his family. In planning care for patients with urologic conditions, it has been found that each patient has his own special problems and that it does not help him to meet other patients with the same or similar conditions. There should be a referral system between the hospital and the public health agency, and when it can be arranged the public health nurse should visit the patient in the hospital before he goes home. Information should be available to the public health nurse concerning the care needed and the instructions given the patient. When the patient returns home, the public health nurse will visit him to supervise or assist with the necessary care. The continuity of care between the hospital and the home provides a feeling of security for the patient and facilitates the process of rehabilitation.

NURSING THE PATIENT WITH DISEASES AND DISORDERS OF THE URINARY SYSTEM
Noninfectious diseases
Glomerulonephritis No cure

Glomerulonephritis was first recognized and described by Richard Bright in 1876, and it is often referred to as _Bright's disease_. The term encompasses several conditions affecting the nephrons of the kidney. All of the disorders are characterized by albuminuria, hypoproteinuria, and renal failure. Glomerulonephritis may be acute, subacute, and chronic. It generally affects

affects both kidneys

children and young adults and affects males more often than females. Most children are under 7 years of age, and the disease appears most often in the springtime.[3] During the acute stage of the disease severe inflammation of the glomeruli, edema caused by water retention, and oliguria are present. Frequently hypertension occurs. If the disease becomes subacute, large amounts of protein are lost *(proteinuria)* and albuminuria and edema are present, whereas in chronic glomerulonephritis hypertension and renal failure may be anticipated.

Pathophysiology. Glomerulonephritis affects the glomeruli of both kidneys, causing inflammation of the glomeruli, reduced glomeruli filtration because capillary vessels become obstructed, atrophy of the nephrons, and renal failure. The disease follows a streptococcal infection, and it has been thought that the disease was caused by the streptococci. However, since the invasion of the glomeruli by the bacteria cannot be demonstrated, and because of the interval between the initial infection and the onset of the disease, it is now believed that an antigen-antibody reaction is the cause. The onset of glomerulonephritis is usually abrupt, with fever, nausea and vomiting, edema about the eyes, weakness, loss of appetite, pallor, and abnormal urinary constituents. The type of red blood cell found in the urine is considered to be of diagnostic value. Blood pressure may be elevated, and convulsions may occur in children. The disease may progress rapidly to renal failure and death. With prompt and adequate treatment, recovery may be expected in 85% to 100% of children, whereas 35% to 65% of adults may be expected to recover.[5] If there is a continuation of symptoms, the disease becomes subacute and ultimately becomes chronic. In chronic glomerulonephritis the damage to the nephrons is permanent, and kidney function is reduced as normal tissue is replaced by fibrous tissue.

Treatment and nursing care. Bed rest is essential, and convalescence will extend over a long period of time. The patient should not be allowed to become chilled, and it is best if an even room temperature can be maintained. The patient must not be exposed to respiratory infections through contact with visitors or other patients. The diet is prescribed on the basis of symptoms.

If suppression of urine or a significant decrease in the urinary output occurs, fluids, protein foods, and potassium are restricted, and the diet is high in carbohydrate. If edema is present, sodium will be restricted, and patients with severe cases may be given glucose orally or by a drip method through a nasogastric tube to provide the necessary carbohydrate. All urinary output or vomitus must be accurately measured and recorded. The patient is weighed daily to determine the increase or decrease of edema fluid. Edematous areas should be supported with pillows; frequent massage and change of position are important. Warm baths and special mouth care should be given, and small enemas or mild laxatives may be ordered for elimination. Vital signs are checked and recorded every 4 hours, and any sudden elevation in blood pressure or decrease in pulse rate should be reported to the physician.

Several laboratory tests and examinations may be done, including blood cultures, renal function studies, and immunoglobulin levels (p. 40). Symptoms vary with the individual patient, but a generalized edema is present and may continue for months or years. The course of the disease is variable, with periods of remission when the patient may feel well followed by periods of exacerbation. Although the patient may live for years, renal failure eventually develops (p. 351). During periods of exacerbation, bed rest is indicated, and the patient receives a diet that is low in sodium. Hypertension, anemia, or congestive heart failure may be present, and the patient is treated according to the severity of the symptoms. Convalescence must be a slow, gradual process.

Since acute glomerulonephritis is a disease of children and young persons, their needs will vary. Rest and decreased physical activity are important, and activities that will interest and keep a young child quiet must be provided. There are many simple games and toys that provide limited activity; cutting, pasting, and drawing materials will provide amusement. A variety of activities is necessary to prevent monotony. The nurse in the hospital or the parents in the home must plan to spend many hours with the child if he is to be kept quiet.

The problems of the adolescent are different. He worries about his absence from school, and falling behind his class is a traumatic experience. At times it is possible to continue with some schoolwork while in bed. The physician must determine the amount of activity that the individual may have. The adolescent is curious, and he wants to know. He may be expected to cooperate better if he is given the reason why each aspect of his treatment is necessary. He should be given details concerning the various tests, why some must be repeated, and why he must follow a certain diet. He should be made a partner in his treatment who can be depended on to participate in many aspects of his care because he wants to be respected and treated as a mature individual.[15]

Nephrotic syndrome

The nephrotic syndrome is a functional disorder causing tubular degeneration. It is characterized by increased amounts of protein in the urine *(proteinuria)*, abnormally low albumin in the blood *(hypoalbuminemia)*, excessive amount of fat in the blood *(hyperlipemia)*, and generalized edema. The disorder affects both children and adults but is most common in children. There are numerous causes, including some infectious diseases, poisoning from chemical substances, toxemia of pregnancy, shock resulting from external burns, or coronary occlusion, and the condition may follow transfusion with incompatible blood.

Treatment. Treatment usually consists of administration of diuretics to decrease the edema. Dietary restraints depend on the severity of symptoms, and the individual is encouraged to continue normal activity. Bed rest is not required. The disorder is generally chronic, and consideration must be given to the precipitating cause.[14]

Nephrosclerosis

Nephrosclerosis is due to sclerosis of the blood vessels in the kidney and is accompanied by hypertension. The disease usually progresses slowly, and only a small number of patients develop renal failure. However, it may occur as a result of heart failure. In patients with malignant hypertension, kidney function is rapidly impaired, and renal failure develops.

Treatment and nursing care. The treatment and nursing care of patients with nephrosclerosis is the same as that for patients with hypertensive heart disease (p. 268).

Infectious diseases
Cystitis

Cystitis is an inflammation of the lining of the bladder. It may be acute or chronic and is more common in the female than the male. The female urethra is shorter and straighter than the male urethra and therefore is more easily traumatized or contaminated. Cystitis may be caused by bacteria that enter through the urinary meatus, or it may occur through catheterization, during which organisms in the urethra are carried into the bladder. Infections may also be carried from the upper urinary tract, beginning with the kidney and involving the ureters and the bladder. In this instance the infectious organism gains entrance to the kidney by way of the bloodstream. Cystitis may result from nonbacterial factors such as injury to the lining of the bladder caused by instruments or a catheter, or it may be caused by certain drugs that are excreted by the kidneys and eliminated in the urine.

The symptoms are frequent urination, with severe pain in the urethra occurring after urination. Examination of the urine may show the presence of pus and may reveal blood. Frequently specific pathogenic organisms are not found.

Treatment and nursing care. The first criterion of treatment is to establish the cause of the problem. Antispasmodic drugs, sulfonamide or antibiotic drugs, and preparations to alkalize the urine may be ordered. The patient should be encouraged to drink water freely. Hot sitz baths and the application of heat to the abdomen may relieve pain. Phenazopyridine (Pyridium), a urinary antiseptic, may be given to relieve discomfort.

Cystitis may be caused by the gonococcus bacteria, in which case treatment of the primary infection (gonorrhea) with penicillin is indicated.

Pyelonephritis

Pyelonephritis is a pyogenic infection involving the parenchyma and the collection system of the kidney. One or both kidneys may be involved. The disorder occurs as an acute infection, and the possibility of it becoming chronic has been questioned. Although pyelitis (infection of the kidney pelvis) may occur alone, it is considered rare.[2]

Pathophysiology. Pyelonephritis is caused by bacterial infection. Pathogenic organisms that may be responsible for infection include the *Proteus* group, *Escherichia coli,* and *Pseudomonas* (p. 68); less common are the streptococcus and the staphylococcus bacteria. The infection may be brought to the kidney by the bloodstream or the lymphatic system from infection elsewhere in the body. It may also spread upward from the bladder. Infants under 18 months of age frequently develop the condition that results from fecal soiling of the urinary meatus. Women between 18 and 40 years of age are affected more often than men. Factors that contribute to the disorder include obstructions that restrict urinary flow, examinations such as cystoscopy, and catheterization. Pyelonephritis may occur in persons with some neurologic diseases or with conditions that require long periods of immobilization during which urinary calculi may develop.

The kidney becomes edematous and inflamed, and the blood vessels are congested. The urine may be cloudy and contain pus, mucus, and blood. Small abscesses may form in the kidney. Diagnosis is made by microscopic examination of the urine and urine cultures; an intravenous urogram may be done.

The symptoms may occur abruptly with fever, chills, elevated leukocyte count, aching, urinary frequency, and dysuria. There may or may not be pain in the back.

Treatment and nursing care. The treatment of the patient depends on locating and eliminating the cause. Sensitivity tests are done, and the appropriate antibiotic is administered. Antibiotics often used include nitrofurantoin (Furadantin), penicillin, chloramphenicol (Chloromycetin), and streptomycin. Sulfonamide agents may also be used. Bed rest is required during the acute period. Fluid intake is encouraged, and all intake and output should be recorded. The patient should be observed for any difficulty in voiding such as pain and burning. Urine should be observed for color. Bowel elimination should be provided by enemas or laxative agents ordered by the physician. The patient should be kept warm, should not be exposed to drafts or chilling, and should be protected from respiratory infections.

Perinephritic abscess

Abscess in the soft tissue of the kidney may be single or multiple. The infection may be brought to the kidney by the bloodstream. Symptoms may vary, depending on the extent of the infection; however, chills, fever, tenderness over the kidney region, and increased leukocyte count may be present.

Treatment. The treatment is usually surgical, with incision and drainage and administration of the appropriate antibiotic drugs. There may be considerable drainage, and dressings will need changing frequently.

Obstructions of the urinary system

Obstructions of the urinary system may result from many different causes and may be located anywhere from the kidney to the urinary meatus. Any prolonged obstruction will lead to serious pathologic conditions, since the filtration rate will be reduced, pressure within the kidney or the bladder may cause dilation, and excretion of creatinine and urea will be reduced.

Renal calculi

The formation of stones is called *lithiasis,* and the presence of stones in the kidney is called *nephrolithiasis.* When stones occur in any other part of the urinary system, the location determines the term used, as in ureteral calculi. The exact cause of the formation of renal calculi is unknown, but some factors that contribute to their formation are known. Patients who are required to remain on a regimen of bed rest for long periods and paraplegic patients are likely to develop calculi because of stasis of urine and the release of increased amounts of calcium from bone. Some common organisms that cause infection of the bladder and kidney cause the urine to become alkaline. Calcium phosphate, a compound readily excreted by the kidneys, cannot dissolve in the alkaline urine and will form crystals around a shred of tissue or other substance in the kidney, resulting in stone formation. Patients requiring continuous urinary drainage often will develop kidney or bladder stones as a complication. Pathologic disorders such as senile osteoporosis, gout, infection, hyperparathyroidism, and disorders affecting the pH and concentration of the urine are believed to be contributing factors.[2]

Stones may be tiny "gravel," and the patient may be asymptomatic. Large stones with irregular branches may be present in the kidney pelvis; they are known as *staghorn* calculi and require surgical intervention. When stones occur in the kidney, pain is present on the involved side and usually radiates from the flank to the crest of the ileum. Pus may be present in the urine, resulting from infection at the back of the stone. Hematuria, usually microscopic, results from injury to the mucous membrane from the rough jagged edges of the stone.

Medical and nursing care. Most (90%) stones are small and they are usually passed in the urine; thus all urine should be strained through gauze and carefully inspected in patients with renal calculi. The patient is encouraged to drink at least 3000 ml. of fluid in 24 hours, since increasing urinary output will facilitate passage of the stone. If infection is present, the appropriate antibiotic may be ordered. The patient is encouraged to remain active because stones are more likely to be passed if the patient is ambulatory. Patients confined to bed should be turned regularly every 2 hours. The use of the tilt table, CircOlectric bed, rocking bed, and overhead trapeze provides exercise for the patient and helps in the prevention of stone formation. The nurse must be sure that the patient receives adequate hydration.[21]

Ureteral colic

Ureteral colic is caused by a stone passing down or becoming lodged in the ureter. The pain is excruciating and radiates down the ureter and may extend to the thigh and the urethra. Nausea, vomiting, and sweating occur, and the patient feels weak and faint.

Treatment. Narcotics are required to relieve the pain, and an antispasmodic drug such as methantheline (Banthine) or propanthedine (Pro-Banthine) may be ordered to relieve spasm. If stones are not passed,

any of several surgical procedures may be required to remove the stone. The physician may catheterize the ureters by passing a ureteral catheter through the cystoscope and into the ureteral orifice. This will drain the kidney and relieve the pain, and often the stone will be pulled out when the catheter is removed. If the stone is in the lower third of the ureter, it sometimes can be removed by manipulation of special catheters, which are passed through the cystoscope and into the ureter. If these methods are unsuccessful, surgery is done. X-ray films must be taken just prior to surgery to determine the exact location of the stone.

Hydronephrosis

Obstruction within the urinary tract may lead to dilation of the kidney pelvis and wasting of kidney tissue. The obstruction may be caused by stones, tumors, kinking of a ureter, congenital anomaly, or an enlarged prostate gland in the elderly male patient.

Treatment. The treatment is based on locating the obstruction, which may be done by a series of x-ray studies and tests. Depending on the cause, correction may be made and the condition cured. However, if the kidney has undergone considerable destruction, a nephrectomy may be necessary.

Traumatic injuries

Injuries to the urinary system often occur in connection with injuries to other parts of the body. Injuries may be caused by gunshot wounds, penetrating wounds from sharp objects, and crushing injuries with fracture of the pelvis, which may cause rupture of the bladder or the urethra. Injuries resulting from external violence such as falls or blows may result in simple injury to the kidney or may completely shatter the kidney. Many injuries are the result of automobile accidents, and on admission to the hospital the patient may be in shock. The initial concern is to stabilize the vital signs. Assessment of the extent of injury determines the method of treatment, which may be conservative, or surgical intervention may be required.

Tumors of the urinary tract

Tumors of the kidneys are generally malignant. The malignancy is often spread to the lungs and bones by the bloodstream. The primary symptom is blood in the urine. The treatment is nephrectomy and may be only palliative, since metastasis may have occurred. Wilms' tumor is one of the most frequent types of malignant tumors seen in children. It may often be detected during the first year of life, and if it is not discovered, it may reach a considerable size. It may be diagnosed by an intravenous pyelogram, and treatment is surgical removal, followed by irradiation. Metastasis has usually occurred, and the prognosis for such children is generally poor. However, recent research using the antibiotic dactinomycin (Cosmegen) combined with surgery and irradiation has more than doubled the survival rate. When metastasis is extensive throughout the body, however, a sufficient amount of the drug cannot be given to achieve cure.[19]

Cysts may occur in the kidney and often exert pressure against and destroy kidney tissue. Congenital polycystic kidney involves both kidneys and may present no symptoms until adult life. There is no known effective treatment, and death usually occurs from renal failure.

Tumors of the bladder may be benign or malignant. A complete urologic examination, including cystoscopy and biopsy, is done, and surgery is indicated, depending on complete diagnosis.

Renal failure

Renal failure may be acute or chronic and occurs when the kidneys can no longer perform their normal function. *critically ill*

Pathophysiology. Acute renal failure may develop insidiously or suddenly, occurring in several stages. The initial phase includes the causal factors, which are numerous. Postoperative shock may occur, during which the hypotension prevents the kidney from filtering the blood adequately. The decreased blood flow and lack of oxygen to the kidneys may cause acute renal failure. Other causes include burns, blood transfusion reactions, serous infections, antigen-antibody reactions, and obstructions. During the stage of oliguria the urinary output may drop to 400 ml. or less in 24 hours. The oliguric phase may last for only a day or two, or it may last for as long as 2 weeks. After the oliguric

stage the kidney begins to recover, and the diuretic stage begins when the urinary output starts to increase. Changes that occur in the kidney include necrosis and a sloughing of the lining of the renal tubules. There are areas of the nephron membrane that rupture, resulting in the formation of scar tissue. In renal failure resulting from glomerulonephritis or chronic renal disease, the nephrons have been permanently damaged, and the kidneys will not recover.

The blood chemistry shows an increase in the blood urea nitrogen (BUN) and the nonprotein nitrogen (NPN) levels. The serum potassium level is increased. Generalized edema, pruritus, headache, disturbance of vision, hypertension, and vomiting occur, and there is an odor of urine on the breath. The patient appears acutely ill.

Treatment and nursing care. Treatment for acute renal failure often begins with determining the cause and may involve many of the procedures reviewed earlier in this chapter. Treatment is designed according to the severity of the condition and is directed toward both preventing a fatal outcome of anuria and altering the course of the existing condition. The treatment of choice for many of these patients is dialysis, which many physicians believe should be started early. The diet is low in protein and high in carbohydrate to prevent the breakdown of proteins and decrease the possibility of ketosis. If the level of serum potassium continues to increase and becomes dangerously high, the sodium form of an exchange resin is administered to release the excess potassium. Conservative treatment may be continued; however, if there are indications that irreversible damage to the kidney has occurred, dialysis should be considered.[4, 14] *caused most often by glomerulonephritis*

Chronic renal failure occurs when four fifths of the kidney tissue has been destroyed and has been replaced by fibrous tissue, with no chance for repair or replacement of normal kidney tissue. The most common causes are pyelonephritis, chronic glomerulonephritis, and glomerulosclerosis. Terminal renal failure is inevitable, and the objectives of treatment are to keep the patient comfortable and to prolong life, which may be for a few weeks or several years.[23] *causes of chronic renal failure*

The patient with chronic renal failure will have failing vision, often with rentinal edema and hemorrhage. Other symptoms are severe edema, dyspnea, loss of appetite, failing heart action, mental confusion, and disorientation. If there is little edema, fluids may be given freely to provide for excretion of waste materials. However, they must be restricted if edema or anuria is present. Diet is not restricted and should be well balanced, with a minimum of salt. The protein intake may or may not be restricted. Blood transfusions may be given when the anemia is severe.

Frequent blood studies and determinations are done as well as electrocardiographic studies, daily weighing, and maintenance of electrolyte balance.

There is no cure for chronic renal failure. The damage to kidney tissue is irreversible, and kidney function cannot be restored to normal. Approximately 50,000 persons die each year as the result of renal failure, and although hemodialysis may prolong life, it is estimated that only one in ten persons would benefit from dialysis.

The nurse should be alert for the signs that may indicate renal failure; one of the most significant is a decreased urinary output of less than 400 ml. a day. When the kidneys cannot excrete the water, the fluid intake is decreased. The physician will specify how much fluid the patient may have, which may be less than 500 ml. a day. The patient often complains of thirst, and the thirst associated with renal failure cannot be relieved by ordinary means. Factors that the nurse must consider in relation to the patient's thirst include the total amount of fluid allowed, condition of the patient's mouth, fluid output, diet, physical activity, and the patient's mental state. There are ways in which the nurse can space the fluid without giving more fluid than the amount permitted. The following methods of administering medications should be considered: (1) giving several medications at mealtime, (2) giving small pills and capsules rather than large ones that may require larger amounts of water to swallow, (3) using solid forms of medications rather than liquid forms, (4) using small glasses rather than large glasses (a small glass full of water has a better psychologic effect than a large glass with a small amount of water), and (5) remembering that a small amount of cold water will be more satisfying than warm water.

Patients with renal failure develop a nonbacterial stomatitis as a complication. The more critical the patient's condition the more mouth care will be required, and in some cases it may have to be given hourly. Whatever method is used must meet the needs of the patient. The mouth may be dry because of dyspnea, or when the patient is receiving oxygen. Humidification of the air will provide moisture and relieve dryness. The patient may be allowed to chew gum, which will increase salivation and relieve dryness.

All fluid output must be accurately measured and recorded, including urine, vomitus, liquid stools, and perspiration. Weighing the patient each day at the same time helps to determine fluid loss. The diet may not be palatable, and the patient may need encouragement to accept it. Protein must be limited or omitted and the caloric intake reduced. The hospital dietitian may be helpful in suggesting moist foods rather than dry foods, which require more liquids. It should be kept in mind that salty foods, candy, and sweetened foods tend to increase thirst. Patients who are ambulatory must understand their disease and the reason for restriction of fluids. Otherwise they may take advantage of their ambulation and go to drinking fountains or secure water from other sources such as a tap in the bathroom. If the patient has some activity to keep his mind off himself, he will be less likely to be conscious of thirst. The nurse can be of assistance in helping to supply diversional activities for the patient.[8]

In the treatment of patients with chronic renal failure in which dietary restrictions may be less severe, the patient should be allowed to select foods of choice, and the family may be encouraged to bring foods from home that appeal to the patient's appetite. Fruit juices may be restricted to reduce the intake of potassium. Ginger ale may be given to reduce nausea. The patient should be protected from chilling, drafts, and exposure to respiratory infections. Insulin may be administered to some patients, and the nurse should be familiar with the

Diet very impt. in renal failure.

symptoms of insulin reaction (shock) and observe the patient carefully.

Patients who are on a regimen of bed rest may develop decubiti or pulmonary complications and should be turned regularly and encouraged to breathe deeply. The use of the Airmass alternating pressure pad may provide comfort for some patients. (See Chapter 6.) Skin care is extremely important in the care of patients with chronic renal failure, and frequent bathing is indicated. Sponging with a weak solution of vinegar (2 tablespoons to 1 pint of water) will often help to relieve itching. Edematous areas should be supported with pillows and circulation stimulated through active or passive exercises. Edematous extremities should be elevated above the level of the heart. Proper bowel function should be maintained to provide for the elimination of waste products. If the patient's vision is failing, care should be taken to prevent injury. Padded side rails should be used for patients who are confused or disoriented. The nurse should be sure that a padded mouth gag is kept at the bedside or nearby in case convulsions should occur.

Patients with chronic renal failure should be encouraged to participate in self-care activities and to remain active as long as their condition permits.[21]

Hemodialysis

Extracorporeal hemodialysis. Hemodialysis is a mechanical method of removing waste products and establishing equilibrium of electrolytes and water when the kidneys are unable to perform their function because of disease. Hemodialysis is accomplished by the use of the artificial kidney and may be used in (1) chronic renal failure caused by disease of the kidneys, (2) acute renal failure resulting from injury, infection, or surgery, and (3) drug poisoning. Hemodialysis will not cure the damage caused by these conditions but will remove waste products from the body and prevent damage to other organs until further treatment can be instituted and healing takes place.

The artificial kidney is a machine that is connected to the patient by cannulas, which have been placed in an artery and a vein (arteriovenous shunt). The machine must be primed with blood or plasma prior to the treatment, and when the treatment is begun, the patient's blood flows into the machine from the artery, through the machine, and back to the patient by way of the vein. The machine consists of a semipermeable membrane, much like cellophane, which separates the patient's blood from the dialyzing solution, or "cleansing bath." This solution is chemically equivalent to normal blood plasma. As the blood and the dialyzing solution circulate on the two sides of the semipermeable membrane, waste products leave the bloodstream, cross the membrane, and enter the dialyzing solution, which can be replaced periodically. Some dialyzers have pumps, which ensure that the blood will be moved effectively through the machine. When the treatment is finished, the cannulas are connected with a sterile piece, forming the arteriovenous shunt.[24] Occasionally, a patient on long-term hemodialysis will have an internal arteriovenous shunt performed. This surgical procedure involves the anastomosis of an artery to a vein.

Selected patients may be maintained on dialysis therapy and their lives prolonged pending the possibility of a kidney transplant. When long-term dialysis is necessary for chronic renal failure, the patient may come into the hospital, usually twice weekly, and remain approximately 8 hours for the treatment. Some patients secure their treatment at night and go about their normal activities during the day. Treatment is costly, and few patients can afford it. Considerable progress has been made in the development of equipment for home use, and about 40% of dialysis patients are now receiving treatment in their own home.[11]

Patients receiving dialysis therapy need a great deal of psychologic support and encouragement. Most patients realize the seriousness of their condition. They may become depressed and question why they are being kept alive. The patient's family play a most important role by constantly reassuring the patient of their need for him.

Personnel who work with hemodialysis patients must be specially trained in anatomy, physiology, pathology of the kidney, and pharmacology. Usually each dialysis center has its own training program, which may last for 6 to 12 weeks.

Peritoneal dialysis

The peritoneal form of dialysis can be used in small hospitals and can be managed by the nursing staff. The technique is similar to abdominal paracentesis, but a catheter is inserted through the trocar and remains in the peritoneal cavity after the trocar is withdrawn. Two thousand milliliters of dialyzing solution is allowed to run rapidly into the peritoneal cavity and to remain for 1 hour. The solution then drains out by gravity. When 100 to 200 ml. of solution remains in the cavity, additional bottles of solution are connected, and the process is repeated. The treatment may be continued for more than 24 hours. The principle of peritoneal dialysis is the same as that behind extracorporeal dialysis. By the process of osmosis the waste products in the blood are transferred to the dialyzing solution, and electrolytes needed to maintain normal balance are transferred from the solution to the blood.

The patient should be watched closely during the procedure, and signs of abdominal or respiratory distress should be brought to the attention of the physician. The amount of fluid involved should be recorded and the rate of administration regulated as ordered. Vital signs should be observed and any sign of bleeding should be reported at once. Often the patient may move about during the treatment, but he may need assistance.

Renal homotransplants

A renal transplant is the procedure of replacing a diseased kidney with a normal kidney from a donor. The procedure was first attempted in 1962, and since then considerable progress has been made. The basic problem that has to be overcome is that the human body rejects anything that is not of itself. Therefore the patient's body may reject the transplanted kidney, and the procedure is unsuccessful. A renal transplant must still be considered a pioneering procedure; however, medical science has made progress in matching the tissue of the donor and the recipient and in developing drugs to decrease the rejection of the transplanted kidney. The number of successful transplants is increasing, and some day renal transplantation promises to become a routine procedure. The

nursing care of the patient requires the nurse's skill and understanding. The psychologic care of the patient may be more important than the physiologic care. The nurse should not discuss the procedure with the patient lest false hope and misunderstanding occur but should refer all questions to the physician.

NURSING THE PATIENT WITH OPERATIVE CONDITIONS OF THE URINARY SYSTEM

Many conditions affecting the urinary system require both medical and surgical treatment, and operative procedures are seldom done until a thorough urologic examination has been completed. The preoperative care of patients does not differ greatly from that of other surgical patients. When surgery involves the kidney, the physician may wish to have the patient's blood typed and cross matched in case transfusion should be necessary. The postoperative care differs from other kinds of surgery in that drains, tubes, or catheters are placed to remove urine.

Cystectomy

Cystectomy is the surgical removal of the bladder and may be partial or complete. The surgery may be necessitated because of malignant tumors involving the bladder and adjacent structures (Fig. 15-1). When the bladder is removed, the ureters are transplanted by one of the methods discussed in the following section to provide for urinary drainage. The nursing care is the same as that for patients having abdominal surgery or ureteral transplants. The prostate gland may have been removed through a perineal wound, and such wounds must be observed for evidence of hemorrhage. The patient will have a nasogastric tube connected to suction siphonage and will be given nothing by mouth for several days. During this time the patient should receive special mouth care at frequent intervals. If a partial resection of the bladder has been done, a catheter will be inserted into the remaining bladder, and precautions must be taken to prevent any pulling on the catheter. The tubing should be pinned to the sheet and sufficient slack allowed to permit the patient to turn.

Urinary diversion (ureteral transplants)

Under certain conditions it is necessary to remove the bladder and to transplant the ureters elsewhere to provide for urinary drainage. Several types of procedures exist. The ureters may be transplanted into the sigmoid colon (ureterosigmoidostomy), brought out through the abdominal wall to the skin (cutaneous ureterostomy), transplanted into a resected segment of the ileum or colon, which in turn is sutured to the skin (ileal or colonic conduit) (Fig. 15-5), or a neobladder may be created. Removal of the bladder and the transplanting of the ureters may be done at one time or in two operations, in which the ureters are transplanted first and the bladder is removed in the second operation.

Ureterosigmoidostomy. The preoperative care of the patient who is to have a ureterosigmoidostomy is directed toward reducing the bacterial content of the intestinal tract. Several days prior to the surgery the patient is given a chemotherapeutic drug for its bacteriostatic effect. The patient receives a low-residue diet and is allowed only liquids for 2 or 3 days before the surgery. Cleansing enemas are given on the evening before and the morning of the surgery. A large rectal tube may be inserted into the rectum and secured with adhesive tape.

Postoperatively the rectal tube is left in place for several days and attached to free drainage. The drainage must be measured at hourly intervals, and if no drainage occurs during the 1-hour period, the physician must be notified immediately. The physician may order the rectal tube irrigated with physiologic saline solution to maintain its patency, and the physician may remove the tube or may order it removed for cleansing or to permit defecation. The tube should never be reinserted more than 4 inches. The patient must be watched care-

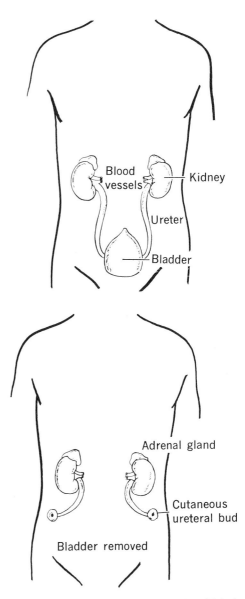

Fig. 15-6. Cutaneous ureterostomy in which the ureters are brought through the skin on the abdomen.

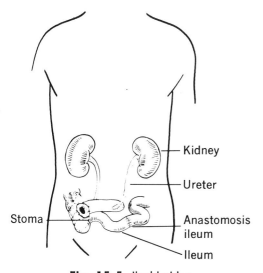

Fig. 15-5. Ileobladder.

fully for abdominal distention, which may occur if there is leakage around the anastomosis. Leakage of urine into the abdominal cavity may cause peritonitis and may not be readily observed. The patient should be observed for nausea, vomiting, and elevation of temperature. The patient will receive intravenous infusions for several days, and food is withheld to allow for healing of the anastomosis. The diet is low in residue, and the patient is not given any enemas or cathartics. A Levin tube may be inserted and connected to suction siphonage, and the nurse should check the apparatus frequently to be sure it is working properly.

When the ureters are transplanted into the sigmoid colon, the danger of ascending infection is always present. The patient should be watched for elevation of temperature, headache, loss of appetite, and drowsiness. After the rectal tube has been removed the patient will use the bedpan for urination, and until he learns to control the sphincter and rectal distention, accidents may happen. As the patient gradually gains control, he will be able to hold approximately 200 ml. of urine and may not need to urinate more often than every 2 or 3 hours. The urine will be mixed with feces so that the stools will be soft.

Cutaneous ureterostomy. When a cutaneous ureterostomy is done, the ureters are brought out through the abdominal wall, where they are secured (Fig. 15-6). When healing is complete, a ureterostomy cup is attached to the skin over the ureteral buds and connected to a rubber leg urinal (Fig. 15-7).

The care of the skin is important, and

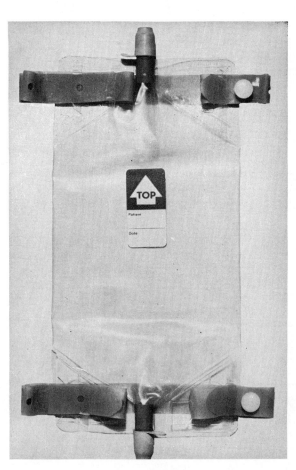

Fig. 15-7. Rubber leg urinal is attached to a ureterostomy cup covering the ureteral bud. The urinal is fastened around the leg with straps. (Courtesy Sterilon Corp., Buffalo, N. Y.)

the patient must be taught how to apply the cup and how to care for it. The hospital may have printed instructions for the patient, and the public health nurse may visit the patient in the home at intervals to assist or instruct the patient in the care of the skin and the appliance. This procedure is not commonly used, since infections occur frequently, causing a series of complications.

Ileal or colonic conduit (ileobladder). The ileal conduit is the most common method of urinary diversion at present. In this procedure a section of the ileum is resected from the small bowel, and its blood supply is preserved. The remaining small bowel is then anastomosed so that normal bowel function will be maintained. The segment of ileum is sutured closed at one end, and the other end is sutured to the skin forming an ileostomy. The ureters are transplanted into the segment of ileum, which will serve as a passageway for urine to flow from the body[16] (Fig. 15-5). This procedure results in fewer fluid and elec-

trolyte problems and provides an added barrier to infection. A section of colon can also be used in a similar manner.

Preoperatively, the patient may or may not be given a bowel preparation. After the surgery a catheter is usually placed in the ileostomy opening to provide for drainage until sufficient healing has occurred. The section of ileum will secrete mucus, and the catheter may have to be irrigated. If a catheter is not used, an ileostomy bag will be placed over the opening (Fig. 15-8). The bag will have to be changed, and the physician may do this for the first few postoperative days. When complete healing has occurred, a permanent ileal bag is fitted for the individual patient. Proper application of the bag will prevent leaking and irritation of the skin. The ileostomy stoma is covered with a cotton ball or gauze while the area about the stoma is being cleaned. After cleaning ether may be applied to the skin, followed by tincture of benzoin. A special skin cement may be used to attach the bag to the skin. In changing the bag, ether or a cement solvent may be used to remove the cement from the skin and the bag. Rubber bags should be washed with mild soap and warm water, dried, and powdered.

The nurse must watch closely for low abdominal pain and decreased urinary output. The segment of ileum may become distended with urine and cause back pressure on the kidneys or rupture the suture lines. Symptoms of peritonitis should be reported at once. A nasogastric tube will be in place until peristalsis returns. The stoma may need to be dilated for several days after surgery and is the responsibility of the nurse or physician. The care of a urinary ileostomy is similar to that for a small bowel ileostomy (pp. 305 to 307).

The psychologic problems that result from urinary diversion are similar to those occurring from diversion of the intestinal tract. The necessity for the surgery has been a traumatic experience, and the patient must adapt to an altered body image. He must be supported and reassured when learning to care for his ileostomy and encouraged to continue his everyday activities once he has recuperated from surgery.[16] An ileostomy need not change a person's life-style.

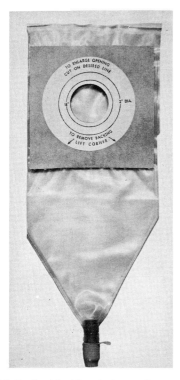

Fig. 15-8. Ileobladder drainage bag, which is cemented to the skin over the ileostomy stoma. (Courtesy Sterilon Corp., Buffalo, N. Y.)

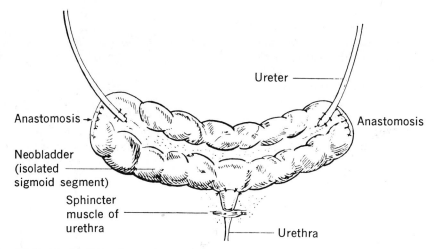

Fig. 15-9. Neobladder. A new bladder is constructed from a segment of the sigmoid, and the ureters and urethra are attached.

Neobladder. Neobladder, or colocysto-plasty, is a surgical procedure in which an artificial bladder is constructed from a segment of the sigmoid (Fig. 15-9). The newly constructed urinary reservoir is placed in the same position as the bladder before its removal. The ureters and urethra are attached to it, and the patient voids normally. The new bladder will hold approximately 140 ml. of urine, and many of the problems encountered with other ureteral transplants are eliminated.

The patient requires extensive preoperative preparation similar to that given prior to a sigmoid transplant. The postoperative care of the patient is essentially the same as for other types of major abdominal surgery. The procedure is relatively new in the United States but has been used successfully in other countries. Not all patients are suitable candidates, and the selection of patients for the procedure is made only after careful examination and study.[22]

Cystotomy

A cystotomy is a surgical incision into the bladder and may be performed for various reasons, including the correction of prostatic hypertrophy in connection with suprapubic prostatectomy. It may be performed to remove tumors or stones from the bladder.

The preoperative care of the patient is the same as that for other abdominal surgery. When the patient returns from surgery, a drainage tube will have been inserted into the bladder, which may be connected to drainage. The dressings will have to be changed frequently to keep the patient dry and comfortable. The skin must be kept clean, and a protective ointment may be used to prevent irritation. Often the patient is elderly and in poor physical condition, and the nurse must be alert to symptoms of shock. Blood pressure and pulse must be checked frequently during the immediate postoperative period, and the patient must be turned from side to side to prevent pulmonary complications.

Ureterotomy

Surgery on the ureter is generally performed to remove a stone, to repair the severed ureter, or to do plastic repair of a stricture. If the stone is in the ureter, a *ureterolithotomy* is performed. Removal of the stone from the kidney is a *nephrolithotomy*. Patients having a stone removed from the lower third of the ureter will have an abdominal incision, and care is similar to that for any patient with abdominal surgery. However, the incision will drain urine for several days after surgery, since the ureter cannot be closed with watertight sutures or strictures will form. Stones removed from the upper two thirds of the ureter and the kidney will necessitate a flank or kidney incision (p. 359).

The postoperative care of the patient is directed toward the care of tubes and maintaining drainage. Occasionally a catheter is inserted into the ureter, which serves as a splint while healing occurs. It is important that the catheter be kept in place at all times. When there is urinary drainage onto the skin, there must be frequent change of dressings and cleansing of the skin to prevent irritation and maceration. All urinary drainage should be measured and recorded.

Nephrectomy and nephrostomy

Nephrectomy is the surgical removal of the kidney, and when the kidney is removed, drainage is unnecessary; however, a small drain may be placed in the wound. Nephrostomy is an incision into the kidney pelvis for the purpose of drainage. When the patient has had a nephrectomy, there may be a minimum amount of drainage from the wound for the first 24 to 48 hours, gradually diminishing.

Dressings should be checked frequently for evidence of fresh bleeding, since hemorrhage is always a possibility. Vital signs are watched, and any significant change in the pulse rate with restlessness should be reported to the physician. Gastrointestinal complications with nausea, vomiting, and abdominal distention may occur. Fluids by mouth may be restricted and a nasogastric tube inserted, which should be connected to suction drainage. The most important postoperative concern is that good urinary drainage be established from the remaining kidney. The patient may have a retention catheter in place, which is connected to gravity drainage, or if the patient does not void, catheterization may be ordered. All intake and output must be carefully measured and recorded. The patient will find it difficult to breathe deeply because of the location of the incision (Fig. 15-10). In some cases the thoracic cavity may have been opened, and the patient will have chest tubes connected to underwater drainage. Medication for pain should be given, after which the incision may be splinted and the patient encouraged to breathe deeply. The patient should be positioned according to the physician's directions after surgery. The patient is usually out of bed on the first postoperative day and ambulatory soon after. Most patients are able to tolerate a regular diet by the fourth postoperative day, with a fluid intake of approximately 3000 ml.

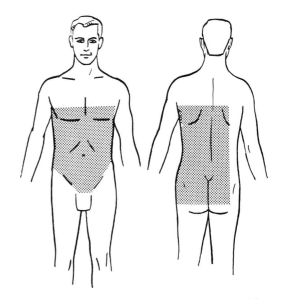

Fig. 15-10. Area of the skin to be prepared for a nephrectomy.

When the patient leaves the hospital, he is advised to avoid heavy lifting and straining for approximately 6 weeks to maintain his fluid intake, and to avoid alcohol. The patient should be advised to avoid respiratory infections, and if the person is young, he should be advised against activities that might result in injury to the other kidney.

The postoperatve care of the patient with a nephrostomy or pyelostomy is the same as that for nephrectomy except for the presence of catheters, which are attached to drainage (Fig. 15-11). The nurse should watch carefully to be sure that the catheters do not become plugged with a blood clot. The physician's orders concerning turning the patient onto the affected side should be clearly understood. Drainage must be accurately measured and recorded, and dressings about the tubes or wound may have to be changed frequently. The skin must be kept clean by washing with mild soap and water and dried to prevent irritation. If tubes have been placed in both kidneys, both tubes should be placed on one side of the bed. (For instructions for irrigating these tubes, see the discussion for catheter care on p. 345.)

Urethral stricture

A narrowing of the urethra that interferes with the passage of urine may result from infection or the formation of scar tissue

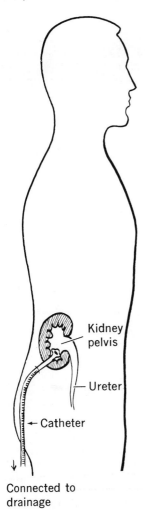

Kidney
pelvis

— Ureter

← Catheter

Connected to
drainage

Fig. 15-11. Nephrostomy with the catheter in the kidney pelvis. The catheter is brought out through a skin incision and connected to tubing and gravity drainage.

after injury or surgery. Surgery may be required to relieve the condition, and the type of procedure will depend partly on the location of the stricture.

The postoperative care of the patient is directed toward the care of the catheter, which may be in the urethra or in the bladder, as in a cystotomy.

Congenital malformations

Congenital malformations may be present in any part of the urinary system, and their seriousness depends on the extent of the defect. Malformation involving both kidneys usually results in death soon after

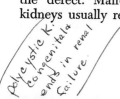

birth. Some conditions involving the bladder may be corrected by surgery when the child is between 2 and 4 years of age. The mother will need to be taught how to care for the child during the years prior to surgery, and follow-up observation by the public health nurse is advisable. Any anomaly of the urinary system is extremely serious if it obstructs the flow of urine.

PSYCHOSOCIAL ASPECTS

The patient with a urinary tract disease or disorder faces many problems, some of which are not easily resolved. The average person views the loss of a kidney as a threat to his life. Since the function of the urinary system is considered to be extremely personal and private, the patient often feels embarrassed, keeping his fears and anxieties to himself. The male patient may often be reluctant to let the nurse irrigate a urethral catheter. When the physician tells the patient that extensive urologic surgery is necessary, the patient may experience an emotional anesthesia, and even though he may know what to expect, he fails to comprehend its significance. When the patient recovers from the immediate postoperative period and begins to convalesce, the realization of what has happened to him may cause the patient to become irritable, depressed, and difficult. The odor of urine, wet dressings, and draining catheters contribute to his fears, apprehensions, and feelings of rejection. It is at this time that the patient needs emotional support, and he may be helped if the hospital environment provides an atmosphere of acceptance and understanding. The nurse, by using skill in skin care and in keeping the patient dry, clean, and free of odor, will do much to encourage and provide support for the patient.

Summary outline

1. Structure and function of urinary system
   A. Organs of urinary system—two kidneys, two ureters, one bladder, and one urethra
   B. Functions
      1. To filter materials not needed by body or of which it has excess
      2. To maintain water and electrolyte balance
      3. To maintain acid-base balance
2. Causes of urinary disease and disorder
   A. Infection
   B. Obstructions

C. Tumors
D. Trauma
E. Allergy
F. Degenerative changes
3. Urinary output
    A. Normally urinary system should filter, concentrate, and excrete 1500 to 2000 ml. in 24 hours
    B. Retention—inability to void because of various factors
        1. Delayed ambulation after surgery
        2. Obstruction
        3. Trauma
        4. Childbirth
        5. Emotional factors
    C. Suppression (anuria)—indicates that kidneys are failing to do their work; may be caused by:
        1. Nephritis
        2. Shock
        3. Cardiac decompensation
        4. Extreme dehydration
    D. Residual urine—urine left in bladder after patient has voided
    E. Incontinence—inability to retain urine in bladder
        1. True incontinence—occurrence of continuous dribbling
    F. Enuresis (bed-wetting)
        1. Nocturnal enuresis—bed-wetting at night
        2. In children may be symptomatic of emotional or behavior problems
4. Diuretics
    Drugs to increase urinary output
    A. Effects—increased excretion of water and sodium
    B. They do not cure disease, but relieve symptoms
5. Composition of urine
    A. Normally urine is 95% water, slightly acid, clear, pale yellow to amber, with specific gravity of 1.003 to 1.030, and contains urea and various electrolytes
    B. Abnormal constituents—blood, pus, glucose, acetone, albumin, casts, and bile
6. Diagnostic tests and procedures
    A. Urinalysis
        1. Routine collection of specimens from adult and child
        2. Sterile specimens collected by catheterization
        3. Washed, or "clean-catch," specimens
        4. Commercially prepared test materials
        5. Fractional (two-glass) test—used for male patients to diagnose disorder in upper or lower urinary tract
        6. Urine culture—sterile specimen for bacteriologic study for specific organisms
    B. Tests of kidney function
        1. Nonprotein nitrogen (NPN) or blood urea nitrogen BUN)—increased when rise in blood urea occurs
        2. Concentration and dilution tests
        3. Phenolsulfonphthalein (PSP) test—determines excretory ability of kidney tubules

        4. Serum creatinine—measures kidney function and is elevated in blood when renal function is impaired
    C. Nursing responsibilities
    D. Other tests and procedures
        1. X-ray examination (KUB)—flat x-ray film of kidneys, ureters, and bladder, often used as screening procedure
        2. Pyleography
            a. Intravenous pyelogram—dye is injected into vein, and x-ray films are taken
            b. Retrograde pyelogram—radiopaque substance is injected into kidney pelvis through ureter, and x-ray films are taken
        3. Cystography—x-ray films of bladder are taken after injection of radiopaque material
        4. Cystoscopic examination—allows direct visualization of bladder with lighted instrument
    E. Radioisotope studies
        1. Renography
        2. Renoscan
        3. Renovascular studies
7. Specific aspects of nursing the patient with diseases and disorders of urinary system
    A. Intake and output
        1. Adequate and accurate measurement of both intake and output of fluid is important in all urologic conditions
    B. Provision for urinary drainage
        1. Closed gravity drainage
        2. Collection sets
        3. Tidal drainage
    C. Catheter care—retention catheters should provide free flow of urine and be comfortable for patient
        1. Pyelostomy, nephrostomy, uretrostomy, and cystostomy catheters and their care
        2. Catheter irrigation—may be performed for urethral catheters with 30 ml. of physiologic saline solution when necessary to maintain patency and on physician's order
            a. Separate equipment must be maintained for irrigation of bilateral pyelostomy catheters
            b. Separate equipment is kept for pyelostomy and urethral catheters
            c. All equipment and solution for catheter irrigation must be kept sterile
    D. Patient care after catheter removal
        1. Observe patient for voiding and retention
    E. Dressings over draining wounds—should be changed frequently and kept dry, clean, and free from urinary odors
    F. Follow-up care by public health nurse
8. Nursing the patient with diseases and disorders of urinary system
    A. Noninfectious diseases
        1. Glomerulonephritis—acute, subacute, chronic
            a. Recognized by Richard Bright in 1876

b. Characterized by albuminuria, hypoproteinuria, and renal failure
c. Affects children and young adults
d. Pathophysiology
e. Treatment and nursing care
2. Nephrotic syndrome—functional disor-
   order causing tubular degeneration
3. Nephrosclerosis—sclerosis of blood vessels in kidney
B. Infectious diseases
1. Cystitis—inflammation of bladder
2. Pyelonephritis—pyrogenic infection affecting parenchyma and collecting system of kidney
   a. Pathophysiology
   b. Treatment and nursing care
3. Perinephritic abscess—single or multiple abscesses in soft tissue of kidney
C. Obstructions of urinary system
1. Renal calculi
   a. Lithiasis—formation of stones
   b. Nephrolithiasis—formation of stones
      in kidney
   c. Small stones may pass in urine
   d. Large stones may require surgery
   e. Medical and nursing care
2. Ureteral colic—caused by stone passing
   down or lodged in ureter; causes excruciating pain
D. Hydronephrosis—dilation of kidney pelvis
   from obstruction; results in wasting of kidney tissue
E. Traumatic injuries—may result from gunshot wounds, penetrating wounds from
   sharp objects, and crushing injuries
F. Tumors of urinary tract
1. Tumors of kidney are usually malignant
2. Wilms' tumor is seen in children and is
   malignant
3. Congenital polycystic kidneys—respond
   to no known treatment and are ultimately fatal
4. Tumors of bladder may be benign or
   malignant
G. Renal failure—inability of kidneys to perform their function
1. Pathophysiology
2. Treatment and nursing care
3. Dialysis
   a. Extracorporeal hemodialysis
   b. Peritoneal dialysis
4. Renal homotransplants
9. Nursing the patient with operative conditions
   of the urinary system
A. Cystectomy—partial or complete removal
   of bladder with transplantation of ureters
B. Urinary diversion (ureter transplants)—
   removal of bladder and transplant of ureters elsewhere in body
1. Ureterosigmoidostomy—transplant   of
   ureters into sigmoid colon
2. Cutaneous   ureterostomy—ureters
   brought out through abdominal wall
3. Neobladder (colocystoplasty) may be
   constructed
4. Ileal or colonic conduit (ileobladder)
C. Cystotomy—incision into bladder

1. Performed with suprapubic prostatectomy
2. To remove tumor or stones
D. Ureterotomy—incision into ureter
1. To remove a stone
2. For repair after injury
3. Plastic repair of stricture
4. Ureterolithotomy—removal   of   stone
   from ureter
5. Nephrolithotomy—removal   of   stone
   from kidney
E. Nephrectomy and nephrostomy
1. Nephrectomy—surgical removal of kidney
2. Nephrostomy—incision into kidney pelvis for purpose of drainage
F. Urethral stricture—narrowing that interferes with passage of urine
1. May be caused by infection
2. May be caused by scar tissue after injury or surgery
G. Congenital malformations
1. Involvement of both kidneys results in
   death soon after birth
2. Conditions involving bladder may be
   surgically corrected when child is between 2 and 4 years of age
3. Obstruction of urinary flow is extremely
   serious condition
10. Psychosocial aspects
A. Patient will face many problems and will
   need emotional support, acceptance, and
   understanding

Review questions

1. What is the name for urine left in the bladder
   after the patient has voided?
   a. *residual*
2. What are drugs called that are used to increase the urinary output?
   a. *diuretics*
3. What is the name for one group of synthetic
   agents commonly used to increase urinary output?
   a. *chlorothyazides*
4. What is the approximate normal value for the
   blood urea nitrogen test (BUN)?
   a. *1.003 - 1.030*
5. When a urinary retention catheter has been
   removed, dribbling may occur for the following reason:
   a. *loss of sphincter control (dilation*
6. What very important observation should the
   nurse make after the patient has had a nephrectomy? *signs of hemorrhage*
7. List three ways in which the nurse may help
   to space fluid when the patient is receiving
   limited fluid intake.
   a. *give meds c meals*
   b. *give solid meds rather than pills*
   c. *small full glass rather than 1/2 glass*
8. What is one method that would help the nurse
   to determine fluid output?
   a. *closed catheter system*
9. When a patient has had a nephrostomy, what
   specific nursing procedures are important?

a. *watch for hemorrhage*
b. *catheters can't be blocked*
c. *meas. drge. accurately*
d. *care in turning to affected side*

10. If a patient is confined to bed, what measures may provide exercise and help prevent the formation of renal calculi?

a. *trapeze*
b. *exercises*
c. *turning side to side*
d. *tilt table or rocking bed.*

Films

1. Arteriovenous shunts in chronic dialysis (27 min., sound, color, 16 mm.), Baxter Laboratories, Inc., 6301 Lincoln Ave., Morton Grove, Ill. 60053. Shows the surgical implantation, use, and care of shunts related to chronic dialysis.
2. Dialysis procedures (27 min., sound, color, 16 mm.), Eli Lilly Co., Audiovisual Library, Indianapolis, Ind. 46206. Describes techniques and procedure involved in hemodialysis, also surgical procedures and purpose of peritoneal dialysis. Home dialysis, kidney transplantation, and the need for more dialysis centers are discussed.
3. Kidney function in health (38½ min., sound, color, 16 mm.), Eli Lilly and Co., Audiovisual Library, Indianapolis, Ind. 46206. Describes normal kidney function. Amend as necessary.
4. Pyelonephritis—WSU (32 min., sound, color, 16 mm.), Audio-Visual Utilization Center, Wayne State University, Detroit, Mich. 48202. Relates modern-day bacteriology to the problem of pyelonephritis. Shows patient demonstrations. Danger during pregnancy and hazards of catheterization are discussed. Methods of obtaining urine specimens and the bacteriology associated with examination and analysis of the specimen are shown.
5. Rendezvous with life (27 min., sound, color, 16 mm.), Baxter Laboratories, Inc., 6301 Lincoln Ave., Morton Grove, Ill. 60053. Reviews the treatment of patients with chronic renal failure on home dialysis basis with the family operating the artificial kidney.
6. Peritoneal dialysis: a bedside procedure (25 min., sound, color, 16 mm., free loan), Abbott Laboratories, Abbott Park, North Chicago, Ill. 60064. Describes peritoneal dialysis procedure in detail, along with the structure and function of the peritoneum in relation to dialysis.
7. Catheter care and use (15 min., sound, color, 16 mm., free loan), Eaton Medical Film Library, 17 Eaton Ave., Norwich, N. Y., 13815. Illustrates principles and techniques of catheter care and use.

References

1. Beaumont, Estelle: Urinary drainage systems, Nursing 74 4:52-60, Jan., 1974.
2. Beeson, Paul B., and McDermott, Walsh, editors: Cecil-Loeb textbook of medicine, ed. 13, Philadelphia, 1973, W. B. Saunders Co.
3. Beland, Irene L.: Clinical nursing pathophysi-ological and psychosocial approaches, ed. 3, New York, 1975, The Macmillan Co.
4. Brunner, Lillian S., and Suddarth, Doris S.: Textbook of medical-surgical nursing, ed. 3, Philadelphia, 1975, J. B. Lippincott Co.
5. Conn, Howard F., editor: Current therapy 1976, Philadelphia, 1976, W. B. Saunders Co.
6. Davis, Joseph E.: Drugs for urologic disorders, American Journal of Nursing 65:107-112, Aug., 1965.
7. Delehanty, Lorraine, and Stravino, Vincent: Achieving bladder control, American Journal of Nursing 70:312-316, Feb., 1970.
8. Fellows, Barbara: Hemodialysis at home, American Journal of Nursing 66:1775-1778, Aug., 1966.
9. Fenton, Mary: What to do about thirst, American Journal of Nursing 69:1014-1017, May, 1969.
10. Grollman, Arthur: Diuretics, American Journal of Nursing 65:84-89, Jan., 1965.
11. Gutch, C. F., and Stoner, Martha H.: Review of hemodialysis for nurses and dialysis personnel, ed. 2, St. Louis, 1975, The C. V. Mosby Co.
12. Holden, Helen M., Skerry, Vilda M., and Quinlan, John J.: Peritoneal dialysis, The Canadian Nurse 62:40-43, March, 1963.
13. Ingram, Mary B.: Incontinence and decubitus ulcers, The Journal of Practical Nursing 20:24-26, April, 1970.
14. Keuhnelian, John G., and Sanders, Virginia E.: Urologic nursing, New York, 1970, The Macmillan Co.
15. Monroe, Jewel M., and Komorita, Nori I.: Problems with nephrosis in adolescence, American Journal of Nursing 67:336-340, Feb., 1967.
16. Murray, Barbara S., Elmore, Joyce, and Sawyer, Janet R.: The patient has an ileal conduit, American Journal of Nursing 71:1560-1565, Aug., 1971.
17. Nesbill, Lynda: Nursing the patient on long-term hemodialysis, The Canadian Nurse 63:40-41, Oct., 1967.
18. Pask, Eleanor G.: Collecting urine specimens from children, The Canadian Nurse 65:35-39, Oct., 1969.
19. Progress against cancer 1969, a report of the national advisory Council, Washington, D. C., 1969, Government Printing Office.
20. Santora, Delores: Preventing hospital-acquired urinary infection, American Journal of Nursing 66:790-794, April, 1966.
21. Shafer, Kathleen N., Sawyer, Janet R., McCluskey, Audrey M., Beck, Edna L., and Phipps, Wilma J.: Medical-surgical nursing, ed. 6, St. Louis, 1975, The C. V. Mosby Co.
22. Shebelski, Dorothy I.: Nursing patients who have had renal homotransplants, American Journal of Nursing 66:2425-2428, Nov., 1966.
23. Shepro, David, Belamrich, Frank, and Levy, Charles: Human anatomy and physiology—a cellular approach, New York, 1974, Holt, Rinehart & Winston, Inc.

24. Soffer, Rae-Ann: The nurse and hemodialysis, Nursing Care 6:14-18, Oct., 1973.
25. Walsh, Michael, Edner, Marian, and Casey, William: Neobladder, American Journal of Nursing 63:107-110, April, 1963.
26. Winter, Chester C., and Barker, Marilyn Roehm: Nursing care of patients with urologic diseases, ed. 3, St. Louis, 1972, The C. V. Mosby Co.

CHAPTER 16

Nursing the patient with diseases and disorders of the reproductive system

STRUCTURE AND FUNCTION OF THE REPRODUCTIVE SYSTEM

The female reproductive system is divided into the external and the internal parts. The external parts include the mons veneris, a pad of fat that lies over the pubis; the labia (minora and majora); the clitoris, which is covered with a foreskin; and the perineum, a muscular area between the anus and the vaginal opening. There are two sets of secretory glands with ducts opening to the outside, the Bartholin's glands and Skene's glands. The urinary meatus opens to the outside above the vaginal opening. The region of the external organs is usually referred to as the vulva. Dividing the external parts from the internal parts is a thin fold of mucous membrane called the *hymen*. The internal structures consist of the vagina, located between the urinary meatus and the anus; the uterus; two fallopian tubes; and two ovaries. During the childbearing period the epithelium that lines the vagina is arranged in transverse folds called *rugae*. After menopause the walls of the vagina become thin and smooth, resembling those of childhood. The uterus is a pear-shaped hollow organ with a bulging upper part called the *fundus*. The lower portion extends downward, with the internal os opening into the cervical canal. The cervical canal extends into the vagina, where its opening forms the external os. Two fallopian tubes (oviducts) open into the upper part of the uterus. The distal end of the tubes has a fimbriated opening into the abdominal cavity. There are two ovaries, each located near the distal end of the fallopian tubes. The white,

365

almond-shaped ovaries are attached to the uterus by a ligament. Each ovary consists of a cortex and a medulla. The ovarian follicles form within the cortex. The entire internal structures are attached to and supported by several ligaments.

The male organs of reproduction include the testes, which produce the male sperm and hormones. The testes are enclosed in and supported by the scrotum. The epididymis is located along the upper side of the testes. There are two seminal ducts, two seminal vesicles that secrete a portion of the semen, two ejaculatory ducts, two spermatic cords, and the penis. The urethra, which serves a dual purpose, passes through a small opening in the prostate gland. Enlargement of the prostate gland may compress the urethra, causing a disturbance of the urinary flow. Below the prostate gland are two secretory glands known as the bulbourethral glands. The glans penis, located at the end of the penis, is a bulging structure over which a loose retractable skin, called the *prepuce* (foreskin), covers the glans. Sometimes this skin cannot be retracted, and a surgical procedure called circumcision may be necessary (p. 387).[2]

The overall function of the reproductive system is the production of the female ova and the male spermatozoa, the manufacture of certain endocrine secretions, and the retaining and nurturing of the fertilized ovum until the mature fetus is ready for expulsion.

PUBERTY, MENSTRUATION, AND MENOPAUSE

Puberty. Puberty is the period during which secondary sex characteristics begin to make their appearance. The size of the external reproductive organs increases, growth of axillary and pubic hair occurs in both the male and the female, the female breasts become larger, and the male voice deepens. In the female the first menstrual period (menarche) signifies the end of puberty. Some variation in age at onset of puberty and the menarche exists. The first menstrual period usually occurs between the twelfth and sixteenth year; however, it may occur anytime from the tenth to the eighteenth year. Studies have shown that the onset of menstruation is not influenced

to any extent by climate, race, or nationality.[23]

All children need preparation for puberty through sex education. From the moment of birth the infant begins to respond to and reflect the attitudes of others who care for him. Parents are usually the most influential people through the developing years, and they should have healthy attitudes regarding sexuality. Young children are curious and need direct and truthful answers to their questions. Although sex education in schools still arouses controversy, it is generally being accepted and incorporated into elementary and junior high schools. Often nurses are requested to teach basic sex education to small groups of children.

As the boy and girl approach maturity, they encounter many problems at a time when the physiologic organism is already required to make many adjustments, and they need guidance and wise counseling to help them establish patterns that will prepare them for parenthood.

Menstruation. Menstruation is a cyclic process occurring at fairly regular intervals between puberty and menopause that spans a period of approximately 30 to 35 years. It is a normal physiologic process and does not indicate a state of illness or disability. Some persons, particularly adolescent girls, have been negatively conditioned by the emotional climate surrounding them and may complain of exaggerated or fancied menstrual pains and complaints throughout their lives.

A wide variation exists in the cycle and duration of the menstrual flow. A cycle of every 28 days may be normal for some persons, but for others it may be shorter or longer. Ovulation usually occurs approximately 2 weeks before the onset of menstruation. The flow usually lasts from 3 to 5 days, but for some women 6 or 7 days may be normal. In the beginning an initial period may occur and then a skip of 2 or 3 months, followed by a normal period, after which the function proceeds in an orderly fashion. Brief periods with slight flow may occur and be perfectly normal, but if this pattern is continued over an extended amount of time, medical consultation should be secured.

Each individual should be encouraged

to lead a normal life at the time of menstruation. The regular program of personal hygiene, including sleep, rest, proper diet, exercise, and bathing should be continued. Exercise with few exceptions is considered helpful in relieving minor discomfort. Although many taboos still exist concerning bathing and washing the hair, there is no valid evidence that harmful results occur from such procedures. A daily warm shower is important, since there is often increased activity of the sweat glands during this period. Douches should not be taken unless ordered by the physician. Coitus is usually objectionable to women during their periods and is avoided for esthetic reasons.

Occasionally slight discomfort may occur on the first day of the menstrual period, including low back pain, a feeling of heaviness or aching of the legs, and varying degrees of pelvic discomfort. However, many persons experience no discomfort. There has been considerable investigation into the problem of premenstrual tension, which is characterized by irritability, depression, weight gain, edema, anxiety, and nervousness occurring 4 or 5 days prior to the beginning of the menstrual period. Not all women experience the syndrome, and all the symptoms may not occur in those who do. With the beginning of menstruation the symptoms usually disappear. The exact cause of the condition is not known but is believed to be due to some imbalance of hormones. Treatment for the disorder depends on the severity of the symptoms. Although opinions differ and results are variable, some physicians prescribe a diuretic such as chlorothiazide (Diuril) to relieve the edema resulting from water and sodium retention and sedatives and tranquilizing agents to relieve the emotional symptoms.

Many girls reach puberty with little or no understanding of or preparation for the function of menstruation. Too often they are faced with embarrassing situations that may have serious emotional effects. Every mother should prepare her daughter for the event before it occurs. The girl should be supplied with the proper pads and belt and instructed in their care. She should also be provided with protection to relieve fear of soiling clothing. The consolidation of schools requires that girls ride buses long distances and be away from home all day. Schools have the responsibility of providing proper facilities and privacy as well as emergency supplies for the adolescent girl. Proper attitudes and good mental health should be established early and may have far-reaching effects when the reproductive period comes to an end.

The reproductive years. All couples contemplating marriage should have complete physical examinations, including a serologic test for syphilis. At this time possible problems can be eliminated, and both people can be given the opportunity to discuss any questions concerning married life. Common questions concern birth control and family planning.

As a result of energy crises and a variety of other environmental problems, the world has been forced to realize that continued population expansion can only lead to a decrease in life style standards. There has been much discussion about zero population growth as a means to ensure survival in the future. This in addition to the desire to live a comfortable life without hardship and to provide the best for their children has caused many couples to limit the size of their families.

There are several methods of birth control available: the diaphragm, oral contraceptives ("the pill"), rhythm, intrauterine devices, and the newer injectable medications. Tubal ligations for the female and vasectomy for the male are the current means of permanent contraception.

Menopause (climacteric). The menopause is often referred to as "the change of life"; however, for the well-adjusted person there should not be any appreciable change in the normal pattern of living. Menopause is a normal, physiologic process and simply means that the period of reproductivity has come to an end. Marital relationships continue, people do not lose their minds, and the host of other conditions so often attributed to menopause may be unrelated to the physical process.

In the majority of women menopause occurs between 45 and 55 years of age. Occasionally it may occur earlier or later. Artificial menopause may be induced by the surgical removal of the ovaries or by deep external x-ray radiation and radium placed in the vaginal canal. The amount of radiation required to destroy the function of the ovaries may vary with the individual. Although some women may stop menstruating abruptly, the usual pattern is a gradual tapering off. The flow may gradually decrease, with some irregularity of periods, and when the production of the ovarian hormone (estrogen) falls below the level necessary to stimulate the endometrium, menstruation ceases. Several changes in the epithelial cells occur in the postmenopausal woman that affect the vagina, urinary tract, and oral cavity. These changes are believed to be due to the loss of estrogen. It has not been well established that other disorders such as cardiovascular disease, hypertension, osteoporosis, arthritis, and mental illness are related to the menopause—they may be simply coincidental.

With the cessation of menses most women do not experience any symptoms severe enough to require medical care. A few persons may complain of hot flashes, which are warm feelings about the face and neck accompanied by sweating. The condition may be more severe in persons in stress situations or who are emotionally unstable. A few persons may also complain of headache, nervousness, palpitation, dizziness, insomnia, and irritability. When the symptoms are severe enough to require medical care, some form of estrogen therapy may be advised. Estrogens may be administered by injection or given by the oral route. One form in common use is a naturally occurring estrogen (Premarin) derived from the urine of pregnant mares. Some form of mild sedation may also be ordered.[23] The vaginal mucosa may atrophy and cause an irritating discharge. Vaginal creams with estrogens are effective in eliminating this discomfort. Emphasis should be placed on the normalcy of menopause, and women should be encouraged to seek new interests and hobbies. There are many kinds of community volunteer services and activities in which women can render valuable service and which also help to relieve tension and stress.

DISTURBANCES OF MENSTRUAL FUNCTION

Dysmenorrhea. Painful menstruation is the most common complaint associated with the menstrual process, and at least one half of all women experience some degree of physical discomfort. The discomfort may occur with or without the presence of a pathologic condition. When pain and discomfort are severe enough to incapacitate the individual, medical examination should be secured to rule out disease. Sometimes pain may result from fibroid tumors of the uterus, ovarian cysts, chronic inflammation of the fallopian tubes, or displacement of the uterus.[19] The discomfort of cramplike pain, backache, and aching of the legs can often be relieved by rest, a heating pad or hot-water bottle applied to the abdomen, and a few simple exercises (Fig. 16-1). If the flow is not profuse, a hot sitz bath may be taken. The physician may advise a simple pain-relieving drug such as aspirin, but under no circumstances should the individual resort to narcotics for menstrual pain because of the habit-forming possibilities of such drugs. Bowel function should be regular and, if necessary, aided by the use of a mild laxative.

Amenorrhea. Amenorrhea is an absence of menstruation, which is normal during prepuberty, after menopause, and during pregnancy and lactation. Amenorrhea may occur with some diseases such as tuberculosis, nephritis, and certain endocrine disturbances. It may also occur as a result of change of climate or emotional factors. Amenorrhea that exists prior to the beginning of menses is usually referred to as primary, whereas suppression of menstruation once it has occurred is called *secondary amenorrhea.* The treatment is based on the underlying cause and must be determined on an individual basis.

Menorrhagia. Menorrhagia refers to excessive menstrual flow, either in amount or duration. The condition is usually associated with some pelvic pathologic condition such as uterine fibroids or with endocrine disturbance or some other disease. Medical examination is always indicated, and if bleeding is severe, the individual should remain in bed with the foot of the bed elevated.

Metrorrhagia. Metrorrhagia is bleeding that occurs between regular menstrual periods and usually indicates the presence of some abnormal pathologic condition. It is often associated with a malignant con-

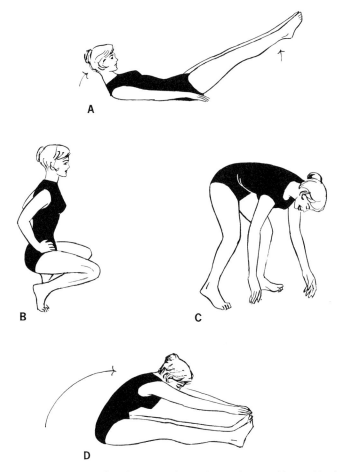

Fig. 16-1. Sitting-up exercises for dysmenorrhea. **A,** Supine position with the head and legs raised simultaneously; the arms should be kept at the side and the legs straight. **B,** Deep knee bends; the back should be kept straight. **C,** Monkey walk; keep the hands flat on the floor and walk around on the hands and feet. **D,** Toe touching; keeping the back straight and the legs straight, bend and touch the toes with the hands.

dition of the reproductive system but may result from benign lesions of the cervix or the uterus.

DIAGNOSTIC TESTS AND PROCEDURES
Examination of the female patient

Most female patients are seen in the gynecologist's office and are treated on an outpatient basis. Since the reproductive system of the male patient is so intricately related to the urinary system, such patients are usually cared for by the urologist.

Physical examination. Examination of the patient begins with a complete history, which includes the menstrual history, history of any pregnancies, or past illness, and history of the present illness. The physical examination of the patient will include palpation of the breasts for evidence of cysts or tumors and examination of the pelvis. Nurses are employed in many physicians' offices, and it is important for them to be familiar with the procedure for pelvic examination and their responsibilities in assisting the physician. The nurse also must understand that the examination may not be easy for the patient and may have been long delayed. The nurse should be thoughtful and try to relieve the patient's anxiety, fears, and embarrassment.

Often children have gynecologic problems and are brought to the physician by the parent. Young children are likely to have a profound sense of modesty and may resist exposure for examination. Efforts should be made to secure the child's confidence and cooperation, and care should be taken to see that she is carefully draped for the examination. The child should not be restrained if it can be avoided, since this may cause traumatic results that can affect future behavior.

The physician will determine the position in which the patient should be placed for the pelvic examination; it may be the lithotomy position, the Sims' position, or the knee-chest position. (Refer to a textbook on basic nursing.) The patient should be carefully draped and any unnecessary exposure avoided. The examination includes inspection of the external genitals, a bimanual examination through the vagina with two gloved fingers, and a rectal examination using the index finger. An examination with a vaginal speculum is usually done to permit the physician to see the cervix and the walls of the vagina. This examination may be omitted in young girls if the hymen is intact. The nurse should remain in attendance during the examination. After the examination the nurse should protect herself in caring for instruments and gloves or other articles used during the examination because some conditions may be infectious.

The nurse who assists the physician in the gynecologic examination has a professional and moral responsibility to refrain from discussing the examination with any person. No other type of disease or examination is regarded as so personal and private as that involving the reproductive system in both male and female.

Laboratory examination. The laboratory examination will include urinalysis, the Papanicolaou cytologic test for cancer, and smears and cultures from the vagina, cervix, and urethra, which may be examined for both infectious and noninfectious organisms. A complete blood count and a serologic test for syphilis are usually done. Examination of the male patient may include prostatic smears secured through massage of the prostate gland by the gloved finger placed in the rectum. A urine specimen is then secured for laboratory examination.

Schiller test. The Schiller test is used for the early detection of cancer cells and to guide the physician in doing a biopsy. Usually the test involves the cervix, which is painted with an iodine solution. Glycogen, which is present in normal cells, will stain brown when the iodine solution is applied, but in the presence of cancer and some other conditions the cells do not contain glycogen and will not stain when the iodine is applied. Thus the physician will be able to determine the exact areas from which biopsy should be taken.

Breast examination. The physician will palpate the breast during the examination. In recent years emphasis has been placed on teaching women to palpate their own breasts monthly. Early cancer of the breast is curable, and if every woman would take time to carefully examine her own breasts at regular intervals, many benign and malignant tumors would be discovered early. Nurses should become familiar with the procedure of breast self-examination so that they may teach patients, friends, or members of their families. (See a basic nursing text for technique.)

Huhner test. The Huhner test is used to study the effect of vaginal secretions on the spermatozoa and is generally used when sterility is suspected. The test must be made within 1 hour after coitus. The patient is instructed to remain lying on her back for 5 minutes after coitus, apply a vulva pad, and report immediately to the physician's office. Tampons should not be used, and no douche should be taken prior to the test. Vaginal secretions are aspirated and examined microscopically to determine the motility, viability, and number of abnormal forms in the spermatozoa.

Rubin test (tubal insufflation). The Rubin test is done to determine if the fallopian tubes are open when sterility is suspected. The test consists of injecting carbon dioxide gas into the uterine cavity under controlled pressure. If the tubes are open, the gas escapes through the tube into the peritoneal cavity, where it is absorbed. The test is usually done about 8 days after the end of the menstrual period. The test is contraindicated if pregnancy is suspected, if any infection is present, or if the patient has recently had a dilation and curettage. When the examination is completed and the patient sits up, she will experience discomfort in the right shoulder and neck. This pain is referred to the shoulder and neck from irritation of nerves under the diaphragm where the gas collects. The patient should be assured that the discomfort will last only a few minutes because the gas absorbs quickly. An absence of pain or discomfort indicates that the tubes are not open.[23]

Hysterosalpingogram. A radiopaque substance is injected into the uterus and through it into the fallopian tubes, and x-ray films are taken. The examination will show the extent and location of an occlusion if present and will enable the physician to study the exact location of the pelvic organs.

The patient is generally given a laxative on the evening before and an enema on the morning of the examination. A mild sedative may be given before the procedure. The patient usually has some minor discomfort similar to gas pains and abdominal cramps. Occasionally nausea, vomiting, or faintness may occur. Positioning the patient with the head low may provide relief from the pelvic discomfort.

Culdoscopy and laparoscopy. A culdoscope is a long, metal, lighted instrument that can be inserted into the cul-de-sac of Douglas, a pouch between the uterus and the rectum. Through the instrument, diseases or conditions affecting the pelvis can be observed. A similar instrument, the laparoscope, can be used in the same manner, although an incision is made in the abdomen rather than entering by way of the vagina. The patient is usually hospitalized, and the procedure is performed in the operating room. After the surgery the patient should be observed for signs of infection such as increased temperature and pain in the lower abdomen.

Pregnancy tests. Several pregnancy tests are essentially the same. The Aschheim-Zondek test uses mice, and the Friedman test uses rabbits. Because rabbits are used, the individual often refers to having a "rabbit test." The patient is instructed to restrict fluids on the day before the test so that the urine specimen will be as concentrated as possible. The first voided urine in the morning should be collected in a sterile container and taken to the laboratory. For the Aschheim-Zondek test urine is injected into mature mice, and at the

end of 96 hours the ovaries of the mice are examined. If changes have occurred, the test is considered positive. The Friedman test uses virgin rabbits, and at the end of 48 hours the abdomen is opened with the rabbit under anesthesia and the ovaries of the animal examined for changes. Although positive reactions are expected to occur in pregnancy, a positive reaction may occur in other conditions. A positive test in a male patient may indicate a malignant condition of the testes.

Immunologic tests. A group of immunologic tests to detect pregnancy that use urine or serum have been developed and are distributed commercially. Immunologic tests are based on finding human chorionic gonadotropin in the urine. The hormone is secreted by the placenta and is always present in the urine from 3 to 5 days after a missed menstrual period. Since these tests may be performed in the physician's office with the results available in minutes, they are largely replacing the tests using animals or rodents.[18] As with all tests, false positive or negative reactions can occur.

Dilation and curettage (D and C). Dilation and curettage is a procedure in which the cervical os is dilated and the inside of the uterus is scraped with a curette. There are three basic reasons for this procedure: (1) to secure tissue from the lining of the uterus (endometrium) for examination, (2) to control uterine bleeding, and (3) to clear the uterine cavity of any residue left after incomplete abortion (p. 383). D and C is a surgical procedure requiring an anesthetic. Preoperative preparation of the patient is the same as that for most other surgical patients. Postoperative care includes observation of the patient for excessive bleeding and urinary retention. The patient may have packing in the vaginal canal, which is removed in 24 hours. The patient is usually ambulatory on the first day, and little or no analgesic is required. The patient is generally discharged from the hospital on the second day with instructions to report to her physician for follow-up care.

Examination of the male patient

Examination of the male reproductive system is usually done by the physician without the nurse in attendance. The external genitals are examined for abnormalities of structure, signs of infection, or skin lesions. If sterility is suspected, several examinations may be carried out, including examination of semen to determine the presence and characteristics of spermatozoa and examination to locate obstructions along the tubal route. A voided specimen may be collected after massage of the prostate gland for examination for cancer cells or tubercle bacilli. A biopsy of the prostate gland or the testicles may also be done.

NURSING THE PATIENT WITH DISEASES AND DISORDERS OF THE REPRODUCTIVE SYSTEM
Conditions affecting the external genitals and vagina
Vulvitis

Vulvitis may be either an acute or chronic inflammatory condition of the vulva. There are many causes, including an irritating vaginal discharge, infectious diseases, untreated diabetes, contraceptive pills, and trauma caused by scratching. There usually is severe itching and burning with redness and, in some patients, ulceration. Treatment consists of identifying and treating or removing the cause. Clothing that may rub or irritate the condition should be eliminated.

Vaginitis

Vaginitis is one of the most common disorders affecting the female. The condition affects infants and young children and may occur any time to old age.

Pathophysiology. Vaginitis is an inflammation of the vagina. There are many etiologic factors associated with its occurrence. When vaginitis occurs after menopause, it is usually caused by the *Trichomonas vaginalis*, a parasitic flagellate protozoa (p. 7). It may also be caused by *Candida albicans*, a yeastlike fungus. The disorder occurs in persons with diabetes, during pregnancy, and in some persons after antibiotic therapy. When vaginitis occurs in these persons, the etiologic agent is usually the *Candida* fungus. Atrophic vaginitis may be found in elderly persons and adolescent girls. Although the vaginal discharge may cause

concern, it may not be pathologic unless there is secondary infection. When vaginitis occurs in children, it is generally caused by pinworms, poor hygiene, or gonorrhea. A bloody vaginal discharge in women past menopause may be the first sign of malignancy of the cervix or uterus.

In the presence of vaginitis there is burning and itching about the vulva, a vaginal discharge, and occasionally pelvic pain. If the etiologic agent is *Candida albicans*, the discharge may be thin and watery. Examination of the vaginal walls may show a white exudate, and microscopic examination reveals the fungi. When the disorder is acute and caused by *Trichomonas vaginalis*, the vaginal discharge is foamy and greenish yellow in color. The vaginal walls are very red, and minute hemorrhagic areas may be observed. Vulva irritation may be severe, and the person has considerable discomfort.

Treatment. Most persons with vaginitis caused by *Trichomonas* organisms are treated with metronidazole (Flagyl), 250 mg. orally three times a day for 10 days. Both marital partners should be treated at the same time. Douches using 1 tablespoonful of vinegar to 1 quart of warm water may be ordered to help remove excessive discharge and provide local comfort. During the first trimester of pregnancy Flagyl vaginal inserts, 500 mg. twice a day for 10 days, may be ordered. The treatment for vaginitis caused by *Candida albicans* is nystatin (Mycostatin) tablets for vaginal insertion twice daily for 7 days, followed by 1 tablet a day for 7 days. Meticulous vaginal cleansing with povidone iodine (Betadine) should precede inserting the tablet. A cream such as gramicidin (Gramoderm) may be ordered to relieve the vulvar irritation. Resistance to treatment may be encountered, and an adjustment in treatment may be necessary. When gonorrheal vaginitis occurs, treatment is with aqueous procaine penicillin (p. 562). Infection by pinworm infestation may be treated with piperazine (Antepar) or pyrvinium pamoate (Povan) (p. 10). Atrophic vaginitis in women past menopause is designed to restore the normal epithelium of the vagina. An estrogen cream used vaginally and the oral administration of Premarin, 0.625 mg. once a day, are given. Any unusual vaginal discharge that cannot be identified as caused by pathogenic organisms should always be investigated to rule out disease.[8, 10]

Leukorrhea

Leukorrhea is an abnormal white or yellow discharge from the vagina. Under normal conditions there may be some increase in vaginal secretions at the beginning and ending of the menstrual period, and this should not be confused with the increased discharge that occurs at other times. Leukorrhea is usually the result of some infection of the vagina or the cervix and may occur in cancer of the uterus. Medical examination and treatment should always be secured.

Vulvovaginitis (Bartholinitis)

Vulvovaginitis is an inflammation of the vulva and vagina or of Bartholin's glands, which are located on either side of the vaginal opening. The condition may result from any of several pathogenic bacteria and is frequently seen in untreated gonorrhea. The ducts from the glands may become occluded by the inflammatory condition, and abscess formation occurs. The abscess may rupture spontaneously, or incision and drainage may be necessary. Treatment includes administration of the appropriate antibiotic and hot sitz baths. The patient is usually treated in the physician's office or in an outpatient clinic.

Vesicovaginal and rectovaginal fistula

A vesicovaginal fistula is an abnormal opening from the bladder to the vagina often caused by obstetric injury at the time of delivery. The condition rarely occurs in the practice of modern obstetrics, but should it occur, surgical correction is indicated.

Rectovaginal fistula is an abnormal opening between the rectum and the vagina caused by laceration through the rectal sphincter at the time of delivery. Most lacerations are repaired at the time of delivery, but if they fail to heal completely, a fistula may remain and will result in some degree of fecal incontinence. Further surgical repair is necessary to correct the condition.

Relaxation of the pelvic musculature

Rectocele, cystocele, and uterine prolapse are conditions often seen in older women. All three conditions may be present at the same time. Formerly it was not uncommon for women to have severe lacerations of the cervix or the perineum, often extending through the sphincter muscles into the rectum. These lacerations resulted from childbirth and occur less frequently now because of the practice of modern obstetrics; today lacerations that do occur are generally repaired at the time of delivery.

Rectocele is a protrusion of the rectum into the vagina, and cystocele is a displacement of the bladder toward or into the vagina. Uterine prolapse permits the uterus to drop downward, and in severe cases the downward descent may cause the cervix to protrude through the external vaginal opening.

These conditions may result from injury during childbirth, changes resulting from weakening or stretching of supporting structures, and loss of muscle tone. The condition causes a feeling of downward pressure, especially when standing or walking, and urinary incontinence with frequency or urgency. There may be fatigue and constipation, and in cases of complete laceration through the sphincter muscle of the rectum, feces will be expelled through the vagina. Patients are generally worried, apprehensive, and likely to delay medical examination and treatment. Surgery is required to correct these conditions.

Preoperative care is especially important in assuring as clean an operative area as possible. Patients may be admitted to the hospital 2 or 3 days prior to surgery and given a cathartic, followed by enemas to be sure the bowel is completely empty. A liquid diet for 48 hours prior to surgery will help to keep the bowel empty. The surgeon may or may not order a cleansing vaginal douche on the evening before and the morning of surgery. The entire vaginal area is shaved, including the pubis and the rectal area.

The postoperative care of the patient includes checking vital signs and frequent observation for hemorrhage. A retention catheter is usually inserted into the urinary bladder to keep it empty and prevent pressure on sutures. It is important to keep the fecal residue as soft as possible, and for that reason some physicians order only liquids for several days, or they may order mineral oil to be given every night. An oil retention enema may be ordered, but cleansing enemas should not be given. A small, soft rubber tube should be used for the oil retention enema, and the patient must be instructed not to strain when defecating. External sutures may or may not be present, depending on whether perineal repair has been done. The nurse should understand the physician's orders concerning perineal care, since some physicians wish the area to be kept completely dry. The heat lamp may be used two or three times a day for periods of 20 to 30 minutes. If a solution is to be used in giving perineal care, the physician will order it; all equipment and supplies must be sterile to prevent infection.

The patient is usually kept in low Fowler's position to prevent pressure or strain on sutures. When ambulation is allowed, the patient should be taught to roll out of bed. On discharge from the hospital the patient should be advised against standing for long periods or lifting heavy objects for several weeks.

Malignant lesions

Malignant lesions of the vulva and vagina are relatively rare. The most common complaint of patients with early vulvar cancer is pruritus (itching). This usually accompanies the precancerous condition of leukoplakia, which is thickened white patches on the mucous membranes.[3] These cancers grow slowly, metastasize late, and if malignancy does occur, radical surgery is usually indicated. X-ray therapy may be used when the disease has progressed beyond the operable stage.

Vulvectomy includes the removal of the external female genitals. It may be a partial procedure for biopsy purposes, a simple procedure for removal of a benign lesion, or a radical procedure for malignant lesions. The conditions necessitating vulvectomy are peculiar to older women: The average age of such patients is 62 years. The rather typical situation is one in which the patient has tried various salves, ointments, and lotions before finally seeking medical care. When a radical vulvectomy is

necessary, the inguinal lymph nodes in the groin on both sides are removed. The age factor may present both medical and surgical problems, since patients are at an age when cardiovascular and other degenerative diseases may be present.

Preoperative care includes the same care as reviewed in Chapter 9. Wide areas of skin preparation should include the inguinal regions, vulva, and pubic and perineal area. The emotional preparation of the patient is important, and the nurse should listen to any apprehensions or fears that the patient expresses. Fear of disfigurement and loss of a body part are common. Both before and after surgery the patient may show signs of a grief reaction such as depression, anger, denial, or withdrawal. The patient may be assured that after recovery from the surgery her normal life patterns will not be altered.

When the patient returns from surgery, a Foley catheter will be in the urinary bladder. Dressings may have to be changed frequently for several days because of the serous drainage from the wounds. A T binder may be used to hold dressings in place. The patient is placed in low Fowler's position to prevent strain on the sutures. The patient should be turned every 2 hours, and when on her side a pillow should be placed lengthwise between her legs to support the upper leg and prevent strain. The wound is cleansed daily according to the physician's orders. Solutions often used for cleansing include hydrogen peroxide, warm physiologic saline solution, benzalkonium chloride (Zephiran chloride) solution, and solutions that contain hexachlorophene. The surgeon may prefer that wounds be exposed and that a heat lamp be used, since it stimulates circulation and promotes healing. Some physicians may order sitz baths, whereas others may believe that such baths increase the danger of wound infection. The patient is usually given a low-residue diet. Analgesics will be required for several days, and recovery is generally slow. The patient may be ambulatory by the third day, but the nurse should remember that ambulation must be gradual for the older person. Leg edema is common after surgery, and some patients may develop chronic leg edema. Elastic stockings, elevation of the legs frequently, and avoidance of long periods of sitting or standing will help to provide better venous return. An important nursing function is the prevention of wound infection. Care should be taken to provide privacy when caring for the wound and to avoid any unnecessary exposure of the patient.[5, 21]

Conditions affecting the cervix and uterus
Cervicitis

Cervicitis may be the result of an acute inflammatory condition of the vagina, or it may be a chronic condition resulting from lacerations occurring at the time of delivery, erosion, cysts, or a specific infection such as gonorrhea. The cause of erosions is not always known and is often believed to be congenital. It appears to be more common in women who are taking oral contraceptives. Cervicitis may occur in any woman, often producing no symptoms, and is detected only on a routine pelvic examination. Most physicians believe that untreated chronic cervicitis predisposes to cancer of the cervix. Treatment includes examination and studies to exclude cancer of the cervix. If lacerations exist, they should be repaired surgically, and erosions may be cauterized. If the condition does not respond to conservative treatment, the patient may be admitted to the hospital and under general anesthesia have a cone-shaped portion of the cervix removed (conization).

Uterine displacement

Retroversion is a displacement of the uterus backward from its normal position. It frequently occurs as a congenital condition and may result from laceration at the time of delivery followed by lack of proper postpartum exercises. It may be caused by large tumors or cysts that tend to weaken the uterine supports or contribute to the formation of adhesions. The condition may present no symptoms, or it may be evidenced by backache, fatigue, a feeling of pelvic pressure, and leukorrhea. Treatment may be confined to exercises or to the placement of pessaries to hold the uterus in a normal position. Pessaries are inserted by the physician and should not cause the person any difficulty or discomfort. They may be worn for several months; however, they must be removed at intervals by the

physician, cleaned, and reinserted. The patient may be advised to use a douche several times a week, since there may be some vaginal irritation and discharge. For some persons abdominal surgery is needed to correct the condition.

Endometriosis

The uterus is an organ that sheds cells periodically. These are endometrial cells, and occasionally they become seeded throughout the pelvis and other organs. The exact cause is unknown, but possibly it is of congenital origin. Although these endometrial cells are not in the uterus, they are stimulated by the ovarian hormones and bleed into the nearby tissue, resulting in an inflammatory process. Adhesions, strictures, cysts, and infertility can result.[16, 21]

The patient is usually asymptomatic until she is between 30 and 40 years of age. Symptoms that gradually begin to occur are pain during menstruation, which becomes progressively worse, fatigue, pressure in the pelvic organs, and general discomfort. Treatment with drugs that suppress ovulation for a period of time delays the stimulation of the cells and increases the chance of fertility when administration of the drug is stopped. When endometriosis in severe, removal of the uterus, fallopian tubes, and ovaries may be necessary.

Tumors

Cancer of the cervix is the most common form of malignancy affecting the female reproductive organs. It is much more common than cancer of the uterus. Unfortunately, cancer of the cervix does not cause any symptoms during the early stages, and the condition is usually far advanced before any signs appear. Although cancer of the cervix may occur in young adults, the incidence increases with age, with the greatest incidence in patients between 30 and 50 years of age. The Papanicolaou smear test (p. 78) is being used widely and has had a primary effect on the decreasing mortality rates for cervical cancer. Carcinoma in situ is a preinvasive, asymptomatic carcinoma that can only be diagnosed by microscopic examination.[14] Once it is diagnosed, it can be treated early without radical surgery and a cure results. Carcinoma in situ of the cervix is essentially 100% curable. Therefore all women over 20 years of age should have a yearly pelvic examination and Pap smear.

Cancer of the uterus occurs somewhat later in life, usually being postmenopausal. The most common symptom is vaginal bleeding, and no relationship exists between the amount of bleeding and the existence of cancer. Sometimes only a slight spotting occurs.

Treatment of cancer of the cervix and uterus varies with the extent of the cancer and age of the patient. For cancer in situ a conization may be performed, which removes a portion of the cervix. Other patients may have a simple hysterectomy. Radical surgery and radiation therapy (Chapter 5) are used for more advanced cancer.

A frequently occurring type of benign tumor is commonly called a *fibroid*, which is an abnormal growth of uterine muscle tissue. These tumors are usually localized and may grow slowly, but they may become extremely large. Vaginal bleeding is the characteristic symptom; however, if they become large enough to cause pressure on other structures, there may be backache, constipation, and urinary symptoms. Uterine fibroids may be treated with radium if the individual is near menopause; however, if tumors are large, surgery is usually the treatment of choice.

Conditions affecting the ovaries and fallopian tubes
Cysts and tumors

Many different kinds of ovarian tumors and cysts are benign; however, some may be malignant. Ovarian cysts may cause no symptoms, or they may result in a disturbance of menstruation, a feeling of heaviness, and slight bleeding. If a pedicle (a stemlike structure) is present, the cyst may become twisted on the pedicle, cutting off the blood supply. If this occurs, immediate surgery is indicated.

Carcinoma of the ovary is most common in women 50 years of age or older. It may be primary but often is the result of metastasis from a lesion somewhere else in the body. Sites from which metastasis may spread include the gastrointestinal tract, uterus, or breast. The occurrence of a ma-

lignant ovarian tumor alerts the physician to look for malignancy elsewhere in the body. Carcinoma of the ovary is usually bilateral, and the surgical procedure generally includes a complete hysterectomy and bilateral removal of the ovaries and the fallopian tubes. X-ray therapy may be used as an adjunct to surgery, and some patients may be treated with chemotherapy.[4]

Salpingitis

Salpingitis is an inflammation of the fallopian tube caused by bacteria. The gonococcus is frequently the invading organism, but other bacteria such as the streptococcus or staphylococcus may be responsible for the infection. The causative organism usually enters the uterine cavity and from there finds its way to the tubes. The ovaries and the pelvic peritoneum may become involved, resulting in what is called *pelvic inflammatory disease*. The condition may become chronic, and recurrent attacks may occur. The inflammatory process frequently gives rise to the formation of adhesions, and the tubes may be completely occluded. Atresia of the tubes, whether from a congenital condition or from disease, may result in sterility or a tubal pregnancy (ectopic pregnancy).

Abdominal pain may be severe, and an elevation of temperature, nausea, vomiting, vaginal discharge, and backache occur during the acute stage of the illness. Chronic pelvic inflammatory disease may result in menstrual disturbances, including dysmenorrhea. Conservative treatment includes bed rest, placing the patient in Fowler's position, hot vaginal irrigations at a temperature of 120° F., heat to the abdomen, hot sitz baths, and antibiotic drugs. If the condition does not respond to conservative treatment, surgery may be done to remove the tubes (salpingectomy).

Surgical treatment

Hysterectomy. Hysterectomy is the surgical removal of the uterus. A hysterectomy may be performed through an incision into the abdominal cavity (abdominal hysterectomy), or the uterus may be removed through the vagina (vaginal hysterectomy). In premenopausal women the ovaries are usually not removed unless some abnormal condition exists. Depending on the existing condition, the physician may consider it necessary to remove one or both ovaries or one or both fallopian tubes. Removal of both ovaries is called *bilateral oophorectomy*, and removal of both fallopian tubes is called *bilateral salpingectomy*. When the entire uterus, tubes, and ovaries are removed, the operation is called *panhysterosalpingo-oophorectomy*. A hysterectomy does not necessarily mean that any organs will be removed other than the uterus. However, if there is evidence of disease affecting other organs, they will be removed at the same time as the uterus.

Surgery involving the female reproductive tract is upsetting to most women. Often the patient perceives the procedure as a threat to her femininity. If the patient is of childbearing age, she may be disappointed because she can no longer have children. Often patients will worry about the process of healing and the resumption of sexual activity.[24] If cancer is suspected or found, thoughts of death may occur. The more thoroughly the patient is prepared for the surgery, the more satisfactorily she will recover, both physically and emotionally.

Preoperative care. Preoperative care is the same as that for patients having other kinds of abdominal surgery. The surgical preparation of the skin includes the abdomen, pubis, and perineum. The physician may or may not order a douche preoperatively.

Postoperative care. Postoperative nursing care is concerned with the prevention of urinary retention, intestinal distention, and venous thrombosis. The incidence of urinary retention is greater after hysterectomy than after other types of surgery because some trauma to the bladder unavoidably occurs. Urinary retention leads to discomfort from distention and increases the danger of urinary tract infection. Before administering drugs for pain, the nurse should be sure that the discomfort is not from an overdistended bladder. Most patients are given intravenous fluids for 1 or 2 days, and the additional fluid may contribute to bladder distention. Every method should be used to assist the patient to void prior to catheterization; efforts should be instituted early, not delayed until the pa-

tient is miserable because of an overdistended bladder. For some patients a retention catheter may have been inserted into the bladder and should be connected to closed drainage (p. 343). If the patient does not have a catheter and is unable to void, catheterization every 8 hours may be necessary.

A nasogastric tube is usually inserted and is connected to suction siphonage to help prevent abdominal distention. A small tap water enema or saline enema may be ordered to help prevent distention, and administration of neostigmine (Prostigmin) may be ordered by the physician. As soon as bowel sounds have returned and flatus is being expelled, the patient is allowed liquids by mouth with a gradual return to solid food.

Patients undergoing pelvic surgery are more susceptible to venous stasis and phlebitis because of trauma to blood vessels. Patients who have varicose veins in the extremities must be carefully observed. The nurse should remember the admonitions that have been given previously: do *not* raise the knee gatch, place pillows under the knees, or place the patient in high Fowler's position. Active exercise should be started as soon as the patient is fully conscious, and early ambulation helps to prevent venous stasis. Some surgeons order the patient's legs wrapped with elastic bandages, which should be removed several times a day for inspection of the legs and then rewrapped.

Sedation such as meperidine hydrochloride (Demerol) may be ordered for relief of pain. Slight vaginal drainage may occur for a day or two, but any unusual bleeding should be reported to the physician. Checking vital signs and observing the abdominal dressing for evidence of bleeding should be routinely carried out. Most patients without complications are dismissed from the hospital in about 1 week.

If the vaginal approach is used for a hysterectomy, the postoperative nursing care is essentially the same as that for repair of relaxed muscles[5] (p. 373).

Before the patient is discharged she should know what changes she can expect. She will no longer menstruate, and she should not have coitus until her physician permits. She may have worries concerning her ability to continue to please her partner sexually. When a hysterectomy is done, the vaginal floor is reconstructed with ligaments, and the majority of women should have the same sexual relations after surgery as before. Light housework may be done when she returns home; however, lifting heavy objects and more difficult housework must be avoided for a few weeks. Most women may return to work within 6 weeks.[24]

Isolation perfusion (intra-arterial perfusion). Isolation perfusion is a technique for administering chemotherapy to a malignant tumor in amounts that would not be possible to place in the patient's general system. Reports have indicated that some patients have benefited, but this type of therapy is still regarded as a research procedure.[20] A pump-oxygenator is used, and a closed system is established so that the tumor area may be exposed to large doses of a chemotherapeutic agent without the drug entering the general system. When therapy is applied to the pelvic area, the abdominal aorta and the vena cava are used. For intra-arterial perfusion other vessels such as the brachial, femoral, axillary, or carotid vessels are used, and a catheter is inserted using the fluoroscope to guide its introduction.

Patients who are to receive pelvic perfusion are admitted to the hospital several days prior to the procedure. Extensive studies and tests, especially blood studies, are completed because, as in open heart surgery, large amounts of blood are used. Careful and efficient preparation can be reassuring to the patient, who may be apprehensive and discouraged; thus emotional support is extremely important.

Postoperative care includes the same care given to all surgical patients. In addition, the patient must be observed carefully for failure of kidney function, and accurate intake and output records must be maintained. The diet should be high in calories. Blood samples are collected every day and checked for the white blood cell count, which may show a significant drop on about the tenth day. Depending on the extent of decrease in the number of white blood cells, medical aseptic technique and reverse isolation may be established to protect the patient from infection. The patient should be observed for venous stasis and evidence of thrombophlebitis, and the color, temperature, and pulse in the extremities should be checked. Skin care is especially important because these patients are likely to develop decubitus ulcers.[11] One of the primary factors in the care of the patient who undergoes pelvic perfusion is the necessity for continuous encouragement and support by all personnel who participate in any aspect of the patient's care.

Conditions affecting the breast
Acute mastitis

Mastitis is an inflammation of the mammary gland (breast) that often occurs during lactation but may occur any time. It is the result of the entrance of bacteria through a crack or fissure of the nipple. The infection may block one or more of the milk ducts, causing the milk to stagnate in the lobule. The infection may spread throughout the breast tissue and cause abscess formation. The infection usually causes an elevation of temperature, with pain and tenderness of the breast. The treatment consists of administration of antibiotic drugs, application of heat or cold, and support of the breast. Incision and drainage of an abscess may be necessary. Although uncommon, mastitis may occur in both the male and female as a complication of mumps. Since the invading organism in mastitis is frequently the staphylococcus, isolation and care as outlined in Chapter 4 should be followed.

Chronic cystic mastitis

Chronic cystic mastitis is characterized by the formation of a nodular type of benign cyst in the breast. The exact cause is unknown but may be related to some hormone imbalance. Many women go through life unaware of the condition or neglect diagnosis and treatment. The disease is not malignant and does not produce an inflammatory condition; although it may involve both breasts, it is generally accentuated in one breast. The cysts may occur singly or may be numerous and vary in size and tenderness. Pain may be present and may become worse during the menstrual period. Treatment is usually conservative after cancer has been ruled out; however, the patient should examine her own breasts at monthly intervals and remain under medical supervision.

Tumors

Tumors of the breasts may be benign and are often found in young persons. This type of tumor is not tender and is freely movable, and its removal should not be delayed. Although such tumors may appear to be benign, an exact diagnosis can be made only by careful microscopic examination.

Cancer (carcinoma) of the breast is one of the most frequently occurring malignancies in the white female, and any breast tumor occurring past menopause should be viewed as potentially malignant. Time is an important factor in the diagnosis and treatment of breast cancer, since in the early stages the possibility of cure is good. The development of the disease is insidious, and pain is usually absent in the early stages. The only sign that may be present is a small firm lump in the breast, not well defined or movable, which may be discovered only by careful examination. As the tumor increases in size, it attaches itself to the chest wall or to the skin above. A dimpling of the skin may be present, the nipple may be retracted or inverted, and discharge from the nipple may be present. In some cases reddening of the skin may be present, and if the tumor is large, change in the contour of the breast may be present. Without treatment the axillary lymph nodes become involved, ulceration may occur, and metastasis to the lungs, bones, liver, and brain may occur. A gradual state of ill health occurs with weight loss and poor appetite.

The American Cancer Society has outlined a program for self-examination of the breasts and through films and printed material has sought to encourage women to detect any abnormal lump in their breasts. Cancer of the breast is the leading cause of cancer deaths in women and the leading cause of all deaths in women today. It has been estimated that 33,000 women will die from breast cancer during 1974.[7] When the disease is localized in the breast, 85% of women affected will survive 5 years or longer. The 5-year survival rate is decreased to 53% when the cancer has spread to the surrounding tissues.[20] The single woman is more likely to have cancer of the breast than the married woman, and married women who do not bear children are more likely to have cancer of the breast than married women who have children. There also appears to be a lower incidence of breast cancer among women who breast-feed their babies for the first 3 months. However, some authorities question this factor. It should be remembered that cancer of the breast is not hereditary but is based on family histories; some families do have a greater incidence of breast cancer than others.[15]

Diagnosis is based on mammography, thermography (p. 79), and incision of the tumor for laboratory microscopic examination. This is followed by a simple or radical mastectomy if cancer is present.

Mastectomy. The surgical removal of the breast may be simple or radical. In simple mastectomy the breast is incised and sutured without removal of lymph nodes, whereas a radical mastectomy includes removal of the breast and the underlying tissues, including the muscles, axillary lymph nodes and vessels, and perhaps the entire mammary lymph node chain and supraclavicular nodes. The extent of surgery depends on the extensiveness of the neoplasm. When the malignant tumor is localized and examination of the lymph nodes is negative, most surgeons believe that a radical mastectomy should be done.[6]

Recently there has been a belief among some surgeons that a less radical procedure should be considered for mastectomy patients. Such a procedure would decrease the amount of muscle tissue under the gland that would be excised and the number of lymph nodes removed. This modified procedure does not have unanimous approval among surgeons at this time. Therefore no broad recommendations have been made. Each patient will continue to be evaluated on an individual basis, and the procedure best suited for her will be performed.

Most mastectomies are performed because of cancer, and irradiation may precede or follow the surgical procedure. Often patients have delayed medical care and surgery too long so that the cancer has become invasive and therefore inoperable.

Although treatment may be only palliative at this stage, the patient must be assured and convinced that something can be done.

Preoperative care. The emotional preparation of the patient may be even more important than the physical preparation. The patient may go to surgery believing that only a biopsy is to be done, and although the physician may have explained the possibility of more extensive surgery, the patient may not comprehend its real significance. When she awakens and finds her side enclosed in tight bandages and realizes what has happened, the shock may be profound. The female nurse can help provide emotional preparation and support for the patient. The woman-to-woman understanding between nurse and patient is not easily conveyed by the physician to the patient, and even the patient's husband may be unable to provide the understanding that the patient needs. The Reach to Recovery program sponsored by local chapters of the American Cancer Society, Inc., will send volunteer women who have had mastectomies to speak to individuals or groups on request. Providing an opportunity to discuss the effects of a mastectomy often gives needed reassurance to the patient facing or recuperating from such surgery.

The physical preparation of the patient requires that a wide area of skin be shaved, including the axilla (Fig. 16-2). Frequently a radical mastectomy requires skin grafting, and if the nurse understands this possibility, the anterior surface of the thigh should be shaved, since the donor skin may be taken from this area. For some patients blood transfusion or intravenous fluids may be administered preoperatively. Other preparation is the same as that for other types of major surgery.

Postoperative care. Postoperative nursing care should include checking vital signs and observation for symptoms of shock or hemorrhage, since many large blood vessels are involved in the procedure. Drains may be placed in the axilla to facilitate drainage, and some surgeons attach them to low suction. Other physicians use the Hemovac for drainage. Dressings are usually applied rather tightly and may tend to embarrass respiration and cause some pain and dis-

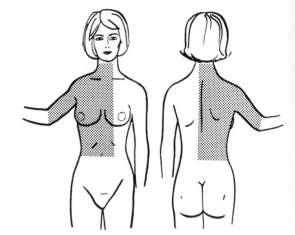

Fig. 16-2. Area of the skin to be prepared for a mastectomy.

comfort. When the vital signs are stable, the patient is placed in a 45-degree Fowler's position to promote drainage. The position should be changed frequently and deep breathing and coughing encouraged. The patient may have considerable pain and should be given pain-relieving medication, but care must be exercised to prevent oversedation so that the patient will be able to cough and breathe deeply. Physicians differ in opinion concerning the best positioning of the affected arm. Some physicians include the arm in the dressing. If the arm is not included, it may be elevated on a pillow with the hand and wrist higher than the elbow and the elbow higher than the shoulder joint. This will facilitate the flow of fluids by the lymph and venous routes and prevent lymphedema. The arm should be observed for signs of circulatory disturbance such as coldness, lack of radial pulse, cyanosis, or blanching. If the arm is left entirely free, it should be observed for edema, numbness, or inability to move the fingers, which should be reported immediately. The patient is allowed out of bed on the first or second postoperative day. The nurse must remember that balance may be poor and that the patient may need assistance to prevent falling. Fluids are permitted as soon as nausea ceases, and diet is usually ordered as tolerated. The patient will need help in cutting meat and in arranging food conveniently, since use of the arm on the affected side may be difficult.

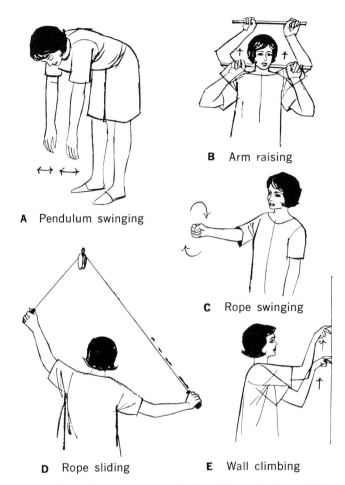

A Pendulum swinging

B Arm raising

C Rope swinging

D Rope sliding

E Wall climbing

Fig. 16-3. Arm exercises after mastectomy. **A,** Pendulum swinging with the arms relaxed and swinging free. **B,** Arm raising from back of the neck over the head. **C,** Rope swinging with a length of rope tied to the doorknob and swinging with shoulder motion. **D,** Rope sliding by placing a length of rope over a pulley and sliding the rope up and down. **E,** Wall climbing by standing with the face to the wall and climbing the wall with the hands, with the fingers reaching as far as possible.

Any intravenous fluids should be administered or blood pressure readings should be taken using the unaffected arm.

Rehabilitation. One of the aims of rehabilitation is to restore the use of the affected arm as soon as possible to prevent contracture. The physician will determine the time at which exercises may be started, depending on the presence of sutures and whether skin grafting has been done. If the donor site for skin used in grafting is the thigh, it must be carefully protected from infection. Often these areas are very sore and may cause the patient some pain and difficulty in walking. Care for the patient remaining in the hospital for x-ray therapy was outlined in Chapter 5.

When the patient is discharged home, the public health nurse may visit the patient to encourage and to reassure her and to supervise exercises. Some exercises that will help the patient regain use of the arm are shown in Fig. 16-3. The public health nurse may follow up suggestions made in the hospital concerning a breast prosthesis. Whatever type of prosthesis is selected by the patient should be comfortable and meet her needs. The physician will determine when the prosthesis may be used.

Conditions of pregnancy
Abortion

Abortion exceeds the sum of all other complications of pregnancy. On January 22, 1973, the United States Supreme Court ruled that all antiabortion laws were unconstitutional in the United States. In general, the court made the following ruling concerning abortion:

1. During the first trimester, the abortion decision is a matter between the woman and her physician.

2. During the second trimester, states can regulate abortion procedures but not the grounds for abortion.

3. After fetal viability (about 24 weeks) the state may regulate abortion, except that abortion must always be allowed if appropriate medical judgment deems the abortion necessary to preserve the life or health of the woman.

In 1973, twenty-three states and thirty-nine abortion laws had been enacted. However, 260 bills were introduced by state legislatures with only thirty-nine enacted into law. The laws passed by the states differ widely, and as of January 1, 1973, there were twenty-five states in which abortion was allowed only when necessary to preserve the life of the pregnant woman. Many of these state laws are now being challenged in the courts. During 1972, the last year that statistics are available, 586,760 legal abortions were reported to the Center for Disease Control. Because of the laws in some states, women are still unable to secure an abortion in their home state.

Exact data for illegal abortions are not available. Before abortion was legalized estimates placed the number of illegal abortions between 200,000 and 1 million annually. In 1972, seventy-one maternal deaths related to abortion occurred, of which thirty-four deaths were attributed to criminal abortion.[1, 12]

However, spontaneous abortion may result from an emergency situation, and the possibility of death of both fetus and mother is present. Legalized abortions have brought about rapid changes in maternity nursing, which has always been focused on bringing new life into the world. Many nursing personnel have had difficulty accepting these changes, and many hospitals have used in-service education to help nurses to verbalize their feelings. Whatever the feelings of the individual nurse, the patient entering the hospital seeking an abortion should never face hostility or discrimination. The decision to seek an abortion may be a difficult one, and these patients have problems and worries similar to those of any other hospitalized patient.[9]

The patient hospitalized because of abortion needs sympathy and understanding without assurance that a wanted pregnancy will not fail. The nurse should provide any assistance to help alleviate problems created by the emergency. A social worker, the public health nurse, or the patient's religious counselor may be able to provide assistance.

The term *abortion* is frequently applied to any expulsion of the products of conception prior to full-term delivery. More correctly, abortion means expulsion of the fetal contents before viability (approximately 24 weeks). Thereafter, loss of the fetus is considered as premature birth. Nonprofessional persons may refer to loss during any stage of the pregnancy as *miscarriage*. There are two main categories of abortion: spontaneous and induced. Abortion may be classified as follows:

1. Spontaneous abortion
   a. Habitual
   b. Threatened
   c. Inevitable
   d. Incomplete
   e. Complete
   f. Missed
   g. Septic
2. Induced abortion
   a. Therapeutic
   b. Criminal, or illegal
   c. Legalized

Abortion may also be classified according to weight of the fetus. This method separates the product of conception that is not viable or is unable to sustain life outside the uterus from the fetus, which is premature or mature and will live in view of modern methods of infant care.

The exact cause of spontaneous abortion is unknown, but some evidence indicates that some abortions are the result of defective germ plasm. It is not believed that falls are significant as a cause of abortion.

Habitual abortion is a term applied when three or more successive pregnancies are spontaneously interrupted. The situation frequently creates a severe emotional problem when a woman wants to have children.

Threatened abortion is indicated when vaginal bleeding or spotting occurs during the first 20 weeks of gestation. The cervix is not dilated, and with conservative treatment the pregnancy may continue uninterrupted. The patient is placed on a regimen of bed rest for 48 hours and is given a mild sedative. All pads should be saved for the physician's inspection, and the patient is instructed not to take an enema or a laxative.

In *inevitable abortion* the vaginal bleeding may be only spotting, or hemorrhage may occur with passing of clots. The cervix is dilated, and mild pelvic cramping occurs with gradual increase until all or part of the uterine contents are expelled. In inevitable abortion there is no chance of saving the pregnancy.

In *incomplete abortion* only a portion of the products of conception has been expelled; bleeding continues and may cause severe hemorrhage. The part retained is usually fragments of the placenta. It is necessary to hospitalize the patient and place her on a regimen of bed rest. Sedative drugs are administered and blood transfusions given if hemorrhage has been severe. Oxytocin may be administered to stimulate contractions of the uterus. If the residue is not expelled and bleeding continues, the patient is prepared for surgery, taken to the operating room, and given a light anesthetic; dilation and curettage is done. Recovery is rapid, and the patient may be dismissed from the hospital in 2 or 3 days.

In *complete abortion* the entire products of conception are expelled. It is probable that many complete abortions occur without any major difficulty, and a physician does not see the patient.

In *missed abortion* the fetus dies and is retained for 8 weeks or more prior to the twentieth week of gestation. Weekly examinations of the fibrinogen level in the blood are done. No attempt is made to empty the uterus unless the level of fibrinogen begins to fall. Oxytocin may be administered to stimulate contractions and cause the fetus to be expelled.

Evidence of *septic abortion* includes an elevation of temperature to 104° F. or more, with threatened or incomplete loss of the products of conception. The presence or absence of any other focus of infection is ruled out prior to establishing a diagnosis of septic abortion. The sepsis may be caused by any of several pathogenic organisms. If caused by *Clostridium perfringens*, a spore-forming organism, a powerful exotoxin is liberated. The patient is critically ill with a temperature of 104° F. or more, the pulse is rapid, and headache, malaise, abdominal tenderness, and indications of pelvic peritonitis occur. The patient is isolated, and medical aseptic technique is carried out. Cultures from the cervix and the uterus are taken, and the appropriate antibiotics are administered. Intravenous fluids and blood transfusions may be given, hydrocortisone and oxytocin (Pitocin) may be ordered. Septic abortion frequently results in serious complications, including acute renal failure, congestive heart failure, hemorrhage, and severe shock. The patient's condition will be considered in the physician's decision to do a dilation and curettage; however, opinions differ concerning the time when a dilation and curettage should be done. In some cases a hysterectomy may be performed.

Therapeutic abortion is the termination of pregnancy by a physician during the first trimester of pregnancy. Therapeutic abortion is usually indicated only when the life or health of the mother must be protected. It is considered when there is a hazard to the fetus such as rubella (German measles) in the mother during the first trimester of pregnancy (p. 553). Reputable physicians secure medical consultation or approval by an established committee before performing a therapeutic abortion.

Legalized abortion, the termination of a pregnancy at the request of the woman, is now available in all states, the result of a recent Supreme Court ruling.

Criminal or *illegal abortion* is performed without medical or legal approval. Many are self-induced, or they may be performed by midwives, nonprofessional persons known as "doctors," or other lay persons.

Since abortion has been legalized in many states, the incidence of illegal abortion has decreased significantly. It should be noted that the number of illegal abortions cannot be estimated, since they are not reported. Only if the woman encounters problems and is forced to consult a physician or clinic may the abortion be known. When serious complications develop such as hemorrhage, renal failure, or sepsis, medical care will be sought. The maternal mortality rates are higher in illegal abortion than in spontaneous abortion. The treatment of the patient is essentially the same as that for septic abortion.

Nursing care. Patients admitted to the hospital after illegal abortion should be isolated, or precautionary measures should be taken until the existence of sepsis and the specific organism has been established. All patients with known or suspected septic abortions should be isolated. All patients admitted for abortion in any stage must be carefully observed for hemorrhage. The exact number of pad changes and whether they are only spotted or soaked should be recorded. If hemorrhage occurs in the absence of the physician, the nurse may elevate the foot of the bed as an emergency measure. The physician is always notified of the condition. All urinary output is measured hourly, and the color is noted and recorded. Administration of medications, fluids, or blood transfusions is carried out according to the physician's orders.

Everything that the patient expels must be saved for the physician's inspection. The nurse must also be sure of the hospital policy concerning the disposal of the products of conception. A few years ago a lawsuit was threatened against a hospital because a nurse's aide had placed the products of conception resulting from an abortion in a trash can.

Preparation of the patient for dilation and curettage is the same as that for nonpregnant women. The patient having a legal abortion should be made aware of the signs of possible complications such as a foul discharge, fever, or hemorrhage. They also should receive advice concerning birth control before discharge. Nurses should remember that their function is to provide nursing care, support, and encouragement, regardless of the conditions surrounding the abortion.

Ectopic pregnancy

Ectopic pregnancy is gestation anywhere outside the uterus. Rarely, but occasionally, it may be in the abdomen or the ovary; however, the most common site is the fallopian tube. When the ovum becomes implanted in the fallopian tube, it is referred to as *tubal pregnancy*. Infrequently, a tubal pregnancy may be palpated in the area near the uterus, but the first indication of tubal pregnancy occurs when the tube ruptures. Tubal pregnancy results from some condition within the tube that slows or prevents passage of the ovum through the tube to the endometrium of the uterus. Conditions such as inflammation from disease, narrowing of the tube, and an elongated or immature tube create a situation conducive to tubal pregnancy.

As the embryo increases in size, the tube stretches until it can no longer remain intact. The tube may rupture, releasing the entire products of conception into the abdominal cavity (ectopic abortion), or the rupture may be small, and the embryo remains within the tube, but severe bleeding occurs from damage to the blood vessels. The length of time the tube remains intact with the developing embryo is variable and may be from 3 to 4 weeks or as long as 8 to 12 weeks.

Frequently the patient has missed one period and has noted slight spotting but may not know that she is pregnant. In the majority of patients rupture results in acute abdominal pain that occurs suddenly. The pain may extend to the shoulder and the rectal area. The patient becomes faint and pale and may be in shock. Hemorrhage may be severe, and acute secondary anemia results.

A ruptured tubal pregnancy is always an emergency and requires immediate surgery. There may be little time for preoperative preparation. The shock is treated immediately by blood transfusions or intravenous infusion of lactated Ringer's solution. The nurse must anticipate the physician's needs and work quickly and efficiently.

Postoperative care of the patient is the same as that for other abdominal surgery. Transfusions with whole blood may be necessary to combat the anemia. Uterine bleeding will occur for several days, and the patient must be observed for any unusual bleeding from the abdominal incision or from the vagina.

Cesarean section

Cesarean section is a surgical procedure providing for delivery by a method other than through the normal birth canal. The oldest method is through an abdominal incision into the peritoneal cavity. This method is still used by many physicians. In recent years several methods have been developed by which the uterine cavity is entered through the abdomen, but without entering the general peritoneal cavity. In situations in which abnormality or a pathologic uterine condition exists, a cesarean hysterectomy may be done.

There are various indications for cesarean section, among which are severe toxemia of pregnancy, contracted pelvis and a large baby, certain pathologic conditions such as a tumor that interferes with normal passage, and avoidance of rupture of the uterus when the patient has had a previous cesarean section. In addition, several other complications may prevent normal delivery or threaten the life of the mother or the baby or both.

In some situations cesarean section may be an emergency, but most often it is an elective procedure. When it is to be done as an elective procedure, the physician indicates the time that the patient should enter the hospital. It is generally as near full term as possible but prior to onset of labor. The patient should enter the hospital a couple of days prior to the surgery.

The preoperative preparation includes the usual preparation for abdominal surgery. A retention catheter is placed in the urinary bladder, fetal heart tones are taken, and the only preoperative medication generally ordered is atropine. It is necessary for the operating room staff to provide for the baby as well as the mother. A warm bed and resuscitation equipment should be available for the baby, and a nurse or a pediatrician should be available to give undivided attention to the baby. Drugs, sterile syringes, and needles should be on a tray available for emergency.

Postoperative nursing care of the patient after cesarean section is largely the same as that after other abdominal surgery. In addition, the patient must be observed for signs of internal hemorrhage or excessive vaginal bleeding. If there is excessive vomiting, unusual bleeding, or signs of shock, the physician must be notified immediately. Postoperatively the physican may order oxytocin to keep the uterus contracted, and the nurse must remember that the uterus is not to be massaged. The retention catheter may be left in place for a day or two, and sterile technique should be observed in its care (p. 344). Intravenous fluids may be administered, and records of intake and output should be maintained. Pain-relieving drugs will be needed for a day or two, but if no complications occur, the patient progresses rapidly and may be ambulatory by the first or second day. Routine postpartum care can usually be given after 3 or 4 days.[11, 13]

Toxemias of pregnancy

Toxemias of pregnancy are responsible for both maternal and infant deaths. The cause is not completely understood, but the indications are that toxemia is in some way related to the influence of the pregnancy state. The condition is always serious because of its life-threatening potential, and it requires skilled medical and nursing care.

Toxemias are classified as either preeclampsia or eclampsia. Both actually belong to the same symptom complex; the primary differentiation is that convulsions occur in eclampsia, whereas they are uncommon in preeclampsia. In addition, eclampsia may be imposed on an already existing hypertension and after eclampsia, hypertension may continue to exist, posing problems in subsequent pregnancies.

Preeclampsia. Preeclampsia usually develops during the first trimester of pregnancy and is more common in first pregnancies and multiple births. Eclampsia is most characteristic of the last trimester of pregnancy, and in each situation the condition may be mild or severe.

The first consideration is prevention, and here the nurse has the opportunity to play an important role. Every pregnant woman should place herself under the care of an obstetrician at the beginning of her pregnancy. In addition, teaching the woman and observing her for early signs of preeclampsia are important. Most women visit the physician every 2 or 3 weeks until the last months of pregnancy and then weekly.

The nurse should encourage each woman not to delay or omit the regular visits. Every woman should be taught to recognize and report to the physician immediately any of the following signs: sudden or severe headache, disturbance of vision, vomiting if persistent, edema of face or hands, decreased urinary output, or pain in the epigastric region. When the woman comes into the physician's office, one of the most important observations that the nurse can make is to observe for edema of the eyelids; another observation is to note if the woman's wedding ring appears tight. This can be done in a casual manner without the woman even being aware of it.

There are three important aspects of the medical visit: (1) urinalysis for the presence of albumin, (2) blood pressure readings, and (3) weighing the patient. Each should be done with accuracy, and the information should be made available for the physician, together with any objective observations that the nurse may have made.

Symptoms. There are four significant signs of preeclampsia: (1) elevation of blood pressure in which the systolic pressure is elevated 30 mm. Hg or more and the diastolic pressure is elevated 15 mm. Hg or more above the normal base pressure, (2) the continued presence of 2+ or more albumin in the urine, (3) edema of the face and hands that persists, and (4) a sudden unexplained gain in weight of 2 pounds or more. The presence of any two of these signs is regarded as preeclamptic.

Treatment. Most patients with preeclampsia are first treated on an outpatient basis, but failure to obtain reversal or a worsening of symptoms usually requires hospitalization. Conservative outpatient treatment may include restriction of physical activity with as much bed rest as possible and low-sodium diet with restriction of calories. Fluid intake of 2500 to 3000 ml. in 24 hours is recommended (cola drinks should be avoided because of their sodium content). If the patient fails to respond, she is hospitalized and placed on a regimen of complete bed rest.

Nursing responsibilities include blood pressure readings every 4 hours, maintaining accurate records of intake and output, and collecting urine specimens, as requested by the physician. Frequently a re-

tention catheter is placed in the urinary bladder, and aseptic technique must be maintained in its care (p. 344). Calculations of urinary output may be required every hour. A quiet, restful environment should be provided for the patient. Administration of medications may include sedation such as phenobarbital, ½ grain every 4 hours, and a diuretic, usually a chlorothiazide (p. 337). The patient should be reassured and anxiety relieved. She should be watched for convulsions, and a mouth gag should always be in readiness. In most cases the patient will recover and return home, but careful and regular medical supervision will be needed.

Eclampsia. In the eclamptic state the same symptoms are present as in preeclampsia, but they are more severe and convulsions occur. The blood pressure is elevated to 160/110 mm. Hg or more, albumin in the urine is greatly increased, and anuria may occur. Severe visual disturbances, pulmonary edema, cyanosis, and convulsions followed by coma are characteristic.

Treatment and nursing care. There is no uniform treatment for eclampsia. Many older practices are now being questioned, and more conservative measures by a skilled obstetrician are being instituted. However, basic treatment usually falls within the following areas: (1) dietary regulation, (2) sedation, (3) diuretics, (4) regulation of fluid and electrolyte balance, and (5) preparation for delivery if indicated.

Nursing responsibilities include (1) control of the environment, (2) carrying out the physician's orders and procedures related to them, (3) providing safety for the patient, and (4) critical observation of the patient. The patient should be placed in a single room in a quiet area. All noise of any kind must be eliminated. There must be no loud talking, jarring of the bed, noise in handling equipment, or bright lights. The slightest noise or even a slight draft may precipitate a convulsion. All traffic into the room should be eliminated and a nursing care plan instituted to provide uninterrupted periods of rest for the patient. Provision should be made for emergencies, such as oxygen, tracheotomy tray, suction equipment, tray for cardiac arrest, and a tray of emergency drugs. Although equipment should be available, it should not clutter a room in such a manner as to cause undue anxiety for the patient.

During a convulsion the patient will thrash about and may injure herself unless protected. All dentures, including bridges, as well as eyeglasses should be removed and cared for in a safe place. A mouth gag must be available and should be inserted between the teeth at the onset of the convulsion. The nurse should guard against the patient biting the fingers while the mouth gag is being inserted. Bed rails, headboard, and footboard should be padded to prevent injury. The patient should not be restrained during convulsions, but movements may be guided to prevent injury. The patient with true eclampsia must never be left unattended.

Care must be taken to prevent aspiration of secretions, and suctioning may be necessary. A retention catheter will be inserted into the urinary bladder, and catheter care with accurate records of intake and output must be maintained. Intravenous fluids should be administered slowly, and oxygen by mask may be necessary. All vital signs are checked and recorded regularly. Medication and diet orders are carried out promptly as requested by the physician. If possible, the patient's position should be changed frequently.

The patient should be carefully observed during convulsions for the duration, pulse rate, cyanosis, and respiratory difficulty, which are recorded. The patient must be observed for signs of pulmonary edema and labor. The usual signs of labor are absent in eclampsia, and the only visible evidence may be a slight groan or grunt by the patient. Unless the patient is watched carefully, the baby may be born in the bed without the nurse's knowledge. The obstetrician should always be notified immediately if there is the slightest indication of approaching labor.

Most patients will show improvement in 24 to 36 hours. If no recovery occurs after 72 hours, the obstetrician may consider delivery of the patient. All eclamptic patients should be observed for 10 to 14 days post partum, since they are still under the influence of the pregnancy state and convulsions or even eclampsia may occur during this period.[11, 13]

Conditions affecting the male external genitals
Congenital malformation

Congenital malformations involve the bladder, the urethra, and the penis. Exstrophy of the bladder is the most important of the defects. In this condition the abdominal walls have failed to come together, and the anterior surface of the bladder is open on the abdomen. Urine flows continuously from the ureters, and it is impossible to keep the patient dry. Epispadias is frequently associated with exstrophy of the bladder. In epispadias the male urethra is open somewhere along its upper surface, whereas in hypospadias the urethra is open at some point along the undersurface. However, patients with hypospadias are able to control urination. These defects require plastic surgery. When surgery for exstrophy of the bladder is done, a long hospitalization is usually necessary. The surgery is not always successful and is associated with some risk.

Phimosis

Phimosis is a condition in which the orifice of the prepuce is too small to allow retraction of the glans penis. The condition is often congenital but may be acquired as a result of local inflammation or disease. The condition is rarely severe enough to obstruct the flow of urine but may contribute to local infection because it does not permit adequate cleansing. A surgical procedure (circumcision) may be performed in which part of the foreskin is removed, leaving the glans penis uncovered. The operation is usually routinely performed on newborn infants before they leave the hospital. The procedure is also a rite performed in the Jewish religion. After circumcision a sterile petroleum gauze dressing is applied and changed after each voiding. Although excessive bleeding is unusual, the nurse should always observe the infant for more than normal bleeding.

Cryptorchism (undescended testicle)

In embryonic life the testes are in the abdomen, and during the last 2 months before birth they descend into the scrotum. In some instances they fail to do so and remain in the abdomen or in the inguinal canal. One or both testicles may be involved. They sometimes descend during the first few weeks of life, and most will descend before puberty or soon afterward. If the testicles fail to descend, treatment with certain hormones is usually initiated, and if results are not secured, surgery may be done; however, surgery is not always successful. Although the condition is fairly common in the newborn infant, only a small number of adults are seen with an undescended testicle, indicating that the condition is generally self-correcting.

Ectopic testis means that undescended testicles are outside the normal path for descent. Since their location may subject them more readily to injury, intervention to place them into the scrotum is done early. Hormone treatment has no effect on ectopic testis.

Penile ulceration

Ulceration on the penis may result from many conditions, among which are syphilis, chancroid, and tuberculosis. Examination should be made as soon as possible so that proper diagnosis and treatment may be started immediately. (See Chapter 23.)

Conditions affecting the testes and adjacent structures
Epididymitis

The epididymis is a coiled tube approximately 20 feet long that lies in the scrotum and collects the spermatozoa. Any of several bacteria may cause an infection, including the streptococcus, staphylococcus, and colon bacillus. It may occur after prostatitis or infection of the urinary tract. It often occurs as a complication of gonorrhea. The patient may be ill with fever, chills, headache, nausea, and vomiting. Painful swelling of the scrotum, which may be unilateral or bilateral, occurs.

Treatment is to place the patient on a regimen of bed rest and support the scrotum. Heat or cold may be applied, and the appropriate antibiotic is administered. If abscess formation occurs, incision and drainage may be required.[22]

Orchitis

Orchitis, an infection of the testicle, may result from injury or any one of several infectious diseases such as influenza, pneu-

monia, or gonorrhea. It may also occur as a complication of mumps. Symptoms include fever, nausea, and painful swelling of the testicle. The treatment is the same as that for epididymitis.

Hydrocele and varicocele

A hydrocele is a collection of fluid between the testicles and their lining. The condition is often associated with some other disease or injury. Several methods of treatment are used, including aspiration of the fluid; injection of a sclerosing solution, which causes the walls of the sac containing the fluid to adhere; and surgical removal of the sac, which often is the best method of treatment to ensure cure. The scrotum should be supported with bandages or a commercial suspensory.

A varicocele is a form of varicosity that involves the veins of the spermatic cord. It is usually a painless and harmless condition, but if it causes pain, the scrotum should be supported; if support fails to relieve the discomfort, ligation of the veins may be done.

Tumors

Tumors may occur in any part of the male reproductive system. Malignant tumors of the penis account for a small percentage of skin cancer. Malignant tumors of the testicles are rare and when present, metastasize to distant parts of the body. By the time the individual seeks medical care, extensive metastasis may have occurred.

Treatment includes the surgical removal of the testicle and lymph nodes at the back of the perineum, followed by irradiation therapy. Regional perfusion with chemotherapeutic drugs may be used. Cancer of the penis is treated with radium or x rays, and surgical amputation may be required. A primary nursing concern in caring for these patients is providing emotional support.

Conditions affecting the prostate gland
Acute prostatitis

Inflammation of the prostate gland may be the result of a gonorrheal infection; however, it may occur as the result of invasion by other types of bacteria from the bloodstream. The condition may become chronic. During an acute episode the individual may have pain in the perineal area with fever, nausea, vomiting, frequent urination, or retention of urine.

Treatment consists of administration of the appropriate antibiotic or sulfonamide agent, bed rest, and the application of heat. Warm sitz baths and rectal irrigations may provide relief.

Cancer of the prostate gland

The prostate gland is one of the most common sites of cancer among men in the United States. Approximately 54,000 men are affected each year, and 18,000 deaths occur annually. Few persons under 35 years of age are affected. Thorough rectal examinations made at frequent intervals may detect the disease early; however, only a small percentage may be in a curable stage. Hematuria is usually the only early symptom.

When the malignancy is found while it is a small nodule within the gland, surgical removal of the gland may provide cure. Treatment of localized cancer of the prostate with surgery and radiotherapy has been found to increase the 5-year survival rate over that when only surgery is done. When cancer of the prostate gland is extensive, treatment may be only palliative. Treatment is designed to slow the rate of growth of malignant cells and to provide relief from pain. Several procedures may be used, including cryosurgery (freezing prostatic tissues) and radiation therapy. The surgical removal of the testes (orchiectomy) eliminates the male sex hormones that contribute to growth of cancer cells. The administration of estrogen (stilbestrol) in small doses also helps to slow the growth of malignant cells.[6, 17]

Benign prostatic hypertrophy

Simple enlargement of the prostate gland is a nonmalignant disorder that affects men who are past 50 years of age. As the gland enlarges, it presses the urethra, causing urinary symptoms to develop. The condition is slowly progressive, and eventually the surgical removal of the gland will be necessary to provide relief.

Prostatectomy. There are several methods by which the prostate gland may be removed. The method used is determined by the physician and will be the method best suited for the particular patient. Nursing care will be determined by the type of surgery. There are four ways by which a prostatectomy may be done.

1. Suprapubic prostatectomy is accomplished by an incision through the abdomen; the bladder is opened, and the gland is removed with the finger from above.

2. Transurethral prostatectomy is done with the use of instruments introduced through the urethra.

3. Perineal prostatectomy requires an incision through the perineum between the scrotum and the rectum.

4. Retropubic prostatectomy is the method in which an incision is made into the abdomen above the bladder, but the bladder is not opened. The gland is removed by making an incision into the capsule encasing the gland.[21]

Each situation will present certain special problems of nursing care. Additional problems may occur, since most patients are men well past 50 years of age who may have other diseases from degenerative changes.

Prostatectomy may be done because enlargement of the prostate gland obstructs the flow of urine, or it may be necessary to remove benign or malignant tumors. The characteristic symptoms experienced by the patient are (1) slowing of the urinary stream, (2) urinary frequency, (3) painful urination, and (4) complete urinary retention.

The patient is usually admitted to the hospital several days before surgery. Because of the urinary frequency, the patient should be shown the location of the bathroom immediately on admission to the clinical unit. A series of laboratory tests, including kidney function tests and blood tests, are completed. Acid phosphatase is an enzyme that is normally present in large concentrations in the prostate gland. If a disease such as metastatic carcinoma of the prostate gland ruptures the capsule surrounding the gland, the enzyme will be released into the bloodstream. Therefore a high serum acid phosphatase level indicates a strong possibility of carcinoma of the prostate gland in the male. An electrocardiogram, as well as a cystoscopy examination with biopsy, may precede a prostatectomy. Since blood loss may be extensive, blood typing and cross matching are usually ordered in case transfusion therapy is necessary The nurse should be sure that the physician's orders for the various examinations are understood and that the request forms are properly completed and routed to the proper departments. Catheter drainage may or may not be ordered prior to surgery, but accurate records of urinary output must be maintained, including the interval and the amount of urine voided. Many patients may be instructed to help with maintaining the record.

When a suprapubic prostatectomy has been done, the surgeon may place some agent such as gauze packing or a hemostatic bag into the depressed area where the gland was located to prevent hemorrhage. In addition, there will be some provision for urinary drainage through the abdominal incision. Drains or tubes such as a cystostomy tube may be used. Not all urologists use this method. If only small drains are used, a ureterostomy cup may be employed to collect urine and to keep the patient dry, whereas in other cases large abdominal dressings may be used. Abdominal dressings may have to be changed frequently to keep the patient dry, and enclosing them in some type of impervious material may help. In any procedure used the patient must be watched closely for hemorrhage. The patient will need medication for pain, since bladder spasms may be severe and painful. The patient should be assisted and encouraged to turn frequently, and deep breathing and coughing are especially important to prevent pulmonary complications. Ambulation for these patients is delayed, and several weeks of hospitalization are usually required.

A transurethral prostatectomy has the advantages that the patient is ambulatory soon after the surgery, recovery is generally rapid, and a shorter period of hospitalization is required. Postoperatively the patient will have a Foley catheter connected to sterile closed drainage. He should be advised not to try to void around the catheter since it will contribute to bladder spasm. Hemorrhage is always a possible complication, and the patient must be observed closely for it. Some bleeding will occur

after the procedure; urinary drainage bottles changed every 2 hours will provide a better guide to the amount of bleeding, which should gradually diminish. The catheter must be kept open and draining. Gentle irrigation with 20 or 30 ml. of solution as ordered by the physician may remove blood clots that occlude the catheter. The tubing should not be pinched or milked because this will tend to stir up clots. If the nurse is unable to be sure that proper catheter drainage is occurring, it should be reported immediately to the physician. The patient will require medication for pain resulting from bladder spasm. He should be encouraged to drink fluids freely, and the diet is usually given as tolerated.

The patient having a retropubic prostatectomy has less discomfort than when other methods are employed. He will have a retention catheter and should be observed for hemorrhage. There are few or no bladder spasms, and there is no urinary drainage on the abdominal dressing.

Perineal prostatectomy may be performed because of benign prostatic hypertrophy, or a radical procedure through the perineum may be used for cancer of the prostate gland. When the surgery is for cancer, the intact prostate gland is removed as well as the seminal vesicles and the regional tissue. The portion of the ureters remaining is connected to the bladder neck. After this radical procedure the patient may have total permanent urinary incontinence.

The preoperative preparation of the patient for perineal prostatectomy is essentially the same regardless of the purpose. The bowel is prepared by giving a laxative and enemas. Frequently an antibiotic or sulfonamide drug may be administered preoperatively, and only clear liquids may be allowed on the day before surgery.

When the patient returns from surgery, he will have a retention catheter, which should be connected to sterile closed drainage. Extreme care should be taken to be sure that the catheter does not become obstructed or displaced. There is less possibility of hemorrhage and bladder spasms in the perineal approach to the prostate gland. Urinary drainage may occur on the perineal dressings, which will gradually decrease over a few hours. In perineal prostatectomy temporary fecal incontinence may occur. The patient should be taught perineal exercises, and beginning them early will strengthen the rectal and urethral sphincter muscles. Patients having simple perineal prostatectomy for benign prostatic hypertrophy have no problem with urinary control.

In caring for patients with prostatectomy, the nurse should be familiar with the care of the patients after removal of the catheter (p. 345). For some patients the catheter may be removed in about a week, whereas for others it may be several weeks. All patients should receive at least 3000 ml. of fluid daily. After the first 24 to 48 hours most patients are allowed solid food except for those having perineal prostatectomy. During the immediate postoperative period the patient receives nothing by mouth, and liquids or a low-residue diet may be given until there has been time for healing.[25]

Nursing care

Many of the diseases and disorders of the reproductive system will be treated as medical disorders in the physician's office or in an outpatient clinic, whereas others will at times be treated in the hospital. Most patients with tumors will be hospitalized for diagnostic purposes or treatment. Many of the diseases have their beginning as medical problems, but final treatment may necessitate surgical intervention. Surgery will vary from simple incision and drainage to radical operative procedures. The reproductive system in the male is so intimately related to the urinary system that treatment and nursing care may be directed to both systems.

The nurse should also realize that conditions affecting the reproductive system span all age groups from birth to death, with significant differences related to age. The nurse should understand the basic nursing care of infants and children, as well as elderly patients. The nurse who has some basic understanding of the physical and emotional problems of the patient will be a valuable member of the team. The care of the patient with medical or surgical disorders of the reproductive system involves some of the most intimate, personal,

and confidential relationships that will be encountered in nursing.

The technical procedures for the care of the patient will vary little from the nursing skills necessary for all patients.

Summary outline

1. Structure and function of the reproductive system
   A. Female reproductive system
      1. External parts—include pubis, labia, clitoris, perineum, and two sets of secretory glands; urinary meatus opens above vaginal opening
         a. External parts region called *vulva*
      2. Hymen divides external and internal parts
      3. Internal parts include vagina, uterus, two fallopian tubes, and two ovaries
         a. Attached and supported by ligaments
   B. Male reproductive system
      1. Testes supported in scrotum, epididymis, two seminal ducts, two ejaculatory ducts, two spermatic cords, and penis; urethra passes through prostate gland; two secretory glands below prostate
      2. Glans penis covered by prepuce, or foreskin
   C. Function of reproductive system
      1. Production of ova and spermatozoa
      2. Manufacture of endocrine secretions
      3. Nurturing and retaining fertilized ova
2. Puberty, menstruation, and menopause
   A. Puberty—development of secondary sex characteristics
      1. Menarche—end of puberty
      2. First menstruation between twelfth and sixteenth year, with slight variations
   B. Menstruation—cyclic process occurring at fairly regular intervals of every 28 days for period of 30 to 35 years
   C. The reproductive years
      1. All couples contemplating marriage should have physical examination
      2. Consideration of limiting family size
      3. Several methods of birth control available
   D. Menopause (climacteric)—end of reproductive period, characterized by cessation of menses
      1. Occurs between 45 and 55 years of age
      2. Artificial menopause induced by radiation or surgical removal of ovaries
3. Disturbances of menstrual function
   A. Dysmenorrhea—painful menstruation
   B. Amenorrhea—absence of menstruation
   C. Menorrhagia—excessive menstruation
   D. Metrorrhagia—irregular bleeding between menstrual periods
4. Diagnostic tests and procedures
   A. Examination of female patient
      1. Physical examination—includes history, examination of breasts, and pelvic examination
      2. Child should be carefully draped and confidence and cooperation secured
      3. Laboratory examination—include urinal-

ysis, cytologic test for cancer, complete blood count, serologic test for syphilis, smears and cultures
  4. Schiller test—employs iodine solution to detect areas from which biopsy should be taken
  5. Breast examination
  6. Huhner test—sterility test to determine effect of vaginal secretions on spermatozoa
  7. Rubin test—consists of injecting carbon dioxide into uterine cavity under controlled pressure and amount to determine patency of fallopian tubes
  8. Hysterosalpingogram—x-ray examination of pelvic organs after injection of radiopaque substance through uterine cavity into fallopian tubes
  9. Culdoscopy and laparoscopy—methods of visually examining pelvic organs for disease
  10. Pregnancy tests
     a. Aschheim-Zondek test uses mice
     b. Friedman test uses rabbits
        (1) Patient's urine is injected into virgin rabbit, and after period of time ovaries are examined for changes, which indicate positive test
     c. Immunologic test is based on finding human chorionic gonadotropic hormone in urine
  11. Dilation and curettage (D and C)—procedure to dilate cervix and scrape inside of uterus
     a. To secure specimen of endometrium for examination
     b. To control uterine bleeding
     c. To remove residue from incomplete abortion
  B. Examination of male patient
     1. Physical examination of external genitals for abnormalities, infection, or skin lesions
     2. Examination of semen when sterility is suspected
     3. Massage of prostate gland, and urine specimen collected for cytologic examination
     4. Biopsy of prostate gland or testicles
5. Nursing the patient with diseases and disorders of reproductive system
  A. Conditions affecting external genitals and vagina
     1. Vulvitis—acute or chronic inflammatory condition of vulva
     2. Vaginitis—most common disease affecting females
        a. Pathophysiology
           (1) Affects postmenopausal women
           (2) Occurs in persons with diabetes, during pregnancy, and after antibiotic therapy
           (3) Atrophic vaginitis in elderly women and adolescent girls
           (4) May affect children
           (5) May be first sign of cancer
           (6) Symptoms

(7) Treatment depends on causal factors
  3. Leukorrhea—abnormal white or yellow discharge from vagina that may result from infection or from cancer of uterus
  4. Vulvovaginitis—infection of vulva, vagina, and Bartholin glands, usually by gonococcus, with possible inflammation and abscess formation
  5. Vesicovaginal fistula—abnormal opening from bladder to vagina, caused by obstetric injury at time of delivery
  6. Rectovaginal fistula—abnormal opening between rectum and vagina caused by laceration through sphincter at time of delivery
  7. Relaxation of pelvic musculature
     a. Rectocele—protrusion of rectum into vagina
     b. Cystocele—displacement of bladder toward or into vagina
     c. Uterine prolapse—uterus drops downward; cervix may protrude through vagina
     d. Preoperative care—includes cathartic, enemas, liquid diet, cleansing vaginal douche, shave of vaginal area, pubis, and rectal area
     e. Postoperative care
        (1) Avoid pressure on sutures
        (2) Observe for hemorrhage, check vital signs
        (3) Retention catheter in bladder
        (4) Liquid diet
        (5) Perineal care if external sutures —may use heat lamp
        (6) Low Fowler's position
  8. Malignant lesions—relatively rare in vulva and vagina but may require vulvectomy if they occur
     a. Vulvectomy—removal of external female genitals
        (1) Conditions requiring procedure are peculiar to older women
        (2) Partial procedure may be done for biopsy
        (3) Simple procedure is done for benign lesions
        (4) Radical procedure is done for malignant lesions
  B. Conditions affecting cervix and uterus
     1. Cervicitis—may be acute or chronic, resulting from lacerations at time of delivery, erosions, cysts, or specific infections
        a. Erosions—common and may be congenital
        b. Conization—removing cone-shaped portion of cervix
     2. Uterine displacement—usually displacement backward (retroversion)
        a. Treatment consists of exercise and support with pessary
        b. Surgery may be needed to correct condition
     3. Endometriosis—endometrial cells become seeded throughout pelvis and other organs; stimulated by ovarian hormones

a. Inflammatory process occurs outside uterus
b. Symptom is pain with menstruation
c. Treatment is to suppress ovulation
4. Tumors—occur usually as cancer of cervix, most common form of cancer affecting reproductive organs; treatment is with radium, x-ray therapy, and surgery
   a. Papanicolaou smear test is used widely to detect cancer
      (1) All women over 20 years of age should have yearly pelvic examination and Pap smear
   b. Greatest incidence in patients between 30 and 50 years of age
   c. Fibroid tumors are benign abnormal growth of uterine muscle tissue
C. Conditions affecting ovaries and fallopian tubes
1. Cysts and tumors may be of different kinds; when pedicel is present, cyst may become twisted, cutting off blood supply; immediate surgery indicated
   a. Carcinoma of ovaries—usually bilateral and produces no early symptoms; generally due to metastasis
      (1) Treatment is surgery, radiation, and chemotherapy
2. Salpingitis—inflammation of fallopian tubes caused by bacteria; frequent cause is gonorrhea
   a. Pelvic inflammatory disease occurs when ovaries and pelvic peritoneum are involved
3. Treatment and nursing care
   a. Hysterectomy—surgical removal of uterus; may be abdominal or vaginal
      (1) Bilateral oophorectomy—surgical removal of both ovaries
      (2) Bilateral salpingectomy—surgical removal of both fallopian tubes
      (3) Panhysterosalpingo-oophorectomy —surgical removal of uterus, both ovaries, and both tubes
      (4) Preoperative care—same as that for other surgical patients
      (5) Postoperative care—prevention of complications
         (a) Prevention of urinary retention
         (b) Prevention of intestinal distention
         (c) Prevention of venous thrombosis
   b. Isolation perfusion (intra-arterial perfusion—technique for administering large doses of chemotherapeutic drug to part of body isolated from general circulation)
      (1) Regarded as research procedure
      (2) Utilizes pump-oxygenator to establish closed separate system in pelvis
      (3) Preoperative care—emotional support very important
      (4) Postoperative care
         (a) Observation for kidney function failure

(b) Daily blood studies to watch for drop in white blood cell count
(c) Observation for venous stasis and thrombophlebitis
(d) Continuous encouragement
D. Conditions affecting the breast
1. Acute mastitis—inflammation of mammary gland caused by entrance of bacteria through nipple
2. Chronic cystic mastitis—formation of nodular type of benign cyst in breast, cause of which is unknown
3. Tumors
   a. Benign tumors—often found in young women and should be surgically removed
   b. Carcinoma of breast—develops insidiously and is treated by x-ray or radium therapy and simple or radical mastectomy
   c. Mastectomy—surgical removal of breast
      (1) Simple mastectomy—incision and skin sutured, lymph nodes not removed
      (2) Radical mastectomy—removal of skin, lymph nodes, and muscles
      (3) Preoperative care—emotional preparation: radical procedure may need skin grafting, donor skin usually from anterior thigh
      (4) Postoperative care
         (a) Observation for hemorrhage
         (b) Fowler's position—45 degrees to promote drainage
         (c) Elevation of hand and arm on affected side
         (d) Observe hand and arm for edema, coldness, cyanosis, lack of radial pulse, numbness, or inability to move fingers
         (e) Give intravenous fluids in unaffected arm and take blood pressure in unaffected arm
      (5) Rehabilitation—objective is to restore use of affected arm as soon as possible
         (a) Physician will determine when exercises may be started
         (b) Physician will advise when prosthesis may be used
E. Conditions of pregnancy
1. Abortion
   a. United States Supreme Court ruling in 1973
   b. In 1973, twenty-three states passed thirty-nine abortion laws
      (1) Many being challenged in courts
   c. Habitual abortion—abortion occurring in three or more secessive pregnancies
   d. Threatened abortion—vaginal spotting or bleeding in first 20 weeks; no dilation of cervix

e. Inevitable abortion—vaginal spotting or bleeding; cervix dilated; no chance to save pregnancy

f. Incomplete abortion—only part of products of conception expelled

g. Complete abortion—all of products of conception expelled

h. Missed abortion—fetus dies before twentieth week and is retained

i. Septic abortion—serious infection of uterus with incomplete or complete abortion

j. Therapeutic abortion—induced by physician to save life of mother, baby, or both

k. Legalized abortion—termination of pregnancy at request of woman

l. Illegal abortion—induced without medical or legal approval

2. Ectopic pregnancy (tubal pregnancy)—gestation occurs anywhere outside of uterus

   a. Rupture of tube causes hemorrhage and serious emergency; immediate surgery indicated

3. Cesarean section—abdominal

   a. When there is contracted pelvis and large baby

   b. If pathologic condition interferes with normal passage of baby

   c. To avoid rupture of uterus if there has been previous cesarean section

4. Toxemias of pregnancy—causes unknown

   a. Preeclampsia—during first trimester without convulsions

   b. Eclampsia—later in pregnancy with convulsions

   c. Treatment varies; skilled nursing care necessary

F. Conditions affecting male external genitals

1. Congenital malformations

   a. Exstrophy of bladder—anterior surface of bladder open on abdomen

   b. Epispadias—urethra open on upper surface of penis

   c. Hypospadias—urethra open on undersurface of penis

   d. Phimosis—condition in which orifice of prepuce is too small to allow retraction over glans penis

     (1) Circumcision is required; removal of part of foreskin leaves glans uncovered

2. Cryptorchism (undescended testicle)—condition in which testicles (one or both) remain in abdomen; most descend by puberty

3. Penile ulcerations—may occur from many causes, but frequently result from syphilis and chancroid

G. Conditions affecting testes and adjacent structures

1. Epididymitis—inflammation of epididymis, tube that collects spermatozoa and lies in scrotum

2. Orchitis—inflammation of testicle resulting from injury or disease

3. Hydrocele—collection of fluid between testicle and its lining

   a. May be from disease or injury

   b. Treated by aspiration, injection of sclerosing solution, or surgery

   c. Varicocele—form of varicosity involving veins of spermatic cord; usually harmless and causes no symptoms

4. Tumors

   a. Usually malignant and metastasize to distant parts of body

   b. Condition is usually far advanced before medical care is secured

H. Conditions affecting prostate gland

1. Acute prostatis—may also be chronic; inflammation may be caused by gonococcus organism

2. Cancer of prostate—characteristically occurs in older men; is often highly malignant and far advanced before medical care secured

3. Benign prostatic hypertrophy

   a. Nonmalignant enlargement of prostate gland occurring in men past 50 years of ·age

   b. Causes urinary tract symptoms, is progressive, and usually requires surgery

4. Prostatectomy—may be done by several methods, and most patients are men past 50 years of age

   a. Reasons for prostatectomy

     (1) Obstructed urinary flow

     (2) Benign or malignant tumors

   b. Characteristic symptoms leading to surgery

     (1) Slowing of urinary stream

     (2) Urinary frequency

     (3) Painful urination

     (4) Complete urinary retention

   c. Surgical methods for removing all or part of prostate gland

     (1) Suprapubic—incision through abdomen; bladder is opened

     (2) Transurethral—instruments are introduced through urethra

     (3) Retropubic—incision through and into abdomen; bladder is not opened

     (4) Perineal—incision through perineum between scrotum and rectum

   d. Postoperative care

     (1) Observation for excessive bleeding or hemorrhage

     (2) Relief of bladder spasm

     (3) Urethral catheter care

     (4) Dressings to keep patient dry

     (5) From 3000 to 4000 ml. of fluid daily

I. Nursing care—may be both medical and surgical

1. Many patients will be treated in physician's office or in outpatient clinic

2. When conditions are infectious, nurses must be careful to protect themselves and other patients

Review questions

1. List four disturbances of normal menstrual function.
   a. dysmenorrhea - painful
   b. menorrhagia - excessive slow
   c. amenorrhea - absence
   d. metorrhagia - between periods
2. What two signs should the nurse observe the patient for after a dilation and curettage?
   a. hemorrhage
   b. urinary retention
3. Why should the patient be placed in low Fowler's postion after surgical perineal repair?
   a. prevent strain on sutures
4. What is the surgical removal of both ovaries called?
   a. oophorectomy (bilateral)
5. What three postoperative complications should the nurse seek to prevent in the patient who has had a hysterectomy?
   a. blood stasis
   b. urinary retention
   c. abdominal distension
6. What three procedures should be avoided postoperatively when the patient has had a hysterectomy?
   a. raising legs of bed
   b. no pillow under knees
   c. no high Fowler's pos.
7. What is the purpose of placing a patient who has had a mastectomy in a 45-degree Fowler's position?
   a. drainage
8. List five observations that the nurse should make of the affected arm in the postoperative mastectomy patient.
   a. edema
   b. numbness
   c. coldness
   d. inability to move fingers
   e. lack of radial pulse
9. Why does enlargement of the prostate gland cause urinary tract symptoms?
   a. it interferes c passage of urine normally
10. When a patient has had a transurethral prostatectomy and has a Foley catheter in the bladder, why is it inadvisable to pinch or milk the catheter?
    a. stirs up clots

Films

1. Female pelvic examination (8 min., sound, color, 16 mm.), Eli Lilly & Co., Audio-visual Library, Indianapolis, Ind. 46206. Female examination procedure demonstrated in live photography and discussed in animated diagrams.
2. The menstrual cycle (12 min., sound, color, 16 mm.), Eli Lilly & Co., Audio-visual Library, Indianapolis, Ind. 46206. Describes changes that occur in the ovaries, uterus, and other organs and tissues during the normal menstrual cycle and their significance in reproduction.
3. X-ray, ultrasound, and thermography in diagnosis (22 min., sound, color, 16 mm.), Upjohn Professional Film Library, 7000 Portage Rd., Kalamazoo, Mich. 49001. Explains and demonstrates the significant advantages of thermography in mass screening for breast cancer.
4. Urinary obstruction in the elderly male (28 min., sound, color, 16 mm.), The Pfizer Laboratories Film Library, 267 West 25th St., New York, N. Y. 10001. Discusses the etiology, pathology, diagnosis, and treatment of the more common causes of obstruction in the male urinary tract. Shows various tissues as filmed through the cystoscope and shows techniques for transurethral and suprapubic prostatectomy.
5. A special kind of care (13 min., sound, color, 16 mm., rental), The American Journal of Nursing Company Film Library, Educational Services Division, 10 Columbus Circle, New York, N. Y. 10019. Shows the emotional impact of a diagnosis of advanced cancer on the family of a dying woman.
6. Sex in today's world (52 min., sound, color, 16 mm., rental), The American Journal of Nursing Company Film Library, Educational Services Division, 10 Columbus Circle, New York, N. Y. 10019. Explains changing sexual attitudes in the United States today.

References

1. Annual summary 1972, Abortion surveillance, Atlanta, 1974, Center for Disease Control.
2. Anthony, Catherine P., and Kolthoff, Norma J.: Textbook of anatomy and physiology, ed. 9, St. Louis, 1975, The C. V. Mosby Co.
3. Avery, Wanda, Gardner, Carolyn, and Palmer, Suzanne: Vulvectomy, American Journal of Nursing **74:**453-455, March, 1974.
4. Brewer, John I., Molibo, Doris M., and Gerbie, Albert B.: Gynecologic nursing, St. Louis, 1966, The C. V. Mosby Co.
5. Brunner, Lillian S., and Suddarth, Doris S.: Textbook of medical-surgical nursing, ed. 3, Philadelphia, 1975, J. B. Lippincott Co.
6. Brunner, Lillian S., and Suddarth, Doris S.: The Lippincott manual of nursing practice, Philadelphia, 1974, J. B. Lippincott Co.
7. Cancer facts and figures, New York, 1973, American Cancer Society, Inc.
8. Carbary, Lorraine J.: Vaginitis—the common female complaint, Nursing Care **7:**29-31, Sept., 1974.
9. Clancy, Barbara: The nurse and the abortion patient, Nursing Clincs of North America **8:**469-477, Sept., 1973.
10. Conn, Howard F., editor: Current therapy 1976, Philadelphia, 1976, W. B. Saunders Co.
11. Davis, M. Edward, and Rubin, Reva: DeLee's obstetrics for nurses, ed. 18, Philadelphia, 1966, W. B. Saunders Co.
12. Family Planning Population Reporter **2:**133-160, Dec., 1973, Washington, D. C., 1973, Family Planning Program Development.
13. Fitzpatrick, Else, Reeder, Sharon R., and Mastroianni, Luigi, Jr.: Maternity nursing, ed. 12, Philadelphia, 1971, J. B. Lippincott Co.
14. Fitzpatrick, Genevieve: Care of the patient

with cancer of the cervix, Bedside Nurse 4:11-18, Jan., 1971.

15. Fitzpatrick, Genevieve: Caring for the patient with cancer of the breast, Part 1, Bedside Nurse 3:20-24, Feb., 1970.

16. Iorio, Josephine: Childbirth: family-centered nursing, ed. 3, St. Louis, 1975, The C. V. Mosby Co.

17. Keuhnelian, John G., and Sanders, Virginia E.: Urologic nursing, New York, 1970, The Macmillan Co.

18. McLennan, Charles E.: Synopsis of obstetrics, ed. 8, St. Louis, 1970, The C. V. Mosby Co.

19. Menaker, Jerome: When menstruation is painful, American Journal of Nursing 62:94-96, Sept., 1962.

20. Progress against cancer 1969, a report of the National Advisory Cancer Council, Washington, D. C., Government Printing Office.

21. Shafer, Kathleen N., Sawyer, Janet R., McCluskey, Audrey M., Beck, Edna L., and Phipps, Wilma J.: Medical-surgical nursing, ed. 6, St. Louis, 1975, The C. V. Mosby Co.

22. Smith, Dorothy W., Germain, Carol P. Hanley, and Gips, Claudia D.: Care of the adult patient, ed. 4, Philadelphia, 1975, J. B. Lippincott Co.

23. Taylor, E. Stewart: Essentials of gynecology, ed. 4, Philadelphia, 1969, Lea & Febiger.

24. Vernon, Audree: Explaining hysterectomy, Nursing 73, 3:36-38, Sept., 1973.

25. Winter, Chester C., and Barker, Marilyn Roehm: Nursing care of patients with urologic diseases, ed. 3, St. Louis, 1972, The C. V. Mosby Co.

Nursing the patient with diseases and disorders of the endocrine system

KEY WORDS

atrophy *waste away/marked inadequacy*

calibrated *graduated*

cretinism *absence of thyroid*

diabetic *deficiency of insulin/sugar in urine*

glycosuria *sugar in urine*

goiter *enlarged thyroid gland*

homeostasis *stable, normal body environment*

hormone *secretion of ductless gland*

hyperglycemia *excess sugar in blood stream*

hyperplasia *enlargement due to increased # of cells*

ketosis *acetone or ketone acidosis - diabetic process*

metabolism *body processes*

syndrome *group of symptoms*

tetany *type of spasm - extremities*

ENDOCRINE GLANDS AND THEIR FUNCTION

The endocrine glands, or ductless glands, are sometimes called glands of internal secretion because they do not have ducts or tubes to carry their secretions to the outside but pour them directly into the tissue fluid, from which they are picked up by the blood. The secretions of the endocrine glands are chemical substances called *hormones.* Some of these hormones have been reproduced synthetically in the laboratory, whereas others are extracted from the glands of animals. The nurse who administers medications will be giving many of these commercially prepared hormone products, which are marketed under various trade names. Although the overproduction or underproduction of certain hormones may result in serious disease, the very life of the individual may depend on an adequate supply of a particular hormone. When for some reason the gland fails to supply the normal requirement, a commercial preparation must be given to compensate for the deficiency. The most significant example of this situation is provided by diabetes.

The endocrine glands have many functions, and they are so interrelated and interdependent that to separate their activities and their importance would be extremely difficult. They regulate the metabolic processes that control energy production, fluid and electrolyte balance, growth, development, reproduction, and lactation. They help to maintain homeostasis and regulate blood pressure and neuro-

397

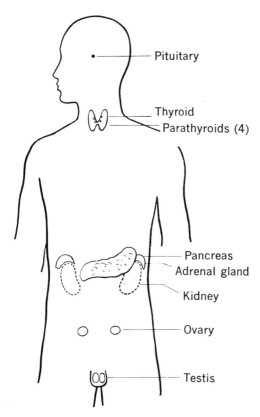

Pituitary

Thyroid
Parathyroids (4)

Pancreas
Adrenal gland

Kidney

Ovary

Testis

Fig. 17-1. Location of the endocrine glands. The testes are the male sex glands, and the ovaries are the female sex glands.

muscular contraction. They assist in maintaining electrolyte, fluid, and acid-base balance. The secretion from some glands stimulates other glands to activity. A description of the endocrine glands (Fig. 17-1) and their chief hormones follows.

The thyroid gland is the largest of the endocrine glands and is located in the neck in front of the trachea, with one lobe on each side of the trachea. The two lobes are connected with a strip of thyroid tissue called the *isthmus*. The gland secretes thyroxin and stores iodine. Its primary function is to help regulate metabolism, the rate at which nutrients are oxidized to provide energy for the body. Any disturbance in the secretion of thyroxin may result in hyperthyroidism or hypothyroidism. A congenital absence of the thyroid gland causes cretinism in the infant, and a deficiency of secretion may result in myxedema in the adult. Calcitonin is a re-

cently discovered hormone that is believed to be secreted by the thyroid gland. It acts rapidly to decrease the level of calcium in the blood by increasing the movement of calcium from the blood into the bones.[1]

The parathyroids are small glands, which are usually four in number but may be more or fewer, arranged in pairs and embedded in the posterior lateral lobe of the thyroid gland. The parathyroids secrete parathormone, which helps to maintain the homeostasis or relative consistency of the calcium levels in the blood and body fluids. The presence of this hormone tends to increase calcium in the blood and to increase the excretion of phosphates.

The adrenal (suprarenal) glands are small bodies located above each kidney. Each gland is divided into two parts, the medulla and the cortex, and each part secretes a different hormone. One hormone secreted by the medulla is epinephrine, prepared commercially as Adrenalin. The other hormone secreted by the medulla is norepinephrine. In medicine epinephrine (Adrenalin) has many uses, such as elevating the blood pressure, acting as a vasoconstrictor, and relaxing the bronchioles as in asthma. Epinephrine is sometimes called the *fight hormone* because in stress situations and anger an increased amount of epinephrine is poured into the bloodstream. The adrenal cortex secretes hydrocortisone (cortisol), corticosterone, aldosterone, and small amounts of sex hormones. Hydrocortisone and corticosterone have many functions in the body, but they primarily function to promote normal metabolism and resist stressful situations. Aldosterone regulates the level of sodium in the blood and body fluids. When a deficiency of these hormones occurs, Addison's disease results, and a hypersecretion causes Cushing's syndrome (p. 413).

The pituitary body (hypophysis) is often referred to as the master gland, since it is important in regulating many of the functions of the other glands. The pituitary gland is located in the sphenoid bone in the skull and secretes several hormones; in fact, the exact number is not definitely known. The pituitary gland consists of two lobes, the anterior lobe and the posterior lobe. The anterior lobe is known to secrete seven different hormones, each of which stimulates other glands and affects the growth process, as well as affecting the pigmentation of the skin. The posterior lobe secretes two hormones, an antidiuretic hormone and oxytocin. The antidiuretic hormone affects the amount of urine excreted because it causes a faster reabsorption of water from the kidney into the blood. When extremely large amounts of urine are excreted, this indicates an inadequate amount of the antidiuretic hormone. Oxytocin affects uterine contractions and lactation; it is prepared commercially and used in obstetrics to promote uterine contraction after delivery.

The gonads, or sex glands, include the ovaries in the female, which secrete estrogen and progesterone, and the testes in the male, which secrete testosterone and androsterone. These hormones are important in the development of sex characteristics and in the reproductive process.

The pancreas has more than one function. Scattered throughout the organ are small, specialized cells called the *islands of Langerhans,* which manufacture and secrete a hormone called *insulin.* These cells function independently of the pancreas as a whole and do not pour their secretion into the pancreatic ducts. Insulin is necessary for the proper utilization of sugar by the body, as the study of diabetes will demonstrate.

DIAGNOSTIC TESTS AND PROCEDURES

Many of the tests used in the diagnosis of endocrine disease and disorder and in following its course are performed on blood and urine. The amount and kind of specific hormones can be estimated through chemical analysis of the blood and urine. When an excess or deficiency is found, further tests and procedures may be done to determine the effect on the body as a whole. Procedures common to many of these tests are nursing functions and include withholding food and fluids and collecting urine specimens. If results from tests are to be significant, it is important that nurses perform their duties accurately and conscientiously.

Blood chemistry. Common tests include the blood glucose test, the insulin tolerance test, the glucose tolerance test, and the Thorn test. However, many other tests may be performed for which the patient must be in a fasting state. No food is allowed after midnight, and breakfast is withheld until the blood specimen has been taken. The patient may or may not be allowed water after midnight. In certain emergency situations such as suspected diabetic coma, blood may be taken at any time. It is most important to explain to the patient with endocrine disease why food or water is withheld, since many of these patients are nervous, irritable, and often excitable. Precautions must be taken to identify the room and bed, as in all tests of blood chemistry, and provision should be made to serve the patient's meal as soon as the specimen has been collected.

Urinalysis. A 24-hour urine collection is necessary for hormone analysis. The collection may start at any hour. The nurse should secure a clean container sufficient to hold all urine voided for the 24-hour period. The procedure should be explained to the patient to avoid error, and the hour at which the collection was started should be carefully noted. The patient is asked to void, and the specimen is discarded, but all urine voided from that hour is saved. The collection is completed at exactly the same hour the next day, at which time the patient voids and that urine becomes a part of the specimen. It is the responsibility of the nurse to see that the patient voids the last specimen exactly 24 hours from the time the collection started. The container holding the urine should be kept in the refrigerator and properly labeled with the patient's name, the room number, and the hour the collection began. It must be remembered that the omission of a single voiding will destroy the validity of the test. All persons concerned with the patient's care should be thoroughly familiar with the procedure and should cooperate fully if successful results are to be achieved.

Basal metabolic rate (BMR). The test for basal metabolic rate measures the amount of oxygen consumed by an individual at rest who is in a fasting condition. The test is useful in determining activity of the thyroid gland. A level considered normal for the individual is determined; significant elevation above that rate indicates hyperthyroidism, and a rate significantly below, hypothyroidism. It is usually considered that a –10% to a +10% is the average normal range of value for basal metabolism. However, many factors enter into the reliability of the test, and since the development of more accurate measurements of thyroid activity, the BMR is used less frequently. When it is used, it serves as a screening procedure and is followed with other tests.

The preparation of the patient is a nursing responsibility, and a clear explanation of what to expect should be given to the patient. The patient should be told that it is a breathing test in which a clip will be placed on his nose and that he will breathe and exhale oxygen for a few minutes. He should be assured that the test is painless and that he should inhale and exhale normally and be relaxed. The test may be done on an outpatient basis; however, conditions may be controlled more effectively when the patient enters the hospital on the evening before the test. The patient is allowed no food or fluid after midnight, and breakfast is held until after the test. A sedative may or may not be given to ensure a good night's rest. The patient is instructed to remain in bed until after the test in the morning. If the test is done in the outpatient clinic, the patient reports without breakfast and is made comfortable in bed for 1 hour before the test. Nurses should be familiar with the procedure in the hospital in which they are employed because there may be some variation in details of procedure.

Protein-bound iodine (PBI). The test for protein-bound iodine is another test of thyroid function and is done on the serum from venous blood. It is not necessary to restrict food or fluids prior to the test; the blood specimen may be taken at any time. Prior to the test, however, iodine in any form must have been restricted. This includes food (iodized salt), any of a large number of drugs that contain iodine, and all radiologic procedures that use a contrast medium.

Radioactive iodine uptake. The test for radioactive iodine uptake is to determine thyroid activity. A small amount of radioactive iodine is administered orally to the patient, either in capsule form or in a colorless, odorless drink. The amount is called a *tracer dose.* After 24 to 48 hours the amount of iodine stored in the thyroid gland is measured by an instrument called a *scintillator* held near the thyroid gland. Persons with overactivity of the gland will be found to store a high percentage of the iodine, whereas those with underactivity will take up a small amount of the iodine.

Another method of determining the radioactive iodine uptake is by measuring the amount of radioactive iodine excreted in the urine. All urine voided for 24 to 48 hours is saved and sent to the laboratory. The amount of iodine excreted is subtracted from the amount administered; the difference is the amount taken up by the gland. The same care should be exercised in collecting the urine as previously outlined.

In the triiodothyronine (T_3) resin uptake test a blood specimen is secured from the patient, and iodine 131 is added to the blood in the laboratory. Normally the red blood cells will take up from 11% to 19% of the iodine.[17] In hypofunction of the gland less will be taken up, whereas in hyperfunction more will be taken up by the red blood cells. The advantage of the test is that the patient does not have to be given the iodine 131.

Scanogram. The patient is given radioactive iodine 131, and the uptake is quantitatively measured by the external passing of the scintillator over the throat. The scintillator is connected to a recording device that provides a record of the activity. The scan is used in connection with other tests and is used to differentiate between a nonmalignant condition and a possible malignancy of the thyroid gland.

Nursing responsibilities. Several other thyroid function tests utilize iodine 131. The nurse may not be directly concerned with the test but may have important functions related to the various tests. These responsibilities include reassuring the patient and encouraging him to cooperate. The collection of urine specimens must be absolutely correct or the test results will not be valid. Care must be taken to be sure that the patient does not receive iodine prior to the test. Some drugs contain various iodine preparations; contrast mediums used in x-ray examinations, iodine used as a skin antiseptic, and iodized salt are all forms of iodine that should be avoided.

NURSING THE PATIENT WITH DISEASES AND DISORDERS OF THE ENDOCRINE SYSTEM

Diseases and disorders of the thyroid

Simple (endemic) goiter

Any enlargement of the thyroid gland is called a goiter. Inadequate amounts of iodine cause the thyroid gland to grow larger as it attempts to make more thyroid hormones. Goiters may occur as a result of altered metabolism or a deficiency of iodine in food or water. Such a deficiency exists in certain areas of the United States, and it has been in those areas that the occurrence of endemic goiter has been greatest. The marketing and use of iodized salt has reduced the incidence of this type of goiter. Endemic goiter is more common in girls and usually occurs just before puberty, after which it may completely disappear. Usually these types of goiter produce no symptoms unless they grow large and exert pressure on adjacent structures. Large goiters may be surgically removed to relieve pressure or for esthetic reasons.

In studying family nutrition the nurse should become familiar with foods rich in natural iodine, such as leafy vegetables and seafood. While caring for patients, the nurse should emphasize the importance of these foods in the diet, especially if any enlargement of the thyroid gland is noted. Persons living in areas where there is a known deficiency of iodine in the water and soil should be encouraged to use iodized salt.

Hyperthyroidism

Hyperthyroidism is caused by an overactive thyroid gland that produces an excess of thyroxin. Specific causes are unknown, but the condition often follows infections or emotional stress. The disease is known by several names, including toxic goiter, thyrotoxicosis, exophthalmic goiter, and Graves' disease. The increase in hormone production increases all metabolic processes of the body and gives rise to a characteristic set of symptoms.

The appetite is increased, although there is weight loss and the individual is thin. There is an increase in the systolic blood pressure, and the pulse rate is greatly increased, even while the individual is at rest. The skin is warm, and the patient perspires freely and is sensitive to heat. Palpitation, tachycardia, and atrial fibrillation may occur. When the fingers are extended, a fine tremor may be observed. Fatigue, weakness, disturbance of menstruation, and constipation or diarrhea may exist. Profound personality changes may be present, with irritability, excitability, and crying episodes, which may occur spontaneously. There may be a bulging of the eyeballs known as exophthalmos, which gives the patient a startled expression and may not be relieved even after treatment.

The diagnostic tests will show an increase above normal in the metabolic rate. A rapid and increased iodine uptake will be indicated in the radioactive iodine uptake test.

Medical treatment and nursing care. The treatment of patients with hyperthyroidism is directed toward reducing the activity of the thyroid gland and the excessive production of thyroxin. The disease may be treated with antithyroid drugs, the surgical removal of the gland, or therapeutic doses of radioactive iodine. Surgery is usually indicated if the patient's condition will permit it, but when symptoms are severe, the patient may be given antithyroid drugs to relieve symptoms before surgery is done. Drugs being used are propylthiouracil, methimazole (Tapazole), iothiouracil and carbimazole, which depress the production of thyroxin. The drug is administered orally in tablet form, and the nurse should be alert for toxic symptoms that may occur. The patient should be observed for evidence of a skin rash, sore throat, fever, coryza, and malaise. An iodine solution known as Lugol's solution may be used; a few drops are placed in milk or fruit juice and administered through a straw, since iodine will stain the teeth.

Each patient must be considered as an individual, and patience and tact may be required in meeting nursing needs. If exophthalmos is present, the eyes will need to be protected from irritation. The environment should provide rest and quiet and be free from annoying distractions. Since the patient is sensitive to warmth, the room should be private, well ventilated, and cool. Visitors should be limited to members of the family, and efforts should be made to interpret the patient's erratic behavior as a part of his disease. The patient needs emotional as well as physical quiet and should be protected from situations that increase emotional tension and anxiety. Psychotherapy is occasionally beneficial.

The diet should be high in calories and vitamins, with carbohydrate supplements. Extra servings should be available, and between-meal feedings may be given if sufficient calories are not taken with the regular meals. Patients should be permitted choice of food, especially if the appetite is poor, and a visit from the dietitian may be helpful in ascertaining the patient's likes and dislikes.

If the patient is to be cared for at home, the public health nurse may visit the home and help the family plan the patient's care.

When the patient is treated with radioactive iodine, it is administered using the same procedure as for the radioactive iodine uptake test, and the same precautions are followed on the clinical unit for the patient's care. It is important to observe the patient for rapid pulse and severe apprehension, as well as restlessness, irritability, and prostration, which may precede coma and death.

Thyroidectomy. The surgical removal of part or all of the thyroid gland may be done because of malignancy, exophthalmic goiter, or any other severe condition affecting the gland and adjacent structures. Thyroidectomy is not an emergency procedure, and the patient may have been in the hospital for several weeks or may have been receiving outpatient care in a clinic or physician's office.

Preoperative nursing care. Preoperative care of the patient is directed toward reducing the environmental factors that contribute to restlessness and nervousness. A mild sedative such as phenobarbital may be ordered to provide rest. The diet should be high in proteins and calories—often as much as 5000 calories may be required, with the addition of vitamins such as thiamine and ascorbic acid. The use of tea and coffee is avoided because of their stimulating effect. Surgery is usually not done until drug therapy has reduced the basal metabolic rate to nearly normal.[9] (See Fig. 17-2.)

Postoperative nursing care. Postoperative nursing care of the patient includes careful observation for hemorrhage, edema of the larynx, nerve paralysis, and tetany. Tetany is the continuous spasm of a muscle or a group of muscles and is commonly a result of a decreased level of calcium in the body fluids. This may occur after injury to the parathyroid glands during surgery. Early indications of this complication are apprehension and tingling of the fingers, toes, and around the mouth. The facial muscles may twitch as the cheek is stroked, or flexion spasms of the hands and feet may be observed as the condition progresses (carpopedal spasm). Often spasms of the hand can be noticed when the blood pressure is taken, and this is a warning sign of impending tetany.

When the patient returns from surgery, he may be placed in a low or semi-Fowler's position, with his head supported at all times to prevent strain on the suture line. Dressings must be observed for bleeding, and the nurse's hand should be slipped under the back of the neck and shoulders, since blood may trickle back and not be observed. Bleeding may occur internally in the tissue, and the patient should be observed for hoarseness, fullness or tightness about the neck, irregular breathing, and dyspnea. The nurse should report any of these symptoms to the physician immediately.

The patient should be encouraged to breathe deeply and to cough and expectorate the thick mucus from the throat and bronchi. A vaporizer is sometimes used to

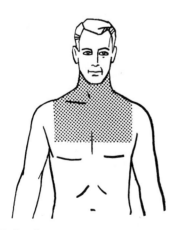

Fig. 17-2. The area of skin to be prepared for a thyroidectomy.

help thin secretions and facilitate their removal. Occasionally it may be necessary to suction secretions to maintain a free airway. Vital signs are checked every 15 minutes for several hours and then at intervals specified by the physician. Talking should be discouraged, but it is desirable to have the patient speak every 30 minutes, since injury to the nerves may cause paralysis of the vocal cords. Signs of nerve injury are hoarseness or a crowing sound resembling croup and retraction of tissue about the neck, and they must be reported immediately. If nerve injury has occurred, an emergency tracheotomy may be necessary.

Intravenous fluids may be administered for a day or two until the patient is able to take sufficient oral fluids. Swallowing may be difficult for a few days, but the patient should know that it is to be expected. Speech may be limited for a few days. Diet is usually given as tolerated. Meperidine hydrochloride (Demerol) may be ordered for pain or discomfort. The patient is allowed out of bed on the first or second postoperative day and is ambulatory thereafter. Recovery is generally rapid, and the patient is dismissed from the hospital from 5 to 7 days after surgery.

Although thyroidectomy is a safe surgical procedure and complications are rare, preparation should be made to provide for any emergency that might occur. A tracheotomy tray, suction machine, and calcium gluconate should be placed in the room ready for emergency use if necessary. Thyroid crisis (storm) is a rare complication that can occur before surgery or during the initial postoperative period. Increased amounts of thyroid hormones are released into the bloodstream, resulting in a sudden increase of metabolism. The heart rate, pulse rate, and temperature are elevated, and the patient is apprehensive, restless, and may finally become comatose and die. The patient is given oxygen, intravenous fluids, and sedatives and is placed on a hypothermia blanket to control temperature. The administration of cardiac drugs may be indicated if heart failure is imminent.

Hypothyroidism

Hypothyrodism is the result of an undersecretion of thyroxin by the thyroid gland or in some cases a complete lack of secretion. It may occur after surgical removal of the gland if too much thyroid tissue is removed. When the production of thyroid hormones is decreased, the symptoms are almost the reverse of those characterizing hyperthyroidism. Three conditions are recognized as resulting from hypothyroidism: myxedema, juvenile myxedema, and cretinism, all of which are actually forms of the same deficiency occurring at different ages.

Myxedema is the term applied to hypothyroidism in adults. The symptoms usually occur gradually and include sensitivity to cold, dryness of the skin and hair, gain in weight, loss of appetite, and a gradually appearing dull facial expression, with thickening of the lips and puffiness about the lips and eyes. The individual becomes lethargic and may fall asleep at intervals; the speech is slurred, and the individual responds slowly. The pulse is slow, the basal metabolic rate is well below normal, and the protein-bound iodine level is decreased.

The treatment is to replace the hormone deficiency by administering desiccated thyroid. Although remarkable improvement may be noted in a few days, the nurse must be alert for signs of hyperthyroidism and myocardial infarction that may occur as a complication. It should be remembered that patients with hypothyroidism do not tolerate sedative drugs well, and if given, only a fraction of the usual dose should be administered, and the patient should be carefully observed. When the condition is diagnosed early, replacement therapy reverses it rapidly. Eventually a maintenance dose of thyroid, which must be continued throughout life, will be calculated for each individual patient.

The nursing care of the patient is the opposite of that in hyperthyroidism. The environment should be warm, and super-fatted soaps, creams, and lotions should be used to overcome the dryness of the skin. Caloric intake may be reduced to prevent gain in weight, and an iron preparation may be ordered to correct anemia that may be present. The diet may have to be high in roughage when there is constipation.

Juvenile myxedema is similar to adult myxedema and varies in degree of severity. When the disease is moderately severe, both physical and mental growth is retarded. Puberty is delayed, and the child tends to be lethargic. The treatment is administration of thyroid, which is well tolerated by the child. The dose administered is sufficient to relieve the symptoms but not large enough to result in hyperthyroidism. These children are usually treated in an outpatient clinic or in a physician's office.

Cretinism is the result of complete absence of thyroid secretion from birth, which may be caused by absence of the gland or its failure to secrete thyroxin. Intrauterine development is usually normal, and the characteristics of the condition do not begin to appear until between the third and fifth month. The infant's growth is stunted, and characteristic conditions are present, including a short neck, broad hands with short fingers, and a thick tongue that protrudes from the mouth. The skin is dry, the abdomen is large and protruding, and mental development is greatly retarded and may even be imbecilic. If treatment is given early, some improvement may be obtained; however, not all the defects will be relieved.

Tumors of the thyroid

Tumors occurring in the thyroid gland may be benign or malignant and may be associated with hyperthyroidism. Enlargement of thyroid from benign tumors is referred to as nodular goiter, and the tumors may be single or multiple. Some of the tumors secrete thyroxin, since they consist of the same kind of cells as those found in normal thyroid tissue. If they secrete appreciable amounts of the hormone, hyperthyroidsm will develop, and the symptoms will be the same as those generally associated with hyperthyroidism. Surgical removal is generally indicated for the nodular type of tumors. Carcinoma of the thyroid may be any of several types. Some types grow slowly and metastasize first to the lymph nodes, then to the lungs and bones. This type, occurring in older persons, is more likely to be fatal. One type, termed *benign metastasizing struma,* closely resembles normal thyroid tissue, and its first appearance may be in the metastasis to distant parts of the body, including the pelvis, hips, spine, and skull. This type of thyroid tumor will take up fairly large

amounts of radioactive iodine and may be treated with radioactive iodine. Other types progress rapidly, and some may be fatal within a few weeks. Surgery has proved to be the most satisfactory method of treatment, although radioactive iodine and x-ray therapy may be used in conjunction with surgery for some types.[3] Approximately 1150 persons may die from carcinoma of the thyroid in 1974.[5] The nurse may care for patients for whom treatment is only palliative. The same physical care and emotional support are necessary as for all patients with terminal cancer. (See Chapter 5.)

Diseases and disorders of the pancreas
Diabetes mellitus

Diabetes mellitus is the most common endocrine disorder in the United States. It is a chronic metabolic disease resulting in abnormal metabolism of carbohydrates. It has been estimated that diabetes mellitus affects one in fifty individuals in the United States, and it is found most frequently in persons over 40 years of age who are obese and have a family history of diabetes.[17]

Pathophysiology. The cause of diabetes mellitus is a deficiency of the hormone insulin, which is secreted by the beta cells that comprise most of the islands of Langerhans in the pancreas. The deficiency may result because the cells do not produce enough insulin, the body's needs are greater than the amount normally produced, or insulin may be destroyed by some body tissues. The predisposition to diabetes is a hereditary trait, and if persons who both have diabetes marry, all their offspring will develop diabetes at some time during their lifetimes. However, if only one of the marital partners has diabetes, providing the other partner does not carry the trait, none of their offspring will develop the disease, but they will carry the trait to the next generation.[17]

An adequate supply of insulin in the body is necessary for the body cells to combine oxygen and glucose to produce the energy necessary for body functions. In the absence of insulin several metabolic changes occur. Glucose accumulates in the blood and is excreted in the urine, and the body is required to use proteins and fat for energy, which under certain conditions contributes to acidosis.

The nurse will care for more patients with diabetes than with any other endocrine disease. At any given time care may be given to at least one diabetic patient, who may be a child, a middle-aged person, or an elderly person. Often a distinction is made between *juvenile-onset* and *maturity-onset diabetes.* In juvenile diabetes there may be an absence of insulin production because of a pathologic condition of the islands of Langerhans. In maturity-onset diabetes the rate of insulin secretion may be slower than normal, and often the diagnosis is preceded by a weight gain, which places a greater demand on the pancreas to produce insulin. The individual may be a *prediabetic* who is at risk because of the hereditary predisposition. The person may have one or more family members with diabetes. The patient may have *latent diabetes,* in which glucose may appear in the blood and urine only when the individual is exposed to stress situations such as illness, surgery, pregnancy, or injury. After recovery the blood and urine return to normal. The usual symptoms are lacking, and diagnosis of diabetes is often difficult. However, damage to the blood vessels may occur in the absence of overt symptoms. *Clinical diabetes* is indicated when one or more of the classic symptoms are present.[15]

Symptoms. Five symptoms are considered to be characteristic of diabetes: (1) excretion of sugar in the urine (glycosuria), (2) excessive concentration of sugar in the blood (hyperglycemia), (3) increased urinary output (polyuria), (4) excessive thirst (polydipsia), and (5) increased appetite with weight loss. Although some of these symptoms may occur in nondiabetic conditions, their presence should always call for a thorough investigation. Diabetes occurring in children is often abrupt in onset and severe, whereas its occurrence in adults is gradual and may not be detected for years. When diabetes exists for a considerable period of time and is untreated, symptoms of varied severity may occur, including skin infections such as boils and carbuncles and arteriosclerotic conditions, particularly of the eyes, kidneys, lower extremities, and coronary and cerebral blood vessels.

The nurse should understand that diabetes is not curable but controllable and that the patient with well-controlled diabetes can live a happy and productive life. The care of the diabetic patient must be concerned first with his immediate nursing needs and second with his long-range needs, since diabetes is a lifetime disease.

Diagnostic tests

Urine testing. When the patient is in the hospital for regulation of diabetes, the urine is usually tested every 4 hours or before meals and at bedtime. Specimens should be collected approximately 30 minutes before mealtime. Clinitest, one test for detection of sugar, is often used on the clinical unit because of its convenience. The Tes-Tape (Chapter 15) may also be used to test for sugar. When the urine contains sugar, the physician usually requests a test for acetone. Directions for the use of these tests are supplied with each test.

The amount of sugar present in the urine is important in regulating the insulin dosage, and the physician may order 5 units of regular insulin, which may be given before the meal, for each plus of sugar indicated on the color chart. A word of caution should be given concerning insulin ordered on the basis of a voided specimen of urine. Although sugar may be found in the voided specimen, residual urine may be negative for sugar. If this is the case, the administration of insulin may precipitate an insulin reaction. Therefore unless insulin is ordered on the basis of residual urine, the patient should be observed closely after the administration of insulin.[15] The best procedure for testing urine is to have the patient void and discard the urine. One hour later a specimen should be collected for testing. In this way the urine being excreted by the kidneys will be tested and will not contain urine that has been pooled in the bladder for several hours. Specimens should always be examined before meals and before administering insulin.[19]

When the patient is taught to test his own urine, stress should be placed on testing at least once a day and preferably four times. The patient should always be instructed to test a second voided specimen to avoid testing urine that has been allowed to pool in the bladder. The patient may

Test fresh residual urine

not be required to test for acetone unless sugar is present in the urine consistently or there is severe illness. A 24-hour quantitative test is usually done every 3 or 4 weeks on diabetic children.

Blood glucose. The laboratory examination of the blood requires that the patient be in a fasting state. The patient should be told that his breakfast will not be served until the blood specimen has been taken. If the patient is receiving insulin, it also is withheld until after the blood has been obtained. In case of diabetic acidosis and coma, blood for examination may be taken at any time.

Glucose tolerance test. The glucose tolerance test is used to discover any abnormality of the carbohydrate metabolism. The test is done with the patient in a fasting state. In the morning a blood sample is taken, and a urine specimen is obtained and sent to the laboratory. The patient is then weighed, and a measured amount of glucose, based on the patient's weight, is added to water with a few drops of lemon juice and given to the patient to drink. Blood and urine samples are then collected at 30-minute, 1-hour, and 2-hour intervals. The nurse may secure the urine specimens and should be sure that they are collected at the proper time, correctly labeled, and sent to the laboratory. If glucose remains in the blood for longer than 2 hours, it indicates some disorder of carbohydrate metabolism.

Approximate normal values of tests to determine diabetes are as follows:

Blood glucose test	80 to 100 mg./100 ml blood
Glucose tolerance test	Peak, 150 mg./100 ml. serum; at 2 hours return to normal in fasting state Peak in elderly persons may be 200 mg./100 ml. serum

Diet. Many patients with mild diabetes are maintained on diet alone. However, success depends on the seriousness and conscientiousness with which the patient accepts and follows his diet. This is true whether the patient is taking insulin or is on a diet without insulin. The diet is calculated for each individual patient on the basis of his needs and requirements, and any change in the diet must be made by the physician. While the patient is in the hospital, the dietary prescription goes to the therapeutic dietitian, who assumes the responsibility for preparing the food. The nurses' responsibility is to see that the patient eats all the food on the diet and nothing else. If for any reason the food or any part of it is not eaten, this must be reported, and a record must be kept so that the adjustments can be made. The nurse should know that the insulin covers the diet and that when food is not eaten and the patient has received insulin, complications may occur.

The diabetic patient must be given thorough instruction about his diet, and this responsibility does not end until it has been ascertained that he or some member of his family is competent to follow the dietary formula.

Usually the food exchange lists that were prepared jointly by the American Diabetes Association, the American Dietetic Association, and the United States Public Health Service are used in planning the patient's therapeutic diet. Seven lists of exchangeable foods have been defined: foods allowed as desired, vegetables, fruits, bread, meat, fats, and milk. Each food on a specific list is interchangeable with another and is equal in nutritional value, permitting patients their likes and dislikes. A specified number of exchanges is allowed for each meal and at bedtime, according to the caloric intake prescribed by the physician. Persons responsible for teaching the patient must be thoroughly familiar with diabetic diets and must be competent to teach the patient and to answer any question he may ask. The chief responsibility rests with the dietitian and the nurse. Numerous aids are available for helping the patient understand his diet, including a booklet *Meal Planning and Exchange Lists.**

Insulin. More than one half of the patients with diabetes require insulin. Insulin is commercially derived from pork or beef pancreas, although it has recently been synthesized in the laboratory. The amount of insulin needed depends on the individual patient and will vary at different times in the same patient. The type of in-

---

*Obtainable from The American Dietetic Association, Inc., 620 N. Michigan Ave., Chicago, Ill. 60611.

Table 17-1. Types of insulin

Type of insulin	Action	Duration (hours)	Peak of action (hours)
Regular	Fast acting	6 to 12	2 to 4
Crystalline zinc	Fast acting	6 to 12	2 to 4
Semilente	Fast acting	12 to 16	6 to 10
Globin zinc	Intermediate acting	12 to 24	6 to 10
NPH	Intermediate acting	About 24	8 to 12
Lente	Intermediate acting	About 24	8 to 12
Protamine zinc	Long lasting	24 to 36	16 to 24
Ultralente	Long lasting	24 to 36	16 to 24

sulin needed by the patient will also vary, depending on his specific requirement. The nurse must be familiar with the different kinds of insulin in current use, their action, and the method of administration. The purpose of administering insulin is to replace the deficiency, and its action is to lower the blood glucose level and to enable the body to metabolize carbohydrates. Insulin is designated as fast acting, intermediate acting, or long lasting. Insulin that is fast acting has to be administered more frequently than insulin that is long lasting. Several kinds of insulin are available, and the physician will order the type best suited for the individual patient (Table 17-1).

The NPH insulin has been found suitable for many patients because it requires only one injection a day. This preparation has a milky white precipitate and must be rotated between the palms of the hands before use (Fig. 17-3).

The distribution of meals varies for the individual patient who is receiving insulin. Some patients can be maintained on a regimen of three meals a day, whereas others require a midmorning, midafternoon, and bedtime feeding. Some patients must also be given a feeding during the night. When the physician calculates the daily food requirement, it will be apportioned to provide for between-meal feedings if they are necessary.

Insulin is administered in units that have been standardizd so that no matter where it is purchased or from which pharmaceutical manufacturer it comes, it will be the same. To help in identifying types of insulin and the number of units in each cubic

centimeter, various colored labels are used on the vials. The nurse should become familiar with the various types of syringes used for giving insulin. Needles should be 26 gauge and from ⅜ to ½ inch in length. Syringes are calibrated and labeled U-40, U-80, or U-100, each scale corresponding to the strength of the insulin to be used. U-40 insulin contains 40 units of insulin in 1 ml., U-80 insulin contains 80 units in 1 ml., and U-100 insulin contains 100 units in 1 ml. One type of syringe has a double scale and is calibrated for both U-40 and U-80 insulin. A separate U-100 syringe must be used for U-100 insulin. Most insulin is now available in U-100, and it is hoped that the majority of diabetic patients will be using this strength in the future and that the U-40 and U-80 concentrations will be phased out. The U-100 insulin is based on the decimal system and is therefore easier to understand. In addition, U-100 insulin is a stronger solution, and less volume is introduced with each injection.

A method now in use for the administration of insulin is to place the insulin in the

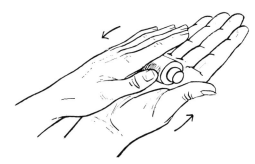

Fig. 17-3. Method of mixing insulin. Roll the vial between the palms of the hands.

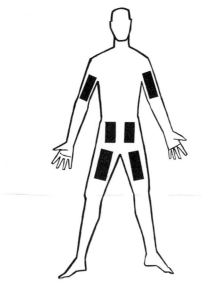

Fig. 17-4. Injection sites for insulin. By dividing each site into twelve areas, the same site will not be used more often than once in 12 weeks.

Injecting insulin

space between the subcutaneous tissue and the muscle. The correct dose of insulin is prepared, the skin is disinfected, and a large fold of skin and fat is carefully pinched up. Holding the syringe in a perpendicular position, the needle is quickly inserted all the way to the hub with a dartlike technique. Pinching the tissue leaves a loose space into which the insulin is injected. The needle is withdrawn and an alcohol sponge used to exert slight pressure over the injection site for a couple of minutes. This technique prevents the discolored lumps that usually occur on the skin after repeated injections. It avoids the necessity of aspirating the syringe and eliminates the problem of injection into blood vessels, and the procedure is essentially painless.[7, 16] The sites for injection should be rotated with each injection to prevent lumps from forming at the injection sites, which will interfere with absorption and may predispose to abscess formation (Fig. 17-4). If insulin is given in the same site for a period of time, it may slow absorption, and then a change in the site of injection may cause a more rapid absorption, predisposing the patient to insulin reaction.

The patient should be taught to administer his own insulin as soon as his condition permits. He should observe the administra-

tion, then participate by assisting the nurse, and finally be able to measure the correct dose and administer it. If the patient will be unable to administer his own insulin, a member of the family should be taught and given practice in the technique.

Oral agents. The oral hypoglycemic agents fall into two groups: (1) sulfonylureas and (2) biguanide compounds. The sulfonylureas are all similar in action but differ in their duration of action and side effects. The sulfonylureas act primarily by assisting the pancreas to secrete insulin, whereas the biguanide compounds have no effect on the release of insulin from the pancreas. Exactly how the biguanide agents act is unknown. Among the sulfonylurea preparations are tolbutamide (Orinase), chlorpropamide (Diabinese), acetohexamide (Dymelor), and tolazamide (Tolinase). Biguanide compounds include phenformin (DBI) or a long-lasting form (DBI-TD). Not all patients will benefit from oral hypoglycemic agents. Patients who develop diabetes after 40 years of age and who do not require more than 40 units of insulin or who do not have a tendency toward diabetic complications may be given the oral agents. Children and young diabetic patients usually require insulin. During periods of stress, such as infections, injuries, surgery, or pergnancy, the oral agents are not recommended. All the sulfonylurea preparations may produce hypoglycemia, and jaundice has been reported as a side effect from some of them. The biguanide agents may cause nausea, vomiting, weakness, and drowsiness and therefore are commonly given after meals. Some oral agents have been scrutinized by the Food and Drug Administration and their value questioned. Recently the medical director of a large diabetic clinic stated that the condition of a patient receiving an oral hypoglycemic agent could be controlled by diet alone. The problem is that physicians and nurses do not take the time to teach the patient about dietary planning.

Hygiene. Patients with diabetes have a lowered resistance to infection, and open abrasions or wounds are slow in healing. Care of the skin is of the utmost importance, and if the nurse gives proper care while the patient is in the hospital, it will help to impress on him its importance. One of the most important aspects of hygiene is proper care of the feet. They should be washed daily with warm water (avoid hot water) and soap and dried well, particularly between the toes. Nails should be trimmed straight across and not too short. Corns and calluses should be smoothed with an emery board or pumice stone and should never be cut by anyone except the podiatrist. Corn plasters or corn removers should never be used. The use of lanolin after bathing will help to keep the skin soft and prevent the nails from becoming dry. Clean socks or hose (preferably undyed) should be worn daily. Iodine or other strong antiseptics should not be applied to the feet, and they should not be soaked in commercially prepared foot soaks. Shoes should be well fitting, and new shoes should be broken in gradually to avoid pressure on any part of the foot. House slippers should be made of leather, and the practice of going barefooted should be avoided because of the danger of injury to the feet. The feet should not be exposed to extremes of temperature; bed socks should be worn at night rather than using hot-water bottles or heating pads. Round garters should not be worn, and the patient should be cautioned about sitting with the knees crossed. The patient should be advised to consult the physician about any injury to the feet, even though it may seem trivial.

Moderate exercise is important for the diabetic patient and should be planned for each day. Exercise utilizes sugar for energy, and if the patient knows that he will engage in any unusual activity, he may need to plan for more carbohydrate intake.

Provision should be made for adequate sleep and rest, and if necessary, mild sedatives may be ordered by the physician. Although the patient with diabetes must learn to live with the disease the rest of his life, adjustments should follow his normal pattern and habits of living as nearly as possible.

Diabetic acidosis (ketoacidosis). Diabetic acidosis, or diabetic coma, is a serious complication of the disease and must always be considered as an emergency. It may occur in an individual with undiagnosed diabetes and may be the first indication of the disease. In the patient with diagnosed diabetes

it usually results from neglect or ignorance, such as dietary excesses, failure to check urine, omission of insulin, infection with elevation of temperature, or some condition within the body that has caused resistance to insulin. It may sometimes occur after ether anesthesia. It may also occur because the patient has not received proper instruction. The immediate cause is always lack of insulin.

The onset of diabetic acidosis is a gradual process, the duration of which may be from hours to days. A gradual loss of appetite, increased thirst, and nausea and vomiting occur; the skin becomes dry, and the face is flushed. A fruity odor may be detected on the breath, headache and weakness are present, and the patient looks and feels sick. Examination of the urine shows large amounts of sugar and acetone, and the blood glucose level is elevated. Difficult, deep, rapid breathing and air hunger may occur, the blood pressure drops, and the pulse becomes rapid and weak. Without prompt treatment, fluid and electrolyte losses can lead to coma and death.

The patient may be brought into the hospital in a state of coma, and diagnosis must be established before giving insulin. The patient should be catheterized immediately to secure a urine specimen to test for sugar and acetone, and a retention catheter is usually inserted into the urinary bladder and connected to gravity drainage. A blood sample is obtained for blood glucose examination. The physician may order several additional tests that will be made on the blood. An infusion of 1000 ml of isotonic saline solution may be administered. When the diagnosis of diabetic acidosis has been confirmed, insulin will be given. The patient will be placed in the intensive care unit because continuous nursing care must be provided. The nurse must keep accurate records of all intake and output on an hourly basis, and the urine is checked hourly for sugar and acetone. All urine is saved for a 24-hour analysis. A rectal temperature is taken hourly for 6 hours or longer, and the patient is kept warm with extra blankets. Hot-water bottles should not be used because of the danger of burning an unconscious patient. A warm cleansing enema may be given, and

Insulin reaction

Blood sugar ↓
missing a meal
physical exertion
occurs quickly

a gastric lavage may be done to decrease the chance of aspiration of vomitus. Nothing is given by mouth until ordered by the physician. The patient may be given intravenous infusions with replacement of electrolytes. If infection is present, antibiotics may be administered.

Insulin reaction. Insulin shock, or hypoglycemic reaction, is the result of a drop in blood glucose level. Several factors may be responsible, including the omission of a meal, nausea and vomiting after the meal with loss of the food eaten, excessive physical exercise, exposure to extremes of cold, or too much insulin. With the present types of insulin it is important to understand the time at which the maximum insulin effect occurs and to meet that time with proper food supplements.

Insulin reaction (shock) may be mild to severe and occurs quickly. The most common symptoms are a trembling sensation, profuse perspiration, irritability, and dizziness. Additional signs may be weakness, headache, blurring of vision, pallor, and hunger. Without immediate treatment the patient may become confused and comatose and have convulsions.

The immediate treatment is to give some form of carbohydrate. A specimen of blood should be taken before sugar is given. If the patient is conscious, 4 ounces of sweetened fruit juice or carbonated drink may be given, to be repeated in 1 hour. Several small candies, fruit, or 1 or 2 teaspoons of jelly may be given. Corn syrup may be given to the stuporous patient, since it is swallowed slowly. The conscious patient in insulin shock may be resistive, stubborn, and difficult to manage; if so, 1 or 2 teaspoons of sugar may be added to the fruit drink[15] If the patient is unconscious, 20 to 50 ml. of 50% glucose solution intravenously, 0.3 to 0.5 ml. of a 1:1000 solution of epinephrine subcutaneously, or 1 to 2 ml. of glucagon intravenously may be given.[15] Each will elevate the blood glucose level long enough for the patient to return to consciousness and enable him to take a drink of sweetened fruit juice.

Every diabetic patient should be familiar with the signs of insulin reaction and should know what to do. The patient should always carry some form of carbohydrate such as sugar or a candy bar and a special identification card or Medic Alert tag. It is not uncommon for a diabetic person to be picked up on the street unconscious, believed to be intoxicated, and taken to jail. The nurse caring for the diabetic patient in the home should be thoroughly familiar with the signs of insulin reaction and should know what to do. The nurse should be able to help teach the patient to recognize approaching signs of insulin reaction and diabetic coma as well as the preventive aspects.

Diabetic acidosis and insulin reaction are preventable. Many patients are cared for in the physician's office or in an outpatient clinic. Prevention is based on thorough teaching of the patient and his family and the willingness and readiness of the patient to accept his disease, to accept the teaching, and to profit from it. Teaching the patient is a joint responsibility of the physician, the nursing team, and the dietitian. When there are economic problems relating to the purchase of insulin, a social worker may give assistance. Diabetic patients may be referred to the public health nurse for follow-up care in the home, and the patient should understand the importance of regular medical supervision.

Other complications. Several complicating conditions may accompany diabetes, and most are related to changes in the vascular system. Although any part of the body may be affected, the eyes, kidneys, nervous system, and skin are most frequently involved. The diabetic person is likely to develop atherosclerosis earlier than the nondiabetic person, and when infections occur, they are more severe than they are in other individuals. Diabetic gangrene of the toes or the feet may result from injury, and even slight abrasions or scratches may result in gangrene. Gangrene may also be due to vascular changes resulting from atherosclerosis. Frequently the only help that can be offered the patient is amputation of the affected extremity.[2]

What the diabetic patient should know. The diabetic patient must be willing to accept the fact that he has a chronic disease, and he must learn to live with it for the rest of his life. This may be especially difficult for the older person, and it may mean that a younger individual will have to make changes in his pattern of daily living.

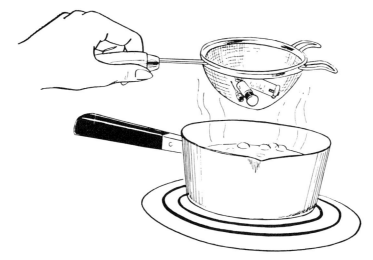

Fig. 17-5. A method of sterilizing the insulin syringe and needle in the home.

Nurses in hospitals, clinics, and physician's offices are often responsible for teaching the diabetic patient what he should know. Evidence indicates that the patient frequently makes mistakes and is confused, and some errors are potentially serious. Nurses must realize that although they may be familiar with the procedure of administering insulin, the patient is being asked to learn a technique that is entirely unfamiliar to him. Often a poorly controlled case of diabetes may be the result of the patient's confusion and misunderstanding. The following have been cited as causes for errors made by diabetic patients:

1. Failure to understand diet exchange lists
2. Confusion over the different syringes and how to match the right syringe with the right insulin
3. Failure to understand why the glass syringe should be sterilized and how to keep it sterile (Fig. 17-5)
4. Ignorance of the reason why plastic disposable syringes should not be reused
5. Failure to understand that the second urine specimen is the one that should always be tested
6. Ignorance of the fact that urine specimens should always be tested before eating or taking insulin[19]

These points may serve as a guide for the nurse who is teaching the patient. It is better for only one person to teach the patient to avoid confusion. The public health nurse can provide follow-up instruction and supervision for the patient in the home. Observation of the patient's performance is better than asking him how he carries out procedures, since he may be likely to say what he thinks the nurse wants to hear.

Diabetes and pregnancy. The pregnant woman with diabetes should be under the care of both the obstetrician and an internist from the beginning of pregnancy. Complications such as diabetic acidosis, infections, toxemia, abortion, and intrauterine or perinatal death are more likely to occur in the pregnant patient with diabetes. The insulin needs will vary, and frequent evaluation is necessary. Diet must be rigidly controlled, and salt is usually restricted from the beginning. The patient often retains water and may become edematous, requiring diuretic medications. The risks in pregnancy are greater in the diabetic than in the nondiabetic woman. Since the incidence of diabetes is greater after 35 years of age, the occurrence of pregnancy with diabetes is increased during the late childbearing years. The diabetic woman often has a large baby, resulting in a difficult delivery.

The infant of the diabetic mother must be considered as prediabetic. In many instances a pediatrician may be in attendance at delivery to assume responsibility for the infant. The infant may have unexplained episodes of cyanosis and may require oxygen. The nursing care of the infant is essentially the same as that for the premature infant, and close observation for evidence of respiratory distress or convulsions is important. Most perinatal deaths occur during the first 48 hours, after which the infant's prognosis is improved.[10, 11]

Diabetes and surgery. With the increased knowledge about diabetes, insulin, improved surgical techniques, and anesthesia, surgical procedures may be safely performed on the patient with diabetes. The preoperative withholding of food and the postoperative vomiting will disturb the metabolism of carbohydrates, and treatment must be established both preoperatively and postoperatively to minimize or overcome the metabolic upset.

The patient will be admitted to the hospital 1 or 2 days prior to surgery, and a careful evaluation will be made of his diabetic status. Blood chemistry, including blood glucose level and urine analysis for sugar and acetone will be done. Frequently an electrocardiogram may be ordered. In the event of emergency surgery the physician will take into consideration the patient's condition and the time element when deciding on tests. The nurse should be certain that all laboratory reports are available for the surgeon and on the patient's record before the patient goes to surgery. Surgery for the diabetic patient is usually scheduled in the morning. In some instances in which the blood glucose value is negative, insulin is omitted on the operative day, whereas in other cases half the usual amount is given. When surgery is prolonged and intravenous infusion of glucose solution is administered, many physicians order insulin added to the solution; however, there is not general agreement on this procedure. Postoperatively frequent blood glucose determinations are made until the patient's diabetes is stabilized.[9]

The nurse caring for the surgical patient with diabetes must be constantly alert for the early signs of diabetic coma and insulin reaction. Aseptic technique in the care of wounds must be exacting, since the patient is highly susceptible to infection and wounds heal slowly. The nurse should be familiar with the physician's orders concerning the administration of insulin, urine testing, and diet. Other care follows the same plan as for all surgical patients.

Hypoglycemia

An abnormally low level of blood glucose may also occur in the absence of diabetes. It may be caused by disease of the liver or pancreas or disease of the pituitary or adrenal glands. The symptoms include hunger, weakness, anxiety, pallor, headache, sweating, and rapid pulse. One type known as functional hypoglycemia has an unknown cause. The symptoms are variable and frequently occur several hours after meals or after exercise. The attacks may last from minutes to days. Treatment is based on relieving the immediate attack, followed by removing the cause when it is known. In mild attacks orange juice or hard candy may relieve the symptoms, whereas for patients with severe cases glucose may be administered intravenously.[13, 18]

Diseases and disorders of the parathyroid glands
Hyperparathyroidism and Hypoparathyroidism

Excessive secretion of parathormone may be caused by a benign tumor of one of the glands. Since the purpose of the hormone is to maintain a constant calcium balance in the blood, oversecretion of the hormone results in the removal of calcium from the bones. The bones become weak, tender, and painful, and spontaneous fractures may occur. The appetite may become poor, constipation may be present, and there may be fatigue, depression, weight loss, and loss of muscle tone, making walking difficult. An increase in the blood calcium level occurs, and renal calculi composed chiefly of calcium salts may form in the kidney. Small tumors, which are detected by x-ray examination, may form in the bones. The treatment is surgical removal of the tumor or removal of all but one of the glands.

When too little parathormone is secreted, the level of blood calcium decreases, and phosphorus increases in the blood. The deficiency of the hormone may result from injury to the glands or the removal of too much parathyroid tissue during a thyroidectomy. The primary symptom is tetany resulting from the decreased level of blood calcium. There is muscular incoordination with tremor and muscular spasm. Laryngeal spasm and convulsions may occur. The treatment is to elevate the blood calcium level by the administration of calcium salts, parathormone extract, and vitamin D. Depending on the severity of the condition, calcium lactate in physiologic saline solution, parathormone solution, and vitamin D may be administered intravenously.[9]

Diseases and disorders of the adrenal (suprarenal) glands

Each adrenal gland consists of two lobes, which function as separate glands. One lobe, the adrenal cortex, produces several different hormones that are essential to life. These hormones regulate much of the cell activity of the body and maintain an optimum internal environment for the body cells. They also regulate the body's ability to adapt to constant changes in the external environment. From the other lobe of the adrenal glands, the medulla, two hormones are secreted that affect various functions of the body but are not essential to life. These two hormones are epinephrine and norepinephrine.

Addison's disease

Hypofunction of the adrenal cortex resulting in insufficient secretion of hormones causes Addison's disease. The specific cause for the atrophy, or wasting away, of the gland is unknown, but it often is diagnosed after the patient has undergone stressful situations such as injury, infection, or surgery.

Symptoms result from inadequate amounts of adrenal cortical hormones in the blood and body fluids. Common gastrointestinal symptoms are nausea, vomiting, anorexia, diarrhea, and abdominal pain. The patient may fatigue easily and show signs of hypoglycemia such as nervousness, increased perspiration, headache, and trembling. These symptoms result from inadequate amounts of circulating cortisone and hydrocortisone. The normal fluid and electrolyte balance is interrupted, and the patient will have a deficiency of sodium and chloride and an excess of potassium because of insufficient aldosterone. Often

the skin will develop a bronze color, and the patient will appear tanned.[17]

Care of the patient with Addison's disease involves replacement therapy. Hydrocortisone (cortisol), 20 to 40 mg. a day, and 9 alpha-fluorohydrocortisone (Florinef), 0.1 mg. a day, are often given after meals.[8] The patient should realize the importance of taking the medicines and should avoid undue stress, which could cause serious complications. Addison's crisis is a serious exacerbation of the disease and can produce a severe drop in blood pressure, leading to shock, coma, and death. When this occurs, hydrocortisone is given intravenously, and drugs such as phenylephrine (Neo-Synephrine) are given to elevate the blood pressure. The patient often is put in reverse isolation, since he has a low resistance to infection.

Cushing's syndrome

Hyperfunction of the adrenal cortex produces an excessive secretion of hormones from the gland and results in Cushing's syndrome. The cause is usually an overgrowth (hyperplasia) of one or both glands; however, a tumor in the anterior pituitary gland can stimulate the adrenal cortex and also result in Cushing's syndrome.

Characteristic symptoms of Cushing's syndrome include weakness with muscle wasting, fat accumulation in the face, neck, and trunk, hemorrhagic tendencies, changes in secondary sex characteristics, and symptoms of fluid and electrolyte imbalance. Irritability and hypertension may also be present. The patient's appearance may be upsetting, especially to a woman, and the patient may withdraw from others.

Nursing care should convey acceptance and reassurance. Treatment usually involves surgical removal of the adrenal cortex. However, if the pituitary gland is involved, a hypophysectomy (removal of the gland) or irradiation of the pituitary gland may be performed.

A variety of chronic diseases are treated with adrenal steroids, although no adrenal disease is present. Examples of such diseases are rheumatoid arthritis, leukemia, emphysema, and ulcerative colitis. Drugs such as prednisone have potent anti-inflammatory effects, which can be of great therapeutic value. However, most patients treated with adrenal steroids will develop Cushing's syndrome to a variable degree, and serious complications and side effects can occur.[4] The nurse should be familiar with the untoward effects of the steroid preparations, and they should be reported if they are observed. (See Table 2-3).

Pheochromocytoma

Pheochromocytoma is a tumor of the adrenal medulla. These tumors are generally small and benign, with only a tiny number being malignant. A malignant tumor (neuroblastoma) may occur in children and is usually fatal. Pheochromocytoma occurs most often in women of middle age. It is believed that causal factors may be hereditary in some cases, whereas stress situations and pregnancy may be causal factors in other cases.

Symptoms result from the hypersecretion of epinephrine and norepinephrine. The characteristic symptom is hypertension. However, the hypertension may be variable, being persistent and chronic or occurring in intermittent attacks. Because of the elevated blood pressure, it is often confused with essential hypertension (p. 268). Other symptoms may include severe headache, excessive sweating, nausea, vomiting, palpitation, and nervousness with acute anxiety. During an acute attack, tachycardia, hyperglycemia, and polyuria may occur.

Provisional diagnosis is made by tests on the urine and the blood to detect the presence of catecholamines. Injection of certain drugs to determine the behavior of the blood pressure is gradually being replaced by the urine tests. Various x-ray procedures are used, including pneumography in which air is injected into the rectoperitoneal areas and x-ray films are taken. Arteriography and intravenous urogram may also be used to confirm the diagnosis. The treatment is surgical.

Adrenalectomy

Adrenalectomy is the surgical removal of the adrenal gland, usually because of a pathologic disorder such as a tumor. The preoperative preparation of the patient is the same as that for other abdominal surgery. The postoperative care may require the administration of hydrocortisone if the

adrenal cortex has been removed. When surgery has been done because of pheochromocytoma, the patient's condition may be critical for the first 48 hours. Shock may occur because of the abrupt fall in the blood pressure. Blood pressure must be monitored continuously and the patient observed for hemorrhage, which may be external or internal. Central venous pressure is monitoried, and the urinary output must be observed for signs of oliguria. Vasopressor drugs are administered intravenously. Caution should be used when administering narcotic drugs for pain, since some have a tendency to cause hypotension. After the critical period, recovery progresses normally. If both adrenal glands are removed, the patient will have to take corticosteroids for the rest of his life.

Diseases of the pituitary gland

The pituitary gland has been called the *master gland* because it exerts some control over the other endocrine glands. The pituitary gland has a posterior and an anterior lobe. The anterior lobe secretes several hormones. The exact number of hormones secreted by this gland is probably unknown. The posterior lobe secretes two hormones. The hormones from the anterior lobe stimulate other glands to produce their hormones.

A hypersecretion of the anterior lobe of the pituitary gland may result from a tumor affecting certain cells. The condition causes acromegaly in the adult and is characterized by the following: the features become coarse, the bones become large and heavy, the hands and feet become broad and massive, the chin protrudes, and the tongue enlarges. Surgical removal of the tumor is extremely difficult, and radiation therapy may be used in treatment of the condition. A congenital deficiency of the growth hormone results in dwarfism (midget), whereas a tumor affecting the growth hormone in childhood or adolescence causes the individual to grow extremely tall. This is known as gigantism.

Since the pituitary gland regulates many functions of the body and controls other functions through its influence on other glands, many disorders may result from an oversecretion or an undersecretion of its various hormones. Since many of these conditions occur only rarely, a discussion of them is not included in this book. If the nurse is interested in further study, materials may be secured from other books and from journals.

Summary outline

1. Endocrine glands and their function
   A. Thyroid gland—secretes thyroxin and stores iodine
   B. Parathyroids—secrete parathormone
   C. Adrenal (suprarenal) glands—secrete epinephrine (Adrenalin), hydrocortisone, and corticosterone
   D. Pituitary body (master gland)—secretes several hormones
   E. Gonads—secrete estrogen and progesterone hormones in female and testosterone and androsterone in male
   F. Pancreas (islands of Langerhans)—secrete insulin
2. Diagnostic tests and procedures
   A. Blood chemistry—includes blood glucose, insulin tolerance, glucose tolerance, and Thorn test
   B. Urinalysis—performed with 24-hour collection for hormone determination
   C. Basal metabolic rate—used to determine activity of thyroid gland
      1. Test measures amount of oxygen consumed by individual at rest and in fasting state
      2. Increased rate indicates hyperthyroidism
      3. Decreased rate indicates hypothyroidism
   D. Protein-bound iodine (PBI) test
   E. Radioactive iodine uptake—performed to determine activity of thyroid gland
      1. Oral administration of tracer dose of radioactive iodine and uptake measured 24 to 48 hours later with a scintillator
      2. Oral administration of tracer dose of radioactive iodine and uptake measured by amount secreted in urine during period of 24 to 48 hours
      3. Triiodothyronine resin uptake test—uses blood sample from patient; radioactive iodine 131 is added to blood in laboratory
      4. Scanogram—patient is given iodine 131, and scintillator connected to recording device is passed externally over throat; used to differentiate between malignant and nonmalignant condition
      5. Nursing responsibilities—reassuring patient, collection of urine specimens, and avoiding administration of any drugs containing iodine prior to tests
3. Nursing the patient with diseases of endocrine system
   A. Diseases of thyroid
      1. Simple (endemic) goiter—caused by deficiency of iodine in food and water or by altered metabolism
      2. Hyperthyroidism—also known as toxic goiter, thyrotoxicosis, exophthalmic goiter, and Graves' disease
      3. Medical treatment and nursing care—directed toward reducing activity of gland and production of thyroxin
         a. Antithyroid drugs to relieve symptoms
         b. Quiet restful environment
         c. High-caloric diet
      4. Thyroidectomy—surgical removal of part or all of thyroid gland
         a. Preoperative care—follows same patterns as medical care
         b. Postoperative care
            (1) Observation for hemorrhage
            (2) Observation of edema of larynx
            (3) Observation for nerve paralysis
            (4) Observation for tetany
            (5) Preparation for emergency
      5. Hypothyroidism—results from undersecretion of thyroxin
         a. Myxedema—hypothyroidism in adult
         b. Juvenile myxedema—hypothyroidism in child or adolescent
         c. Cretinism—complete absence of thyroxin at birth
      6. Tumors of thyroid
         a. Nodular goiter
         b. Carcinoma of thyroid
   B. Diseases of pancreas
      1. Diabetes mellitus—caused by deficiency of insulin
         a. Pathophysiology
            (1) Prediabetes
            (2) Latent diabetes
            (3) Clinical diabetes
         b. Five basic symptoms
            (1) Glycosuria
            (2) Hyperglycemia
            (3) Polyuria
            (4) Polydipsia
            (5) Increased appetite with weight loss
         c. Diagnostic tests
            (1) Urine testing—should be done every 4 hours or 30 minutes before meals and before administration of insulin
               (a) Discard first specimen and test second specimen
               (b) Test for sugar and test for acetone if sugar is present
            (2) Blood glucose determination
               (a) Patient must be in fasting state
               (b) Insulin and food held until blood is taken
            (3) Glucose tolerance test
               (a) Patient must be in fasting state
               (b) Blood and urine specimens taken
               (c) Patient weighed, then drinks solution containing glucose
               (d) Blood and urine samples collected at 30-minute, 1-hour, and 2-hour intervals
         d. Diet—calculated for individual patient
            (1) Patient must eat all of diet and nothing else
            (2) Failure to eat must be reported

(3) Loss of food through vomiting should be reported

(4) Patient must have thorough instruction concerning diet

e. Insulin—used to replace deficiency, to lower blood glucose levels, and to enable body to metabolize carbohydrates

(1) Regular, crystalline, zinc, and semilente insulin are fast acting

(2) Globin, NPH, zinc, and lente insulin are intermediate acting

(3) Protamine zinc and ultralente insulin are long lasting

(4) Insulin is measured and administered in units per milliliter; U40, U80, U100

(5) Needle should be 26 gauge, ⅜ to ½ inch in length

(6) Syringe should correspond to units per milliliter

(7) Rotate sites of injection

f. Oral hypoglycemic agents

(1) Sulfonylureas

(a) Tolbutamide (Orinase)

(b) Chlorpropamide (Diabinese)

(c) Acetohexamide (Dymelor)

(d) Tolazamide (Tolinase)

(2) Biguanide compounds

(a) Phenformin (DBI)

(b) DBI-TD long-lasting form of phenformin

(3) Not all patients will benefit from oral hypoglycemic agents

g. Hygiene—important because of lowered resistance to infection

(1) Care of feet should have particular attention

(2) Moderate daily exercise

(3) Adequate sleep and rest

h. Diabetic acidosis—has gradual onset, is serious complication and always an emergency; may have various causes

(1) Ignorance or neglect

(2) Failure to check urine

(3) Omission of insulin

(4) Infection with elevation of temperature

(5) Some condition within body causing resistance to insulin

(6) Not receiving proper insulin

i. Insulin reaction—has rapid onset and is result of drop in blood glucose level caused by one of following:

(1) Omission of meal

(2) Loss of food through vomiting

(3) Excessive physical exercise

(4) Exposure to extremes of cold

(5) Too much insulin

j. Vascular complications may occur in following parts of body:

(1) Eyes

(2) Kidneys

(3) Nervous system

(4) Skin

k. What diabetic patient should know

(1) Acceptance that he has chronic disease and will live with it for the rest of life

(2) Nurses often responsible for teaching patient

l. Diabetes and pregnancy

(1) Patients with diabetes are more likely to have complications

(2) Diet and insulin must be rigidly controlled

(3) Close medical supervision necessary from beginning of pregnancy

(4) If complications are present, delivery is usually complicated

m. Diabetes and surgery

(1) Surgery may be safely performed on many diabetic patients

(2) Nurse must be alert for signs of diabetic acidosis and insulin reaction

(3) All wounds must be protected from infection

C. Hypoglycemia—may occur in absence of diabetes

1. Cause may be disease of liver, of pancreas, or of pituitary or adrenal glands

2. Functional hypoglycemia may occur with unknown cause

D. Diseases of parathyroid glands

1. Hyperparathyroidism—excessive secretion of hormone parathormone

a. Results in removal of calcium from bones with increase of calcium in blood

b. Small tumors may form in bones, and spontaneous fractures may occur

2. Hypoparathyroidism—result of too little secretion of parathormone

a. Affects nerves and muscles, with loss of coordination and muscle spasm

E. Diseases of adrenal (suprarenal) glands

1. Adrenal cortex—produces several hormones

a. Steroids in form of cortisone preparations used to treat many diseases

2. Medulla—produces two hormones, epinephrine and norepinephrine

3. Addison's disease—hypofunction of adrenal cortex

a. Produces gastrointestinal disorders, hypoglycemia and fluid and electrolyte imbalances

b. Addison's crisis may occur

4. Cushing's syndrome—hyperfunction of adrenal cortex

a. Causes weakness and muscle wasting, abnormal fat accumulation, hemorrhagic tendencies, changes in sex characteristics, and fluid and electrolyte imbalances

b. Many chronic diseases treated with adrenal steroids; Cushing's syndrome may occur

5. Pheochromocytoma—tumor of adrenal medulla

a. Symptoms caused by hypersecretion of epinephrine and norepinephrine

b. Treatment surgical

6. Adrenalectomy—surgical removal of adrenal gland
F. Diseases of pituitary gland (master gland)
   1. Anterior lobe secretes several hormones; exact number unknown
   2. Posterior lobe secretes two hormones
   3. Oversecretion of growth hormone from anterior lobe results in gigantism in child or early adolescent; acromegaly in adult caused by tumor of certain cells
   4. Undersecretion of growth hormone from anterior lobe results in dwarfism (midget) in young child
   5. Pituitary body exerts control over and influences other endocrine glands

Review questions

1. Why should calcium gluconate be placed in the room of the postoperative patient who has had a thyroidectomy?
   a. *in case of po tetany*
2. What five signs are characteristic of diabetes mellitis?
   a. *polyuria*.
   b. *glycosuria* -
   c. *hyperglycemia*
   d. *polydipsia (thirst)*
   e. *incl. appetite c wt. loss*
3. If two diabetics should marry, how many of their children would develop diabetes at some time during their life?
   a. *All*
4. When the diabetic patient is receiving the oral hypoglycemic agent phenformin, what side effects should the nurse watch for?
   a. *nausea*
   b. *vomiting*
   c. *weakness*
   d. *drowsiness*
5. What hormone secreted by the adrenal medulla is prepared commercially?
   a. *Adrenalin (epinephrine)*
6. What are three effects that epinephrine may have on the body?
   a. *↑ BP*
   b. *vasoconstriction*
   c. *relaxing the bronchioles*
7. Where would you expect to find the pituitary gland?
   a. *in the brain (skull)*
8. Why are the endocrine glands called the glands of internal secretion? *bloodstream -*
   a. *release secretions into no ducts*
9. What two important points would you teach the diabetic patient about testing of urine?
   a. *Test second voided urine—fresh*
   b. *Test daily—sometimes 4X daily*
10. How would you compare the onset of diabetic acidosis with that of a hypoglycemic reaction?
    a. *slow reaction   ↑ rapid occurance*

Films

1. The critical balance (25 min., sound, color, 16 mm.), The Pfizer Laboratories Film Library, 267 West 25th St., New York, N. Y. 10001. Stresses the urgent need for patient education in diabetes. Demonstrates how the program is carried out at Joslin Clinic in Boston. Gives particular attention to the emotional aspects of diabetes.
2. Quiet victory—M-1522-X (32 min., sound, color, 16 mm.), Media Resources Branch, National Medical Audiovisual Center (Annex), Station K, Atlanta, Ga. 30324. Portrays the basic responsibility of the nurse in instructing the diabetic patient and his family in vital elements of self-care. Shows nurses's follow-up care. Shows patients and their families in hospital, outpatient department, school, industry, and home.
3. Understanding diabetes—M-1523-X (35 min., sound, color, 16 mm.), Media Resources Branch, National Medical Audiovisual Center (Annex), Station K, Atlanta, Ga. 30324. Presents basic scientific concepts about diabetes, clinical and public health aspects, epidemiologic factors, and modern concepts and methods of management. The prevention of acute problems and degenerative complications is discussed. Uses live photography and animation.

References

1. Anthony, Catherine P., and Kolthoff, Norma J: Textbook of anatomy and physiology, ed. 9, St. Louis, 1975, The C. V. Mosby Co.
2. Arnold, Helen M.: Elderly diabetic amputees, American Journal of Nursing 69:2646-2649, Dec., 1969.
3. Beeson, Paul B., and McDermott, Walsh, editors: Cecil-Loeb textbook of medicine, ed. 13, Philadelphia, 1971, W. B. Saunders Co.
4. Blount, Mary, and Kinney, Anna Belle: Chronic steroid therapy, American Journal of Nursing 74:1626-1631, Sept., 1974.
5. Brunner, Lillian S., and Suddarth, Doris S.: Textbook of medical-surgical nursing, ed. 3, Philadelphia, 1975, J. B. Lippincott Co.
6. Brunner, Lillian S., and Suddarth, Doris S.: The Lippincott manual of nursing practice, Philadelphia, 1974, J. B. Lippincott Co.
7. Burke, Elizabeth L.: Insulin injection, the site and the technique, American Journal of Nursing 72:2194-2196, Dec., 1972.
8. Cancer facts and figures 74, New York, 1974, American Cancer Society, Inc.
9. Conn, Howard F., editor: Current therapy 1976, Philadelphia, 1976, W. B. Saunders Co.
10. Fitzpatrick, Elise, Reeder, Sharon R., and Mastroianni, Lugi: Maternity nursing, ed. 12, Philadelphia, 1971, J. B. Lippincott Co.
11. Iorio, Josephine: Principles of obstetrics and gynecology for nurses, ed. 3, St. Louis, 1975, The C. V. Mosby Co.
12. Luckman, Joan, and Sorensen, Karen C.: Medical-surgical nursing, Philadelphia, 1974, W. B. Saunders Co.
13. Jay, Arthur N.: Hypoglycemia, American Journal of Nursing 62:77-78, Jan., 1962.
14. Martin, Marguerite M.: Diabetes mellitus: current concepts, American Journal of Nursing 66:510-514, March, 1966.
15. Martin, Marguerite M.: Insulin reaction, American Journal of Nursing 67:328-331, Feb., 1967.
16. St. James, Peter: Insulin injection—a new

technique, The Canadian Nurse **65:**32-33, July, 1969.

17. Shafer, Kathleen N., Sawyer, Janet R., Mc-Cluskey, Audrey M., Beck, Edna L., and Phipps, Wilma J.: Medical-surgical nursing, ed. 6, St. Louis, 1975, The C. V. Mosby Co.

18. Taif, Betty: Hypoglycemia, a symptom not a disease, The Journal of Practical Nursing **24:**16-18, March, 1974.

19. Watkins, Julia D., and Moss, Fay T.: Confusion in the management of diabetes, American Journal of Nursing **69:**521-524, March, 1969.

Nursing the patient with diseases and disorders of the nervous system

KEY WORDS

aphasia *inability to speak*
ataxia *lack of coordination of motor movements*
coma *deep sleep — unarousable*
concussion *violent shaking of the brain against the skull*
confusion
convulsion *involuntary contracture of muscles*
delirium *disorientation*
flaccid *limp*
hemiplegia *one sided paralysis*
lethargic *abnormal drowsy*
meninges *brain + spinal cord covering*
opisthotonos *arching of the body*
paraplegia *lower body paralysis*
quadriplegia *paralysis of all 4 extremities*
seizure *sudden loss of consciousness*
spastic *involuntary muscular contractures*
stimuli
stuporous *deep sleep*

STRUCTURE AND FUNCTION OF THE NERVOUS SYSTEM

The human body is a highly organized structure with the various systems performing specific functions. However, all systems are interdependent and must be coordinated into a closely integrated whole. The part of the body responsible for coordinating the various functions is the nervous system.

The nervous system consists of the brain, spinal cord, and nerves, with their related structures. The brain and spinal cord are known as the *central nervous system.* There are twelve pairs of cranial nerves that arise from under the surface of the brain and carry messages to and from the brain. Thirty-one pairs of nerves (spinal nerves) arise from the spinal cord and are distributed from the cervical area to the coccyx. The spinal nerves carry messages to and from the spinal cord. The cranial nerves and the spinal nerves are called the *peripheral nervous system.* Several functions within the body are automatic to a large extent and go on without the individual being conscious of them. Some of these functions involve the glands, heart, lungs, and stomach. Nerves that are responsible for these automatic functions are a part of the peripheral nervous system and are called the *autonomic nervous system.* The autonomic nervous system is divided into the sympathetic nervous system and the parasympathetic nervous system. The sympathetic nervous system speeds up body activities, such as increasing the heartbeat, whereas the parasympathetic nervous system slows down activities and helps to maintain the body in a state of equilibrium.

The brain is a vital organ; to protect it from injury, nature has enclosed it in a bony framework known as the *skull,* or *cranium.* The brain is divided into several parts, the largest of which is the cerebrum. The cerebrum is divided into the right and left hemispheres; each hemisphere is divided into lobes. The lobes have the same names as the bones that comprise the cranium. The cerebrum is the center for all mental activities; for example, when you decide to go shopping or to retire, it is the cerebrum that is responsible for your decision. The next largest part of the brain is the cerebellum, which assists in the coordination and integration of voluntary movement. The vital part of the brain is the medulla, which controls vital functions. The medulla is essentially an extension of the spinal cord. It contains the vital control centers for respiration, heart action, vasoconstriction, and several reflex activities. Many of the nerve pathways from the brain cross in the medulla. This is the reason that an injury to one side of the brain may affect the opposite side of the body.

The brain and spinal cord are enclosed in membranes called *meninges.* Located within each hemisphere of the brain are small irregular spaces (ventricles) filled with clear fluid known as *spinal fluid.* The spinal fluid extends into the spinal canal and bathes the entire surface of the brain and cord. It provides moisture, lubricates, and helps to protect the brain and spinal cord. The spinal cord passes through the spinal canal and terminates just above the hip line. When the physician does a lumbar puncture, the needle is inserted below the cord, usually between the third and fourth lumbar vertebrae. The entire spinal cord and canal are enclosed in the vertebrae.

The brain and its related structures comprise a highly complex system, and the nurse will find it helpful to review its structure and function in more detail to gain a better understanding of the patient with nervous system disease.

DIAGNOSTIC TESTS AND PROCEDURES
Basic neurologic examination

The diagnosis of disease of the nervous system includes a thorough neurologic examination performed by a physician known as a neurologist. The cranial nerves are responsible for impulses to and from many of the special senses, and the procedure will include examination and testing of the eyes, the ears, the action of certain muscles, the senses of smell, touch, and temperature, and the pain sensation of the skin. Most of the reflexes are tested by the use of the percussion hammer. During the examination the physician will observe the patient for certain signs that are characteristic of specific disease conditions and aid in diagnosis. After the physical examination the neurologist may order special examinations, which may involve x-ray films or laboratory examinations.

Lumbar puncture. The lumbar puncture may be performed to diagnose many illnesses in which a neurologic involvement is present. The procedure consists of withdrawing a small amount of spinal fluid, usually 8 to 10 ml., which is sent to the laboratory for examination. The nurse may frequently be asked to assist the physician with this examination. The procedure is usually performed in the patient's room, and the patient should be given information about what to expect. The patient should know that a local anesthetic will be used but that there may be slight pain, possibly extending into the leg. The patient will be less apprehensive and feel more secure if he knows that the needle is inserted below the spinal cord. The nurse should assemble the equipment for the physician and should remember that the procedure is performed under strict surgical asepsis.

The patient is positioned on the side near the edge of the bed with the knees pulled up, the back bowed, and the chin and knees close together (Fig. 18-1). Some physicians prefer to have the patient sitting up and bending forward. The patient should be instructed not to move. The nurse should observe the patient during the procedure. The procedure may be performed in the outpatient clinic with the patient allowed to go home after it is com-

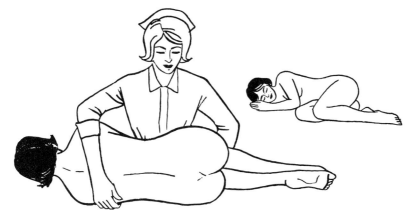

Fig. 18-1. Position of patient for a lumbar puncture.

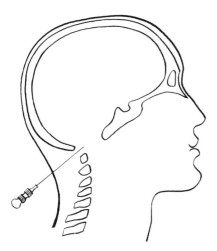

Fig. 18-2. Cisternal puncture, showing the location for insertion of the needle.

pleted. Some patients complain of severe headache after a lumbar puncture, and although many theories exist, the exact cause is unknown. The spinal fluid specimens should be correctly labeled and sent to the laboratory.

Cisternal puncture. Cisternal puncture is another method of securing spinal fluid for examination. The back of the neck is usually shaved, and the needle is inserted just below the occipital bone. The patient is positioned on the side with the head flexed forward, and the nurse should hold the head securely in position to avoid injury. This method is frequently used for small children, and some physicians prefer it to the lumbar puncture method for all patients. (See Fig. 18-2.)

Special neurologic examinations

Several special neurologic examinations may be performed for the purpose of detecting pathologic disorders affecting the brain and spinal cord. Some examinations require the use of a radiopaque substance and x rays. Some may be done in the x-ray department, whereas others are performed in the operating room. Most procedures require only a local anesthetic preceded by mild sedation, but in some cases a general anesthetic may be required. The nurse may not be directly concerned with the examination but may help to provide care of the patient before and after the examination.

Cerebral angiography. Injection of a radiopaque substance into the cerebral circulation followed by x-ray examination of the cranium is called cerebral angiography. Generally an artery such as the carotid artery is used, and the procedure is called arteriography. The purpose of the examination is to detect the presence of tumors or cranial aneurysms and their location, size, and shape. The examination may be done with the patient under local anesthesia, or a general anesthetic may be given. The patient may be given a bedtime sedative and preoperative medication of atropine and meperidine hydrochloride. A permission form signed by the patient must always be on the patient's chart.

Ventriculography. Ventriculography is x-ray examination to visualize the spaces within the brain. Small openings are made through the skin and skull over the area of the ventricles. Spinal fluid is aspirated and replaced by a gas, after which x-ray films are taken. The procedure may be done in the x-ray department or in the operating room. The examination is usually done while the patient has local anesthesia, and a sedative and analgesic are administered in the morning before the patient reports for the examination.

Pneumoencephalography. Examination by pneumoencephalogram consists of the introduction of air or gas into the spinal canal through a lumbar or cisternal puncture to outline the ventricular and subarachnoid space for possible cerebral abnormalities. Approximately 8 ml. of air are slowly injected prior to the removal of any spinal fluid, and x-ray films are taken. The procedure continues, and small amounts of cerebral spinal fluid are withdrawn and air injected until a total of 25 to 30 ml. of air have been introducd. A series of skull films are then taken with the patient placed in various positions. The procedure usually is done under local anesthesia, although general anesthesia may be used. Patients may be given a sedative in the evening before to ensure a good night's rest, and a sedative and analgesic may be administered in the morning prior to the examination. The patient may complain of nausea and a severe headache after the examination. His bed must be kept flat for 12 hours, intake of fluids should be forced to 3000 ml., and vital signs should be taken frequently for the first 24 hours.[6]

Myelography. The myelography procedure is done to identify tumors of the spinal cord or ruptured intervertebral disks. A lumbar puncture is done, and a few milliliters of spinal fluid are aspirated, followed by the injection of air or a contrast medium into the subarachnoid space. X-ray films are then taken, after which a second lumbar puncture is made, and the dye is removed. It is important for all the dye to be removed to prevent irritation. The test is done less frequently than formerly because of the irritation from the dye.

Electroencephalography (EEG). Examination by electroencephalography may be compared to electrocardiography. It is a graphic recording of brain waves from the cerebrum. The purpose of the electroencephalogram is to detect abnormal conditions in the brain, including existence of

tumors or the presence of convulsive disorders. The test is not considered conclusive but is generally used as an adjunct to other diagnostic methods. The EEG test is done by placing small electrodes at specific locations on each side of the scalp. The electrodes are connected to wires leading to a machine. All tracings are made simultaneously. The procedure is painless, requires no preparation, and takes from 1 to 2 hours. The test can be made on persons of any age, including infants.

Attention has been given to the use of the electroencephalogram in determining when death occurs (p. 113). It has been an accepted belief that death does not occur until the heart stops beating and respiration ceases. It is now believed that death may take place when all brain waves cease as indicated by the EEG, although the heart may still be beating.

Caloric test. The caloric test is done to evaluate equilibrium by testing the vestibular branch of the eighth cranial nerve. Lesions in the brainstem and the cerebellum can be differentiated. Cold or hot water is allowed to drip into the ear and is stopped the moment that the patient complains of dizziness or nausea or if the physician observes any symptoms such as nystagmus. If no signs or symptoms occur within 3 minutes, the irrigation is terminated. Each ear is irrigated separately, and the entire procedure usually takes from 30 to 40 minutes.[6]

Queckenstedt's sign (lumbar puncture with dynamics). Queckenstedt's test is done in connection with the lumbar puncture. A manometer is attached to the lumbar puncture needle, and the cerebrospinal fluid pressure is measured. Digital pressure is placed on the jugular veins of the neck. Normally the cerebrospinal fluid pressure rises rapidly but falls rapidly as the digital pressure is released. If there is a block in the canal, the cerebrospinal fluid pressure will scarcely be affected or will rise and fall slowly. The patient should be told about the test in advance so that he will not be frightened.

Brain scan. A solution of the radioactive material is injected intravenously, and after 4 hours a Geiger counter or scintillator is used to determine the uptake. If tumors are present in the brain, they tend to retain the radioactive material. Minute amounts of radioactive material are used, and the patient is not considered to be radioactive. When used with other tests and examinations, the isotope has been found to give good diagnostic data.[18]

Nursing care. The procedures just outlined are among the most common used, although several new ones are being developed. There are probably few instances in which the nurse will assist with them; however, the nurse may care for the patient before and after the test. The success of neurologic examinations depends on the patient's understanding and willingness to cooperate. The patient is apprehensive, and if neurológic disease is present, personality changes may contribute to the problems. The nurse can be of most assistance in reassuring the patient and in helping to relieve his anxiety.

In many instances the patient will be given a bedtime sedative to ensure a good night's rest. Food and fluids may be omitted after midnight, and breakfast may be withheld in the morning to avoid nausea and vomiting. Sedatives and analgesics ordered in the morning should be administered promptly. The patient should void before reporting for the examination, and a signed permission form must always be on the patient's record. When the patient returns to his room, he may complain of severe headache and may require an analgesic. Vital signs should be checked at frequent intervals, and the patient should be observed for intracranial pressure, respiratory distress, or convulsions. After ventriculography and pneumoencephalography a mouth gag, oxygen, and side rails should be available for emergency use.

PAIN

Pain is the result of experiences—external or internal—that are transmitted through complicated nerve pathways to the brain, in which they are interpreted as pain. Pain may be superficial, involving the skin and mucous membrane, where pain receptors are numerous. The skin is vulnerable to a variety of external stimuli that give rise to sensations of pain, which may be interpreted as burning, pricking, or pinching. Deep pain produces an aching sensation and is poorly localized because of the few pain receptors in internal organs. The stretching, retracting, and tension associated with some surgery eventually reach the brain and are interpreted as pain. Referred pain may reach the brain but not from the site that was stimulated. The stimulus for pain from acute appendicitis may occur in the appendix but reach the brain from the umbilicus. Therefore the sensation of pain is interpreted in the region of the umbilicus.

To the patient, pain means something that hurts for which he wants relief as quickly as possible. It is not always possible to relieve all pain completely, but it is possible to reduce it to a tolerable degree. Pain may be a warning signal, as in cancer, but the warning comes too late. However, pain may mean survival when it signals disease that can be cured; modern medicine and surgery have made it possible to remove the causes of some pain completely. All patients do not perceive pain in the same way. One person may disregard pain from an injury, whereas another patient with a similar injury may find the pain intolerable. Because of differences in the perception of pain and the cultural attitudes concerning it, it is difficult for the physician to treat pain on an individual basis; often a routine drug in a routine dose is prescribed for all patients. With an increasing older population with more chronic diseases and degenerative disorders, pain will be an increasing problem that physicians and nurses must find ways of alleviating.[15]

The nurse must realize that pain is a subjective symptom and must depend on what the patient describes and what is observed. Regardless of the cause or what the nurse may think, pain is always real to the person who experiences it. The nurse does not have the right to judge the presence or absence of pain or its intensity. Good nursing care requires that the nurse provides nursing measures such as changing the patient's position, giving a soothing back rub, washing the face and hands, loosening a bandage that may be too tight, emptying the bladder, and adjusting room temperature. The presence of the nurse doing something for the patient may be sufficient to relieve pain. When simple nursing measures fail to provide relief, medication should not be withheld. If the physician has failed to leave an order, the nurse should, if the situation requires it, call the patient's physician. Sometimes there is a tendency to withhold medication that is habit forming. The nurse should report the problem to the physician, who will make whatever adjustments are necessary.

LEVELS OF CONSCIOUSNESS

To understand what is meant by consciousnesses or unconsciousness the nurse must understand that the brain is responsible for storing all things related to memory. Associating, perceiving differences, discerning, and making judgments are functions of the cerebral cortex. Because of injury to the head or certain disease conditions, these functions may be temporarily disrupted or disturbed. The patient may be unable to perceive normally many things that ordinarily would be considered conscious behavior. These may include recognition of persons, location, the time of day, or day and month of the year. The patient may perceive the nurse as a neighbor; when certain centers of the brain are disturbed, the patient may see things that do not exist or hear sounds and voices not heard by others. In some situations the patient's state of awareness may be completely disturbed so that he falls into a deep sleep from which he may be aroused only momentarily.

The nurse should understand that deterioration of brain cells and nerve tissue occurs with the normal aging process. The aged person will exhibit many symptoms characteristic of patients with frank disease but normal for the aging process.

The patient's state of awareness, which is called consciousness, is important to the physician in both diagnosis and treatment. In many situations the physician must depend on nurses to observe and record accurately the patient's level of responsiveness[21] (Table 18-1). By recording exactly what the patient says, the nurse may be most helpful to the physician. Several descriptive terms have been used to explain the deviation from normal conscious behavior. The nurse should become familiar with the terms and be able to apply them correctly.

Confusion (disorientation). The elderly person or the patient with a severe illness who is apprehensive and anxious is often confused. Confusion, which is generally worse at night, is a state in which the patient mistakes the identity of persons and hears their conversation as a confused mixture of dissimilar things, although usually these things are within his experience. This state may be fleeting, occurring only at intervals, or it may exist for several days. A common expression refers to the patient as being "all mixed up."

Delirium. Delirium is a symptom of some major distortion of cerebral function and may result from several causes. The state of delirium fluctuates widely from that of confusion and disorientation and includes the mental state of the raging hyperactive patient who may fatally injure himself. Characteristically, the state of de-

Table 18-1. Levels of responsiveness

Level	Behavior	Movement	Respirations	Pupils
Alert	Normal	Normal	Normal	Normal
Drowsy	Sleepy; lethargic; may be confused; aroused with stimulation	Normal when aroused	Normal	Normal
Stuporous	Inappropriate responses; confused; delirious; very difficult to arouse	Some voluntary; defensive when stimulated	Normal or irregular	Vary in size and reaction
Comatose	No response	No voluntary movement; reflexes only	Irregular, shallow or Cheyne-Stokes	Dilated, unequal, fixed, or pinpoint

lirium involves sight and hearing. The patient may see snakes or worms crawling over the bed and try to get away from them. He may jump through a window, believing that it is a door and that he is fleeing from someone. A patient who owned a grocery store suddenly developed a temporary state of delirium and believed his cash register was in the hospital hall and burglars were robbing it. In a couple of hours the disturbance had passed, and the patient recalled in detail his thoughts and behavior. The patient may understand a part of what is said to him but be unable to comprehend in entirety.

The nurse should watch for signs that may foretell an approaching state of delirium. The patient may be restless and unable to sleep, and impaired memory and inability to concentrate may be present. Administration of a sedative may provide rest and sleep and forestall delirium. Delirium may occur in persons who have used alcohol regularly over a period of years. This type of delirium, known as *delirium tremens* or *alcoholic psychosis*, is most likely to occur when the patient cannot obtain alcohol. When a known alcoholic patient is admitted to the hospital, the nurse should be alert for restlessness, nervousness, insomnia, and momentary states of confusion. When these symptoms are observed, administration of a tranquilizing agent and a sedative may prevent more serious behavior. To protect the patient from serious injury it may be necessary to use restraints; however, they should only be used when other measures fail.

Stupor. The stuporous patient is lethargic and apathetic. The sense of feeling and the degree of responsiveness are diminished. The patient appears to be in a deep sleep and to be unconscious.

It is possible to arouse the patient momentarily, but he immediately lapses into sleep.

Coma. The comatose patient is in an abnormally deep sleep that differs from stupor in that the patient in coma cannot be roused by any external stimuli. Coma may follow severe injuries to the head, or it may occur in serious illness. It is always to be considered a serious condition.

The nurse should know that all these disturbances may occur in the purely psychic state. However, concern in this book is only with the medical-surgical patient whose condition is the result of injury, tumors, infections, disease, or drugs.

Convulsions (seizures, fits). Convulsions are often referred to as seizures or fits and represent some disturbance of cerebral function. They do not always follow a single general pattern, as may be seen in epilepsy (p. 437) or in the case of convulsion in a young child with a high temperature. Convulsions may occur at any age and are associated with a large number of diseases and disorders. Frequently throughout this book the nurse has been cautioned to observe the patient for the possibility of convulsions.

As a rule there is temporary loss of consciousness during a generalized convulsion, although in some situations this may not be true. A convulsion usually occurs suddenly, and an early indication is rolling of the eyes with a fixed stare into space and twitching of the facial muscles. This is the stage at which a padded mouth gag must quickly be placed between the teeth. In a few seconds the entire body becomes rigid in muscular contraction. Pallor usually occurs, the extremities jerk, the facial expression is distorted, hands are clenched, and incontinence frequently occurs. At this stage it will be impossible to insert a mouth gag because of the rigid contraction of the facial muscles. The patient may bite the tongue, and saliva will be blood tinged. The patient will be unable to swallow, and a suction machine must be used to clear the respiratory passages. The pulse is weak and irregular, respirations may appear to have ceased, but suddenly there is a long, deep, snoring type of breath, and breathing is restored. Alternating contraction and relaxation of muscles may be so forceful that the patient may injure himself unless precautions have been taken to prevent injury. Gradually relaxation of the body begins to occur, and consciousness returns, or the patient may remain in a stuporous condition and in some cases may lapse into coma. The duration of the convulsion may be short, from 15 to 20 seconds, or it may continue for more than 30 minutes. Convulsions may be recurring at varying intervals. The patient must never be left alone during a convulsion, and no restraints

Beta lactamase test - for hemophilos
influenza - neg. means use
certain drugs.

should be used. Side rails must be on the bed, and they should be padded to prevent injury of the patient. Depending on age and underlying disease conditions, the physician may order amobarbital sodium (Amytal sodium), 0.25 to 0.5 Gm. administered intravenously.

Once a convulsion has begun to occur, little can be done, but extremely accurate observation of the patient is important. Observation should be made of the behavior of the patient prior to and after the convulsion; the state of consciousness; the muscles affected and which were affected first; the vital signs such as pulse rate, volume, and rhythm, and the presence of cyanosis, incontinence, and eye movements. A careful and accurate recording may help the physician to determine further care and treatment for the patient. Convulsions are one of the most frightening conditions that can occur. The patient's family may be in a near panic stage the first time they observe the patient having a convulsion. The nurse must be able to maintain emotional control and to remain calm and reassuring to the family. There should be no conversation concerning the condition in the patient's room, since the unconscious patient may hear and understand even though he cannot speak.

NURSING THE PATIENT WITH DISEASES AND DISORDERS OF THE NERVOUS SYSTEM
Infectious diseases
Meningitis

Meningitis is an inflammation of the meninges that cover the brain and spinal cord. When only the spinal cord is involved, the condition is called *spinal meningitis,* and when both the cord and the brain are involved, the disease is called *cerebrospinal meningitis.*

The disease is caused by pathogenic bacteria, including the meningococcus, streptococcus, pneumococcus, and tubercle bacillus, or it may occur in certain viral infections such as influenza. The causative organism may reach the meninges by way of the bloodstream. The disease often occurs in sporadic epidemics and is regarded as a threat where crowded conditions exist. During 1970 approximately 2500 cases of meningococcal infections

occurred in the United States, most of which were among the civilian population.

Meningitis may occur after a sore throat caused by the hemolytic streptococcus or after otitis media, paranasal sinusitis, or mastoiditis, in which the bacteria may reach the brain through bones near the base of the skull. The disease may have a sudden onset and may progress rapidly to a fatal termination. In less severe forms the disease may have a sudden onset or may develop gradually. However, the patient is usually extremely sick. The greatest incidence is found in children.

The clinical picture of meningitis is extremely variable. Severe and persistent headache, fever, nausea, and vomiting are generally the initial signs. The temperature may begin with an elevation between 100° and 102° F. but later may be as high as 105° F. as the disease progresses. Stiffness of the neck is present, and there may be a drawing backward of the head with bowing of the back (opisthotonos). Disturbance of respiration may simulate Cheyne-Stokes respiration. Acute urinary retention is characteristic of the disease, and constipation is generally present. Disorientation, delirium, and convulsions may occur quickly.

Treatment and nursing care. The nursing care of the patient is essentially the same as that for any critically ill patient and is demanding and exacting. The diagnosis is confirmed by spinal fluid findings, and the causative organism may be isolated on culture or smear examination. The patient is treated with large doses of penicillin, which may be administered initially by the intravenous route, after which oral administration is continued for about 10 days. If the patient is sensitive to penicillin, other drugs such as tetracycline or cephalothin may be given. Analgesics may be ordered for severe headache, and sedatives are given sparingly. The patient is isolated, and strict medical asepsis is carried out in the care of nose and throat secretions, in drainage from otitis media, and in handling of any laboratory specimens. Gloves should be used for handling highly contaminated articles. The duration of isolation varies. The patient should be placed in a quiet, slightly darkened room. An ice bag may be applied to the head to relieve head-

possible skull fracture

ache, and tepid or alcohol sponges and antipyretic drugs may be used to reduce the temperature. Devices to maintain good body alignment such as a footboard, pillows for support, and bed cradles should be available. Padded side rails should be on the bed. Accurate records of intake and output should be maintained. Since retention with overflow may occur, the nurse should be alert for this condition. The intake of fluids should be encouraged, and intravenous infusions may be given. During the acute stage the diet will consist of liquids, but during convalescence a regular diet may be given, although tube feedings may be necessary for some patients.

The patient should be turned regularly during entire 24-hour periods, and gentleness is important because convulsions may easily occur. The use of flannel gowns or pajamas and cotton sheet blankets may add to the patient's comfort.

The patient should have constant attendance and be observed for evidence of increased intracranial pressure such as a slowing pulse and respiration rate and a widening pulse pressure when the blood pressure is measured. A suction machine should be at the bedside. The outcome cannot always be predicted, and if the patient recovers, there may be residual damage such as blindness, deafness, mental retardation, or paralysis.[18]

Encephalitis

Encephalitis is an inflammation of the brain and meninges that may affect all parts of the nervous system. It may be caused by viruses, bacteria, fungi, chemical substances, toxins, and injury. It may occur with or follow one of the acute infectious diseases of childhood, and may also occur as a complication of smallpox vaccination (postvaccinal encephalitis). Residual neurologic disorders may follow encephalitis, including a slowly developing Parkinson's syndrome. The disease occurs sporadically and in epidemics, with the greatest incidence during the hot summer months. An average of about 500 cases occurs each year in the United States, although during severe epidemics the total number of cases may be greater. Mortality is variable and ranges from a minimum of 5% to 70%.

Viral encephalitis is caused by several viruses, including the herpes simplex virus. Among the viral infections most frequently encountered are those caused by several kinds of mosquitoes (arthropod-borne encephalitis). The virus is transmitted to humans by the bite of an infected mosquito and is not transmitted from person to person. Evidence indicates that the virus is harbored by several species of wild birds from which it is picked up by the mosquitoes. These forms of arthropod-borne encephalitis have been classified as St. Louis encephalitis, Eastern encephalitis, Western encephalitis, and Japanese encephalitis. St. Louis encephalitis is the most common type, and several epidemics have occurred in recent years. The most recent epidemic occurred in 1975 when over thirty deaths from 220 reported cases occurred in Mississippi. Illinois reported approximately 130 cases, and outbreaks also occurred in several other southern and midwestern states. In 1964 in Houston, Texas, thirty-two deaths resulted among 700 clinical cases of the infection. Eastern encephalitis may have a mortality rate as high as 60% to 70%, and very young and elderly persons are most frequently affected, although persons of all ages may contract the disease. Each of the viral types is caused by a different virus, although it is believed that they are all related.

The symptoms are fairly uniform for all types of encephalitis. Onset is sudden, with an elevation of temperature of 104° to 105° F., increased pulse rate, and severe headache that is not relieved by analgesics. Symptoms include nausea, vomiting, tremor of the hands, tongue, and lips, stiffness of the neck, speech difficulty, and drowsiness. In severe cases convulsions, coma, and death may occur suddenly.[13]

Treatment and nursing care. For patients with viral encephalitis there is no specific treatment, and isolation is not required. There is no danger to the nurse. However, as a precautionary measure, some states require isolation for 7 days. The nursing care requires careful observation of the patient, since progress of the disease may be rapid. The patient is critically ill, and nursing care is based on symptoms. Vital signs are checked every 4 hours, and the patient should be in a darkened, quiet environment. Accurate records of intake and output are maintained, and fluids may be administered by intravenous infusion. Diet, which is high in calories and protein, may be given by gavage. Hot moist packs are applied to muscles for spasm. The patient may perspire profusely, and the breath has a disagreeable odor. Total incontinence may be present; thus meticulous skin and oral care must be given.

Considerable variation may occur in the level of consciousness and behavior, and side rails and restraints should be available. A mouth gag should be at the bedside in case convulsions occur. Tracheotomy may sometimes be performed as an emergency, or breathing may be assisted with mechanical ventilation.

Poliomyelitis (infantile paralysis)

Poliomyelitis is an acute disease caused by three different strains of viruses. These strains have been designated as I, II, and III. The disease affects the spinal cord, in which motor pathways are located, and may involve the brain. It is believed to be spread through secretions from the nose and throat and through the feces of infected persons.

One of the outstanding medical advances of this century has been the discovery and production of the Salk vaccine, and Sabin oral vaccine for immunization against poliomyelitis. Through the efforts of physicians, health departments, and public education, this dreaded disease has been almost eliminated. During 1974 only 7 cases, 5 of which were paralytic, were reported to the Center for Disease Control. The nurse may help to maintain an immune population by encouraging mothers to take infants and young children to their physicians or the health department for inoculation.

Symptoms of poliomyelitis begin suddenly with fever, nausea, and vomiting, severe headache, pain in the extremities, and stiffness in the back of the neck. When the motor pathways in the spinal cord are involved, paralysis of the extremities may occur. When the brain is attacked, the cranial nerves may be affected and bulbar poliomyelitis may occur, which is more serious. It is possible for both the spinal cord and brain to be attacked. In bulbar

poliomyelitis the muscles of respiration and of the face and neck become weak so that swallowing is difficult. Speech and voice are affected, and food or liquids may be regurgitated through the nose. When muscles of respiration are paralyzed, the outcome of the disease may be fatal.

Treatment and nursing care. Poliomyelitis is an infectious disease, and the patient is isolated for 7 days or longer. The nurse wears a gown and mask when in contact with the patient, and care should be exercised in the disposal of secretions from the nose, throat, and bowels. There is no specific treatment for the disease other than supportive and symptomatic treatment and care. The nurse should remember that paralyzed muscles are extremely tender and sensitive and that patients should therefore be moved gently. Massage with alcohol should be avoided. Hot packs are used for relief of pain, and training in the method of packing is advisable. Antibiotics may be administered as a preventive measure but have no influence on the outcome of the disease. The patient should be kept warm and should have a quiet environment. Urinary retention may occur, and the nurse should be alert to the need for catheterization; a retention catheter may be ordered. Positioning the patient to support weak muscles and provide for good body alignment is extremely important. Footboard, bed cradle, trochanter roll, and pillows may be needed; when swallowing is affected, tube feeding may be necessary. The foot of the bed is elevated slightly to permit secretions to drain from the mouth and throat.

Provision should always be made for emergency, such as having available a tracheotomy tray, suction equipment, and oxygen. When muscles of respiration are paralyzed, the patient may need mechanical ventilation. As the patient begins to convalesce, reeducation of weakened muscles is started by the physical therapist. Paralysis may completely disappear, or it may remain, with a gradual wasting of muscle tissue.

Central nervous system syphilis

Lesions caused by the syphilis organism (Treponema pallidum) may develop in the central nervous system and cause a wide variety of complex neurologic conditions. These disorders usually make their appearance 15 or 20 years after the primary lesion. The three forms of neurologic disorders most often encountered are <u>meningovascular syphilis, tabes dorsalis, and general paresis.</u>

Meningovascular syphilis. <u>The lesions of meningovascular syphilis are in the meninges of the brain</u> and may be acute or chronic. The acute form resembles meningitis caused by other bacteria, with the significant difference that both the blood and the spinal fluid are reactive for syphilis. Fever, headache, vomiting, and rigidity of the neck may be present; vision may be blurred, and paralysis of facial muscles may occur. In the chronic form of syphilitic meningitis the fever is low grade, and there is loss of weight.

Tabes dorsalis (locomotor ataxia). The <u>lesions associated with tabes dorsalis are in the spinal cord,</u> and the sensory nerve roots are gradually destroyed. The patient's sense of equilibrium is destroyed so that he is unaware of the position of his feet and legs. His gait becomes staggering and unsteady, and he walks with a slapping movement of the feet. The patient must keep his eyes on his feet to be able to walk and is unable to walk in the dark. In the neurologic examination he is asked to close his eyes and stand with his feet together. When tabes dorsalis is present, the patient sways and will fall. This is known as a *positive* <u>Romberg's sign.</u> The patient's vision may be affected. He becomes undernourished and is incontinent and impotent. At intervals he has sudden acute attacks of pain that often involve the stomach and are accompanied by severe vomiting (gastric crisis).

<u>*General paresis.*</u> General paresis is a more common form of neurosyphilis. A condition in which general paresis and tabes dorsalis occur together is called *tabo-paresis.* The <u>lesions of paresis are in the brain cells, and a gradual deterioration and atrophy of the brain occur.</u> Over a period of time a change in personality occurs. There may be outbursts of temper, extreme irritability, impaired judgment, and the development of delusions of persecution or of grandeur. The patient may become paranoid and be dangerous. The con-

dition grows progressively worse until it is necessary to commit the patient to a mental hospital.

Neurosyphilis can be prevented by early and adequate treatment (Chapter 23).

Degenerative diseases

Degenerative diseases of the central nervous system result in chronic disability, which may extend over a period of years. These diseases are marked by periods of remissions and exacerbations, and in some cases the onset is so insidious that the disease process may actually have been going on for years before symptoms become acute enough for medical attention. Nursing care is concerned primarily with the care given any patient with chronic disease (Chapter 6). The second concern is to provide understanding, encouragement, and emotional support for the patient and his family. The third concern is to help the patient be independent and self-sufficient as long as possible. Only three of the degenerative diseases of the nervous system will be reviewed here; <u>multiple sclerosis, Parkinson's disease,</u> and <u>myasthenia gravis.</u>

Multiple sclerosis (disseminated sclerosis)

<u>Multiple sclerosis is a chronic progressive disease,</u> with 95% of all cases beginning in persons under 25 years of age. The disease <u>affects the myelin sheaths</u> (segmented covering around nerve fibers), and the lesions are spaced far apart along the nerve pathways, which results in variation of symptoms.

The cause of the <u>disease is unknown,</u> and research efforts to link the disease with any specific factor have not been entirely successful. The disease predominately affects persons living in cold damp climates, with about sixty cases per 100,000 population occurring, as compared to ten cases per 100,000 population in warmer parts of the country. The onset of the disease may be acute, or the disorder may develop slowly over a period of months. Its course is frequently marked by long remissions and exacerbations. The life-span after onset varies widely and is not predictable but has been estimated to average from about 13 years to more than 25 years. Many persons are able to continue gainful employment for many years before they finally succumb to complications resulting from the disease.[2]

Among the earliest symptoms are weakness and visual complaints. Loss of visual acuity, nystagmus, and double vision may occur. Although all extremities may be involved, the lower ones are most often affected; weakness may be minor, or it may result in complete paralysis. When both lower extremities are affected, urinary complaints will be present. Tremor is usually present, and speech disturbances, dizziness, vertigo, and incoordination may exist in varying degrees. Approximately one third of patients with multiple sclerosis develop mental changes. Symptoms and the severity of symptoms reflect the nerve fibers affected.

Treatment and nursing care. There is no specific treatment for multiple sclerosis. During acute exacerbations the patient may be given corticosteroids and placed on a regimen of bed rest. The patient should not remain in bed longer than necessary, and the continued use of the corticosteroids is not recommended because of their side effects. The patient and his family should understand the disease and should be helped to avoid drugs or treatment that promises a cure. Unless terminally ill, most patients will be cared for in their own homes by members of the family. Therefore the family needs to be taught the importance of a balanced program of activity and rest. The patient should be protected from chilling, cold, and dampness; the use of heating pads and hot-water bottles should be avoided because the patient may easily be burned, and special precautions should be taken to prevent respiratory infections. The patient must be protected from injury by proper lighting and the use of hand rails. Scatter rugs and polished floors should be avoided, and furniture should be placed where the patient will not fall. The patient needs a well-balanced diet high in vitamins. Work and social activities should be continued for as long as possible, although a change in occupation may be necessary to avoid fatigue. The patient or his family should be told about the National Multiple Sclerosis Society,*

---

*Address of home office: 257 Park Ave., S., New York, N. Y. 10010.

which provides printed material that may help the family in caring for the patient.

Parkinson's disease (paralysis agitans, shaking palsy)

Parkinson's disease is a chronic progressive disease that affects the basal ganglia. The basal ganglia are also called *basal,* or *cerebral, nuclei* and consist of islands of gray matter within the cerebrum. Although not completely understood, the basal ganglia are important in motor activities. When degenerative changes occur within the basal ganglia, as in Parkinson's disease, there is a disturbance of motor activity characterized by tremor, rigidity, and involuntary movements. Exactly how many persons in the United States have Parkinson's disease is unknown, but estimates range from 200,000 to 1 million, with approximately 50,000 new cases each year.

In most cases the cause of the disease is unknown; however, it has been demonstrated that patients with Parkinson's disease have a deficiency of the amino acid dopamine in their brains. This substance functions primarily in the transmission of nerve impulses. Parkinson's disease has been found to follow some other disorders, primarily encephalitis, and it may be induced by the use of derivatives of the phenothiazine group of drugs. Characteristic symptoms may be found in arteriosclerotic patients. When the cause is associated with another disease, it is called *secondary Parkinsonism,* whereas when it occurs in the absence of any known cause, it is *primary Parkinsonism.*[2]

Parkinson's disease develops slowly and progresses slowly, with the rate of progression extremely variable. The onset of the disease usually occurs in persons between 50 and 65 years of age. Because of its slow progress and the increase in the life-span, many persons with the disease are in the older age group, in whom other degenerative conditions may be present. The disease progressess so slowly that 20 years or more may elapse before the person becomes incapacitated. Although Parkinson's disease may be contributory to or may be the underlying cause of death, other disorders such as cerebrovascular accident may be the immediate cause of death.

The characteristic signs of the disease include tremor, muscular weakness, and shuffling gait. The tremor may begin slowly and occurs in varying degrees and combinations. The tremor is present whether the patient is sitting quietly or walking with the arms at the side. Muscular rigidity, which offers resistance even to passive exercise, is an outstanding symptom. A disturbance of gait occurs in which the patient walks slowly, stooped forward with the arms quietly at the side. The facial expression becomes masklike; the patient's voice is weak, and his speech is slurred. There may be difficulty in swallowing that results in drooling. There is a disturbance of the heat-regulating mechanism so that sweating and hypersensitivity to heat result. Because of difficulty in swallowing, the patient may be undernourished and dehydrated; thus a high fluid intake is important.

Treatment and nursing care. There is no cure for Parkinson's disease. Treatment is symptomatic, supportive, and palliative. The patient needs encouragement and understanding. Mental faculties are not affected, and fears and anxiety over symptoms and disability may lead to depression. The patient should be encouraged to lead a normal, active, productive life. Dorothy Dent,[9] a nurse who has Parkinson's disease, has written a small booklet on self-exercises and stresses their importance in maintaining an active life. She expresses the philosophy that although we cannot all "swing on the same gate, let us keep swinging."* Several drugs have been used for their symptomatic effects, including trihexyphenidyl (Artane), cycrimine (Pagitane), and benztropine methanesulfonate (Cogentin methanesulfonate). Other drugs found to be useful include antihistamines and antidepressants such as amitriptyline (Elavil) and imipramine (Tofranil). Amantadine (Symmetrel), a drug used for influenza immunization, appears to have some value in the treatment of Parkinson's disease.

The most significant progress in the treatment of the disease has been the discovery of L-*dopa* (dihydroxyphenylalanine), and it is now the treatment of choice. This drug has been characterized as representing the greatest breakthrough in the field of neurology during the past 50 years.[16]

L-Dopa has been under clinical investigation in several medical centers for a number of years, and in June, 1970, the drug was approved and released for use by all physicians for the treatment of Parkinson's disease. The drug is metabolized within the brain to form the deficient amino acid dopamine.[17] Approximately 50% to 65% of the patients treated with this drug are improved 50% or more. The most common side effects of L-dopa include include nausea and vomiting, hypotension, and abnormal involuntary movements. The drug should be taken after eating to reduce nausea, and blood pressure should be checked routinely. Involuntary movements can be partially controlled with small frequent doses of the medication. Occasionally, mental confusion, depression, hallucinations, and difficulties in thinking and memory occur. This usually indicates that the dosage should be reduced.[14]

The patient needs a well-balanced diet with a high fluid intake, and supplementary feedings may be necessary to help maintain good nutrition. Constipation is often a problem, and a routine should be established to help regulate bowel habits. The nurse can do much to teach the patient how to manage and care for his personal hygiene and can assist with and teach a regular program of exercise. The nurse must be patient because slowness of movement is characteristic of the disease, and the patient cannot be hurried. Anything that produces anxiety should be avoided because it will tend to increase symptoms. The objective of medical and nursing care of the patient with Parkinson's disease is to delay disability as long as possible.*

Surgery. In selected patients any of several surgical procedures may be done. However, the number of patients who are suitable candidates for surgery is small. The postoperative nursing care of patients is planned on an individual basis.

Myasthenia gravis

Although myasthenia gravis is a fairly uncommon disease, it is estimated that

---

*Dent, Dorothy: Self-help Parkinson's disease, 265 Daly Ave., Ottawa 2, Ontario, Canada.

*Helpful information for the patient with Parkinson's disease and his family is available from the following organizations: American Parkinson's Disease Association, 147 East 50th St., New York, N. Y. 10022, and Parkinson's Disease Foundation, 640 West 168th St., New York, N. Y. 10032.

there are about 50,000 persons in the United States with the disorder. The disease is neurologic only to the extent that a deficiency in neuromuscular transmission exists at the point where a motor nerve joins a skeletal muscle, causing an improper contraction of the muscle.

Normally nerve endings produce a substance called acetylcholine, which carries the nerve impulse from the nerve fiber to the muscle, causing it to contract. The muscle then produces an enzyme, cholinesterase, which inactivates the acetylcholine. The patient with myasthenia gravis has either too little acetylcholine or too much cholinesterase produced, and the result is insufficient muscle contraction or weakness. The exact reason why the deficiency exists is essentially unknown, although recent investigations have indicated that it might be an autoimmune disease[20] (p. 531). The disease occurs most frequently in women between the ages of 15 and 40 years and in men over 50 years. Women are more often victims of the disease than men. At present the disease can be fairly well controlled with drugs, although there is no cure. The patient must learn to live with it for the rest of his life.[6] With understanding on the part of physicians, nurses, and the patient's family it is possible to formulate a program whereby the patient may live a relatively normal life.

The primary symptom is muscle weakness, which affects almost every muscle of the body except those of the heart, intestines, and bladder. Only the patient understands the extent of the weakness, which may vary from hour to hour. As a result of the weakness, difficulty in focusing the eyes may occur; ptosis of the eyelid is common, giving the patient a sleepy appearance. The patient may have weakness of the muscles of swallowing, chewing, and speaking. All muscles tire quickly on exertion or even normal activity. Shortness of breath may occur when walking, and the patient may be unable to turn over in bed.

Treatment and nursing care. The nurse caring for the patient in the hospital should realize that the simple activities of combing the hair or brushing the teeth may be too fatiguing for the patient. The patient may eat part of his food before weakness overtakes him, or he may refuse a meal because he is too weak to eat and is sensitive about asking for help. The patient may be admitted to the hospital because of a crisis resulting from too little or too much medication. In some cases the muscles of respiration may be affected, and the patient will need mechanical assistance.

Maintenance doses of anticholinesterase drugs have been found effective in controlling symptoms. These include neostigmine (Prostigmin), pyrdostigmine (Mestinon), and ambenonium (Mytelase). A fourth drug, edrophonium (Tensilon) may be given intravenously as a diagnostic test, but it is not effective for treatment purposes. ACTH is sometimes given to patients who do not respond to these drugs. The effect of drugs used in therapy is to strengthen muscles and to prevent muscle fatigue. If the dosage is too large, side effects may occur, inluding abdominal cramping, nausea, diarrhea, and urinary frequency and urgency. The nurse must remember that drugs classified as respiratory depressants, such as morphine, may cause fatal results if administered to a patient with myasthenia gravis.

The condition of a patient with myasthenia gravis may worsen in the presence of a respiratory infection or surgery and may occur without any apparent cause, precipitating myasthenic crisis. An overdose of medication may weaken rather than strengthen muscles and may cause respiratory failure.[20] Medication is prescribed on an individual basis, and the amount may vary from hour to hour or day to day.

Myasthenia gravis is a chronic disease that will affect every aspect of the patient's life. It afflicts young people in the prime of life and can be a terrifying, life-threatening condition. Apprehension and fear may be great, with the patient never knowing when he may lose the ability to swallow, breathe, or move. Patients need the consistent reassuring care that a nurse can give. Helpful information can be obtained from the Myasthenia Gravis Foundation, Inc.*

---

*Address of home office: 2 East 103rd St., New York, N. Y. 10029.

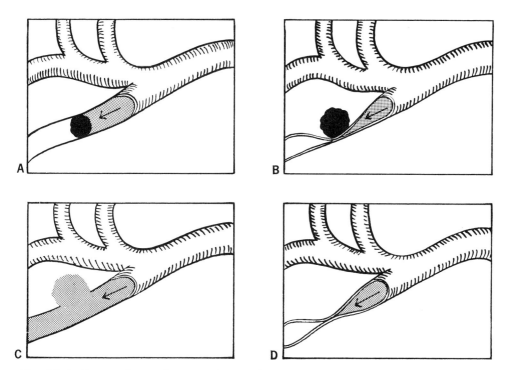

Cerebral vascular accident (CVA), apoplexy or stroke

Cerebral vascular disease continues to be the third leading cause of death in the United States. At the present time several factors tend to make statistical information unreliable; however, evidence indicates that the following trends may be anticipated. The frequency of cerebrovascular disease increases with age. As the number of persons 65 years of age and older continues to increase, an increase in cerebrovascular disease may be expected to occur. Present mortality data show a greater frequency of cerebral vascular accident among men than among women, and the frequency is greater among the nonwhite than the white population. The incidence of hypertension and arteriosclerosis bears a direct relationship to the incidence of cerebrovascular disease.[22] Socioeconomic factors as they affect the nonwhite population and the elderly may contribute to the lack of early and adequate medical care for the hypertension, thus hastening a cerebral vascular accident.

Pathophysiology. There are three major causes of stroke: (1) cerebral thrombosis, ASHD (2) cerebral hemorrhage, and (3) cerebral embolus. Cerebral thrombosis is the most common cause and develops slowly as the blood vessels become occluded because of arteriosclerotic changes. These changes are brought about by increasing age, hypertension, and some disease conditions such as diabetes. Most persons who have a stroke from cerebral thrombosis are between 60 and 80 years of age.[1] Cerebral hemorrhage results from the rupture of a blood vessel in the brain. Hemorrhage occurs suddenly, is severe, and is frequently fatal. About three fourths of the patients have an elevation of blood pressure and some degree of arteriosclerosis. Frequently there is some disturbance of the clotting mechanism of the blood. Cerebral hemorrhage occurs at a somewhat younger age, usually between 50 and 70 years of age.

Fig. 18-3. Causes of a cerebral vascular accident. **A,** Formation of a blood clot in a blood vessel, resulting in occlusion of the vessel. **B,** Pressure on a blood vessel resulting from a blood clot, tumor, or anything that compresses the vessel. **C,** Rupture of a blood vessel in the brain with hemorrhage into the adjacent tissue. **D,** Closing of the blood vessel resulting from spasm or contraction, causing blockage of the flow of blood.

Cerebral embolus is less often the cause of stroke. Its occurrence may be associated with myocardial infarction or rheumatic heart disease. It may be the result of any condition in which an embolus becomes trapped in a small blood vessel in the cerebrum. Strokes caused by cerebral embolus occur in younger persons, in whom recovery is more likely. (See Fig. 18-3.) Strokes can also be caused by arterial spasm, which reduces the blood flow to a specific area of the brain, or by compression of vessels by tumors, edema, large blood clots, or other disorders.

Symptoms. A wide variety of neurologic symptoms can result from cerebral vascular accidents. Warning symptoms seldom occur; however, mental confusion, drowsiness, headache, and dizziness may precede the stroke. Occasionally, transient cerebral ischemic attacks, or "little strokes" may precede the cerebral vascular accident. These attacks are brief (2 to 60 minutes), reversible, and caused by a temporary decrease or interruption of blood flow to an area of the brain. Symptoms of transient cerebral ischemic attacks may include visual or auditory disturbances, abnormal sensations in the extremities, dizziness, headache, slowing of thinking processes or convulsions. Neurologic examinations given between attacks are normal. Patients having transient ischemic attacks may benefit from surgical procedures such as an endarterectomy (p. 276) or a shunting procedure, where the blocked artery is bypassed with an artificial shunt. Patients who are not candidates for this surgery receive anticoagulant therapy to prevent future episodes and a possible cerebral vascular accident.[11]

Usually cerebral vascular accidents are sudden, without warning, and frequently are serious enough to cause loss of consciousness, hemiplegia, or aphasia. These symptoms are related to the location of the defect in the brain. A cerebral vascular accident on the right side of the brain will cause left side hemiplegia and vice versa because the motor nerves cross from one side of the brain to the other before they descend to the spinal cord. Other symptoms that follow a stroke may include headache, vomiting, increased vital signs, confusion, convulsions, and loss of memory.

Treatment and nursing care. Radical changes have taken place in recent years in the medical management and nursing care of patients with cerebral vascular accidents. It is known that many of these patients can be restored to a useful life; rather than being dependent and economic burdens to their families and society, they may become physically, mentally socially, and vocationally independent. The nurse is a team member in the restoration of the patient and in many situations will play a major role in his care. It should be recognized that not all patients will be restored to a useful life; some will remain chronically incapacitated throughout life. The nurse should realize that nursing care after cerebral vascular accident must include the family.

Acute stage. The patient is generally first seen immediatey after the accident has occurred. He is admitted to the hospital and placed in a bed with side rails. He may be conscious or unconscious, and the nurse's first concern is the survival of the patient. His head should be turned to the side and the airway cleared of mucus and secretions that may have collected in the pharynx. A suction machine should be available, and the airway should be cleared by suctioning if necessary. If the patient is unconscious, no effort should be made to arouse him, and dentures should be removed. The vital signs are checked, and the blood pressure is recorded hourly for the first 24 hours, after which it should be checked every 2 to 4 hours. If the patient is conscious, he may be emotionally disturbed, frightened, apprehensive, and anxious, and every effort should be made to reassure him. The environment should be quiet and well ventilated, and visitors should be excluded except for the family and the patient's religious counselor. Intravenous fluids are administered for the first 24 to 48 hours, and records of all intake and output should be maintained. The patient who suffers a mild stroke will usually not lose bladder control, but retention may occur, and the nurse should watch for bladder distention. When the stroke is severe or if the patient is unconscious, urinary and sometimes bowel incontinence is present. Although the physician may order a retention catheter

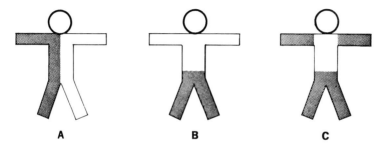

Fig. 18-4. Damage to the central nervous system may result in paralysis of some or all of the extremities. **A,** Hemiplegia. **B,** Paraplegia. **C,** Quadriplegia.

inserted, the nurse must remember the danger of infection from catheterization and be sure that a sterile closed system of urinary drainage is maintained. If the patient remains unconscious, a high caloric feeding is given through a nasogastric tube. If the patient is conscious, swallowing may be difficult, and some physicians prefer tube feeding for a few days to prevent the danger of aspiration. Oral care should be given several times a day. The blink reflex may be absent on the affected side so that secretions do not spread over the eye. The cornea may become dry, and corneal ulcers may occur. Gentle irrigation with physiologic saline solution and the instillation of Tearisol or a preparation ordered by the physician will prevent drying.[10]

Positioning. As soon as the immediate care has been completed, the nurse should institute a program of therapeutic nursing. The extent of damage will depend on the amount of brain tissue destroyed and its location. The patient may have loss of function on one side of the body, and the nurse will discover that the arm and leg are paralyzed (hemiplegia) (Fig. 18-4). Proper positioning of the patient is important to prevent contractures, improve circulation, prevent dependent edema, facilitate breathing, and prevent decubitus ulcers. The following are important points in proper positioning:

1. Board under mattress—to provide firmness and better alignment
2. Footboard—to prevent foot drop
3. Supine position—blanket or pillow between legs, trochanter roll or sandbags on outside of affected leg to prevent outward rotation
4. Side-lying position—affected side for 20-minute intervals four times a day; unaffected side for 2-hour intervals (flex knees and place pillows between legs, place sandbags at feet to keep at 90-degree angle)
5. Affected arm—90 degrees away from body with pillow between arm and body, arm supported on pillow with wrist higher than elbow and elbow higher than shoulder, roll in hand to maintain functional position and prevent contracture
6. Head—elevate 20 degrees with small pillow under head
7. Turn patient onto abdomen with physician's permission, turn head to side, position feet to hang over bottom of mattress

Things that should be avoided are as follows:

1. Do not raise gatch section of bed
2. Pillows should not be placed under knees when patient is in supine position because this contributes to contractures
3. Avoid letting patient's head fall forward onto chest or hyperextension of head to prevent pressure on veins of neck

Aphasia. If the patient is conscious or when consciousness returns, the nurse may discover that he is unable to speak because of damage to the speech areas of the brain. There are various types of aphasia referred to as *receptive* or *expressive.* In receptive aphasia the patient may have difficulty in understanding what is said to him or in reading what may be written, whereas in expressive aphasia he will have difficulty in speaking and in writing. The patient's discovery that he is unable to communicate is a shock to him and one that he does not readily accept. The nurse caring for the patient must provide emotional support and reassurance. The nurse should understand that the patient's inability to speak may cause periods of frustration and depression and must be willing to accept his behavior with complete understanding. The nurse should observe the patient carefully because the type of aphasia will determine to a large extent the kind of directions and help that must be given to the patient. When the patient cannot speak, his needs should be anticipated; questions should be asked to which he may reply yes or no or nod or shake his head. The patient should never be forced into speaking and should not be asked to repeat words after the nurse. Pleasant conversations concerning the present in which the nurse speaks clearly, slowly, and in short sentences may help the patient and encourage him to speak. Sometimes the nurse may be surprised by hearing the patient make a statement such as "good morning" or "how are you." This is called *automatic,* or *primitive,* speech and should not be interpreted as speech progress. The patient will be referred to a speech thrapist when his condition permits, but the nurse can pave the way for speech training.

Rehabilitation. Rehabilitation of the stroke patient begins the day he enters the hospital. Passive joint range-of-motion exercises should be started immediately to maintain muscle tone and prevent contractures. Active exercise should not be started without the physician's permission. After several days the patient may be allowed out of bed into a chair. The physical therapist and the speech therapist should be active participants in the program of rehabilitation. However, in many instances the physician and the nurse will be the only persons to guide and assist the patient to independence and self-assurance. The patient will tend to lean toward the affected side and must be taught balance while sitting. The patient should have a Hi-Lo bed and be taught how to move himself from the bed to the wheelchair and from the wheelchair to the toilet. He should be taught how to use the good hand to move the affected arm and how to use the good leg to move the affected leg. The patient should become a part of his own program of therapy and should participate in passive exercise of the affected arm and leg. As soon as the patient has attained a sense of balance in standing, a walking pattern should be instituted. Some form of a brace or splint may be necessary for the affected leg. The patient should be encouraged to seek independence. Realistic goals should be established that will help the patient have a feeling of accomplishment.

The patient who has suffered a cerebral vascular accident has experienced a sudden drastic change in body function that may be overwhelming. Although intellect is usually intact, the body will no longer react according to the patient's wishes. He may not be able to speak intelligently, move at will, or control the most basic body functions. The individual's perception of himself has suddenly been altered, and emotional reactions are to be expected. Many patients succumb to outbursts of anger, tears, or extreme withdrawal as a means of expressing their fear, anxiety, and frustration. Nursing personnel must understand the needs and feelings of the patient and provide opportunities for the patient to communicate in whatever way possible.[3, 7] Often nursing attitudes play an important part in what the patient accomplishes. The nurse who is calm, reassuring, recognizes small gains, and gives constant encouragement will stimulate the patient to continuous progress.

The nurse shares with other team members the responsibility for preparing the patient for his return home (Chapter 10). The other aspect of nursing is preparing the family to assume responsibility for the patient. Whoever will be caring for the patient should be taught simple nursing procedures and should understand how to let the patient do as much for himself as possible. The patient should have his own room and sleep in his own bed. The room should be located near the bathroom, the dining room, or the family room. He should be allowed to go to the bathroom, and he should eat his meals with the family and be a part of the normal family life. It should be remembered that the patient is a mature adult whose intelligence is not affected. He is likely to be sensitive and easily embarrassed, and all efforts should be made to protect him from embarrassing situations. His memory span may be short, he may have difficulty in concentrating and thinking clearly, and he may show lack of judgment, but he is an adult and should be treated as one. The family should understand that balance may be poor when the patient is sitting or standing or that balance may be good when sitting but poor when standing. The patient may have poor perception and be unable to distinguish between right and left and top and bottom, and he thus becomes tangled in his clothing when he tries to dress himself. Constant and consistent teaching may be necessary for him to learn to put the affected arm into the sleeve of his shirt first or the affected leg into the leg of his pants first. He may have difficulty in judging distance, and as he tries to move about will bump into things. When told to turn right, he may do the opposite. He may be unable to judge the passing of time. When the family understands what may be anticipated, it will help to provide for a smoother adjustment to everyday living for both the patient and the family.[5]

The unconscious patient may never regain consciousness and may die in a few hours or days. In other cases, consciousness will return in hours or 2 or 3 days, and the cerebral vascular accident may leave no residual symptoms.

Convulsive disorders (epilepsy)

Convulsive disorders are periodic disturbances of the nervous system resulting in a temporary loss of consciousness, abnormal motor activity, unusual sensations, or abnormal behavior. It is estimated that approximately 4 million people in the United States have some form of this disorder.[6] Convulsions occur with many illnesses and in some psychologic and neurologic conditions. Children are especially likely to have convulsions with temperature elevation.

Some convulsive disorders occur with no known cause. Other forms may be associated with infections affecting the brain and its covering. Epileptiform seizures may occur as a result of various metabolic disturbances, congenital malformations, cerebral vascular accident, head injuries, and brain tumor.[2] Although causes vary, it is known that convulsions occur from excessive neuron activity. For some reason cells in the affected area overreact to stimuli. There are three basic types of seizures that will be discussed: grand mal, petit mal, and psychomotor.

Grand mal seizures. The patient often has some warning or sign of the approaching attack, which is called an aura, but almost immediately he becomes unconscious, often falling. The attack may be immediately preceded by a cry, which occurs as the thoracic and abdominal muscles go into spasm, forcing air out of the lungs. The body becomes rigid, with legs extended straight, the jaws tightly clenched, and the hands gripped tightly (tonic phase). The eyes are wide open and pupils dilated. In a few seconds the convulsive stage begins, with all the muscles beginning to jerk and twitch violently (clonic phase). Unless a mouth gag is placed between the teeth before the jaws are set, the patient may chew the tongue. There is bowel and bladder incontinence and profuse salivation. The convulsive state is of short duration, but the patient may remain comatose. When the patient regains consciousness, he falls into a deep sleep and may sleep for several hours. On awakening, he may complain of headache, slight nausea, and general malaise. After the convulsive stage some patients may become mentally confused and violent.

Occasionally, typical grand mal seizures are preceded by convulsive twitching in one part of the body, which spreads to affect other areas of the body. This type of seizure is called a focal, or Jacksonian, seizure. Focal seizures may be limited to a specific part of the body, and a grand mal seizure may not occur.

Status epilepticus is a condition in which there are rapid, recurring seizures without recovery between them. The respiration is disturbed, blood pressure is elevated, and sweating and elevation of temperature occur. The condition may continue for hours or days and is serious because brain damage is possible. Emergency treatment is always required.

Petit mal seizures. Petit mal epilepsy is a mild form of the disease in which there is no aura, and only momentary loss of consciousness occurs. Tonic-clonic convulsions do not occur, and only a slight twiching of the face or nod of the head may be observed. A patient with petit mal epilepsy may have several attacks in a day. These seizures are common in children under 10 years of age and often they are outgrown at puberty. Because of the frequency of these attacks, children may have problems in school. Some patients experience both grand mal and petit mal convulsions.

Psychomotor attacks. Psychomotor attacks are frequently associated with brain damage, specifically of the temporal lobe. The patient does not lose consciousness but automatically performs normal actions although he is not aware of what is happening and cannot remember his actions afterward. Behavior may seem purposeless or inappropriate, and the patient may have sensory disturbances. Attacks last from 30 seconds to 2 minutes.

Treatment. Convulsive disorders can be controlled. Treatment must be planned on an individual basis and should include the whole person. A program that includes regulation of rest, diet, activity, fluids, and medication should be followed on a regular basis. Medication is prescribed for the purpose of preventing seizures, and any attempt on the part of the patient to skip, reduce, or otherwise alter the schedule of dosage may cause the return of serious seizures. Drugs in use for the treatment of grand mal epilepsy and some psychomotor attacks include diphenylhydantoin sodium (Dilantin sodium), 0.4 to 0.6 mg. daily, mephenytoin (Mesantoin), 0.3 to 0.5 Gm. daily, ethotoin (Peganone), 2 to 3 Gm. daily, metharbital (Gemonil), 0.1 to 0.8 Gm. daily, and primidone (Myosoline), 0.5 to 2 Gm. daily. All medication is administered in divided doses, and the patient should be observed for toxic effects such as skin rash, nervousness, drowsiness, fatigue, ataxia, and nystagmus. Drugs in current use for petit mal seizures are trimethadione (Tridione), 0.3 to 2 Gm. daily, paramethadione (Paradione), 0.3 to 2 Gm. daily, and methylphenylsuccinimide (Milontin), 0.5 to 2.5 Gm. daily in divided doses. Because of the possible toxic effects from drugs, all patients should be under medical supervision. Periodic blood counts are made because some drugs may cause depression of bone marrow.[4] The patient should understand that conscientious attention to the program planned for him will enable him to lead a normal, happy life.

Social factors. The person with epilepsy lives in a world of insecurity and misunderstanding. He must constantly anticipate and fear a seizure and its embarrassment. He is often rejected, avoided, and discriminated against and becomes a lonely person who needs help. Following are three cases that illustrate these social problems.

A 7-year-old girl enrolled in the second grade at school was diagnosed as having grand mal epilepsy. The child had an aura in which she jumped from her seat and screamed, "I'm going to have a fit." This was followed by an epileptic seizure. The experience frightened the teacher and the children in the room, whose anxiety was transferred to their parents. The parents ultimately demanded the withdrawal of the child from school.

A young woman was employed as secretary in a large governmental agency. One day she had a grand mal seizure while on her job. She was immediately released from her position.

A young man with petit mal epilepsy also had a severe case of psoriasis. He was devoted to his father but felt that he was not treated fairly by a stepmother. His father became ill, and the young man feared his father would die. His anxiety over the possible loss of the father and the realization of what the loss would mean for him resulted in his committing suicide.

Nursing care. If a patient who has a history of epilepsy is admitted to the hospital, the information should be available to the nurse. The first consideration is to protect the patient from injury; padded side rails should be on the bed. If an ambulatory patient has an aura and becomes aware of an approaching seizure, he should lie down on the floor, since there probably will not be time to return him to his room. A blanket may be placed under the patient, and a small hard pillow or folded pad may be placed under his head. A mouth gag or a safe substitute must be available and inserted quickly between the teeth to prevent biting the tongue. As the seizure develops, the teeth will be tightly clenched, and any effort to pry open the mouth may damage the teeth. The nurse should remain with the patient, and no effort should be made to restrain him. During the seizure there are increased oral secretions, and since the patient is unable to swallow, the airway should be kept clear by suctioning. Care must be exercised so that the tongue does not fall back into the throat and obstruct the airway. If possible, the patient should be turned onto the side, which will facilitate drainage of secretions. The patient should be protected from onlookers. If the patient is in a ward, curtains should be drawn around the bed, and if he is in a private room, the door should be closed. The nurse should remember that privacy from public scrutiny is a legal right of the patient. Since incontinence usually occurs, the bed should be protected with a plastic or rubber sheet. After the seizure the bed should be dried, the skin bathed, and the patient made comfortable. The patient should be oriented to his environment and reassured that he is all right.

Observation of the patient during the seizure is important and may help the physician to determine the location of the lesion. Paper and pencil should be kept in the patient's room to be readily available for notes that may later be transferred to the patient's record. Top bedding should be folded back during a seizure so that movement may be observed. Observation of the patient should include the following:

1. Exact time of beginning, duration, and ending of the seizure
2. Presence or absence of an aura—signs observed or anything said by the patient
3. State of consciousness
4. Occurrence of incontinence
5. Postseizure behavior—drowsiness, sleep, loss of speech
6. Presence of cyanosis or respiratory difficulty
7. Condition of pupils
8. Part of body involved and type of movement—clonic or tonic
9. Any injury that may have occurred during the seizure[4, 19]

Patients with epilepsy should carry an identification card or wear a Medic Alert bracelet or tag. There are two agencies that provide assistance to the epileptic patient and his family.*

---

*National Epilepsy League, Inc., 203 North Wabash Ave., Chicago, Ill. 60601 and Epilepsy Foundation of America, 733 15th St., N. W., Washington, D. C. 20201.

Head injuries

Injuries to the head often result in the individual's brain being shaken violently against the skull. This is called a *concussion.* The number of these injuries is increasing, and although many will be cared for in hospitals with large neurologic services, others will be cared for in rural and community hospitals near where they occur. Some patients will die within a few hours or a day or two, and the quality of nursing care during the first 48 hours may mean the difference between life and death. In many situations the nurse will be helping to care for patients with varying degrees of cerebral concussion.

The degree of injury may be classified as minor, moderate, or severe. All patients with concussion will be unconscious, with duration of unconsciousness depending on the severity of the injury. If the injury is minor, return to consciousness may be within an hour or several hours, whereas in severe concussion the patient may remain unconscious for days. However, what appears to be a minor injury may develop into a serious condition that may not be determined until months later. The patient who has suffered a moderately severe or severe injury will present varying symptoms. Often other injuries may be present such as fractures, including chest injuries, and the patient will be admitted in shock. Severe injuries are often accompanied by lacerations of the face or scalp, and there may be bleeding from the nose, ears, or mouth. Since an unconscious patient will not be able to complain of pain, injuries may not be detected immediately. When the head injury is severe, extensive x-ray examinations may be delayed until the patient's condition improves.

Treatment and nursing care. The most important function of the nurse during the first 48 to 72 hours is observation of the patient. If the patient is in shock, he must be immediately treated. The nurse should watch the patient carefully for return to consciousness and record carefully the level and duration of unconsciousness (p. 425). The pulse and respiration rates and blood pressure are taken every 15 minutes until they are well stabilized, and then they may be taken hourly. Rectal temperatures are taken, and if elevation is above

Intracranial pressure
↓ P/BP

Shock
↑ P ↓ BP

102° F., hypothermia measures may be instituted. If there is a decrease in the pulse rate with an increase in the blood pressure, it should be reported immediately to the physician. These are signs of increasing intracranial pressure. If there is an increase in the pulse rate with a drop in blood pressure, it also should be reported. A state of shock is developing. Any significant elevation of temperature or change in the rate or character of the respiration is extremely important. A large number of patients with head injuries die as the result of respiratory failure. A suction machine should be at the bedside so that the airway can be kept clear, but the nurse should not suction through the nose. Many hospitals have an inhalation therapist available who will assist if respiratory difficulties should occur. Mechanical ventilation may be necessary. Intravenous fluids may be administered, and accurate records of intake and output must be kept. The nurse should observe the size of the pupils, and a flashlight may be used to check for their reaction to light. The patient should be observed for any inability to move the extremities or for speech difficulty. Patients with head injuries may have convulsions; therefore a mouth gag should be available and the patient observed during the convulsion as in other seizures (p. 425). There should be padded side rails on the bed. The patient may be kept flat, or the physician may allow the head of the bed to be slightly elevated. If there is indication of cerebral edema, intracranial pressure, or hemorrhage, the head of the bed may be slightly elevated to facilitate venous return of blood to the heart.

The patient should be turned every 2 hours from side to side, using a turning sheet and supporting the head, and should be kept off his back. If the patient is unconscious, there may be bowel and bladder incontinence, and a urinary retention catheter is inserted and connected to sterile closed drainage. Bowel function is disregarded for several days, and enemas are not given if there is intracranial pressure. If the patient remains unconscious, tube feedings may be started after the critical period. Most patients with head injuries will be placed in the intensive care unit, and since all head injuries may be serious,

continuous skilled nursing care is important.

A subdural hemorrhage is bleeding into the subdural space between the dura and the arachnoid layers of the meninges. An epidural or extradural hemorrhage occurs when blood hemorrhages into the space between the dura and the skull. Bleeding may occur from arteries or veins. Symptoms of these complications include those of increasing intracranial pressure. Removal of the hematomas by surgery is the only treatment.

Neuritis and neuralgia

Neuritis and neuralgia are rather vague terms used by lay people to describe a variety of pains believed to be associated with peripheral nerves. Neuritis as a clinical disease does exist in several forms; however, its cause is more often associated with a degenerative disorder than with an inflammatory condition. Therefore the suffix may be misleading in some conditions.

Polyneuritis (multiple neuritis)

Polyneuritis, which involves the roots of peripheral nerves, is the most serious form of neuritis known. The degenerative changes that occur result in both sensory and motor symptoms. The motor symptoms, which cause weakness and flaccid paralysis of the lower and upper extremities, are often more significant than the sensory symptoms.

"Poly" means many, and in this form of neuritis many nerves may be affected. Any of numerous factors may cause polyneuritis, including poisonous substances such as mercury, arsenic, methyl alcohol, and some drugs, and it may accompany some infectious diseases. It may occur in persons whose diet is generally deficient in the required nutrients, especially the vitamin B complex, notably thiamine.

Sensory symptoms such as weakness and tingling of the extremities, increased sensitivity of the skin (hyperesthesia), and decreased sensitivity to heat and cold may be present. Sensory symptoms may occur in the absence of any motor symptoms, but if there is motor involvement, there will always be sensory symptoms. Motor symptoms may begin with weakness, disturbance of gait, and paralysis. The paralysis usually begins in the ankles and wrists and gradually extends up the extremity until complete paralysis results. Pain may occur early in some patients.[4]

Treatment and nursing care. Patients with multiple neuritis are treated with administration of large doses of vitamin B_1 (thiamine). If the cause is known, it should be treated or removed. The patient is placed on a regimen of bed rest and given analgesics to relieve pain. The application of moist heat to muscles (not joints) often provides relief. Proper positioning of the patient, the use of bed boards, and support of covers from tender extremities are important. Passive exercise (daily massage) by the physical therapist or the nurse should be done several times a day until the paralysis improves so that active exercise may be done.[4] Splints are sometimes used to prevent wristdrop and ankledrop, and hot compresses and galvanic stimulation may be employed to help maintain muscle tone and prevent atrophy of muscles.

Neuralgia

Neuralgia is a severe pain along the route of a nerve and may be the result of pressure at some point along the nerve pathway. Tumors, hypertrophic arthritis, and aneurysms are among some of the causes, but the disease may occur with the cause unknown. The more common types of neuralgia are intercostal neuralgia, sciatica, and trigeminal neuralgia.

Intercostal neuralgia. Intercostal neuralgia follows the course of the intercostal nerves, which are branches of the thoracic nerves. It may be from a tumor on the spinal cord or from arthritis. In herpes zoster (Chapter 20) pain usually follows the intercostal nerves. Pain generally begins in the back and radiates toward the front, and only one or both sides may be affected. If the cause is known, it should be treated or removed, and the neuralgic condition is treated with the application of heat and mild analgesics.

Sciatic neuralgia (sciatica). Sciatica is an inflammation and pain along the course of the sciatic nerve. The pain, which may be mild or severe, may be felt in the back and the buttocks and extends down the

back of the thigh and the inside of the leg. In addition to pain the nerve may be sensitive. Sciatica may occur without any known cause, but it frequently occurs from disorders of the sacroiliac joint or the lumbar spine. It may result from a ruptured intervertebral disk. The nerve may be injured by carelessness in the administration of injections in the gluteal muscle. The cause should be located and treated. The patient will be more comfortable if he has a firm mattress with a board beneath it, Moist heat (Figs. 18-5 and 18-6) and analgesic drugs will relieve much of the discomfort; however, the pain is occasionally acute enough to require a narcotic. Traction has also been found helpful in relieving the disorder. Bed rest should be continued until the acute attack is over.

Trigeminal neuralgia (tic douloureux). Trigeminal neuralgia is a facial neuralgia involving one of the branches of the fifth cranial nerve (Figs. 18-7 and 18-8). The condition occurs in persons of middle age and older, and with advancing years attacks increase in frequency. Although there are some theories, in general the specific cause is unknown. The pain comes in paroxysms lasting only a few seconds, but it is believed that it is the most severe pain that can be experienced. The pain is felt only in the skin, and any activity that stimulates the area near the affected nerve will cause a paroxysm of pain. Certain locations on the face are called *trigger points*, and the slightest touch or stimulation of these areas may cause an attack. Many activities of daily living such as brushing the teeth, shaving, washing the face, combing the hair, or eating, as well as environmental factors such as change of temperature, cold air, a breeze or a draft, may precipitate an attack. The patient lives in a constant state of fear and anxiety, afraid to perform any activity that might cause an attack.

Several methods of treatment have been tried. Injections of alcohol or phenol often provide relief for several months. Vitamin B_{12}, analgesics for relief of pain, and sedatives for sleep and rest may be given. Recently anticonvulsive drugs such as diphenylhydantoin (Dilantin) have been used for pain relief. Any of several surgical procedures that divide the nerve fibers and result in loss of sensation in the area may

severe pain

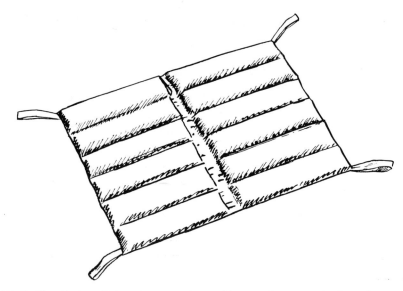

Fig. 18-5. The Hydrocollator steam pack provides continuous moist heat for periods of 30 minutes.

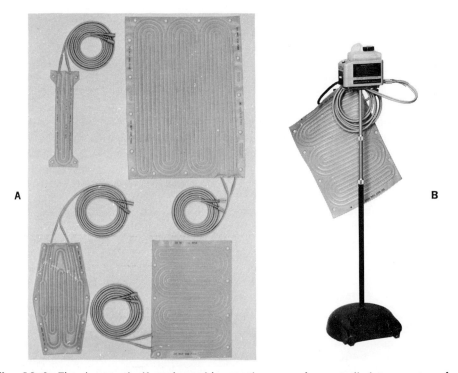

Fig. 18-6. The Aquamatic K pad provides continuous, safe, controlled temperature for warm moist dressings for as long as 8 hours. **A,** Pads are designed to fit and be laced to any part of the body. **B,** The temperature control unit is set to the desired temperature, and a key prevents accidental temperature change. (Courtesy Gorman-Rupp Industries, Inc., Bellville, Ohio.)

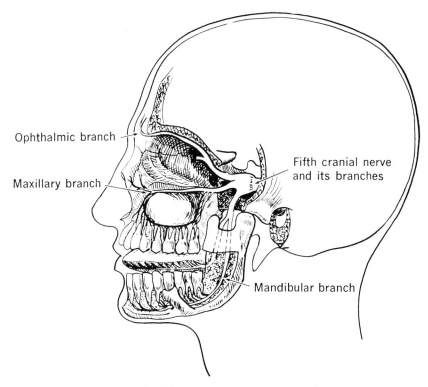

Fig. 18-7. Fifth cranial nerve and its branches.

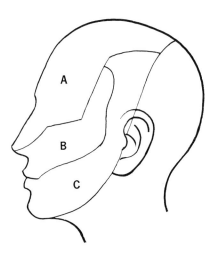

Fig. 18-8. Areas supplied by the three branches of the fifth cranial nerve. **A,** Ophthalmic branch. **B,** Maxillary branch. **C,** Mandibular branch. Any of the branches may be involved in tic douloureux.

provide permanent relief. When caring for patients with trigeminal neuralgia, the nurse should remember that the patient may be completely exhausted from fighting attacks of pain. The patient may be malnourished from lack of food because chewing may cause pain. The patient needs a nourishing diet with food of a consistency that does not require a great deal of mastication. Food should be served tepid rather than extremely hot or cold. The patient should be in a quiet environment and placed where there will not be a breeze blowing on him. Drafts and jarring of the bed should be avoided.[19]

Bell's paralysis (Bell's palsy)

Bell's paralysis, commonly called *Bell's palsy,* affects branches of the seventh cranial nerve and may occur with trigeminal neuralgia. The condition may begin with slight pain and tenderness at the back of the ear and on the side of the neck, followed by paralysis of the muscles on one side of the face. The upper eyelid droops, the lower eyelid sags, and the mouth is pulled to the opposite side of the face. Drooling occurs, and tears from the eyes flow over the face.

Treatment. Treatment consists of faradic intermittent electrical stimulation of the nerve and galvanic steady electrical stimulation of the muscles, which may be used in combination; moist heat is applied, and light active exercises are done. Treatments should be given by a physical therapist. Occasionally, vasodilating drugs may be given to increase circulation to the area, and steroids may be given to reduce edema of the nerve. The paralysis may disappear after several months; however, if after 1 year the paralysis appears to be permanent, plastic surgery may be done. Prostheses are now available to support the sagging corner of the mouth and the eyelid.

Spinal injuries

Injuries to the spine may involve only the vertebrae or the vertebrae and the spinal cord. Injury to the cord may result from tumor growth that presses on the cord, or an intervertebral disk may rupture, allowing its inner part to press against the cord. Accidental or intentional injuries may be from gunshot or knife wounds. The greatest number of serious injuries are the result of motor vehicle accidents, falls, and diving accidents. Metastatic cancer may cause disintegration of the bony framework around the cord. Any injury to the vertebrae is serious, and when the cord is involved, it is extremely serious. Injury to the cord may occur at any place, and body movement below the injury will be impaired or permanently affected. An injury in the cervical region may result in quadriplegia, whereas an injury in the thoracic or lumbar region results in paraplegia (Fig. 18-4). All sensations, including bladder, rectum, and muscles of respiration will be affected.

First aid. Although nurses may not be responsible for first aid, their understanding may be important in informing others, and with the highly mobile population in the United States, one never knows when one may come on the scene of a serious accident. Accident victims may be permanently crippled by improper care given by well-meaning persons at the scene of an accident. Under no condition should an accident victim be put into a car and taken to the hospital. If a spinal injury is suspected, a physician should be called, and the victim should not be moved until the physician arrives. The patient should be handled carefully when placed in an ambulance. He must be placed flat on a firm stretcher with no pillow under the head, but a small roll may be placed under the neck if a cervical neck injury is suspected. If the injury appears to be in the lower thoracic spine or lumbar region, a small roll under the lumbar spine may be more comfortable. At least three to five persons should be available to lift the patient onto the stretcher, with one person holding the head. The head should be supported on either side and should not be turned or allowed to tilt forward or extend backward.

On admission of the patient to the hospital, care will be directed toward relieving specific symptoms and preventing complications. If necessary, the patient is treated for shock. Oxygen, suction equipment, tracheotomy tray, catheterization tray, and a retention catheter should be available. The blood is typed and cross matched, x-ray films are taken, a myelogram may be done, and food and fluids are withheld. Prophylaxis for tetanus and gas gangrene is usually given. The physician will assess the extent of the injury and give directions for the type of positioning he desires.

Positioning. Proper alignment and support of the spine must be maintained. A firm bed is necessary. Hinged boards are placed under the sponge rubber, horsehair, or felt mattress. The Stryker flotation pad or alternating pressure pad may be used. The physician may wish the patient placed on a Stryker frame, Foster frame, or CircOlectric bed. When cervical traction is to be applied, the head is shaved and surgically prepared, and skeletal traction is applied by using Crutchfield, Barton, or Vinke tongs. When the patient is lying face up, the heels must extend over the frame or the mattress with the feet resting against a footboard at a 90-degree angle. Support must be provided to prevent external rotation, and bedding should be supported off the toes by the footboard or a bed cradle. Elastic bandages or stockings may be applied to the lower extremities to improve circulation. Various types of rings and cotton doughnuts should not be used.

Complete severance of the spinal cord is called *complete transverse myelitis,* and the patient with this condition will have no sensory or motor function below the level of the injury. When the injury is to the cervical cord, there will be complete paralysis of all four extremities (quadriplegia). Therefore no hot-water bottles or heating pads should be used because of the danger of burning the patient.

Daily care. The patient should be given a warm bath daily. Immediately after the injury a disturbance of the heat-regulating mechanism occurs so that the patient does not perspire below the level of the injury, which may result in an elevation of temperature. Later, perspiration becomes profuse, and frequent bathing becomes necessary. The skin must have meticulous care; keeping the skin clean and dry and eliminating wrinkles in sheets are important aspects of care. The use of powder is discouraged because it holds moisture and contributes to maceration of the skin. Keeping the body in proper alignment and in functional position through the skillful use of sandbags, trochanter rolls, and hand rolls is important. The range-of-joint motion should be maintained to prevent contractures.

If turning is permitted, the patient should be turned regularly every 2 hours; when the patient is hyperextended, he cannot be turned, and deep-breathing exercises must be done frequently to prevent respiratory complications. Hyperextension is sometimes accomplished with head or neck traction, which should never be released without a physician's order.

The patient with quadriplegia cannot use the bell signal to call for help. Therefore he should not be left alone for any length of time. Special devices are available for use by these patients. The flaccid paralysis present after a severe injury will later change to a spastic type, in which muscle contractions may be violent. The nurse should know that this does not indicate a return of normal function. Every possible consideration should be given to the patient and his family without encouragement or discouragement. The ex-tent of rehabilitation will depend on the extent of injury.

Relief of pain. The administration of pain-relieving drugs depends on the location and extent of pain. Narcotic drugs are not given to patients with cervical cord injuries. The use of narcotics should be avoided whenever possible because of addiction factors. The patient may come to use them as an escape from accepting his condition. Medications should be given orally when possible, and injections should not be given below the level of the injury because desensitized tissue does not have normal circulation.

Elimination. In patients with severe spinal cord injuries above the bladder, urinary retention generally occurs, and a retention catheter is inserted and connected to closed drainage. However, tidal drainage or suprapubic drainage may be instituted later. Since urinary tract infection is a serious complication, citrus fruits and their juices are restricted to prevent alkalinizing the urine, which allows bacterial growth. Cranberry juice tends to acidify the urine, however. The formation of renal calculi is always a possibility in the patient who is immobilized for a long time.

Since bowel function is affected, fecal impaction should be guarded against. One of the wetting agents that soften stools by drawing water into them may be used. They are available under several trade names such as Colace, Peri-Colace, Diovac, and Doxinate. The administration of the wetting agent at night and an oil suppository or a sodium phosphate enema in the morning may give satisfactory results. A well-balanced diet, 3000 ml. of fluid, and the use of 3 ounces of prune juice in the morning will greatly contribute to the prevention of constipation and the need for enemas. It is important that whatever method is used, it should be established on a routine basis.

Diet. The diet should be high in protein, calories, and vitamins. Foods known to be gas forming and those high in roughage should be avoided. The daily fluid intake should be 3000 ml. When the arms are paralyzed, the patient must be fed, and this dependence may be difficult for him to accept. The nurse should remember that attractiveness of food, leisure, and pleasant conversation will make it easier for the patient to accept having to be fed. The patient should be allowed a choice of food, and food brought from home may be enjoyed.

Rehabilitation. Rehabilitation begins immediately, and the primary objective of care is to assist the patient in achieving an optimal level of physical and mental function within the limits of his disability. Bladder and bowel retraining may begin once the patient's condition has stabilized. Immediately after a spinal injury the bladder is atonic; however, later the bladder will empty automatically. When this latter stage is reached, bladder training may be instituted in an attempt to train the bladder to empty at regular intervals. This is begun by intermittently clamping the catheter and then removing the catheter, having the patient make an attempt to void every hour. Bladder retraining may take weeks or months. Hypomobility or paralytic ileus of the bowel may occur directly after the injury, and the patient is incontinent of stool. When the patient has recuperated enough to assume the sitting position, bowel retraining can be initiated. Suppositories or stool softeners are used to establish a routine pattern of elimination. The goal is to achieve regular bowel movements by conditioning the reflex actions of the colon and rectum. If the paralyzed person can attain continence, his self-confidence increases, vocational retraining may be started, and hopefully the patient will be more capable of coping with his altered family and social relationships.

Adjustments to paralysis are very difficult. Extreme changes in body images must be made. The grief process, including such behavior as anger, depression, denial, and withdrawal can be anticipated. Often these patients do well when exposed to others having similar problems, and consequently they are discharged from the acute care hospital to a rehabilitation center where physical and emotional rehabilitation can continue.[12]

Rupture of the intervertebral disk

Between adjacent vertebrae is a flattened disk of cartilage that is slightly compressible and allows for limited flexibility of the spine. Intervertebral disks also act as shock absorbers to protect the vertebrae from jars and jolts. Sometimes these disks rupture, and the soft gelatinous substance in the center (nucleus pulposus) escapes. This mass may escape so that it compresses the spinal cord or exerts pressure on nerves, causing neurologic symptoms. The disks in the lumbar region are those most commonly affected, although cervical disk disorders are not infrequent.

Low back pain is generally the initial symptom, with acute attacks that may occur as the result of some slight movement. The pain eventually radiates over the buttock down the leg to the ankle. Frequently the sciatic nerve or its branches are involved. The patient may experience tingling or numbness in the foot and spasms in the leg, and depending on the amount of pressure on the nerve, gait may be affected.

Treatment is usually conservative until the pain is so severe that the patient cannot bear it or until neurologic symptoms incapacitate the patient, at which time the neurosurgeon advises surgery.

Medical treatment and nursing care. The patient is placed on a regimen of bed rest, and a firm mattress and hinged bedboards are used. Analgesics may be needed for pain. Good body alignment is important, and the patient should be taught to roll in turning over. Physical therapy, applying moist heat to the lumbar area, light massage, or the use of infrared heat with muscle exercises is generally ordered. When pain is severe, pelvic traction is frequently ordered, and when pelvic traction is applied, a small hard pillow or folded sheet should be placed under the back in the lumbar region to provide comfort and help to relieve muscle spasm.

Since the patient may be immobilized for an indefinite period of time, attention should be given to adequate fluid intake and elimination. Mild laxatives may be needed, and since lifting the hips will cause pain, the patient may be taught how to roll onto the bedpan. A pediatric bedpan may be more comfortable for the patient.

Before the patient is allowed up he is generally fitted with some type of support, which is put on before getting out of bed.

The patient should wear well-fitting shoes with a medium heel. The nurse who has learned good body mechanics in basic nursing and practices them can give the patient valuable assistance in learning how to use his body to avoid injury and pain.

A new experimental procedure called chemonucleolysis is being performed in some areas as a final step in the conservative treatment of herniated lumbar disks. In this procedure an enzyme is injected into the disk, and the damaged tissues are dissolved.[11] Conservative treatment of cervical disk herniation consists of bed rest, immobilization of the neck with a Thomas collar, and intermittent cervical traction.

Laminectomy. A laminectomy is a surgical procedure to remove bone, cartilage, the projecting intervertebral disk, or a spinal cord tumor. The posterior arch of the vertebrae is removed so that the spinal cord is exposed and the disk can be removed. A spinal fusion may be done during the operation. A laminectomy may involve the cervical, thoracic, or lumbar vertebrae; however, the thoracic vertebrae are less often involved. A partial or hemi-laminectomy can be performed to remove a herniated disk. A spinal fusion is not necessary, since the defect resulting is negligible.[6]

Preoperative care. Preoperative care of the patient is essentially the same as that for most surgical patients (Chapter 9). The nurse should ascertain the exact areas of the skin to be shaved (Fig. 18-9). If a spinal fusion is to be done, the bone grafts may be taken from the leg or the crest of the ilium, and this area is prepared also. The patient may be apprehensive and needs reassurance. An explanation of what to expect postoperatively will help to relieve anxiety. The patient is usually fitted for a back brace or a bivalved cast is formed prior to surgery, and it is applied immediately after the operation and not removed for 6 weeks.

Postoperative care. Postoperative care includes checking vital signs, maintaining the airway, and observing dressings for bleeding or drainage of spinal fluid. The patient may complain of pain in the back and legs, and urinary retention may be present. Coughing should be kept to a minimum, but the patient should be en-

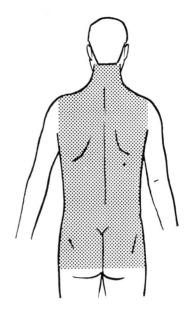

Fig. 18-9. Area of skin to be prepared for laminectomy.

couraged to breathe deeply. If a cervical laminectomy has been done, the respiration and chest expansion must be watched closely, since muscles of respiration may be paralyzed temporarily. The nurse should be sure of the surgeon's orders concerning turning the patient. In some instances the physician may wish the patient to remain flat in bed for the first 8 hours. When turning is permitted, he is turned from side to side every 2 hours. If the patient has been taught how to roll log fashion preoperatively, it will be helpful in postoperative turning. In the beginning the patient should not participate. A turning sheet will help in turning, and a sufficient number of nurses should be available to assist with the procedure. Movement should be slow and even rather than quick and jerky. The back should be supported with sandbags or pillows to keep it straight. Some patients are allowed out of bed on the operative day, whereas others are kept on a regimen of bed rest from 10 to 14 days. When the patient is allowed out of bed, he may be required to wear a back brace or corset while up, and low-heeled shoes are preferred to bedroom slippers. When spinal fusion is performed with laminectomy, recovery is a much slower process, and there is an extra wound to heal. If bone has been taken from the leg, the extremity must be handled carefully. Ambulation of patients who have had spinal fusion should be gradual. The patient should be taught to bend from the hips, keeping the back straight, and he will be more comfortable if he uses a straight chair when sitting.

Tumors of the brain and spinal cord

Tumors of the brain occur frequently at all ages and may be benign or malignant. There are many different kinds of tumors. Malignant tumors may result from metastasis from lesions elsewhere in the body, but primary tumors of the brain do not metastasize outside the brain. Regardless of treatment, the outlook for patients with malignant tumors of the brain is grave. If diagnosis is made early and the site of the tumor mass allows removal, benign tumors may be removed surgically with good results.

Symptoms of brain tumor often do not appear until neurologic signs such as loss or impairment of motor function has developed. Some patients with brain tumor experience headache, nausea, vomiting, increased intracranial pressure from the tumor mass, cerebral edema, changes in personality, aphasia, and convulsions. Depending on the location of the tumor, vision and hearing may be affected, and paraplegia may occur.

The specific symptoms may provide clues to the location of the tumor. Before considering surgery it is necessary to determine the exact location of the tumor. This is done by x-ray examination of the skull, angiography, and any of the special examinations referred to earlier in this chapter. If the neurologic examinations indicate that the tumor is operable, plans for a craniotomy are made. Without surgery most patients will die. If the tumor is inoperable, radiation therapy and in some instances isolation perfusion may be used; however, survival rates after the use of perfusion are still to be determined.

Tumors of the spine may be primary tumors or the result of metastasis. The tumor may be within the cord; it may be outside the cord but cause pressure on it. Pain is generally present and is made worse by movement or activity. The neuro-logic symptoms will develop below the level of the tumor and will cause both sensory and motor changes. A disturbance in gait will occur, and spastic paraplegia may develop. When the tumor affects the cervical spinal cord, quadriplegia will result. One of the early symptoms may be numbness, tingling, and pain in parts of the body supplied by the nerves from the affected area. The diagnosis may be made by lumbar puncture and myelography. Treatment is always surgical.

Craniotomy. A craniotomy is a surgical opening through the cranium for the purpose of removing a tumor or for exploration. The patient is generally admitted to the hospital for a complete neurologic examination, during which time he should be carefully observed for symptoms that may be helpful to the physician in establishing diagnosis. The nurse should be understanding in regard to the patient's anxiety and also that of the family and should give attention to the patient according to his symptoms. The patient may be ambulatory or may have hemiplegia, incontinence, and convulsions.

Preoperative care. Preoperative preparation of the patient may include hypothermia in preparation for surgery (Chapter 9). The head is shaved in the operating room or the evening before in the patient's room, and a surgical dressing is applied. The patient and the family should understand that the hair is to be cut, and long hair is saved and given to the patient. If a women patient is concerned about her appearance, she may be told that inexpensive wigs are available and popular. They may be fashioned to provide a very pleasing appearance. The patient generally is not given an enema, and the usual preoperative drugs are often omitted, although codeine is sometimes given. Sometimes steroids are administered, and a retention catheter is placed into the urinary bladder.

Postoperative care. After craniotomy the patient is placed in the intensive care unit, since constant observation is necessary for the first 48 hours. If the patient is to be returned to his room, the bed should be made from the bottom, and supplies and equipment to meet any emergency should be brought to the room. The nurse is a member of the team caring for the patient, and her most important function during the immediate postoperative period is to assist in observation of the patient. Complications may develop quickly, and early recognition of symptoms may avoid serious problems.

Vital signs are checked at 15-minute intervals. Any change in the blood pressure, pulse, and respiratory rates must be reported immediately. An increase in blood pressure and a decrease in pulse and respiration rates may indicate intracranial pressure. Rectal temperature is taken hourly, and if it reaches 101° F., measures aimed at reduction are taken. These may include administration of aspirin by rectum, hypothermia blankets, or ice packs. Dressings are checked frequently for bleeding, and drainage and sterile pads may be used to reinforce dressings. Unless otherwise ordered, the patient should be positioned on his side and turned at 2-hour intervals. Intravenous fluids are administered and allowed to drip at a rate ordered by the neurosurgeon. They must never be increased, since it may cause intracranial pressure or cerebral edema. Pupils should be checked as previously indicated for head injuries. Urinary output must be watched and measured each hour. Any decrease should be reported. If medications are ordered, they may be given intravenously. Restlessness, failure to move extremities, stiffness of the neck, rigidity of the arms and legs, disorientation, tremor, and convulsions must be watched for and reported immediately.

During convalescence the patient may have neurologic conditions that existed prior to surgery and have not been completely relieved. The physical therapist may help with ambulation and muscle-strengthening exercises. When the patient is dismissed from the hospital, the public health nurse may visit him in his home. The patient needs constant encouragement and reassurance and should be urged to do everything for himself within the limits of his abilities.[4, 8]

Summary outline

1. Structure and function of nervous system
   A. Coordinates various functions of body
   B. Consists of brain, spinal cord, nerves, and related structures
   C. Central nervous system—brain and spinal cord
   D. Peripheral nervous system—cranial and spinal nerves
      1. Twelve pairs of cranial nerves
      2. Thirty-one pairs of spinal nerves
      3. Peripheral nervous system
         a. Autonomic nervous system
            (1) Sympathetic nervous system—accelerates
            (2) Parasympathetic nervous system—slows
   E. Brain
      1. Cerebrum—largest part; includes right and left hemispheres
      2. Cerebellum—next largest
      3. Medulla—some nerves cross in medulla
      4. Ventricles in each hemisphere filled with spinal fluid
   F. Meninges—membrane covering brain and spinal cord
   G. Spinal fluid
      1. Provides moisture
      2. Lubricates
      3. Protects brain and spinal cord
2. Diagnostic tests and procedures
   A. Basic neurologic examination is done by physician known as neurologist
      1. Lumbar puncture—procedure for withdrawing small amount of spinal fluid for examination
      2. Cisternal puncture—another method for securing spinal fluid
   B. Special examinations
      1. Cerebral angiography—x-ray examination of cranium after injection of radiopaque substance into cerebral circulation
      2. Ventriculography—aspiration of spinal fluid from ventricle through small bore hole and replacement by air, after which x-ray films are taken
      3. Pneumoencephalography—introduction of air or gas into spinal canal through lumbar puncture, after which x-ray films are taken
      4. Myelography—consists of lumbar puncture, followed by withdrawal of small amount of spinal fluid, replacement with air or contrast medium, and x-ray films; second lumbar puncture is done to remove dye
      5. Electroencephalography—graphic recording of brain waves
      6. Caloric test—test to evaluate equilibrium; lesions in brainstem and cerebellum can be differentiated
      7. Queckenstedt's sign (lumbar puncture with dynamics)—consists of exerting pressure on jugular veins in neck and observing rise and fall of cerebrospinal fluid pressure
      8. Brain scan—injection of radioactive material and use of Geiger counter or scintillator to determine uptake
      9. Nursing care—importance of reassuring patient
3. Pain
   May be superficial, deep, or referred

A. Each individual reacts to pain differently
B. Pain is subjective symptom and always real to patient who experiences it
C. It is important to provide nursing measures to relieve pain
D. Medication should not be withheld when there is an order for it

4. Levels of consciousness
   A. Confusion (disorientation)—state in which patient mistakes identity of persons, does not understand conversation, and is confused or "mixed up"
   B. Delirium—represents major distortion of cerebral function and involves sight and hearing; patient may understand but be unable to comprehend in entirety
      1. Nurse should watch for early signs, and sedation should be administered
      2. Patient should not be restrained
      3. Delirium tremens (alcoholic psychosis) may occur in persons who use alcohol to excess; may be necessary to restrain these patients
   C. Stupor—state in which patient appears to be in deep sleep but may be aroused momentarily
   D. Coma—abnormal deep sleep from which patient cannot be awakened
   E. Convulsions (seizures, fits)
      1. Once convulsion has occurred, little can be done
      2. Observation of patient during convulsion is important

5. Nursing the patient with diseases and disorders of nervous system
   A. Infectious diseases
      1. Meningitis—inflammation of meninges of brain and spinal cord
         a. Spinal meningitis—only cord is involved
         b. Cerebrospinal meningitis—both cord and brain are involved
         c. Caused by pathogenic bacteria
         d. Symptoms extremely variable
         e. Diagnosis confirmed by spinal fluid
         f. Nursing care same as for any critically ill patient
            (1) Isolation for 24 hours or longer
      2. Encephalitis—inflammation of brain and other parts of nervous system
         a. Pathophysiology—caused by viruses, bacteria, fungi, chemicals, toxins, injury, and some infectious diseases of childhood
         b. Viral encephalitis—anthropod borne and transmitted by bite of infected mosquito
            (1) St. Louis encephalitis—most common
            (2) Eastern encephalitis—highest mortality
            (3) Western encephalitis
            (4) Japanese encephalitis
         c. Symptoms uniform in all types
         d. No specific treatment
         e. Isolation not required—no danger to nurse

f. Nursing care based on symptoms
      3. Poliomyelitis (infantile paralysis)—acute disease caused by three viruses that affect spinal cord
         a. Protection available through inoculation with Salk and Sabin vaccines
         b. Bulbar poliomyelitis occurs when brain and cranial nerves are affected
         c. Patient isolated for 7 days
         d. Provision should be made for emergency by providing tracheotomy tray, suction equipment, and oxygen
         e. Patient may require respirator care
      4. Central nervous system syphilis—disease leading to lesions caused by *Treponema pallidum*
         a. Meningovascular syphilis—affects meninges of brain and may be acute or chronic
         b. Tabes dorsalis (locomotor ataxia)—affects sensory nerve roots in spinal cord
         c. General paresis—consists of lesions in brain cells; deterioration and atrophy occur
            (1) Taboparesis is condition in which both general paresis and tabes dorsalis are present
         d. Prevention through early treatment of syphilis
   B. Degenerative diseases—cause chronic disability
      1. Multiple sclerosis (disseminated sclerosis)—affects myelin sheaths of nerve fibers
         a. Cause is unknown
            (1) Symptoms include loss of visual acuity, weakness, double vision, and nystagmus; may result in complete paralysis
         b. No specific treatment
      2. Parkinson's disease (paralysis agitans)
         a. Chronic progressive disease
            (1) Unknown cause in most cases
            (2) Outstanding symptoms are tremor and disturbance of gait
         b. No cure—treatment symptomatic, supportive, and palliative
            (1) New drug L-dopa may relieve symptoms in some patients but does not cure
            (2) Surgery in selected patients
      3. Myasthenia gravis
         a. Deficiency in neuromuscular transmission
            (1) Patient has too little acetylcholine or too much cholinesterase at nerve endings
            (2) Muscle weakness affects all muscles except bladder, stomach, and heart
         b. No cure
         c. Treatment and nursing care
            (1) Simple activities fatiguing
            (2) Mechanical assistance may be needed
            (3) Anticholinesterase drugs

C. Cerebral vascular accident (CVA), apoplexy, or stroke
1. Pathophysiology
   a. Caused by cerebral thrombosis, cerebral hemorrhage, or cerebral embolus
2. Symptoms
   a. Warning signs seldom occur
   b. Transient cerebral ischemic attacks may occur prior to CVA
   c. Loss of consciousness, hemiplegia, aphasia may occur
3. Treatment and nursing care
   a. Emphasis on restorative care and rehabilitation
4. Acute stage—immediate concern is survival of patient
5. Positioning
   a. Hemiplegia is paralysis of leg and arm on same side
   b. Proper positioning important
      (1) To prevent contractures
      (2) To improve circulation
      (3) To prevent dependent edema
      (4) To facilitate breathing
      (5) To prevent decubitus ulcers
6. Aphasia—when there is damage to speech areas in brain and patient is unable to speak
   a. Receptive
   b. Expressive
7. Rehabilitation—begins day patient enters hospital
   a. Family needs to understand patient and know what to expect
D. Convulsive disorders (epilepsy)—occur with many illnesses and neurologic conditions
1. Temperature elevation in children may cause convulsions
2. Periodic disturbances of nervous system
   a. No known cause for some
   b. Some associated with infections of brain, metabolic disturbances, congenital malformations, CVA, head injuries, or brain tumor
3. Grand mal seizures—severe with loss of consciousness and convulsion
4. Petit mal seizures—momentary loss of consciousness
5. Psychomotor attacks—automatic behavior without memory or loss of consciousness
6. Treatment planned on individual basis
7. Epileptic patient is lonely person who needs help and understanding
8. Social factors
9. Nursing care
   a. Protect from injury
   b. Do not restrain
   c. Ensure privacy
   d. Observe patient during seizure
E. Head injuries
1. Concussion occurs when brain is shaken violently against skull
2. Degree of injury may be minor, moderate, or severe, but all patients with concussion will be unconscious for varying periods of time
3. Treatment and nursing care

   a. Most important nursing function for 48 to 72 hours is observation of patient
F. Neuritis and neuralgia
1. Polyneuritis (multiple neuritis) involves roots of peripheral nerves
2. Neuralgia is severe pain along route of nerve
   a. Intercostal neuralgia follows intercostal nerves in thorax
   b. Sciatic neuralgia is inflammation and pain along sciatic nerve
   c. Trigeminal neuralgia (tic douloureux) is facial neuralgia involving branches of fifth cranial nerve
G. Bell's paralysis (Bell's palsy) affects branches of seventh cranial nerve
1. May be associated with trigeminal neuralgia
H. Spinal injuries
1. Proper first aid at scene of accident is very important to prevent serious complications
2. Position for proper alignment and spine support
3. Care of patient is directed toward specific symptomatic treatment and preventing complications
4. Complete transverse myelitis is complete severance of spinal cord
5. Quadriplegia is paralysis of all four extremities
6. Daily care
7. Drugs for pain relief
8. Elimination
9. Diet high in protein, calories, and vitamins
10. Rehabilitation—assist patient in achieving optimal physical and mental function
I. Rupture of intervertebral disk—may exert pressure on nerves and cause neurologic symptoms
1. Treatment may be conservative
2. If neurologic symptoms are severe, surgery may be done
3. Laminectomy—surgical procedure to remove bone, cartilage, projecting intervertebral disk or tumor
   a. Preoperative care—same as that for other surgical patients; if spinal fusion is to be done, donor site is prepared
   b. Postoperative care—deep breathing, coughing kept to minimum; positioning important
J. Tumors of brain and spinal cord
1. May be malignant with poor prognosis
2. Benign tumors may have favorable prognosis if location allows surgical removal
3. Primary tumors in brain do not metastasize outside brain
4. Tumors of spine may be primary tumors or result of metastasis
5. Craniotomy—surgical opening through cranium for purpose of removing tumor or for exploration
   a. Complete neurologic examination is done

b. Preoperative preparation may include hypothermia
c. Postoperative care similar to that after head injuries
d. Emergency equipment, drugs, and solutions should be available for immediate use

Review questions

1. How many nerves carry messages to and from the brain?
   a. 12 (pr.)
2. When an injury occurs to one side of the brain, why would the opposite side of the body be affected?
   a.
3. What is the state of consciousness when a patient appears to be in a deep sleep from which he cannot be aroused?
   a. coma
4. Why is isolation unnecessary when a patient has St. Louis encephalitis?
   a. not contageous –
5. List three chronic progressive degenerative diseases for which there is no cure.
   a. M.S.
   b. Parkinsons
   c. myasthenia gravis
6. If a patient has had a stroke, how should the affected arm be positioned?
   a. at 90° from body
7. What is the purpose of this positioning?
   a. to prevent contractures
   b. " improve circulation
   c. " prevent edema
8. If a patient has had a severe head injury or a craniotomy, what vital signs may indicate intracranial pressure?
   a. ↑ B/P
   b. ↓ P & R
9. What terms are used for paralysis affecting the body as follows?
   a. Stroke— hemiplegia
   b. Severed cervical spinal cord— quadraplegia
   c. Severed lumbar spinal cord— paraplegia
10. What term is used in neurology when there is a loss of speech?
    a. aphasia

Films

1. Cerebral vascular disease: the challenge of management (38 min., sound, black and white, 16 mm.), Squibb, 745 Fifth Ave., New York, N. Y. 10022 or your local chapter of the American Heart Association. Designed to acquaint physicians and nurses with concepts and techniques basic to the management of persons who have had strokes. Most common premonitory signs, emergency care, physician teaching exercises to the nurse, and the nurse teaching the family shown. Use of splints and slings.
2. Modern concepts of epilepsy (25 min., sound, color, 16 mm.), American Epilepsy Federa-

tion, The Greater Kansas City Epilepsy League, Room 301, Merchandise Mart Building, 2201 Grand Ave., Kansas City, Mo. 64108. Describes different types and problems of epilepsy.
3. My friend Joe (15 min., sound, color, 16 mm.), National Multiple Sclerosis Society, 257 Park Ave., S., New York, N. Y. 10010. The story of one patient's battle against multiple sclerosis.
4. Myasthenia gravis (20 min., sound, color, 16 mm.), Hoffman-LaRoche Laboratories, Department of Education, Nutley, N. J. 17110. Medical version shows diagnosis, course of the disease, and effects of treatment.
5. Physical rehabilitation in hemiplegia—M-1579-X (40 min., sound, color, 16 mm.), Media Resources Branch, National Medical Audiovisual Center (Annex), Station K, Atlanta, Ga. 30324. Shows the role of the physician, physical therapist, occupational therapist, social worker, speech clinician, and nurse in the management of the hemiplegic patient. Includes bed positioning, passive range-of-motion exercises, evaluation of muscle power, wheelchair propulsion, assistive and resistive exercise, standing, balancing, and ambulation.
6. Prevention of disability from stroke (28 min., sound, black and white, 16 mm.), local and state heart associations or AHA Film Library, 267 W. 25th St., New York, N. Y. 10001. Emphasizes that disability is preventable and demonstrates exercises.
7. Seizure (40 min., sound, black and white, 16 mm.), c/o D. J. Chapin, Assistant to the Director of Professional and Trade Relations, Parke Davis & Co., Detroit, Mich. 48232. Reviews social and occupational problems arising from stigma associated with epilepsy. Emphasis on need for making socioeconomic adjustments of epileptics part of their total medical care.
8. The emergency treatment of head injuries—M-1694-X (29 min., sound, color, 16 mm.), Media Resources Branch, National Medical Audiovisual Center (Annex), Station K, Atlanta, Ga. 30324. Shows an accident and gives the details of treatment. Adequate airway, control of bleeding, lessening of shock, and immobilization of head, neck, and broken limbs are included. Discusses various types of head injuries and proper treatment.
9. The stroke patient comes home (28 min., sound, black and white, 16 mm.), local and state heart associations or AHA Film Library, 267 W. 25th St., New York, N. Y. 10001. Series of six films discuss illness, problems, well-being, getting around, self-reliance, and return to community.
10. Treatment of parkinsonism with levodopa (22 min., sound, color, 16 mm.), American Cyanamid Co., Davis and Beck Division, Film Library, 1 Casper Dy., Danbury, Conn. 06810. History, symptoms and treatment are shown.

References

1. Barager, Fletcher: Cerebrovascular accident, The Canadian Nurse **62**:35-37, May, 1966.
2. Beeson, Paul B., and McDermott, Walsh, editors: Cecil Loeb textbook of medicine, ed. 13, Philadelphia, 1971, W. B. Saunders Co.
3. Berni, Rosemarian: Stroke patient rehabilitation: a new approach, The Journal of Practical Nursing **22**:18-20, June, 1972.
4. Brunner, Lillian S., and Suddarth, Doris S.: Textbook of medical-surgical nursing, ed. 3, Philadelphia, 1975, J. B. Lippincott Co.
5. Burt, Margaret N.: Perceptual deficits in hemiplegia, American Journal of Nursing **70**: 1026-1029, May, 1970.
6. Carini, Esta, and Owens, Guy: Neurological and neurosurgical nursing, ed. 6, St. Louis, 1974, The C. V. Mosby Co.
7. Coe, Mary: Understanding the CVA patient, Nursing Care **7**:17-18, May, 1974.
8. Davis, Ruth W.: Postoperative care of the craniotomy patient, Bedside Nurse **2**:23-28, May-June, 1969.
9. Dent, Dorothy: Self-help Parkinson's disease, 265 Daly Ave., Ottawa 2, Ontario, Canada.
10. Large, Helen, Tuthill, Joseph E., Kennedy, F. Bryan, and Pozen, Thomas J.: In the first stroke intensive care unit, American Journal of Nursing **69**:76-80, Jan., 1969.
11. Luckmann, Joan, and Sorensen, Karen C.: Medical-surgical nursing, a psychophysiologic approach, Philadelphia, 1974, W. B. Saunders Co.
12. Mahoney, Mary F.: Treating the spinal cord injured patient, Nursing Care **7**:17-19, March, 1974.
13. McInnes, Mary Elizabeth: Essentials of communicable disease, ed. 2, St. Louis, 1975, The C. V. Mosby Co.
14. Modell, Walter: Drugs of choice, St. Louis, 1974, The C. V. Mosby Co.
15. Pain, National Institutes of Health, Washington, D. C., 1968, Government Printing Office.
16. Recent advances in treatment of Parkinson's disease, Statistical Bulletin, New York, 1970, Metropolitan Life Insurance Co.
17. Robinson, Marilyn B.: Levodopa and parkinsonism, American Journal of Nursing **74**:656-661, April, 1974.
18. Shafer, Kathleen N., Sawyer, Janet R., McCluskey, Audrey M., Beck, Edna L., and Phipps, Wilma J.: Medical-surgical nursing, ed. 6, St. Louis, 1975, The C. V. Mosby Co.
19. Smith, Dorothy W., Germain, Carol P. Hanley, and Gips, Claudia D.: Care of the adult patient, ed. 3, Philadelphia, 1971, J. B. Lippincott Co.
20. Stackhouse, Joan: Myasthenia gravis, American Journal of Nursing **73**:1544-1547, Sept., 1973.
21. Swift, Nancy: Caring for the neurological patient, Nursing Care **7**:17-19, June, 1974.
22. Wylie, Charles M.: Death statistics for cerebrovascular disease: a review of recent findings, Stroke **1**:184-193, May-June, 1970.

CHAPTER 19

Nursing the patient
with diseases and disorders
of the eye and the ear

KEY WORDS

adhesion
astigmatism
audiologist
cataract
cerumen
conjunctivitis
diplopia
eustachian
glaucoma
hyperopia
labyrinthitis
mastoiditis

miotic
myopia
ophthalmologist
otitis media
otologist
otosclerosis
pinna
refraction
stapedectomy
strabismus
tonometry
trephine

STRUCTURE AND FUNCTION OF THE EYE AND THE EAR

The eye

The eye is a highly specialized sense organ, a large portion of which lies protected within a bony cavity, with only the anterior part exposed. The eye has three coats: the outermost is the *sclera,* or white part, the middle coat is the *choroid,* and the inner coat is the *retina.* The portion of the sclera in the front part of the eye is the *cornea,* which is transparent. The colored part of the eye, the *iris,* is circular in shape and located at the back of the cornea. In the center of the iris is a small opening called the *pupil,* and directly behind the pupil is the *lens.* The posterior part of the eye contains a large chamber filled with a soft gelatinous material called *vitreous humor.* A smaller cavity in the anterior part of the eye contains a clear thin fluid called *aqueous humor.* This chamber is partially divided into an anterior and a posterior portion. Entering from the back of the eye are blood vessels and nerves. The optic nerve is concerned with vision, whereas branches of several cranial nerves control muscles. A number of muscles (extrinsic) are voluntary and hold the eye in position and permit the individual to move it. When some of these muscles are unequal in length a condition known as *strabismus* occurs. Involuntary muscles (intrinsic) within the eye are concerned with the shape of the lens and the size of the pupil. The accessory organs of the eye include the eyebrows, eyelids and their muscles, eyelashes, conjunctiva, lacrimal glands and their ducts, and sebaceous glands.

Vision is the result of light rays entering the eye; as they pass through various structures of the eye, they must produce a clear image on the retina. When the image is produced on the retina, visual receptors in the eye are stimulated, thus causing a nerve impulse to be transmitted to the visual center in the brain.

The ear

The ear is the specialized sense organ of hearing composed of external, middle, and internal parts and nerves. The external portion provides a passageway (*auditory canal*) to the *tympanic membrane* (eardrum). The external portion that projects is the *pinna,* which helps to direct sounds toward the auditory canal. The tympanic membrane divides the external and the middle ear. The outside of the membrane is covered with skin, whereas the inside is covered with mucous membrane. A branch of the fifth cranial nerve supplies the membrane. The middle ear is a small bony cavity separated from the internal ear by the oval window (*fenestra ovalis*) and the round window (*fenestra rotunda*). Within the middle ear are three tiny bones: *malleus, incus,* and *stapes.* Because of their shape, they have been called the *hammer, anvil,* and *stirrup.* These three bones are attached to each other, to the tympanic membrane, and to the oval and round windows. They amplify sound vibrations and conduct them to the inner ear. The eustachian tube connects the middle ear with the nasopharynx, and the middle ear is also connected with some of the mastoid cells. The inner ear (labyrinth) consists of the bony or osseous labyrinth, which contains the vestibule, cochlea, and semicircular canals. A membranous labyrinth within the bony labyrinth contains two small sacs, the *utricle* and *saccule,* in which a fluid called *endolymph* is found. *Perilymph* surrounds the utricle and saccule, which are suspended within the vestibule. The cochlea is a snaillike tube containing the cochlear duct with the receptors for the cochlear branch of the eighth cranial nerve and the sense of hearing. The semicircular canals and the utricle contain the receptors for the branch of the eighth cranial nerve concerned with maintaining a sense of equilibrium. Several other structures and sup-porting parts are contained within the inner ear, and students who wish a more detailed review should consult a textbook of anatomy.

The auditory center for hearing is located in the temporal lobe of the cerebrum, and stimulation of this center results in hearing. Sound waves enter the ear through the auditory canal and cause the tympanic membrane to vibrate. The vibrations are transmitted from the tympanic membrane through the middle ear. One of the three small bones, the stapes, moves against the oval window, and its vibrations cause a displacement of the perilymph, which then stimulates the receptors, which in turn transmit the neural impulses to the brain, where they are interpreted as sound.[1, 10]

DIAGNOSTIC TESTS AND PROCEDURES

Physical examination. A complete physical examination is important in the treatment of diseases of the eye and ear. When the underlying cause is diabetes, syphilis, or arteriosclerosis, treatment of the cause must accompany any treatment of the sense organ. The physician may order x-ray examinations, examination of the blood and spinal fluid, or neurologic examination. A thorough eye examination often leads to the discovery of serious diseases in other parts of the body.

Eye examination. Several eye tests are used to detect eye diseases and disorders of vision.

Acuity of vision. Acuity refers to the clearness of vision, or the person's ability to see. The most common method for determining acuity of vision is testing with a Snellen eye chart, a method used in schools, industry, and physician's offices as a screening examination. The chart consists of rows of letters arranged in various sizes that a person should be able to see at various distances from the chart. If the individual is able to read the letters marked 20 at a distance of 20 feet, he is considered to have 20/20 vision, which is normal vision. However, if he reads correctly only the rows of larger letters marked 30, 40, or even 200, he is said to have 20/30, 20/40, or 20/200 vision, indicating a loss of visual acuity. Sometimes the vision in one eye may be 20/20, and the test will indicate a loss of

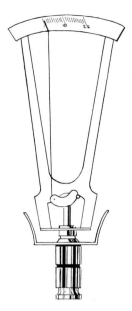

Fig. 19-1. Tonometer used to measure intra-ocular pressure.

vision in the other eye. When the individual is wearing glasses, the test is usually performed both with and without the glasses. One form of the chart consists of the letter "E" arranged in various positions. Very young children may be tested with this chart by having the child indicate with his fingers the open end of the E.

Tonometry. Patients with certain diseases of the eye such as glaucoma have increased intraocular pressure. The tonometer is an instrument for measuring the intraocular pressure (Fig. 19-1). The increased pressure results from some obstruction of the flow of aqueous humor between the posterior and anterior chambers of the eye. When this occurs, tension of the eyeball will increase. To determine the amount of pressure, 1 drop of 0.5% proparacaine (Ophthaine) is instilled into the eye to anesthetize the cornea. The tonometer is then placed on the the center of the cornea and the scale reading taken.

Ophthalmoscope. The ophthalmoscope is an instrument that permits the physician to examine the inside of the eye. The pupil is often dilated to permit a better view. The examination may reveal the presence of tumors, changes in blood vessels, or serious diseases of the eye.

Slit lamp. The slit lamp is an instrument

with a light that throws an intense beam into the eye and, with the attached microscope, permits the physician to visualize its minute structures.

Hearing tests. Several methods exist for determining hearing loss, and the tests vary in accuracy and purpose.

Voice tests. Voice tests may be done by using the whispered voice or a lowered tone of spoken voice. The individual is placed at a distance of 20 feet and turned sideways so that the ear to be tested is toward the examiner, and the other ear is covered. The person is asked to repeat the whispered or spoken words. The method is of value only as a screening test to locate individuals who need more thorough examination.

Audiometer. A more accurate examination is done with the audiometer, which produces tones of varying pitch and intensity. The patient wears earphones that are attached to the audiometer. The individual listens to various tones and indicates when he hears the sound. The audiometer test provides information concerning quantitative and qualitative measurement of hearing and provides the otologist with information that can help to determine the kind of treatment needed.

Tuning forks. Hearing tests may also be done by using tuning forks that are made to vibrate and are placed at various locations near the ear. This type of test is helpful in determining whether deafness is conductive or whether disease of the nerve is present.

Testing hearing in young children. Infants as young as a few days and very young children may be tested for hearing loss. These tests depend on observation of reflex action of the child when exposed to sound stimuli. To administer the tests, a person must be especially trained in the technique. However, the nurse working in the nursery or in pediatrics may contribute to the identification of infants or young children who may have hearing loss by making a few careful observations, such as the following, which should be reported to the physician[13]:

1. Child cannot be awakened unless he is touched
2. Comfort measures fail unless infant is held

3. Child fails to respond to sounds or loud noises
4. Child shows lack of interest in noise-making toys unless they are in his hands
5. Child fails to respond to his name

LOSS OF SIGHT

Loss of vision may be congenital or acquired, and it may occur suddenly or gradually over a period of time. Several pathologic conditions may result in varying degrees of blindness, including diabetes, hypertension, inflammation of the choroid and retina, retinal detachment, infectious diseases such as syphilis, certain poisons such as wood alcohol, and injuries. A gradual loss of vision may be caused by cataracts and glaucoma. Cerebral disorders may affect the optic nerve, as well as malignant lesions that occur in children such as retinoblastoma. Many children were permanently blinded between 1930 and 1950 because of the excessive use of oxygen in the premature newborn nursery, which caused retrolental fibroplasia. Rubella (German measles) occurring in the pregnant woman is implicated as a cause of cataracts and glaucoma in the infant.

LOSS OF HEARING

Hearing loss may be congenital or acquired and may range from minor impairment to complete deafness. Persons are considered to be hard of hearing when their hearing is defective, but they can function without a hearing aid under most situations. The deaf person cannot function satisfactorily without an aid of some type. The deaf may be divided into two groups: those who are congenitally deaf, and those who are born with normal hearing but for some reason become nonfunctional. The deaf person must have assistance such as a hearing aid, auditory training, or speech reading (lipreading).[14]

Types. Hearing loss may be conductive, affecting only the external or middle ear, or it may be sensorineural (nerve deafness), in which the inner ear is involved. Conductive deafness may be caused by an obstruction of the auditory canal that prevents sound waves from reaching the inner ear. The problem may be an accumulation of cerumen (earwax) in the auditory canal,

or it may be due to otosclerosis in the middle ear that prevents transmission of sound vibrations from reaching the inner ear. For these persons, surgery may restore hearing (p. 471). In some cases there may be a congenital absence of the auditory canal or the tympanic membrane. In conductive deafness only the intensity of sound is affected.

In sensorineural deafness the auditory canal and the middle ear may receive the vibrations normally, but they go no further. This is because of degeneration of the nerve fibers of the auditory nerve or the hearing center in the brain. Damage may result from tumors, head injuries, or other causes such as congenital syphilis that affects the eighth cranial nerve. Nerve deafness may occur in babies born to mothers who had rubella during the first trimester of pregnancy. A type of nerve deafness that usually affects the high-frequency sounds may occur as part of the aging process. Persons with nerve deafness talk loudly, and there is confusion and distortion of sounds with poor speech discrimination. When nerve deafness is congenital or acquired during infancy and early childhood, the speech is generally affected. Such children usually need training in lipreading and special education. Nerve deafness cannot be treated medically or surgically. The condition is irreversible and permanent.

Hearing aids. Advertisements for hearing aids appearing in many magazines, newspapers, and television may confuse the hard-of-hearing person. The nurse can be helpful by advising the individual to consult his otologist. After careful examination, if the otologist considers the hearing loss to be irreversible, he will refer the patient to the nearest speech and hearing clinic. Technicians in these clinics evaluate the type of hearing loss and recommend the hearing aid best suited to the individual. The hearing aid is of little value to the individual with total nerve deafness; these persons must be trained in lipreading. The hearing aid is only designed to amplify sound, and in persons with conduction deafness, in which the problem is one of intensity of sound, a hearing aid may help.[16] The hearing aid consists of three parts: a microphone that picks up sound and converts it into electrical signals, an amplifier that intensifies the signal, and a receiver that converts the signal back into an intensified sound. The hearing aid may be used along with auditory training and lipreading. There are various types of hearing aids, including those that may be used about the head. They may be built into the glasses, worn behind the ear, or worn in the auditory canal. Other types may be worn on the torso.

The successful use of a hearing aid depends on the individual and his feelings about his handicap and the use of a hearing aid.[14] Not all persons will be able to adjust to the device, and elderly persons may find it more difficult. Deafness, whether progressive or sudden in onset, produces anxiety and fear within the patient. The possibility of becoming cut off from familiar surroundings, losing friends, losing a job, and becoming isolated often leads to the patient's withdrawal from society. Many patients will deny the defect and refuse assistance. Hearing aids can play an important part in improving residual hearing, thus lessening the emotional impact of approaching deafness.

REFRACTIVE ERRORS OF THE EYE

When light rays enter the eye, they must focus directly on the retina. To reach the retina the rays pass through several structures in the eye, and in doing so are bent so that they will fall directly on the receptors in the retina. This bending of the light rays is called *refraction*. Sometimes an abnormal condition exists in some of the structures so that bending of the light rays may not permit the image to focus directly on the retina (Fig. 19-2). These defects are called *errors of refraction*. The patient may complain of eyestrain, headache, and sometimes nausea. To overcome the error the person must have an eye examination and glasses fitted to correct the refractive error. This examination is also called refraction.

Myopia (nearsightedness). Persons with myopia have a defect that may be in the eyeball or in the bending of the light rays. The rays are brought to focus too soon, or in front of the retina. As a result, distant vision will be blurred rather than clear. Myopia may become progressively worse in some young persons, and it is important for the individual to remain under the care of the ophthalmologist.

Hyperopia (farsightedness). In persons with hyperopia the light rays do not bend sharply enough or soon enough to focus the object on the retina, and the point of focus is behind the retina. The individual will see distant objects clearly, but near vision will be blurred. Examinations such

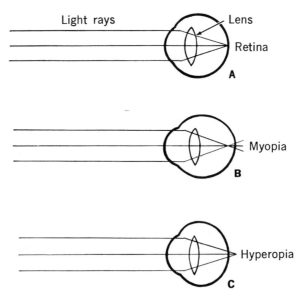

Fig. 19-2. Refractive errors of the eye. **A,** Light rays entering the eye are brought to focus directly on the retina, resulting in normal vision. **B,** Light rays focus in front of the retina, resulting in myopia. **C,** Light rays focus at the back of the retina, resulting in hyperopia.

as those with the Snellen eye chart may not show this condition. However, signs of eyestrain may indicate the need for examination by the ophthalmologist, and eyedrops are usually required to paralyze certain eye muscles to discover the defect.

Astigmatism. Astigmatism is a defect in the curvature of the eyeball surface, usually of the cornea but sometimes of the lens. Exact regularity of the curvature probably does not exist in many persons, but defects may be too slight to cause any trouble. However, when the irregularity is severe, all light rays do not bend equally, and the individual will suffer from eyestrain and blurred vision. When the ophthalmologist fits glasses for astigmatism, the glasses should be worn constantly.

Strabismus (crossing of the eyes). Strabismus is a condition in which the eyes fail to focus in the same direction. Convergent strabismus (esotropia) causes the eye to turn in toward the nose, whereas if the eye turns outward, it is called *divergent strabismus* (exotropia). Strabismus is classified as paralytic or nonparalytic. The disorder may be congenital due to hereditary factors, or it may be acquired; unless diagnosed and treated, it may cause irreversible damage to vision. Paralytic strabismus is the result of damage to the third, fourth, or sixth cranial nerve or to the ocular muscle. The damage may be caused by disease such as tumors or infection, or it may be caused by damage to the eye. The most common symptom is double vision (diplopia). When the eyes are crossed, two different impulses are received by the brain, and the person sees two separate images.

Nonparalytic strabismus is an inherited disorder, in which there is no paralytic condition of the muscles. The child may use the eyes in several different ways but never focuses with both eyes together.[17] The disorder will *not* correct itself as the child becomes older. Early medical treatment should be secured to protect the child's vision. When the condition fails to respond to medical treatment, surgery may be done.

Contact lenses. As more people wear contact lenses, the nurse may be asked about them. The nurse should know that they are constantly being improved and are being worn for many kinds of visual defects and disorders. The individual should have

his eyes examined by an ophthalmologist to be sure that no serious eye disease exists, and contact lenses should be recommended by the ophthalmologist.

Approximately 90% of contact lenses being worn cover only the cornea; the rest cover the entire sclera. A contact lens is a small, thin, polished, plastic disk that is ground on its outer surface to correct vision deformities; its inner surface corresponds to the shape of the eye. It is lightly tinted and is held in place by capillary attraction and the upper eyelid. The lens is moistened before insertion, and the conjunctival secretions provide lubrication and prevent irritation of the cornea. There are many advantages to wearing contact lenses, but the wearer must take precautions to avoid abrasions of the cornea. Causes for abrasions include prolonged wearing of improperly fitted lenses, tilting of the lens when removing or inserting it so that the edge of the lens scratches the cornea, or scratching the cornea with the fingernail. Abrasions are also caused by an inadequate flow of tears under the lenses.[5, 15]

It is important for the nurse to realize that an injured person may be wearing contact lenses, and unless they are removed, serious damage to the cornea may result (Fig. 19-3). A light flashed into the eye

---

1. DETERMINE IF PATIENT IS WEARING CONTACT LENSES:
a. Ask
b. Check I.D. Card
c. Check Medic Alert Medallion
d. Look for contact lenses

2. IF YOU SUSPECT THE LENSES ARE STILL ON THE EYE:
a. Apply adhesive tape strip to patient's forehead or adjacent area and label "Contact Lenses"
b. Consult emergency aid file when time permits

3. IF THE LENSES ARE FOUND:
a. Place in a case or bottle and label with patient's name (Mark "right" or "left," if known)
b. Record on emergency tag

Provided as a public service
by the
AMERICAN OPTOMETRIC ASSOCIATION

Fig. 19-3. Suggested emergency care for patients wearing contact lenses. (Reprinted with permission of the American Optometric Association, St. Louis, Mo.)

from the side will cast a shadow on the iris that will enable the nurse to detect the lenses as the person blinks his eyes. Gentleness must be used when removing the lens to avoid injury to the eye. If the nurse is unable to remove the lenses, an ophthalmologist or an optometrist should be called to remove them. Contact lenses removed from an injured or dying person should be placed in bottles labeled "right" and "left" with the patient's name and protected from loss or damage.

COLOR BLINDNESS

The inability to distinguish colors may be congenital or acquired, and it may be partial or complete. Acquired color blindness may be the result of injury or disease of the nervous mechanism concerned with vision. Partial color blindness is more common in men than in women, is rare in the black race, and is generally a congenital condition. The most common type of color blindness is red-green blindness, a condition in which persons do not see red or green as such but see them as yellow or blue in different intensities of saturation. A person may be color blind in one eye only, in which case he will distinguish colors normally.

Some states require a person applying for a driver's license to be tested for color blindness. When an individual is found to be color blind in both eyes, he is taught to distinguish traffic lights by their location. Awareness of the defect often makes the person with color blindness a more cautious driver than the individual with normal color vision.

SPECIFIC ASPECTS OF NURSING THE PATIENT WITH DISEASES AND DISORDERS OF THE EYE AND THE EAR

Several nursing procedures are often necessary in caring for patients with diseases and disorders of the eye and ear. These include the instillation of eyedrops and ointments, giving eye and ear irrigations, and the application of hot or iced compresses. Absolute cleanliness is essential, and the hands should be washed before beginning any procedure and should be washed after nursing each patient. All equipment must be clean, and in some

situations sterile supplies and equipment may be required. The nurse should review these procedures and understand the precautions necessary in each procedure. (Refer to a textbook on basic nursing.)

NURSING THE PATIENT WITH DISEASES AND DISORDERS OF THE EYE
Inflammatory and infectious eye disorders
Styes (hordeola)

It is commonly but inaccurately believed that styes are a sign of weak eyes; they are small boils or abscesses resulting from infection in the hair follicle of an eyelash. They are characterized by a small inflamed swelling at the edge of the eyelid. The staphylococcus is frequently the causative organism. As the swelling increases, the stye may rupture spontaneously and drain pus, after which healing occurs. Occasionally the condition becomes chronic with the occurrence of repeated infections.

The application of hot moist compresses will relieve pain and facilitate suppuration. Medical care is seldom required, but in some cases incision and drainage and administration of the appropriate antibiotic may be necessary. Precautions should be taken to avoid squeezing or picking of the stye to prevent spread of the infection.[18]

Conjunctivitis

Conjunctivitis is an inflammation of the conjunctiva of the eye, and there are several forms of the disease. Conjunctivitis may be the result of an allergy and will usually clear when the offending allergen is removed. It may also result from bacteria or injury.

Acute purulent conjunctivitis. The most common type, however, is an acute purulent conjunctivitis commonly referred to as *pinkeye.* The infection is caused by the Koch-Weeks bacillus. It is frequently encountered as an epidemic among schoolchildren spread through droplet infection. The conjunctiva becomes red, with burning and a mucopurulent secretion.

The eyelids are usually stuck together in the morning, and hot moist compresses may be applied to soak the crusted lids. Eye irrigations using boric acid or physiologic saline solution may be ordered. The specific organism should be identified, and the disease may be treated with a sulfonamide or antibiotic such as neomycin ointment, 0.1% to 4%. Steroid therapy is contraindicated when infections are present, although it may be of value when the cause is from an allergy. Drops are usually instilled during the day, and an ointment is used at night. Discharge from the eye should always be removed before medication is applied. Persons with the infection should have their own towels and washcloths and should not use public swimming pools. Children with the disease should not attend school until the infection has cleared, which will be in about 1 week.

Gonorrheal conjunctivitis. Gonorrheal conjunctivitis occurs in the adult as gonorrheal ophthalmia' and in the newborn infant as ophthalmia neonatorum; it is caused by the gonococcus bacterium. State laws require that 1% silver nitrate solution or an antibiotic be instilled in the eyes of all newborn infants to prevent the disease. The treatment is so effective that few cases of ophthalmia neonatorum are seen today. Gonorrheal ophthalmia in the adult may result in corneal ulcers with scar formation, which may cause loss of vision. The disease is characterized by thick purulent discharge from the eye, with inflammation of the conjunctiva.

The disease may be treated with penicillin, which is administered intramuscularly and instilled into the eye. The sulfonamide drugs may also be used. Other treatment may consist of placing cold compresses on the eye and cleansing the purulent exudate from the lids. The patient should be isolated and medical asepsis carried out. A gown is worn by the nurse, and precautions should be taken to protect the eyes.

Trachoma. Trachoma is a communicable disease caused by a virus that frequently affects all the members of a family. It is spread through the use of common towels, washbasins, and washcloths, and the incidence is greatest when crowding exists and living conditions are poor. The disease is relatively rare in the United States, although still found in some midwestern states among rural American Indians. The disease begins with inflammation of the conjunctiva, which becomes chronic and is accompanied by formation of granules on the lids; the conjunctiva has a charac-

teristic reddish blue appearance. The disease progresses slowly, with changes in the conjunctival tissue and a tendency to form corneal ulcers. The disease will ultimately lead to blindness. Patients with long-standing cases may develop entropion, which is a turning in of the eyelid that requires surgical correction.

Treatment is sulfonamide drugs or tetracycline drugs administered orally. However, close supervision is necessary because all members of the family must be treated if they are infected, and problems of personal hygiene must be improved, or reinfection may occur.

Blepharitis

Blepharitis is a chronic inflammatory process involving the margin of the eyelids and may be caused by the staphylococcus or other bacteria, allergy, and degenerative diseases. The lids are red and inflamed, and fine, crustlike scales form at the base of the eyelashes. The condition is often associated with excessively oily skin and scalp.

Cleanliness of the hair, skin, and scalp is especially important in controlling the disease. Treatment consists of the application of warm moist compresses to soften the crusts so that they may be removed by gentle rubbing, followed by the application of nitrofurazone (Furacin) or sulfisoxazole (Gantrisin) ointment at bedtime.

Keratitis

Keratitis is an inflammation of the cornea and appears in several different forms; its cause may not always be known. Interstitial keratitis frequently accompanies congenital syphilis. Allergies, viral infections, and diseases such as smallpox or nerve disorders can be causative factors. Keratitis causes pain, sensitivity to light, lacrimation, eyelid spasms, and redness with inflammation. The disease is always serious because it may result in scars on the cornea, and if the scars occur near the pupil, vision will be affected.

Treatment consists of identifying and removing the cause when possible. Antibiotics may be given to treat infection. Hot moist compresses may be employed, with the application of ointments and the use of dark glasses. Present treatment favors the use of cortisone and in some situations the administration of ACTH. Cortisone acetate suspension, 0.5%, may be instilled every hour during the day and 1.5% ointment at night. Hydrocortisone may be administered orally, whereas ACTH is administered intravenously in glucose solution or is given by intramuscular injection. The patient is usually on a regimen of bed rest during the acute stage of the condition, and the eyes are covered to avoid eye movement.

Corneal ulcers

Ulcers on the cornea may result from trachoma, injury, or extension of infection from the conjunctiva and may be present with keratitis. The seriousness of the condition depends on the extent of the ulcer and its location. Superficial ulcers usually heal without complication, but if the ulcer is severe and deep, possibility of perforation is always present, which might be injurious to sight. After healing, a scar will remain, which will interfere with vision if it is near the pupil. Symptoms generally are pain, sensitivity to light, increased lacrimation, and twitching or spasm of certain eye muscles.

Treatment depends on the seriousness of the ulcer. The extent of the ulcer is determined by placing a drop of fluorescein in the conjunctival sac, followed by physiologic saline solution irrigation, which will stain the affected area green. Treatment may consist of instillation of atropine to place the eye at rest, hot compresses to relieve pain, cauterization with silver nitrate or heat, and antibiotic and steroid drugs. Dressings are not used when infected lesions are present, since they favor bacterial growth and limit the flow of discharge from the eye. Corneal ulcers often result in corneal scarring or perforation, which can produce partial or permanent blindness. It has been estimated that these conditions cause 10% of the blindness in the United States.[12]

Corneal transplant (keratoplasty). The corneal transplant operation may be done for certain persons to restore sight. Only the cornea can be used for corneal grafting operations, and the other structures of the eye must function normally. The conditions for which a corneal transplant may be done include scarring as the result of injuries or infection, corneal ulcer, and degeneration of the cornea. Corneal transplants can be done only when a cornea is available that has been willed by a donor or member of his family. The cornea from the deceased person must be removed immediately under aseptic conditions and preserved in a specified way. The ophthalmologist usually has a waiting list, and when the donor cornea is available, the patient is admitted to the hospital immediately because the cornea must be used soon after its removal from the donor.

The postoperative care of the patient is designed to prevent dislocating the graft, the danger of which is great. The patient is returned to his room by stretcher and is carefully lifted by several persons into his bed with his head carefully supported. The patient remains supine with a small pillow under the head and small pillows tucked under on each side to remind him not to turn his head. The foot of the bed may or may not be elevated, and the head of the bed may or may not be slightly elevated, depending on the physician's orders.

The kind of surgical procedure will determine whether one or both eyes are covered, and in some cases they may be left uncovered. Corneal grafts heal slowly because of the lack of blood supply to the area. Infection may occur easily, and strict asepsis must be maintained. The graft will take 3 weeks or more to heal firmly. The amount of activity that is permitted will depend on the procedure and the individual physician. All orders should be clearly written, and the nurse should be sure that they are understood.

Uveitis and iritis

The uveal tract lies between the coats of the eye and includes the ciliary body, iris, and choroid (Fig. 19-4). Inflammation of the uveal tract involving only the iris and the ciliary body is called *iridocyclitis*, but when the choroid is also involved, it is called *uveitis*. Frequently the cornea may be affected; this condition is considered serious and may cause blindness. The inflammation may be from unknown cause, or it may result from diseases such as tuberculosis or syphilis. It may be caused by viruses or by fungi such as *Toxoplasma*. Pain in the eye is a primary symptom, ac-

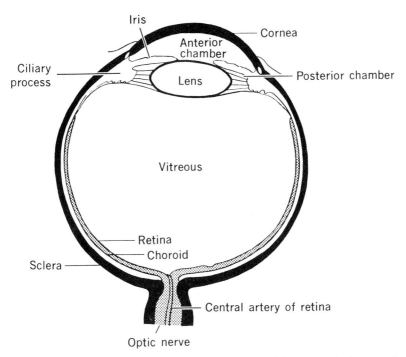

Fig. 19-4. Diagram of the eye showing structures affected by corneal ulcers and uveitis.

companied by sensitivity to light, tearing, disturbance of vision, edema of the upper eyelid, and contraction of the pupil.

Treatment includes keeping the pupil dilated with 1% atropine sulfate. Corticosteroids may be administered, and if a causative organism can be identified, the appropriate therapy is given. Hot moist compresses relieve pain and inflammation, and analgesics may be required for pain. The patient should be on a regimen of bed rest, and the eyes are covered during the acute stage. Dark glasses are worn for protection and sensitivity to light during convalescence.[17]

The nurse should remember that children are more sensitive to atropine than adults are and that poisoning may occur unless care is taken. The nurse should be careful in applying hot compresses to the eye, since the eyelids are particularly sensitive to heat and may be easily burned.

Noninfectious eye disorders
Retrolental fibroplasia

Retrolental fibroplasia is a disease of premature infants caused by excessive use of the oxygen supply in the incubator and is the most frequent cause of blindness in in-

fants. The disease results in partial or total blindness and is seen only in premature infants. The nurse assigned to the premature nursery should be conscious of this relationship and observe very carefully the administration of oxygen to premature babies.

Glaucoma

It has been estimated that one in every eight blind persons in the United States is blind because of glaucoma.[3] The exact incidence of glaucoma is unknown, but it is believed that there may be 1 million persons in the United States with undiagnosed and untreated cases.[6] Glaucoma may occur at any age but is most common in persons 40 years of age and older.

Pathophysiology. Glaucoma may occur as a primary condition without any known cause, or it may be secondary to other disorders such as injuries or infection. In primary glaucoma an inherited predisposition is believed to be a factor.

Glaucoma causes an increase in the intraocular pressure within the eye. Continued pressure may cause damage to the optic nerve. Under normal conditions aqueous humor is formed by the ciliary body and secreted into the posterior chamber from which it flows between the iris and the lens into the anterior chamber. From the anterior chamber it flows through the pupil and drains out over a fine meshwork into the canal of Schlemm located near the angle of the anterior chamber, from which it finally drains into the general circulation. The rate of production of aqueous humor and the outward flow remain constant, and thus normal intraocular pressure is maintained. However, when pathologic changes occur at the angle of the anterior chamber that prevent a normal outflow, the intraocular pressure increases because the balance between production and outflow has been disrupted. There are two types of primary glaucoma: narrow-angle glaucoma and wide-angle glaucoma. Narrow-angle glaucoma results from a narrowing of the angle that leads to the drainage canal. This condition may be acute or chronic. In wide-angle glaucoma the angle is unaffected, but obstruction prevents drainage from the canal. There is no cure for glaucoma, but early diagnosis and treatment will prevent blindness and help to control intraocular pressure.

Symptoms. Acute narrow-angle glaucoma may occur suddenly with nausea, vomiting, dilation of the pupils, pain in the eye, and increase in the intraocular pressure. Without immediate treatment, blindness may occur. Chronic wide-angle glaucoma develops slowly, and the patient may be unaware of any early symptoms. One of the earliest signs is an impairment of peripheral vision. The patient may find that he requires frequent change of glasses, halos appear around lights, vision becomes blurred, there is disturbance of color perception and accommodation to darkness, and the patient complains of fatigue and a tired feeling of the eyes. Chronic glaucoma may appear in one eye, but if untreated, both eyes will become involved.

Treatment and nursing care. The treatment of glaucoma includes the instillation of miotic drugs into the eye. Miotic drugs help to improve drainage of aqueous humor and control intraocular pressure, although they do not cure the condition. Drugs commonly used include pilocarpine in a 1% to 4% solution, eserine salicylate in 25% to 33% solution, and isoflurophate (DFP).

Drugs known as carbonic anhydrase inhibitors are used because they indirectly affect the production of aqueous humor. These drugs include acetazolamide (Diamox) and methazolamide (Neptazane), which are administered orally. When medical treatment fails to control the intraocular pressure, surgery may be done. Any of several surgical procedures may be performed, the objective of which is to provide for the escape of aqueous humor and the reduction of intraocular pressure. In *iridectomy* an incision is made in the iris to provide drainage or to remove an obstruction. *Iridencleisis* is a modified procedure on the iris with the same purpose as iridectomy. In chronic wide-angle glaucoma *corneoscleral trephining* provides a permanent opening between the cornea and the sclera through which the aqueous humor may flow.[6] The patient with glaucoma must remain under medical care, and treatment is continued for life; most patients will be cared for in the ophthalmologist's office. All treatment is planned for the individual patient.

The nurse in the physician's office or in the hospital should be alert for toxic reactions to drugs and should report them. Side effects or toxic reactions may include tingling of the hands, loss of appetite, skin rash, drowsiness, weakness, blood dyscrasias, and central nervous system affection.[4] When a patient is hospitalized, he should have his own individually marked bottles of eyedrops and eyedropper. Extreme care must be taken to be sure that the right medication is given to the right patient. After surgery for glaucoma the patient may be required to remain flat in bed for 24 hours. Analgesics may be given for pain, and the patient may be given a liquid diet. Most patients will be dismissed from the hospital in less than a week.

Persons with glaucoma should wear a Medic Alert tag or carry a card to indicate that they have glaucoma.

Cataract

Pathophysiology. Cataract is a slowly progressive disorder in which there is an opacity of the lens of the eye. Since light must pass through the lens to reach the retina, any opacity will result in impairment of vision. The disorder may occur at any age and may be caused by several conditions. Cataracts are classified as developmental, such as those present at birth (congenital), and degenerative, such as those resulting from aging, injury, allergy, or systemic diseases such as diabetes. Cataract caused by the degenerative changes of aging (senile cataract) develops slowly with advancing years, and patients may be 70 years or older before sight is sufficiently impaired to require surgery. It is believed that there is a hereditary predisposition to senile cataract. A change in the normal metabolism of lens tissue appears to exist. Congenital cataract may be caused by rubella in the mother during the first trimester of pregnancy.

Symptoms caused by cataract may include gradual impairment of vision in varying degrees, blurring, and sensitivity to glare. Some patients may experience double vision and distortions of sight. There is no pain associated with cataract.[9]

Cataract extraction. The only cure for a cataract is surgery, and surgical procedures for the eye have been developed to a high state of perfection. It is no longer necessary to wait for a cataract to mature before its removal. This is determined on an individual basis, dependent on the patient's need for improved vision. If the cataract is present in only one eye and the other eye is normal, surgery may be delayed indefinitely. Generally, senile cataracts are removed when the sight in the better eye is failing and is interfering with the patient's daily routine.

Preoperative care. Most patients admitted to the hospital for surgical removal of cataracts are elderly persons whose vision is impaired in one or both eyes because of the disorder. The patient who has minimal vision may have fears about the success of the surgery and the danger of losing the vision that he has. The nurse caring for the patient should realize that he has poor vision and needs to be oriented to his room and hospital procedures. If the patient feels comfortable and secure in his room and knows what to expect, it will help to relieve his fear and apprehension. Since a metal patch will be worn on one eye and occasionally both eyes after surgery, this should be explained to the patient.

On the day of surgery the patient may or may not be allowed a light breakfast. The male patient is shaved or the woman patient's hair is brushed and combed and, if it is long, braided. Sedative drugs such as barbiturates, tranquilizers, or meperidine hydrochloride may be ordered. The surgical procedure is performed with the patient under local anesthesia.

Postoperative care. With new surgical techniques it is no longer necessary to restrict the patient's activity severely after surgery. Today the average patient can get up and care for himself on the day after surgery, and he is home within a week. He may be on a regimen of bed rest for the first 24 hours, and during this time the head of the bed may be elevated 30 to 45 degrees. The patient should not lie on his operative side. The operated eye is patched and covered with a metal shield for protection. The physician will change the dressings daily. The eye is kept covered for approximately 2 weeks and then covered at night for a period of time.[11] A drop of 1% atropine is instilled daily into the operated eye for 2 weeks, and warm compresses may be used for cleanliness of the eye. The patient is cautioned to avoid straining the eyes and performing heavy work for 4 to 6 weeks after surgery. Reading and light activity are permitted.[9]

After the dressing is removed, the patient should wear dark glasses until temporary lenses are fitted in approximately 3 weeks. Permanent glasses are prescribed in about 2 months. Although they are expensive, plastic cataract lenses can be purchased for the eyeglasses. These lenses can be ground to the edges of the eyeglasses and permit the patient a wider range of vision without distortion.

There are two surgical procedures for the extraction of cataracts: intracapsular extraction, in which the lens is removed within the intact capsule, and extracapsular extraction, in which the capsule is opened and the lens removed through the opening. Intracapsular extraction has become the most common procedure. An enzyme that dissolves the fibers holding the lens in place can be instilled prior to the procedure. This process enables the lens to be lifted out more easily. Other surgical methods such as cryosurgery and ultrasound have proved to be satisfactory methods for cataract removal. Cryosurgery involves inserting a freezing probe into the lens. The lens then reacts and adheres to the probe and is easily removed.[12] The ultrasound technique uses ultrasonic frequencies to emulsify the lens, and it can then be aspirated through a needle inserted through a small incision. In this instance the posterior capsule is left in place.[2]

Retinal detachment

Pathophysiology. The retina is the innermost coat of the eye, and a retinal detachment means that it has become separated from the choroid, the middle coat. Normally the retina and the choroid are in close approximation, although not actually joined together. The choroid provides the blood supply for the retina, and the retina receives the visual stimuli and transmits them to the brain. Injuries, disease, or degeneration may cause small holes or tears to occur in the retina. When this happens, it allows vitreous humor from the large chamber in the back of the eye to seep in between the retina and the choroid, causing the two layers to separate. The blood supply to the retina is reduced, and vision is blurred or lost in that area. Unless the retinal detachment is treated immediately, it will continue to enlarge and become total within 6 months, resulting in blindness in the involved eye.

Symptoms depend on the location and size of the separation. The condition may occur spontaneously with sudden loss of vision, or the person may see flashes of light and have blurring of vision. Often the patient will complain of floaters, which are black spots or lines in his path of vision. One of the first symptoms of vision loss is a shadow appearing in a portion of the visual field of the affected eye. This usually appears in side vision rather than central vision. This is not always immediately recognized by the patient if he has good vision in the opposite eye.[19] Diagnosis and determination of the exact location and extent of the separation is easily made by the ophthalmologist with an ophthalmoscope. Treatment is always surgical.

Preoperative care. Prior to surgery the patient must limit his activities so that the detachment will not become worse. Some patients will be on a regimen of bed rest,

with both eyes patched and positioned so that gravity will help the retina to settle against the choroid. Patching both eyes limits eye movements, which may aggravate the condition. During this period of time the patient must be visited frequently and reassured. Patients must understand the reasons for eye patching, special positioning, and limitation of activity. Elderly patients become apprehensive and confused, especially at night, when they are deprived of their sense of vision. Other patients may be allowed up without eye patches. The physician will order the amount of activity depending on the extent and type of the detachment and the surgery planned.[19]

In case of complications, such as hemorrhage caused by injury to blood vessels in the choroid, surgery may be delayed for several days. However, surgery is usually performed as soon as possible. There are several surgical procedures, and the surgeon will select the one best suited for the patient and the existing disorder. The patient is given a general anesthetic, and the usual preoperative limitation of food and fluids after midnight and breakfast apply. Preoperative medication is administered according to the physician's orders. All instructions concerning care of the patient should be clearly written and understood. This is especially important regarding positioning of the patient both preoperatively and postoperatively.

The patient with retinal detachment may be frightened and apprehensive. The nurse should try to spend some time with the patient and not leave him alone for long periods. A sympathetic understanding of how the patient feels can do much to relieve his anxiety. The nurse should be able to provide comfort, encouragement, and reassurance. If the patient asks questions that the nurse cannot answer, they should be referred to the physician.

In general, existing surgical procedures involve approximating the retina against the choroid and then initiating a treatment that will produce a chorioretinal adhesion, which will seal the holes. The adhesion is usually produced through the use of electrical diathermy, freezing (cryosurgery), or photocoagulation with a laser beam, which will produce burns in the choroid.[12]

Postoperative care. When the patient returns from surgery, both eyes will be bandaged. The patient is required to remain on a regimen of bed rest for 2 days or more. The patient is positioned according to the surgeon's orders, usually so that the area of detachment is in a downward position. The patient is encouraged to exercise the extremities. By the second postoperative day the bandage may be removed from the unaffected eye and the patient allowed to be up in a chair and have bathroom privileges. Cyclopentolate hydrochloride (Cyclogyl hydrochloride), 1%, or atropine, 1%, is used daily for 10 to 14 days to reduce inflammation and dilate the pupil. The same precautions as for cataract surgery should be taken to provide a safe environment for the patient. The patient may be dismissed to his home by the third postoperative day. There will be edema and discoloration about the affected eye, and the patient should be advised to use warm moist compresses several times a day to soften and remove secretions and crusts that form about the eyelashes. At home patients must avoid rapid jolting movements. Light activity and watching television is permitted, but reading is avoided for approximately 2 weeks. The patient is instructed to return to his surgeon in about 10 days and thereafter at frequent intervals for examination. Not all retinal detachments will be corrected by the surgery; surgery may have to be repeated for some patients, and others may develop new areas of detachment.[9]

Injuries to the eye

Injuries to the eye may be the result of foreign bodies, thermal or chemical burns, abrasions, and lacerations or penetrating wounds. Neither the nurse nor the patient can assess the damage resulting from an injury to the eye; therefore all injuries should be seen by the ophthalmologist. If the injury is slight, nothing has been lost, but if it is serious, immediate medical care may mean saving vision or even the eye.

Foreign bodies

Irritation by foreign bodies is one of the most common types of injury and may be from dust particles, loose eyelashes, or cinders, which may lodge in the conjunctiva or become embedded in the cornea. Foreign bodies under the upper lid may cause irritation of the cornea from the movement of the lid and result in considerable discomfort to the patient. Some foreign bodies that have been in the eye only a short time may be removed by gentle irrigation of the eye with physiologic saline solution. A cotton swab dipped in physiologic saline solution may be used to remove a foreign body on the conjunctiva. The patient should be instructed to look up, and the lower lid may be pulled down and the conjunctival sac examined. If the foreign body is under the upper lid, the lid should be everted over a match or applicator. Any person with a foreign body in the eye that cannot be easily removed or that has been in the eye for some time should be examined by the ophthalmologist.

Burns

Burns may be caused by acids, alkalies, hot metal, flashes from acetylene blowtorches, or exposure to the ultraviolet rays of the sun. Whatever the cause, the burn must be considered an emergency. If chemicals are accidentally splashed into the eye, prolonged washing of the eye with plain tap water should be initiated immediately. This first aid measure will prevent formation of permanent scar tissue more effectively than any other treatment. The eyelids should be separated and cool water poured gently over the eyeball for 15 to 20 minutes. Medical care should then be sought. Persons suffering burns caused by heat such as flash burns, burns from overexposure to the sun, and burns from fireworks should be taken immediately to the ophthalmologist. No home or first-aid treatment should be attempted.

Abrasions and lacerations

Superficial abrasions have numerous causes; although painful at the time, they usually do no serious harm. If the abrasion is deep, scarring may result. Antibiotics are generally used to prevent infection, and the eye may be covered with a pad. Lacerations of the eyelids are not serious and are treated like lacerations elsewhere. However, laceration of the eyeball may be extremely serious because it may affect vision and sometimes results in loss of the eye.

Penetrating wounds

Penetrating wounds are especially serious, since they invariably introduce infection into the eye and may destroy eye structures. One child's eye was injured by a hatpin that was thrust into it by another child while playing. Total blindness in the eye resulted, and it was eventually removed. All penetrating injuries of the eye should be treated immediately by the ophthalmologist. Usually it is easy to recognize that an eye has been perforated, although not always. The iris of the eye often will move to plug the wound, resulting in an irregular pupil. Tiny wounds such as caused by a needle or thorn often are self-sealing and cannot be seen. The possibility of infection is high, and occasionally the infection can spread out of the eye and even have fatal consequences. Some wounds can be repaired surgically if the area is clean and relatively free of contamination. If the wound is extensive, enucleation is indicated.[8]

Eye enucleation. Eye enucleation, the surgical removal of the eyeball, may be necessitated because of a severe injury, the need to relieve pain when the patient is blind, the presence of malignant tumors, or for cosmetic purposes when the patient has been blinded from injury or disease. The surgery may include the removal of the entire eyeball, only the contents of the eyeball, or the eyeball and all the related structures.

The preoperative care of the patient is routine. The way the patient feels about the surgery will depend to a large extent on the reason for the surgery and the way he feels about blindness. When a malignancy is present, the nurse may expect that the patient will be depressed and worried. A sympathetic, understanding approach to the patient is essential. Although he may be assured that a prosthesis may be used, an overly optimistic attitude should be avoided. However, when surgery is done to relieve pain, the patient may look forward to its relief, and his emotional reaction will be one of optimism.

When the patient returns from surgery, he will have a pressure dressing over the eye socket. The patient should be observed for any evidence of hemorrhage, pain on the affected side of the head, and headache,

which should be reported immediately. Usually the patient is allowed out of bed and may be ambulatory on the first postoperative day. As soon as the eye socket has healed, generally after 4 to 6 weeks, the patient may begin wearing an artificial eye. Before leaving the hospital the patient should be instructed in the use and care of the prosthesis, care of the eye socket, and protection of the good eye from undue strain.[17]

NURSING THE PATIENT WITH DISEASES AND DISORDERS OF THE EAR
External ear

Certain disorders of the external ear may affect hearing and cause pain and discomfort. Common disorders include infection, obstructions, injury, and perforation of the eardrum. (See Fig. 19-5.)

Infections

Boils are a common type of infection and may be extremely painful. Large boils may obstruct the auditory canal and cause impairment of hearing. They have a tendency to recur unless properly treated. The infectious agents are usually staphylococcal bacteria, which gain entrance to the subcutaneous tissue through a scratch or injury that may occur in removing wax or a foreign body. Relief may be obtained by the application of nonsterile warm compresses, a hot-water bottle, or an electric heating pad. Treatment may include instillation of drops containing antibiotics or cortisone. Also, a solution of aluminum acetate, known as Burow's solution, may be dropped into the auditory canal. If the infection extends to the regional lymph nodes, oral or intramuscular administration of antibiotics may be required. Drugs such as aspirin or codeine may be needed to relieve pain for patients with severe infection.

Other types of infections include those caused by fungi, which are rather uncommon. Various forms of dermatitis may occur, particularly in persons with diabetes. Other generalized infections such as erysipelas or eczema may involve the external ear.

Obstructions

Children frequently put foreign objects into their ears that obstruct the auditory

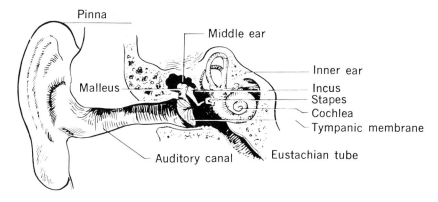

Fig. 19-5. Diagram of the ear.

canal. Parents and nurses should not attempt to remove foreign bodies because of the danger of pushing them farther into the canal. When the foreign body consists of vegetable matter such as corn, peas, or beans, which children are likely to put into the ear, irrigation should not be done. A common cause of obstruction is the accumulation of cerumen (wax), which may plug the canal. Sometimes it pushes against the eardrum and hardens, causing irritation of the drum and pain. Insects such as flies occasionally gain entrance to the canal and cause temporary discomfort. An insect in the auditory canal can generally be removed by instilling a few drops of warm oil to kill the insect and then irrigating with warm water.

Injury

Injury to the external ear may result from many causes and consists of contusions, abrasions, or lacerations. Occasionally there is loss of the pinna without interference with hearing. However, the congenital absence of the pinna may include absence of the canal and eardrum, resulting in total deafness in the ear.

Perforation

Perforation of the eardrum may occur as a result of a fracture of the skull or a severe blow to the ear. It may result from otitis media (infection in the middle ear) in which there is a spontaneous rupture of the drum, with accompanying deafness, dizziness, nausea, and vomiting. Medical care should be secured to avoid or prevent spread of the infection.

Middle ear

The middle ear is connected with the posterior part of the nose by the eustachian tube. Equalization of air pressure on both sides of the eardrum is maintained by air entering the middle ear through this tube. Infection from the nose and throat may reach the middle ear through the eustachian tube. Sometimes the tube may become inflamed or plugged with mucus, resulting in diminished hearing. The middle ear contains the organs for transmitting sound to the inner ear, and if they become diseased, deafness may result.

Otitis media

Infection may enter the middle ear through the eustachian tube as the result of acute upper respiratory infections or infectious diseases such as measles or scarlet fever. Children are more susceptible to otitis media because during the early years of life, the eustachian tube is more horizontal than in later years. This favors the conduction of infection from the respiratory passageways into the middle ear. The infection may cause the formation of an abscess, and the condition is then called *purulent otitis media.* The eardrum becomes red and swollen, and there is severe pain in the ear, with fever and impairment of hearing. The parent may often suspect the disease in infants or young children when crying is accompanied by pulling at the ear and rolling the head from side to side.

Since the mucous membrane lining the middle ear is continuous with parts of the mastoid process, the added danger of extension of the infection into the mastoid cells is always present.

Treatment and nursing care. The patient with acute purulent otitis media is usually on a regimen of bed rest and given penicillin or broad-spectrum antibiotics for a week. The eardrum may rupture from the pressure in the middle ear, or the physician may incise the drum, which is called *paracentesis*, or *myringotomy*. A light general anesthetic is usually necessary when myringotomy is done. Drainage from the ear is generally bloody at first but becomes purulent. Small tissues should be used to remove the drainage, or cotton should be placed loosely at the external opening of the auditory canal. Cotton should not be placed in the canal, since it would obstruct the flow of drainage. The area about the external ear should be kept clean, since the drainage will cause severe irritation if allowed to remain on the skin. After myringotomy the temperature drops and the pain is usually relieved. However, if medication for pain is needed, aspirin is generally given. Purulent otitis media is often caused by the streptococcus or staphylococcus organism, and the appropriate antibiotic is administered. Unless proper treatment is given, the condition may become chronic, and the individual may have a draining ear for months or even years. The patient should be protected from chilling and observed for an increase in pain or temperature, which may indicate need for additional incision or may be a sign of extension of the infection.

Mastoiditis

Mastoiditis is a complication of acute purulent otitis media. Sometimes the infection may extend to the brain, with the formation of brain abscess or the development of meningitis. The infection from the mastoid cells may drain away through the auditory canal. However, if this does not occur, the cells will be destroyed. Symptoms associated with acute mastoiditis are elevation of temperature, increased pain, and tenderness over the mastoid area. There may be swelling, which tends to push the ear forward.

Mastoidectomy. Usually a myringotomy and large doses of antibiotics will cure the condition. If bone destruction has occurred, a simple mastoidectomy may be necessary. Before the development of antibiotics, acute purulent otitis media and acute mastoiditis were common occurrences. However, because of antibiotic drugs, these diseases occur less often today.

Preoperative care. The preoperative care of the patient having a mastoidectomy is the same as that for other surgical patients. A careful explanation should be given to women patients concerning removal of hair, and only the necessary amount of hair should be removed. An area of approximately 1½ to 2 inches around the ear is shaved.

Postoperative care. When the patient returns from surgery, the ear will be covered with a large pressure dressing secured with bandages about the head. When the patient has recovered from anesthesia, he may be placed in semi-Fowler's position. As soon as nausea subsides, oral fluids and diet as tolerated by the patient may be given. Fluids may be administered by the intravenous route if nausea is persistent. Medication is given to relieve pain as necessary. Temperature, pulse, and respiration rates are taken every 4 hours and recorded. Some drainage may occur through the dressing; if necessary, the nurse may reinforce the dressing, but the dressing is changed only by the physician. Antibiotics are usually ordered as indicated.

The patient should be observed for evidence of hemorrhage, which might appear as bright red blood on the dressing. Stiffness of the neck may occur from positioning during surgery, but if stiffness is accompanied by headache, visual disturbance, or signs of facial paralysis, it should be reported to the physician.

Otosclerosis

The middle ear contains three little bones that function in transmitting sound to the inner ear (p. 455). Normally the stapes vibrates against the oval window through which sound reaches the inner ear. In otosclerosis a new growth of bone forms, causing the footplate of the stapes to become fixed in the oval window, preventing it from transmitting sound. Otosclerosis is the most common cause of conductive deafness. The cause of otosclerosis is unknown, but it is believed that there is a hereditary predisposition to the disorder. The loss of hearing may first be detected during the teen years and may be discovered through audiometer testing. Usually the loss affects both ears, although one may be more severely involved than the other. The hearing impairment continues to increase slowly until the person reaches 40 years of age or older, by which time the loss may be great. There is no medical treatment that will cure the disorder or impede its progress. A surgical procedure called *stapedectomy* will restore hearing in approximately 90% of patients.[9]

Stapedectomy. Stapedectomy represents one of the most significant advances in ear surgery. Surgical procedures preceding stapedectomy included stapes mobilization and fenestration, but both provided only temporary restoration of hearing. Today stapedectomy is considered the treatment of choice for otosclerosis. In this procedure the stapes is removed and replaced by a piece of small wire or a plastic piston. This is attached to a graft of fat, vein, or Gelfoam, which covers the oval window. Occasionally, the footplate of the stapes will be left in place and the prosthesis placed through it. Sound then travels from the incus to the wire or plastic piece, which vibrates the tissues of the oval window. Liquids of the inner ear then pick up the vibrations, and nerve impulses are initiated.

Preoperative care. Preoperative preparation of the patient is essentially the same as that for other surgery. The patient should be advised to wash the hair before entering the hospital to avoid the danger of getting water into the ear after surgery. The patient should be given an explanation of the surgery and know what to expect postoperatively.

Postoperative care. Postoperatively the patient is kept flat in bed for the first 24 hours and should not blow his nose or watch television; head movement should be kept at a minimum. After 24 hours the patient may be allowed up but should not get up alone. He should rise slowly, keeping the head level, and should walk slowly with the head and torso in line. There will be a dressing and packing in the auditory canal. Slight drainage may appear on the dressing, but any bright red blood

should be reported. The patient should be carefully observed for signs that might indicate complications such as meningitis or facial paralysis. Symptoms that should be reported if observed include dryness of the mouth, bitter taste, headache, stiffness of the neck, nausea and vomiting, vertigo, disturbance of gait, and a sensation of sloshing in the ear, which may indicate a collection of serous fluid in the middle ear.

The patient may be dismissed from the hospital in 3 or 4 days, and hearing may be expected to return in about 3 weeks. The patient should be advised to avoid getting water in the ear and told how to maintain a sterile technique in changing dressings.[7]

Inner ear
Labyrinthitis

The labyrinth is a system of cavities within the inner ear that communicate with one another. Labyrinthitis is an inflammation of these structures, usually resulting from an extension of infection from the middle ear. The characteristic symptom is severe dizziness, causing a disturbance of equilibrium. In patients with severe cases nausea and vomiting may occur, and there is generally some impairment of hearing.

Treatment and nursing care. The condition is usually treated with antibiotic drugs. The patient is on a regimen of bed rest, and side rails should be placed on the bed. The patient should be instructed not to get up without assistance because of the danger of falling. If nausea and vomiting are severe, intravenous fluids and antiemetic drugs to control vomiting may be administered.

Ménière's syndrome

The symptoms of Ménière's syndrome result from an increase in the endolymph, which causes an increased pressure in the inner ear. An imbalance of the autonomic nervous system results in a spasm of the internal auditory artery, causing the increased pressure. However, the cause is unknown, and there is no specific treatment.

The major symptom is severe vertigo, which is the sensation of seeing and feeling motion that is not present. There may be nausea and vomiting, ringing in the ears, and ultimately loss of hearing.

Treatment and nursing care. The nursing care of the patient should provide for safety by placing side rails on the bed. The symptoms cause the patient anxiety, apprehension, and distress, and any movement may increase the severity of his symptoms. The nurse should explain all procedures to the patient and allow him to move in a way that causes him the least discomfort. Since the appetite is poor, the patient may need encouragement to eat. In severe prolonged attacks intravenous fluids may be administered.

Although some patients may respond to medical treatment, others do not. The patient is usually advised to avoid smoking and may be placed on a low-sodium diet to help control edema. Vitamins have provided relief for some older patients, and meclizine (Bonine) and nicotinic acid have been effective in relieving symptoms in others.

Surgery may be performed to relieve the severe vertigo. If there is considerable hearing loss in the affected ear, and if hearing in one ear is not affected, the destruction of the membranous labyrinth may be done. This type of surgery results in permanent deafness in the ear. When the loss of hearing is minimal, ultrasonic surgery may relieve symptoms and preserve hearing. Bell's palsy may complicate ultrasonic surgery but will clear in several weeks.[6]

Summary outline

1. Structure and function of the eye and ear
   A. The eye—highly specialized sense organ
      1. Coats—sclera, choroid, and retina
      2. Iris—colored part, pupil in center
      3. Lens—behind pupil
      4. Vitreous humor—fills large chamber behind eye
      5. Aqueous humor—fills chambers in front of eye
      6. Extrinsic and intrinsic muscles control movement and hold eye in position
      7. Accessory organs—eyebrows, eyelids, eyelashes, conjunctiva, lacrimal glands and ducts, and sebaceous glands
      8. Visual center in brain
   B. The ear—specialized organ for hearing
      1. External parts—auditory canal, pinna, and tympanic membrane
      2. Middle ear—contains oval and round windows, malleus, incus, and stapes
      3. Inner ear—bony labyrinth, cochlea, semicircular canals, membranous laby-

rinth contains saccule and utricle; fluids in inner ear are endolymph and perilymph
      4. Auditory center for hearing in temporal lobe of cerebrum
2. Diagnostic tests and procedures
   A. Complete physical examination
   B. Eye examinations to determine acuity of vision and eye disease
      1. Snellen eye chart—commonly used screening examination
      2. Tonometry—measurement of intraocular pressure
      3. Ophthalmoscope—instrument to permit visualization of inside of eye
      4. Slit lamp—permits visualization of minute structures of eye
   C. Hearing tests
      1. Voice test—uses whispered or spoken voice and is used as screening test
      2. Audiometer—measures hearing in both pitch and intensity and is both quantitative and qualitative measurement of hearing
      3. Tuning forks—helpful in determining type of hearing loss
      4. Testing hearing in young children
3. Loss of sight
   A. Blindness—may be congenital or acquired
      1. Caused by diseases, poisons, injury, excessive use of oxygen in premature nursery
4. Loss of hearing
   A. Hearing loss—may be congenital or acquired
      1. Classification
         a. Hard-of-hearing
         b. Deaf
      2. Types
         a. Sensorineural (nerve deafness)
         b. Conductive
      3. Hearing aids—contain three parts
         a. Microphone
         b. Amplifier
         c. Receiver
5. Refractive errors of the eye
   A. Refraction—bending of light rays entering eye so that they fall on retina; term also applies to fitting glasses to correct error of refraction
   B. Myopia (nearsightedness)—defect in which light rays focus too soon, or in front of retina
      1. Distant vision will be blurred
      2. Myopia may become progressively worse in young persons
   C. Hyperopia (farsightedness)—defect in which point of focus is behind retina
      1. Near vision will be blurred
      2. Testing with Snellen eye chart may not show condition
   D. Astigmatism—irregularity in curvature of cornea or lens so that all light rays do not bend equally
   E. Strabismus (crossing of eyes)—may be congenital or acquired
      1. Convergent strabismus—eye turns toward nose

2. Divergent strabismus—eye turns outward
3. Classification
   a. Paralytic strabismus—when nerve is damaged
   b. Nonparalytic strabismus—inherited disorder
4. Treatment may be both medical and surgical

F. Contact lenses
1. Eyes should be examined by ophthalmologist to rule out disease
2. Contact lens is small, thin, polished plastic disk that is held in place in eye by capillary attraction and the upper eyelid

6. Color blindness is most commonly red-green blindness
   A. May be congenital or acquired, partial or complete

7. Specific aspects of nursing patient with diseases and disorders of eye and ear
   A. Instillation of eyedrops and ointments
   B. Eye and ear irrigations
   C. Hot or iced compresses
   D. Absolute cleanliness of hands and equipment

8. Nursing the patient with diseases and disorders of the eye
   A. Inflammatory and infectious eye disorders
      1. Styes (hordeola)—small boils or abscesses from infection of hair follicle
         a. May become chronic with frequent recurrence
      2. Conjunctivitis—inflammation of conjunctiva of eye
         a. Acute purulent conjunctivitis ("pinkeye")—may occur as epidemic among schoolchildren
         b. Gonorrheal conjunctivitis—occurs in newborn as ophthalmia neonatorum, in adult as gonorrheal ophthalmia
         c. Trachoma—chronic inflammation of conjunctiva with formation of granules on eyelids; progresses slowly; will ultimately lead to blindness unless treated
      3. Blepharitis—chronic inflammatory process involving margin of eyelids
      4. Keratitis—inflammation of cornea
         a. Interstitial keratitis frequently accompanies congenital syphilis
         b. May result in scar formation near pupil, thus affecting vision
      5. Corneal ulcers—always serious because perforation may occur
         a. Corneal transplant (keratoplasty)—involves only cornea
            (1) Corneal grafts can be done only when cornea is available
            (2) Postoperative care must prevent dislocating graft
      6. Uveitis and iritis—inflammation of uveal tract; may involve all or part of tract
         a. Iridocyclitis—only iris and ciliary body involved
         b. Uveitis—iris, ciliary body, and choroid involved

   c. Condition serious and may cause blindness
   B. Noninfectious eye disorders
      1. Retrolental fibroplasia—disease of premature infants caused by excessive use of oxygen; results in partial or total blindness
      2. Glaucoma
         a. Is characteristic of persons 40 years of age and older
         b. Pathophysiology
            Involves flow of aqueous humor outward from anterior chamber of eye; causes increased intraocular pressure
            (1) Narrow-angle type
            (2) Wide-angle type
            (3) May be primary or secondary
            (4) Cause is unknown
         c. Symptoms
         d. Treatment and nursing care
            (1) Medical treatment with miotics and carbonic anhydrase inhibitors
            (2) Surgical procedures—iridectomy, iridencleisis, or corneoscleral trephining
            (3) Without treatment blindness will occur; there is no cure
      3. Cataract
         a. Pathophysiology
            (1) Slowly progressive disorder causing opacity of lens of eye
            (2) Results in impairment of vision
            (3) Classified as developmental and degenerative
            (4) Senile cataract occurring after 70 years of age is most common form and results from normal aging process
         b. Only cure is surgery by cataract extraction, which is determined on individual basis
            (1) Preoperative preparation—orient to room, provide safe environment, give emotional support, eyedrops, preoperative medication
            (2) Postoperative care—patient may be out of bed on operative day and care for self
            (3) Intracapsular extraction is most common procedure
      4. Retinal detachment
         a. Pathophysiology—separation of retina from choroid
         b. Retinal detachment is corrected by surgical procedure, dependent on extent of detachment
            (1) Wide variation exists in what patient is permitted to do; nurse must have clearly defined orders for care, especially positioning
            (2) Both eyes bandaged; preoperative and postoperative care must be given to patient
            (3) Ambulation depends on type of surgery done

(4) Surgery not always successful; may have to be repeated
9. Injuries to the eye
   A. Irritation by foreign bodies—among most common types of injury and may be caused by dust, loose eyelashes, or cinders
   B. Burns—may be caused by acids, alkalies, hot metal, flashes from acetylene blowtorches, and exposure to ultraviolet rays of sun
      1. Should be considered an emergency
      2. Acid burns may be irrigated with weak solution of sodium bicarbonate
      3. Alkali burns may be irrigated with boric acid solution
      4. Tap water may be used
   C. Abrasions and lacerations may be extremely serious and may affect vision or result in loss of eye
   D. Penetrating wounds are especially serious because they introduce infection
      1. Eye enucleation may be necessary because of injury, pain, malignant tumors, or for cosmetic purposes
         a. Surgery may include removal of eyeball, contents of eyeball, or eyeball and all related structures
         b. Preoperative preparation routine; provide emotional support
         c. Postoperative care—observe for hemorrhage, pain in eye, or headache
            (1) May be out of bed first postoperative day
            (2) Prosthesis may be used in 4 to 6 weeks
            (3) Teach patient care of prosthesis
10. Nursing the patient with diseases and disorders of the ear
    A. External ear
       1. Infections
          a. Boils in auditory canal are common type of infection and may recur unless properly treated
          b. Fungus infections occur rarely
          c. Various forms of dermatitis may cause infection of external ear
       2. Obstructions
          a. May be caused by children putting foreign objects into ear
          b. Frequent cause is accumulation of wax in ear
       3. Injury may result from contusions, abrasions, and lacerations
       4. Perforation of eardrum may result from skull fracture, severe blow on ear, or otitis media
    B. Middle ear—affected by infections reaching it through eustachian tube from nose and throat
       1. Otitis media (purulent)
          a. Formation of abscess in middle ear
          b. Danger of extension of infection to mastoid process
          c. Treatment and nursing care
             (1) Bed rest
             (2) Eardrum may rupture sponta-

neously, or otologist may incise it to permit drainage
       2. Mastoiditis—complication of acute purulent otitis media; surgery may be necessary
          a. Mastoidectomy
             (1) Preoperative care same as that for other surgical patients
             (2) Postoperative care—observe for hemorrhage, headache, visual disturbance, or signs of facial paralysis
       3. Otosclerosis
          a. New growth of bone causing footplate of stapes to become fixed in oval window, preventing sound from reaching inner ear
          b. There is no medical treatment
          c. Surgery will restore hearing in 90% of persons
       4. Stapedectomy—treatment of choice for otosclerosis
          a. Preoperative care same as that for other surgery
          b. Postoperative care
             (1) Patient flat in bed for 24 hours; keep head movement at a minimum
             (2) Ambulation after 24 hours
             (3) Observe for hemorrhage or signs of facial paralysis and meningitis
             (4) Dismissed from hospital in 3 or 4 days; advised not to get water into ear
    C. Inner ear
       1. Labyrinthitis—inflammatory condition of inner ear that may result from extension of infection from middle ear
          a. Treatment usually with antibiotics and bed rest
       2. Ménière's syndrome—caused by increased pressure in inner ear
          a. Severe vertigo is primary symptom
          b. Safety should be provided for patient
          c. Treatment may be medical or surgical

Review questions

1. What is another name for the eardrum?
   a.
2. What is the cause of retrolental fibroplasia in premature infants?
   a.
3. What type of deafness may occur when the auditory nerve is damaged?
   a.
4. What are the three parts of a hearing aid?
   a.
   b.
   c.
5. What are two miotic drugs used to treat glaucoma, and what is their action?
   a.

b.

c.

6. What activities should the patient avoid after surgery for cataract?

a.

b.

7. What are four symptoms that may occur with a retinal detachment?

a.

b.

c.

d.

8. What part of the ear is involved when the patient has otosclerosis?

a.

9. What is the most common procedure for cataract extraction?

a.

10. What emotional reactions would the nurse expect of a patient with retinal detachment?

a.

b.

c.

Films

1. Communication with deaf-blind people (18 min., sound, color, 16 mm.), American Foundation for the Blind, Inc., 15 West 16th St., New York, N. Y. 10011. A demonstration through actual conversation with six blind-deaf people, using the five most commonly used methods of communicating with deaf-blind individuals.

2. Errors of refraction—No. 9154 (21 min., sound, color, 16 mm.), Abbott Laboratories, Abbott Park, North Chicago, Ill. 60064, Professional Services D-384. Illustrates the principles involved in the optical properties of lenses and the refraction errors of the eye. Shows the anatomy of the normal eye and the formation of the image on the retina.

3. Glaucoma—diagnosis and treatment—C-15 (28 min., sound, color, 16 mm.), Film Library, Lederle Laboratories, American Cyanamid Co., Pearl River, N. Y. 10965. Describes the basic physiology of the eye, the flow of aqueous humor, and intraocular pressure. Shows closed-angle glaucoma and simple glaucoma. Discusses treatment by reduction of the intraocular pressure. The use of drugs and the surgical procedure for glaucoma are discussed.

4. The glaucomas (23 min., sound, color, 16 mm., free loan), Prevention of Blindness, Public Information Department, 79 Madison Ave., New York, N. Y. 10016. Describes the mechanism of glaucoma, diagnostic tests, and medical and surgical treatment.

5. Special eye care (for burns)—M-1689-X (11 min., sound, color, 16 mm.), Media Research Branch, National Medical Audiovisual Center (Annex), Station K, Atlanta, Ga. 30324. Demonstrates special eye care of patients suffering second and third degree burns of the face. Shows nursing techniques and procedures before and after burn surgery to prevent eye infection and corneal ulceration.

6. When you meet a blind man (13 min., sound, black and white, 16 mm.), American Foundation for the Blind, Inc., 15 West 15th St., New York, N. Y. 10011. Gives some specific do's and don't's.

References

1. Anthony, Catherine P., and Kolthoff, Norma J.: Textbook of anatomy and physiology, ed. 9, St. Louis, 1975, The C. V. Mosby Co.
2. Arnott, Eric J.: Ultrasonic techniques for removing cataractous lens, Nursing Mirror 136:27-28, Feb. 2, 1973.
3. A special word about cataract and glaucoma, The Journal of Practical Nursing 19:26-28, Feb., 1969.
4. Bledsoe, C. Warren, and Williams, Russell C.: The vision needed to nurse the blind, American Journal of Nursing 66:2432-2435, Nov., 1966.
5. Brueggen, Stella L.: Contact lens, American Journal of Nursing 65:92-95, Sept., 1965.
6. Brunner, Lillian S., and Suddarth, Doris S.: Textbook of medical-surgical nursing, ed. 3, Philadelphia, 1975, J. B. Lippincott Co.
7. Delaney, Ramona E.: Stapedectomy, American Journal of Nursing 69:2406-2409, Nov., 1969.
8. Elkington, A. R.: Perforating wounds, Nursing Times 69:1597-1598, Nov. 29, 1973.
9. Havener, William H., Saunders, William H., Keith, Carol F., and Prescott, Ardra W.: Nursing care in eye, ear, nose and throat disorders, St. Louis, 1974, The C. V. Mosby Co.
10. Leavell, Lutie C., Miller, Marjorie A., and Chapin, Florence M.: Anatomy and physiology, ed. 15, New York, 1966, The Macmillan Co.
11. Ledney, Donna: Understanding the cataract patient, Bedside Nurse 5:10-12, Dec., 1972.
12. Luckmann, Joan, and Sorensen, Karen C.: Medical-surgical nursing, a psychophysiologic approach, Philadelphia, 1974, W. B. Saunders Co.
13. Moore, Mary V.: Diagnosis: deafness, American Journal of Nursing 69:297-300, Feb., 1969.
14. Nilo, Ernest R.: Needs of the hearing impaired, American Journal of Nursing 69:115-116, Jan., 1969.
15. Ruben, Montague: Contact lenses, shells and prosthetics, Nursing Times 68:133-136, Feb. 3, 1972.
16. Rubin, Jack A.: Deafness and its management, The Canadian Nurse 62:32-34, Aug., 1966.
17. Shafer, Kathleen N., Sawyer, Janet R., McCluskey, Audrey M., Beck, Edna L., and Phipps, Wilma J.: Medical-surgical nursing, ed. 6, St. Louis, 1975, The C. V. Mosby Co.
18. Smith, Dorothy W., Germain, Carol P. Hanley, and Gips, Claudia D.: Care of the adult patient, ed. 2, Philadelphia, 1971, J. B. Lippincott Co.
19. Smith, Joan F. and Nachazel, Delbert P.: Retinal detachment, American Journal of Nursing 73:1530-1535, Sept., 1973.

Nursing the patient with diseases and disorders of the skin

KEY WORDS

antipruritic	macule
atrophy	nodule
autograft	papule
bleb	pruritus
comedones	pustule
crust	scale
debridement	scar
dermatologist	sebaceous
dermis	seborrhea
eschar	sebum
excoriation	ulcer
fissure	vesicle
gumma·	vesiculation
heterograft	wheal
homograft	

STRUCTURE AND FUNCTION OF THE SKIN

The skin is the largest organ of the body and is often referred to as the *integumentary system* (Fig. 20-1). It is considered an organ because of its physiologic structure and its many functions. The skin is usually thought of as having two distinct layers: the *epidermis* and the *dermis;* however, a third layer of tissue (subcutaneous tissue) may be included because of its function in helping to protect other body tissues. The epidermis is the outermost layer, and it actually has four layers or regions, sometimes called *strata.* The three outermost regions consist of dead cells that are constantly being pushed to the surface and shed, while new cells are being developed in the innermost region. The principal substance of the outside layer of the epidermis is *keratin,* which provides a waterproof covering and has a slightly acid reaction. Earlier in this book, reference was made to the acidity of the skin as a barrier to invading pathogens. The epidermis also contains the pigment *melanin,* which provides the coloring of the skin. There are no blood vessels in the epidermis, thus it receives its nourishment and fluids through seepage of lymph from blood vessels below.

The dermis, or true skin, is closely attached to the epidermis and consists of two layers: the uppermost layer (superficial layer), which contains small elevations that project upward into the epidermis, and the reticular, or deeper, layer, which contains numerous capillary blood vessels and nerve fibers. (This is why bleeding and

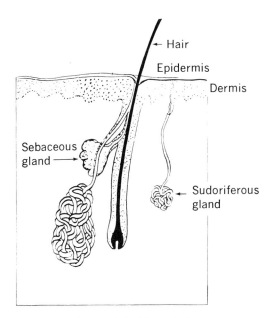

Fig. 20-1. Normal skin.

tion of water from the skin surface. The vernix caseosa seen on the newborn infant is an accumulation of sebum from the sebaceous glands.

The sudoriferous glands originate as blind coiled tubes with ducts that ultimately open on the surface of the skin as pores. The sweat glands are distributed over the entire body but are more numerous on the forehead, palms of the hands, and soles of the feet. The sweat glands are important because they function in regulating body heat through evaporation of water from the skin surface.

The hair and nails are subordinate to the skin. The appearance of the nails will change during illness, and they may become brittle and easily broken, whereas in old age they may be rough and thickened.

The skin functions as a sense organ, it provides a protective covering, it serves as an organ of excretion, it helps to regulate body temperature and provides information about the environment, and it contributes to the psychologic and mental health of the individual.

Because of the numerous nerve endings in the skin, its function as a sense organ is of primary importance. Through the sense of touch the nurse is able to count the patient's pulse, touch the patient's skin and know if it is hot or cool, determine the presence of a draft in the patient's environment, or determine if his room is too warm and in need of improved ventilation. Earlier in the book it was stated that the unbroken skin is the first line of defense against pathogenic organisms, and Fig. 2-2 showed what happens when the skin is broken and pathogens gain entrance to the body. The skin protects deeper tissues from injury and loss of body fluids. The excretory function of the skin is limited, but one of its most important functions is to help regulate body temperature. This is accomplished in two ways: (1) evaporation of sweat from the body and (2) dissipation of excess heat into the air when blood vessels dilate, bringing more blood and thus increased heat to the skin surface.

In health or disease the normal skin tells many things about an individual, and in many situations it may provide valuable diagnostic clues to disease. Nursing personnel should routinely observe the color of

pain occur when a person pricks a finger.) Some of the nerve fibers have receptors for hot and cold, others for touch and pressure, and some are concerned with vasodilation and vasoconstriction. The dermis also contains the sweat glands (sudoriferous glands) and sebaceous, or oil, glands. All the structures are held together by fibrous and elastic connective tissue. The elasticity of this tissue decreases with the aging process, causing the skin to take on a wrinkled appearance.

Beneath the dermis is a layer of subcutaneous tissue, also called *superficial fascia*. The subcutaneous tissue, closely adherent to the dermis, provides support and through small arteries and lymphatics maintains a blood supply to the dermis. Subcutaneous tissue contains large amounts of fat and some sweat glands. The thickness of the skin varies on different parts of the body, and the amount of subcutaneous tissue also varies over the body.

The nails, hair, and sebaceous and sudoriferous glands and their ducts are appendages of the skin.

The sebaceous glands secrete an oily substance called *sebum*, which keeps the hair from becoming brittle. The gland may open into a hair follicle or may open onto the skin. The oil on the skin forms a protective covering that prevents the rapid evapora-

the skin, its texture, presence of rashes or lesions, and characteristics of the hair and nails. Cyanosis, pallor, profuse sweating, and skin rashes are some of the conditions observed that may help to identify disease. In a state of health most persons take their skin for granted and pay too little attention to it, but when disease affects the skin, they become greatly disturbed. A well cared-for skin that is free from disease is a psychologic, social, and economic asset. It contributes to a feeling of well-being, to social acceptance, and to educational and employment opportunities.

CAUSES OF SKIN DISEASES AND DISORDERS

The causes of skin diseases and disorders are numerous, and the number of diseases is so extensive that entire volumes have been written on the subject. Therefore this chapter will only introduce the nurse to a few of the causes and to those skin disorders that are most common. It is known that skin disorders may result from malfunctioning of other body systems. An example is pruritus, which accompanies uremia and certain liver diseases. Allergic reactions to certain substances invariably give rise to skin reactions. The side effects from some drugs cause various kinds of rashes, and exposure to specific chemicals, biologics, or mechanical injury may result in disease of the skin. Extremes of heat may result in blistering of the skin, and extremes of cold may cause frostbite or freezing. Nutritional indiscretions or deficiencies and invasion by pathogenic organisms also affect the skin. The normal aging process brings about changes in pigmentation, as well as loss of elasticity and water from the skin so that wrinkling occurs. Emotional factors also may affect the normal skin.

CHARACTERISTICS OF SKIN LESIONS

Certain types of skin lesions are peculiar to specific disorders and help the dermatologist identify the disease. Some diseases are characterized by an orderly sequence of skin lesions such as that occurring in smallpox, in which there appears a macule, a papule followed by a pustule, and finally a crust. Also, several different types of lesions may be present in the individual at the same time. Following are some of the typical kinds of skin conditions:

atrophy A wasting or thinning of body tissue, typically occurring with the aging process and with some neurologic diseases.

bleb An irregular elevation of the epidermis filled with serous or seropurulent fluid. It may be large in size and is seen in certain forms of severe dermatitis.

crust A dry exudate, commonly called a *scab*, occurring in impetigo, smallpox, chicken pox, and eczema.

excoriation An abraded or denuded area of skin. Unless expert care is given, it may occur where there is drainage, as in colostomy.

fissure A groove, crack, or slit in the skin.

gumma A tumorlike lesion that is similar in appearance to an abcess. It is characteristic of late syphilis.

macule A discolored spot on the skin that may be of various colors and shapes. It is neither raised nor depressed.

nodule A raised solid lesion that is deeper in the skin than a papule.

papule A small, solid elevation varying from the size of a pinhead to a pea. It may be observed in eczema, measles, smallpox, and syphilis.

pustule A small elevation filled with pus. It is characteristic of smallpox and impetigo.

scale A small, thin flake of dry epidermis seen in eczema and psoriasis.

scar The mark left on the skin after repair of tissue.

ulcer An open lesion on the skin with loss of deep tissue. The classic example is the decubitus ulcer.

vesicle A blisterlike elevation on the skin containing serous fluid. It occurs in herpes simplex, chicken pox, and impetigo.

wheal Elevation of varying size and irregular shape. If extensive, wheals may run together. They are characteristic of various allergic reactions and are often referred to as hives.

DIAGNOSTIC TESTS AND PROCEDURES

Most skin disorders can be diagnosed by a carefully taken history, the general appearance, and the distribution of the lesions. Sometimes the dermatologist may wish to make a bacteriologic study, in which case scraping or curetting the lesion is necessary. Various kinds of fungi can be identified by this method of examination. At other times a biopsy may be done for pathologic examination. In certain types of industrial dermatoses, examination of the blood and urine is required for diagnosis.

SPECIFIC ASPECTS OF NURSING THE PATIENT WITH DISEASES AND DISORDERS OF THE SKIN

Nursing care of the patient with skin disorders usually involves several specific nursing procedures, including therapeutic baths, wet dressings, soaks, and the application of various topical medications.

Therapeutic baths. Therapeutic baths are used for several purposes, including disinfecting and deodorizing, relieving pruritus, achieving a soothing effect, and softening and lubricating the skin. Soap, oils, medications, or a variety of substances such as oatmeal, bran, starch, baking soda, or a combination of these may be used. Ordinary laundry starch or cornstarch may be used and is prepared in the same way as for laundry purposes. Several kinds of laundry starch contain bluing and are lightly scented, and these should not be used for therapeutic baths. The starch may be cooked, using 1 cup of starch moistened with cold water and 2 quarts of boiling water. A combination of uncooked starch and baking soda in the proportion of 1 part soda to 4 parts starch may be prepared as a paste and added to the water. Oatmeal may be prepared by placing 2 cups of oatmeal and 1 quart of boiling water in a double boiler and cooking for approximately 45 minutes. The oatmeal mixture is then put in a gauze bag and placed in the tub of water, and the bag is swished in the water. The oatmeal mass may be expressed from the bag and applied gently over the patient's body, but it is washed off before he leaves the bath. Colloidal oatmeal that does not require cooking is available. Bran is prepared in the same way as oatmeal, using 4 cups of bran.

The temperature of the water for therapeutic baths should be about 95° to 100° F., and the tub should be three-fourths full or sufficiently full to cover the involved area. The bath may be given for 20 to 30 minutes several times a day or may last as long as an hour. Occasionally the bath may be continuous. Warm water should be added to maintain a constant temperature.

Since some preparations may cause the tub to be slippery, extreme care should be taken to prevent the patient's slipping in the tub. When the patient is removed from the tub, the skin should be patted dry to avoid damage, and medication, if ordered, is applied. The patient should be prevented from chilling.

Wet dressings. Wet dressings are used in many types of skin disease. Evaporation of the solution provides a cooling effect and relieves the pruritus (itching) that accom-

panies some diseases. The moisture will soften crusts, stimulate drainage, and combat infections, and the dressing will protect the tissues. Dressings may be open or closed and may be warm or cold. Open wet dressings should not be covered with impermeable materials, and because of rapid evaporation, frequent changing is necessary. Pieces of soft old muslin, fluffs, or abdominal gauze is preferred to cotton, which has a tendency to pack down. Closed wet dressings are used most often when warmth is required, and complete changing is required less often. Prior to application of the dressing, normal skin should be protected from the solution with petroleum jelly. The dressing is wet in the prescribed solution and applied to the area. The dressing should be thoroughly saturated but not wet enough to be dripping. Sterile towels are wrapped around the dressing, and the entire dressing is wrapped in thin plastic material and secured with gauze bandage. Because of the danger of burning the patient, external heat should not be used.[2] Wetting the dressing may be done with a sterile Asepto syringe after the outer dressings have been removed; however, it is preferable to remove the entire dressing and saturate as in the beginning. A solution should never be poured through the outside of the dressing. Solutions frequently used for wet dressings include physiologic saline solution, boric acid solution, magnesium sulfate solution, 0.5% aluminum acetate solution, and 1:4000 potassium permanganate solution. The nurse should remember that the bed or pillows must always be protected when wet dressings are used.

Soaks. Soaks may be ordered to loosen necrotic tissue or promote suppuration. When an extremity is involved, a pail or tub large enough to submerge the part should be secured. If open lesions are present, the container should be sterilized. The solution and temperature, as well as frequency and duration of the treatment, will be prescribed by the physician. Burned patients may be placed in physiologic saline soaks for the purpose of debridement. The tub is thoroughly scrubbed and disinfected prior to the soak. Sometimes whirlpool baths are used for the same purpose.

Paste boots. Boots are frequently used for patients with certain kinds of dermatitis and ulcers on the lower extremities. Several commercial preparations containing water, gelatin, glycerin, and zinc oxide are available. One preparation, Dome-Paste bandage, is impregnated with the materials, which simplifies its application. The extremity is elevated about 30 minutes prior to applying the boot. An ointment may be applied to the skin lesions and covered with a thin gauze dressing. The paste bandage is then applied from the ankle to the knee, with greater pressure at the ankle and reduced pressure near the knee. Two layers of stockinette are applied as an outer dressing. The boot is changed every 5 to 8 days.[4]

Emotional support. Patients with skin disorders may have a long road to travel before recovery is complete. Serious skin problems often become chronic, and the patient must learn to live with this disability. When lesions are on the face and exposed parts of the body, the fear of disfigurement is ever present. What the patient believes society thinks is extremely important to him. He often believes that others are afraid he has an infectious disease and that he is shunned and rejected for real or imagined reasons. As a result, he may isolate himself and withdraw into a world of his own. In children and adolescents the impact on personality may be serious. Although few patients with skin disorders may be admitted to the hospital, they are everywhere. Probably few persons escape some type of skin disorder during their lifetimes.

The nurse may be a source of encouragement to patients whether they are in or out of the hospital. First, nurses should know that skin disease is rarely fatal and that few diseases are contagious. Next, nurses should analyze their own feelings toward the patient. If they find the patient repulsive, they will be unable to give him support when he needs it. The nurse must care for the patient with warmth and understanding and convey to him the feeling of acceptance. Gentleness in removing and applying dressings, keeping wet dressings wet, and carrying out treatments on time will help make the patient feel secure. The nurse should avoid the "hurry-up" attitude and should be able to spend some time with the patient to reassure him of interest and acceptance.

NURSING THE PATIENT WITH DISEASES AND DISORDERS OF THE SKIN

Although most diseases and disorders of the skin are treated by the dermatologist as medical or dermatologic conditions, some require surgical treatment. Both the medical and surgical aspects in relation to the disease will be considered in this chapter.

Bacterial diseases
Furuncles, carbuncles, and felons

A furuncle (boil) usually originates about a hair follicle and is caused by the staphylococcus bacterium. The infection begins as a small, red, edematous, painful area on the skin. It may appear as only a tiny pimple and abate spontaneously, or it may continue to increase in size and in a few days give evidence of pus formation. The lesion may rupture spontaneously, drain, and heal (Chapter 2), or surgical incision may be necessary to provide free drainage and to prevent the spread of infection. Furuncles may cause serious complications if the staphylococci get into the bloodstream.

Treatment may consist of warm moist compresses, which promote suppuration; cold compresses are always applied to the face because of the rich blood supply there. Care of the skin surrounding a furuncle is important to prevent spreading of the infection. Antibacterial soaps or alcohol scrubs and an antibiotic ointment may be used, and in some cases the appropriate antibiotic may be given for its systemic effect. The nurse should remember the seriousness of staphylococcal infections and take precautions to dispose of soiled dressings and to prevent spread of the infection.

A carbuncle is similar to a boil, except that the infection infiltrates into the surrounding tissue and results in several boils. Carbuncles are also caused by the staphylococcus bacterium, and the diabetic patient is especially susceptible to them. The most frequent site of the carbuncle is the back of the neck. As the infection gradually comes to the surface from the deeper tissues, there will be several openings discharging pus. Hot wet compresses are applied, and antibiotic therapy is administered. After suppuration begins, incision may be employed to remove the cellular debris.

Most patients with boils and carbuncles

will be cared for in the physician's office, but if admitted to the hospital, they should be isolated and cared for in the same manner as other patients with staphylococcus infections. Recurrent skin infections can be a symptom of a systemic disease such as diabetes.

A felon is an infection of the end of a finger resulting from a puncture wound such as a pinprick, or it may occur without a known cause. The streptococcus bacterium is a frequent cause of the felon. The finger becomes red and edematous, and there is a severe throbbing pain. A radical incision and drainage should be done early, with the patient under general anesthesia. Hot wet dressings may be applied for 24 to 48 hours. Packing or a small drain may be inserted for drainage, and the finger may be immobilized. Antibiotics are usually given to prevent complications. The outcome cannot always be immediately predicted because deformity or loss of the joint may sometimes occur.

Impetigo contagiosa

Impetigo is a superficial contagious skin disease caused by staphylococcus and streptococcus bacteria. The disease occurs primarily on the face and hands but may be transmitted to other parts of the body. It may occur at any age but is most frequently seen in children. The disease begins as a vesicle on the skin, quickly becoming a pustule that ruptures; the exudate forms a crust. The infection may be spread from an existing lesion to other areas on the body so that several lesions may be present at the same time. The disease is spread by both direct and indirect contact.

The treatment consists of removing the crust by soaking with warm physiologic saline solution or hydrogen peroxide. After removal of the crust any of several topical ointments may be applied, including polymyxin (Aerosporin), bacitracin, and Baciguent. Sometimes an antibiotic is administered orally. Children should be provided with individual towels and washcloths.

Most state laws do not require isolation or exclusion from school. However, the local school system may not permit school attendance of children with impetigo. More adequate treatment can be given if the child is kept at home for a few days.

Fungus infections
Tinea (ringworm)

There are four forms of ringworm: tinea capitis, tinea circinata, tinea sycosis, and tinea pedis.

Tinea capitis. Tinea capitis, better known as ringworm of the scalp, occurs primarily in preadolescent children. One type of the disease is transmitted from person to person and another type from animals to humans. The fungus causes several types of lesions, which vary from a single round patch to pustular types of lesions. One type of lesion is called *black dot* because of a small black dot at the site where the hair breaks off. The type transmitted from animals to humans causes a more severe inflammatory reaction, with the formation of pustules similar to boils. This type of lesion is called a *kerion.* The hair in the affected areas becomes dull and brittle and breaks off. When the infection is severe, there may be patches of baldness on the scalp. The loss of hair is temporary, and when the infection subsides, the hair is replaced. The treatment of choice is griseofulvin (Fulvicin, Grifulvin), an antibiotic that is administered orally. This infection is contagious; therefore all members of the family should be examined. The patient's personal toilet articles such as comb and brush should not be used by other members of the family. The individual is usually treated in the physician's office or in a clinic; however, the patient may have been admitted to the hospital for another condition. If tinea capitis is discovered in a hospital patient, it should be called to the physician's attention, and the nurse should take protective precautions. Patients who are receiving cortisone should not be given griseofulvin at the same time.

Tinea circinata. Tinea circinata is a form of ringworm that occurs on the nonhairy parts of the body. It is characterized by congested patches that are slightly elevated and may present a scaly appearance. The lesion increases in size gradually, with the center clearing. Treatment with a topical fungicide is satisfactory if only a few lesions are present. For more extensive cases griseofulvin is used.

Tinea sycosis (barber's itch). Tinea sycosis may result in a serious condition involving the cervical lymph nodes. The disease occurs in the beard and is characterized by a soft nodular type of lesion with edema of the face. The nodules may break down and become suppurative. The hairs of the beard become loose and slip out, leaving bald areas. Several preparations have been used in the treatment of the condition, including ammoniated mercury ointment, griseofulvin, and copper undecylenate.

Tinea pedis. Tinea pedis, or athlete's foot, is a common disorder affecting the feet, although it may be spread to other parts of the body, particularly the hands. The causative fungal organism is often *Epidermophyton floccosum*. It is generally believed that the infection is contracted in showers, around swimming pools, and in similar moist places; however, absolute proof of this method of transmission is lacking. The fungus is widespread in the environment, and there is evidence that some individuals are more sensitive than other persons. If these hypersensitive persons come in contact with the fungus, they may contract the disease. The infection usually begins between the fourth and fifth toe and first appears as small fissures with peeling at the borders. The infection spreads to the other toes, where the epidermis may become macerated. When the dead skin is removed, the new epidermis soon becomes infected. During the acute stage, vesicles may form containing serous fluid, later becoming purulent and eventually drying. If untreated, the infection may become chronic, spreading to the sole, heel, and arch and extending to the top of the foot. In both the acute and chronic stages there is usually severe itching.[5]

Several agents may be used in the treatment, including zinc undecylenate (Desenex); tolnaftate is also reported to be effective, although griseofulvin is not effective in the treament of athlete's foot. Emphasis should be placed on keeping the feet dry and careful drying, especially between the toes; the use of a medicated foot powder with clean socks is recommended.

Dermatitis

Dermatitis is an inflammatory condition of the skin resulting from a wide variety of causes and characterized by varying types of skin manifestations. In most cases it results in redness, itching, and various kinds of skin lesions.

Erythema intertrigo (chafing)

Chafing occurs when two skin surfaces rub together. It results in redness and may cause maceration of the skin. Frequent sites are the areas between the thighs, in the axillae, and under the breasts. In infants chafing may occur in the folds of the skin, particularly about the neck. Obese persons are more likely to be affected. Treatment includes cleansing with mild soap and water, patting dry, and powdering. Good personal hygiene and avoidance of strong or irritating soaps are important.

Miliaria (prickly heat)

The cause of miliaria includes both environmental and physiologic factors. Persons exposed to extremes of temperature and humidity for long periods, those overprotected by clothing, and those with high temperature and obesity are most likely to suffer from attacks of prickly heat. Infants swathed in excessive clothing and blankets are especially susceptible. The condition occurs more frequently during hot weather. The skin manifestation is the appearance of tiny red papules on the trunk, but the lesions may cover the entire body. The lesions are accompanied by burning, prickling, and itching. An infant with prickly heat will be restless and fretful until the condition is relieved. The disorder can be prevented by avoiding extremes of heat and humidity and by wearing absorbent and porous clothing.

Treatment consists of cooling or soothing baths and thorough drying by patting. Emollient baths such as the starch bath may provide relief for persons with severe cases. The application of dusting powders or calamine lotion is generally effective. The condition is of short duration, and efforts to prevent its recurrence should be made.

Dermatitis venenata (plant poisoning)

Allergic dermatitis occurring as the result of contact with certain plants is frequently referred to as ivy poisoning, sumac poisoning, or poisoning by other specific kinds of plants. Individual susceptibility is an important factor in this type of dermatitis. Although many different plants and shrubs may cause the condition, some of the more common ones are poison ivy, poison sumac, poison oak, and poison elder. Symptoms will vary from a mild redness to severe systemic reactions and gangrene. The primary lesions are most frequently on the parts of the body contacted by the irritant, usually the hands, arms, face, and legs. The skin may become erythematous, which may be followed by the formation of papules, vesicles, and pustules. The tissue may be edematous, and severe itching and burning may occur.

When the individual knows that he has been exposed, the exposed parts should be washed immediately with strong soap and water. Washing will not be effective unless it is done soon after contact. After lesions have appeared soap and water should not be used. Wet dressings, using 1:20 solution of aluminum acetate or physiologic saline solution, may be applied three times a day for 30 minutes.[13] Soft pieces of old sheeting are best for wet dressings and should not be wrapped in plastic. After the administration of the wet dressings, corticosteroid ointment or cream may be applied. The steroid ointments are available under several trade names such as Kenalog-S, Neo-Aristocort, Neo-Synalar, and Cordran-N. (See Chapter 22.)

Exfoliative dermatitis

Exfoliative dermatitis may result from several causes, among which is contact with or ingestion of heavy metals such as arsenic, bismuth, and mercury. The disease is characterized by massive desquamation of the skin over the entire body surface. It is a serious disease and may be fatal. Edema, redness, severe itching, and in severe cases, fever may be present because of a disturbance in the heat-regulating mechanism. The patient should be hospitalized and kept warm.

Treatment and nursing care include measures to relieve the itching such as colloidal baths, which are given as warm as can be tolerated, and antihistaminic drugs. Special mouth care, care of the eyes and lips, and prevention of decubitus ulcers are important nursing functions. Lotions and ointments may be ordered, and the nurse should observe the patient carefully for any un-desirable reactions. Patients who are receiving gold salts should be carefully observed, since a form of exfoliative dermatitis may develop among these patients.

This severe form of dermatitis is seen less often today because the use of chemotherapeutic agents has replaced the heavy metals formerly used to treat some diseases.

Dermatitis medicamentosa (drug dermatitis)

The term *dermatitis medicamentosa* is applied to skin eruptions caused by drugs, regardless of the method of administration. Almost any drug may cause a reaction in certain individuals, and with the development of many new drugs and their increased use, the incidence of such reactions will increase. The characteristics of drug reactions may range from mild erythema to severe conditions that may be fatal. Every type of skin lesion reviewed in this chapter may be seen in various reactions to drugs. It is more important than ever that the nurse be aware of the possibility and observe patients for evidence of any skin lesion. It is also important to question patients concerning any undesirable side effects of a drug that they have experienced previously because the same drug given to the same patient again will produce a similar or more severe reaction.

Dermatitis caused by drugs will usually clear up as soon as the drug is withdrawn. However, treatment should be instituted to relieve the distressing symptoms from the skin lesions. Treatment is based on the patient's symptoms and may include antihistaminic drugs, and in some cases corticosteroid agents in the form of lotions may be applied topically. In severe cases the corticosteroid agents may be given orally for their systemic effect.

Psoriasis

Psoriasis is a common skin disease. The exact incidence of the disorder is probably unknown, and estimates vary widely. It has been estimated that approximately 1% of the United States population has had psoriasis at some time.[16] The disease usually begins between the ages of 10 and 35 years but may begin at any age. The exact cause is unknown; however, there is evidence that there may be an inherited tendency to the disease.

The disease is characterized by a reddish brown skin eruption from which silvery white scales are shed. Lesions may vary from a single lesion to multiple lesions. Small lesions may coalesce to form large irregular patches called *plaques*. Lesions make their appearance as small, pinhead-sized bright red spots about the elbows, knees, scalp, lower back, and eyebrows. They may occur about the site of an injury, cut, bruise, or surgical scar. They soon become dry and scaly, and thickening occurs. If the scales are removed, bleeding occurs. The shedding of the epidermis is six to seven times more rapid than the normal shedding of epidermis. In about 10% to 25% of cases a form of arthritis develops. The arthritic condition resembles rheumatoid arthritis; however, opinions vary as to whether it is a form of rheumatoid arthritis or a separate disease. The arthritis may accompany the skin disease, or the skin eruption may exist for several years before the arthritis makes its appearance.[1]

There is no cure for psoriasis, but the disease may undergo long remissions. The disease has a tendency to improve during the summer months when exposed to the ultraviolet rays of the sun. Emotional stress, systemic infections, obesity, injury to the skin, and pregnancy may cause exacerbation of the disorder. There is no specific treatment. Several drugs have been used and frequently bring about a remission. Some of the drugs used include 5% crude coal tar in Vaseline, coal tar and sulfur ointment, 0.25% anthralin (cignolin, dithranol), and cortisone. In many cases ultraviolet light accompanies the topical treatment. Antimetabolites, including methotrexate and 6-mercaptopurine, used in the treatment of leukemia have been used but may produce undesirable toxic reactions.[15] The arthritic condition is treated in the same manner as rheumatoid arthritis. Treatment for each patient must be individualized, and the patient should know that treatment is only palliative. Unless the patient knows, understands, and accepts his disease, he may be led to quacks who continuously advertise cures. The patient needs a great deal of emotional support because

psychologic effects of the disease may be severe.

Eczema

Eczema is a term applied to a group of diseases characterized by many types of skin lesions. The disease may be related to allergic conditions (Chapter 22), hereditary and emotional factors, drugs, and various household detergents. Eczema frequently occurs among industrial employees whose work brings them into contact with various products such as dyes, tars, and other toxic agents, various kinds of cosmetic agents, and metallic fibers in clothing. Whatever the cause, there is always itching, and scratching may cause secondary infection. Lesions may be vesicular in type and tend to rupture, leaving a moist surface (weeping), and they may form crusts. In some types of eczema the skin becomes dry and scaly and has a leathery appearance. If possible, the cause of the disorder should be found and removed.

Treatment is based primarily on relief of itching, and every effort should be made to keep the patient as comfortable as possible. It is also necessary to combat secondary infections. There are many preparations used for these purposes, and every patient must be treated on an individual basis, according to cause and the characteristics of his condition. In most cases of eczema the use of soap is contraindicated. The topical application of corticosteroid creams and ointments has replaced most other forms of treatment. Because of the extreme discomfort and anxiety suffered by many patients with eczema, tranquilizing drugs are frequently given to the patient.

The nurse should be familiar with the methods of applying various topical preparations and should observe each patient carefully for undesirable effects, which should be reported promptly to the physician. The patient also needs sympathetic understanding and reassurance from the nurses who are caring for him.

Acne vulgaris

Acne vulgaris is a distressing skin disease of adolescence, usually occurring between 14 and 30 years of age. Both boys and girls may be affected; however, the condition is more prevalent in boys.

It is fairly well established that increased hormonal activity during adolescence is a causative factor. Increased activity of the sebaceous (oil) glands also may contribute to the condition. This disease is self-limiting and usually disappears by early adult life. The acne generally begins with the appearance of comedones (blackheads) that plug the ducts of the sebaceous glands and are the result of increased secretion of sebum from the glands. The inflammatory process within the duct soon leads to the formation of papules and pustules on the skin.

Treatment for the condition is nonspecific and is directed toward reducing inflammation and infection, reducing blackhead formation, and developing a program of good personal hygiene. The skin should be kept scrupulously clean by washing with soap and water several times a day. A preparation containing hexachlorophene will help to reduce the staphylococcus population on the skin. Agents that cause drying such as salicylic acid and resorcin may be used. The use of 70% alcohol helps to prevent infection. Other agents that have been effective in some cases include the tetracyclines and the corticosteroids. Small doses of estrogens administered to girls just prior to the menstrual period has helped to relieve the oily condition of the skin and retarded the formation of sebum. The patient should be advised against squeezing the lesions, which may worsen the condition and lead to scarring. Stress should be placed on developing a program of adequate diet, sleep, and wholesome physical activity.

The psychologic effects are often more serious than the disease. Acne vulgaris occurs at a period when adolescents are concerned with personal appearance, and the unsightly skin condition may seriously interfere with personality development.

Viral infections
Herpes simplex (fever blister)

Herpes simplex, also known as a cold sore, is a self-limiting condition caused by a virus. It is chacterized by the appearance of a small vesicle at the junction of the skin and mucous membrane of the lip or nose. The disease often occurs when other acute infections are present but may occur in the absence of any other condition. It is believed that similar lesions known as canker sores on the mucous membrane of the mouth or about the external genitals may be caused by the same virus. Herpes simplex is usually of short duration but is a recurring condition.

Treatment generally consists of topical application of alcohol or spirits of camphor. Hot compresses are sometimes used and may provide relief from the discomfort.

Herpes zoster (shingles)

Herpes zoster is often classified as a neurologic disorder because the lesion is located in one or more of the spinal ganglia with involvement of the skin area supplied by the nerve fibers. The disease is believed to be caused by the chicken pox virus and does not recur after one attack. The most common location of the skin lesions is the thoracic region, but the disease may occur in other regions of the body such as the thigh, lower abdomen, or forehead. The patient may have a slight temperature, malaise, and loss of appetite, with severe pain in the skin area prior to development of the rash. After 1 or 2 days an inflammatory edematous area appears, on which papules turning to vesicles are arranged in groups following the sensory nerves from the posterior region to the anterior area. A neuralgic pain occurs in paroxysms and is worse on movement and at night. The pain may persist long after the skin manifestation has subsided. The disease is self-limiting, and there is no specific treatment.

Treatment and nursing care are symptomatic. Analgesics are given for pain, and narcotics may be required for severe pain. Lotions may be used to relieve the discomfort from the skin rash. Methscopolamine bromide (Protamide), a colloidal solution of a proteolytic enzyme, has proved valuable in relieving pain and reducing the rash. It has been reported that patients treated with Protamide have not experienced the postherpetic pain. Some patients may be treated with ACTH to reduce inflammation, and if secondary infection occurs, antibiotics are administered.

Patients with herpes zoster may be hospitalized, and emotional depression frequently accompanies the disease. The nurse may find the patient irritable and uncooperative. Patience and understanding will be needed in caring for these patients. If the rash occurs along the branches of the fifth cranial nerve, the patient should be observed for facial paralysis and eye or ear disturbances.[10]

Disorders of pigmentation
Lentigo (freckles)

So-called freckles are collections of skin pigment that result from quantitative changes in melanin. They may occur in certain persons on exposure to the sun in summer and tend to disappear in winter. Persons with severe cases may have the freckles removed by dermal abrasion, but assurance cannot be given that they will not return.

Chloasma (liver spots)

Patches of pigmentation that may be yellowish brown, brown, or black may occur on various parts of the body. They are more common in women and are often seen during pregnancy or at the time of menopause. The condition is not the result of disease of the liver.

No treatment is necessary, unless the lesions occur on the face and the person is sensitive about them for cosmetic reasons. They may be removed with various bleaching preparations, but the procedure is not recommended.

Disorders of glands
Seborrhea (oily skin)

Some persons have an excessive secretion of oil from the sebaceous glands that is accentuated on the face, neck, and scalp, where the oil glands are most abundant. It is often associated with other conditions such as acne vulgaris, seborrheic dermatitis, eczema, and seborrheic warts. Although the condition is normal for some persons, particularly women, it not only detracts from personal appearance but also predisposes to other more serious skin conditions.

Treatment consists of washing frequently and thoroughly with soap and water and avoiding the use of greasy creams. Preparations containing salicylic acid and/or sulfur may be rubbed into the affected areas several times a day. If the hair and scalp are affected, Sebucare lotion may be applied to wet hair once or twice daily and thoroughly massaged into the scalp.

Sebaceous cyst (wen)

A sebaceous cyst, commonly called a *wen*, is often seen on the scalp and may become large. It is the result of obstruction of the sebaceous duct in the presence of continued secretions from the gland. These tumors contain an accumulation of sebum, which develops an offensive odor. The treatment is surgical incision, with measures to prevent infection.

Hyperhidrosis (excessive sweating)

Excessive sweating occurs in relation to several conditions, including diseases such as tuberculosis and hyperthyroidism, conditions in which severe pain is present as in renal colic, and certain acute heart attacks. It may also occur in some shock states and toxic conditions or after the administration of antipyretic drugs. Under normal conditions excessive sweating usually occurs when a person is exposed to extremes of heat or severe physical exercise. Excessive sweating may predispose the individual to skin disease or irritation.

Treatment is directed toward removing the cause, and nursing care should concern keeping the bed and clothing dry, sponging and drying the skin, and protecting the patient from exposure.

Axillary hyperhidrosis may be controlled by topical application of most of the commercial agents on the market. These preparations act by closing the pores and may occasionally cause a mild irritation. Excessive hyperhidrosis of the feet can be relieved by washing several times daily, drying thoroughly, and dusting with a medicated foot powder.

Anhidrosis (absence of sweating)

Anhidrosis is a normal result of the aging process accompanied by decreased activity of the sebaceous glands, which causes dryness of the skin. The disorder is also characteristic of several skin diseases, may follow the administration of drugs such as atropine, and is characteristic of diabetes mellitus, nephritis, and hypothyroidism.

There is no specific treatment for the condition as such, except the use of superfatted soaps and the application of creams or oils. Treatment of the causative factor may provide relief.

Pruritus (itching)

Pruritus is a symptom that accompanies many disorders, including a variety of skin diseases, systemic diseases, allergic reactions, and anhidrosis in the elderly person. The response of the individual is to scratch, and it is generally useless to tell him not to scratch, since his reply will probably be, "I can't help it." In fact, scratching is almost an automatic unconscious act.

Whenever possible, treatment is based on removing or treating the cause. In treating small children, splinting of the arms or the use of mitts may be necessary to prevent scratching. Cold wet dressings, emollient baths, and emollient lotion containing phenol or menthol may be used, or the physician may prescribe a lotion containing one of the steroid drugs. Some patients may benefit from antihistaminic drugs, whereas others do not find relief in them.

The nurse should do everything possible to provide comfort for the patient and to relieve the emotional tension often associated with pruritic conditions. Maintaining a cool, even room temperature and providing a quiet environment and some diversional activity will help to relieve itching.

Tumors of the skin

Tumors of the skin are among the most common of all tumors and generally affect exposed parts of the body such as the face and back of the hands. Persons whose occupations expose them to wind, sun, and frost are often affected. Most patients with skin tumor are in the older age group. Skin tumors may be benign or malignant, and most malignant tumors can be easily diagnosed and cured. Benign tumors include the keloid, angioma, nevus, wart, and keratoses.[7]

Keloid

The keloid is a tumor mass occurring at the site of a scar that consists of an overgrowth of fibrous tissue. The shape may be irregular and small, or it may increase to the size of the hand. The tumor may develop after inflammation or ulceration from burns or traumatic injuries. It is not known why the condition occurs. It is more common in blacks.

There is no uniform opinion concerning treatment. The lesion may be erythematous, irritated, and painful. Pain may be relieved by injection of a glucocorticoid (Aristocort, Kenakort) diluted 1:5 with lidocaine (Xylocaine). Surgical removal followed by x-ray therapy will be effective in about half the cases.[4]

Angioma

The angioma is a benign skin tumor that consists of dilated blood vessels. There are several types of angiomas—one is congenital, called a *birthmark* by many people. The skin may have an area of purplish color known as port-wine stain. The stain is not elevated and may be large. Port-wine stains frequently are found on the face and may cover an entire side of the face. Treatment may consist of electrolysis, x-ray therapy, or refrigeration, which usually is for cosmetic purposes only.

The spider angioma is an acquired condition often accompanying disease of the liver, which consists of a network of venous capillaries that radiate outward in a spider-like fashion. It generally fades and disappears as the primary condition improves.

Nevus (mole)

The mole is a nonvascular tumor, many of which are pigmented and may be present at birth. There are many different types of nevi, almost all of which are harmless. However, the raised black mole, although benign, may become malignant if it is located where it is subjected to constant irritation. It is generally advisable for these moles to be excised as a precautionary measure.

Verruca (wart)

Warts are common and may occur at any age; however, the largest number are found in persons between 10 and 30 years of age. There are several different types, some of which occur as single lesions, whereas others are multiple. They are caused by a virus, and it is believed that they are contagious, but exactly how they are transmitted is unknown. A common type of wart is found on the hands and arms, including areas about the nails. They occur on the feet, legs, face, and neck and vary in size and color. Another type that appears on the face and neck tends to be elongated. The plantar wart develops on the weight-bearing part of the foot and may be painful. Warts are flat, and removal of the horny epidermis leaves a slightly bleeding surface. Some warts are moist and may occur in persons with gonorrhea; others occuring in infectious syphilis are called *condylomata*. Warts occurring in gonorrhea and syphilis are frequently located about the genital areas. Condylomata tend to coalesce and form large, cauliflower-like lesions.

Treatment of warts depends on the type of wart, the location, and the number. Plantar warts may be especially difficult to treat; they may be treated with preparations containing salicylic acid. In a large number of cases warts disappear spontaneously.[1]

Keratoses

Keratoses are generally considered precancerous lesions, of which there are many types. Some occur in elderly persons as senile keratoses and are most likely to become malignant. Surgical removal is generally indicated. Some forms of keratoses appear in persons who have been exposed to the sun and whose skin has been damaged by it. Others are found in persons past middle age as seborrheic dermatoses. These are less likely to become malignant but should be kept under observation.[7]

Malignant tumors

Several skin lesions may be considered precancerous, particularly if they are located where they are exposed to irritation. Carcinoma of the skin may first appear as a roughened area, gradually increasing in size. As the lesion progresses, ulceration with crusting and destruction of the skin and underlying tissues develops. Prompt treatment of any suspicious lesion should be secured, since skin carcinoma responds readily to x-ray or radium therapy.

Malignant melanoma may be primary, or it may develop from an existing lesion such as a mole. A mole that shows any change such as enlarging, crusting, or bleeding or changes in color should be viewed with suspicion, and medical atten-

tion should be secured without delay. Treatment is usually surgical excision. If regional lymph nodes are involved, they are dissected. Skin cancer can often be prevented by proper protection against or avoiding unnecessary exposure to the sun. Medical advice should be secured for any mole that is located where it is subjected to irritation.[2]

Disorders of the appendages
Alopecia (loss of hair)

Loss of hair may result from several causes, including the normal thinning of the hair as a condition of the aging process. Hair is sometimes lost after long and debilitating diseases such as fevers. A characteristic alopecia occurs in early syphilis and is marked by loss of the hair in round patches; it may progress until the scalp presents a moth-eaten appearance. One type of alopecia areata results in patches of baldness that may appear suddenly and tend to spread from the edges. After several round patches of baldness occur, regrowth of hair begins but may not be permanent. Finally, however, the hair is replaced, and spontaneous recovery takes place after several months.

Hypertrichosis and hypotrichosis

The excessive growth of hair may be congenital or acquired or may result from a hereditary tendency. In congenital hypertrichosis, hair may cover moles or the skin over a spina bifida. Acquired hypertrichosis may be the result of endocrine disturbance and is frequently seen as a growth of hair on the upper lip and on the chin in women. It may also be the result of a hereditary predisposition.

Hypotrichosis is an absence of hair or a deficiency of hair. The condition may be the result of skin disease or endocrine factors. When the cause is endocrine disturbance, correction should be made if possible. The most satisfactory method of removing superfluous hair is by electrolysis.

Nail disorders

Disorders of the nails may be associated with diseases elsewhere in the body or may be caused by congenital defects or infection. The nails may be soft or brittle. Changes in the shape and contour may occur, and nails may grow into the soft tissues at the side (ingrown nails). Paronychia ("run-around") is an infection that begins on the side of the nail, often from a hangnail or injury, and finally encircles it. The infection loosens the nail from the matrix and may become painful. Frequently surgical removal of the affected part of the nail is necessary. Wet dressings, using 1:2000 to 1:10,000 potassium permanganate and the application of neomycin ointment may relieve the condition. Fungus infections of the nails respond poorly to ordinary methods of treatment and may take months for cure.

Infestations
Pediculi (lice)

Three types of pediculi infest human beings: *Pediculus humanus* var. *capitis*, *Pediculus humanus* var. *corporis,* and *Pediculus pubis.*

Pediculus capitis is the head louse, which lives on the scalp and attaches its eggs (nits) to the hair. The nits are attached to the hair by an adhesive substance that makes them difficult to remove. The louse bites the scalp, causing severe itching and scratching. Severe infestations may result in secondary infection, which includes enlargement of lymph glands in the neck. The present recommended treatment is the use of Kwell shampoo, which is applied to the hair and scalp and lathered for 4 to 5 minutes, after which the hair is rinsed and dried. The treatment may be repeated in 24 hours.[20]

Pediculus corporis is a body louse that may be found in the seams of underclothing. Scratch marks may appear on the skin in the area of clothing seams. Treatment consists of boiling the underwear, which kills the louse and the nits. However, all bedding and clothing must be washed and boiled and pillows and blankets treated.

Pediculus pubis is found primarily in the genital area; however, it may infect the axilla, eyebrows, beard, and eyelashes. The lice may be contracted from toilet seats, bedclothes, clothing, and sexual intercourse. Treatment involves shaving the affected areas, bathing, and applying Kwell cream. The cream should be applied over the entire body and left on for 24 hours.

If necessary, the treatment may be repeated.[20]

Scabies (itch)

Scabies, an infectious skin disease, is caused by a parasite that burrows under the skin. The disease is easily recognized by the furrows of dark dots that appear between the fingers, the flexor surfaces of the wrists, and about the breasts. However, the infection may involve other parts of the body. The disease is characterized by itching, which is intensified at night. Neglect in treatment may lead to secondary skin lesions or the development of an eczematous condition. An old but effective treatment is the use of sulfur ointment. The individual is given a hot bath with soap and thorough scrubbing of the lesions. Sulfur ointment is applied, and a suit of long underwear is donned. The ointment is applied each night and morning for 3 consecutive days. A hot bath is then given, and a soothing lotion is applied to the skin. All clothing, towels, and bedding should be washed. If recovery is not complete, the treatment may be repeated. Although old, sulfur ointment is still being used and is effective; however, several other preparations are also effective. These include Kwell lotion or cream, Eurax lotion or cream, Topocide emulsion, and benzyl benzoate. Application must be thorough, all clothing must be washed or dry cleaned, and bedding has to be washed. Individuals are likely to be uncomfortable for several weeks, although the disease is inactive.

NURSING THE PATIENT WITH BURNS

Burns are injuries to body tissue and may be caused by heat (dry or moist), electricity, chemicals, or radiant energy. Burns are classified according to their depth and the extent of body tissue injured.

First-degree burns. First-degree burns are superficial. The dermis is intact, with the injury affecting only the epidermis. There may be erythema, a feeling of warmth, usually sensitivity and pain, and edema but no blisters. First-degree burns generally heal rapidly, since deep layers of the epidermis are usually not involved. Causative factors include brief exposure to hot liquids, gas explosions, or excessive exposure to the sun.

Second-degree burns. In second-degree burns the injury extends through the epidermis and involves the dermis, and vesiculation is usually present. Second-degree burns are referred to as superficial or deep. Superficial second-degree burns have blisters with redness in and around the burned area. They usually heal within 10 to 14 days. Deep second-degree burns have had all layers of the skin destroyed down to the deep layers of the dermis.[11] These burns are slower to heal, taking 3 to 4 weeks.[21] Both types may be extremely painful. Causes of second-degree burns include short exposure to flash heat or hot liquids.

Third-degree burns. Third-degree burns are deep; both the epidermis and the dermis are destroyed, and blistering may be absent. The burned skin may have a brown leathery appearance. All skin structures, including hair shafts and sebaceous glands, are irreversibly damaged. Little pain is present because nerve endings have been destroyed. The destroyed skin must be cleared away before healing can occur. If the area is small, granulation tissue will fill the area, and gradually epithelial tissue will grow from the margins of the injury and cover the wound. However, a scar will result. Large third-degree burns require skin grafting. These burns are caused by more prolonged contact with hot objects, liquids, or flames.

Fourth-degree burns. In fourth-degree burns the full thickness of the skin is destroyed, plus structures underneath the skin, such as subcutaneous tissue, muscle, fascia, tendons, and bones. Causes, symptoms, and the healing process are similar to that for third-degree burns, although prognosis for recovery is more guarded.

Segmental charring. Segmental charring, destruction of the entire extremity, seldom occurs.

"Rule of nine." The extent of the burn, age of the patient, or amount of body surface injured may determine whether or not the patient will live. A method for estimating the extent of a burn is the "rule of nine."[13] Nurses should become familiar with this method because in a major disaster in which large numbers of persons are burned, they may be responsible for making decisions in referring patients for medical treatment (Fig. 20-2).

Head and neck	9%
Anterior torso	18%
Posterior torso	18%
Upper extremities	18%
Lower extremities	36%
Genitals and perineum	1%

When children are burned, these percentages must be adjusted. The percentage of an infant's head is twice that of an adult's, whereas a 10-year-old's head is about one and one half that of an adult. The trunk is considered about two thirds that of an adult.

It is difficult to determine the seriousness of burns covering a large portion of the body. A combination of burns of all degrees may be present. Often the size of the burned area is more important than the depth of the burn. For instance, a large first- or second-degree burn will be more serious than a small third-degree burn.

Treatment and nursing care. Fires and explosions take more than 8000 lives each year in the United States. Elderly persons and children are most frequently the victims of death resulting from fires.[6] Although many persons die at the scene of the conflagration, many more are brought into the hospital, where physicians and nurses work to save their lives. In spite of efforts made by physicians and nurses, all will not survive.

First aid. The only first aid treatment that has shown to be effective in limiting the extent of a burn is the application of cool water. This reduces the temperature, lessens tissue destruction, and may prevent a full-thickness or third-degree burn from occurring. The patient should be wrapped in a clean sheet and blanket and taken to the hospital. No attempt should be made to remove clothes, apply ointment, or give medications.

Initial treatment. Patients who die within the first 72 hours usually do so from shock. It may be expected that an adult with 15% or a child with 10% of the body burned will be suffering from some degree of shock. However, infection is the primary cause of death in severely burned patients.

When a burn occurs, there is damage to the capillary system in the area. This plus the damage to the body cells causes water and electrolytes to shift from the plasma to the interstitial (tissue) fluids. This fluid,

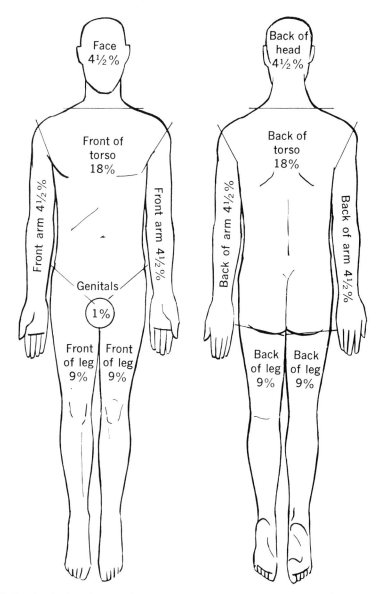

Fig. 20-2. The "rule of nine" for determining the area (in percent) of the body surface burned.

in addition to leakage from the burned surface causes edema, which is particularly noticeable in second-degree burns in the form of blisters. In third-degree burns the same process occurs, but the destroyed layers of the skin may trap the edema fluids beneath it. This may cause acute complications such as tissue ischemia or respiratory distress from pressure on internal organs.

The accumulation of edema fluids in the burned area results in a decrease in the amount of circulating blood plasma. When the volume of the bloodstream falls, blood pressure drops, circulation decreases, and less oxygen is available to all body tissues. This process leads to shock. If treatment is not instituted, metabolic acidosis and acute renal failure will occur.

The nurse caring for a newly burned patient must be constantly alert for symptoms of burn shock. Restlessness is a common sign of hypoxia and may indicate onset of shock. The pulse will increase prior to the

Table 20-1. Priorities for care of the burned patient

1. Stop burning	Patient may be admitted with clothing, blankets, etc. still smoldering
2. Establish patient airway	Consider age and conditions other than burn that may obstruct airway
	Tracheal suctioning to remove aspirated secretions
	Endotracheal intubation
	Tracheotomy may be required
	Edema of face and neck or eschar may constrict neck
3. Intravenous fluids	Type as ordered by physician
	Amount calculated on basis of body surface burned and kilograms of body weight
	Half of total requirements including electrolytes given during first 24 hours
4. Skin care	Method approved by the physician
5. Foley catheter care	Monitor hourly amount and specific gravity of urinary output
6. Reassurance and support of patient	Relieve anxiety and apprehension
7. Analgesics	As required; narcotics may be avoided because they depress the respiratory system
8. Urinalysis	
9. Blood studies	BUN, hematocrit, prothrombin, and electrolytes; CBC
10. Nursing observation	Important to observe for possible shock, pulmonary edema, pulmonary embolism, and dehydration

blood pressure falling, and respirations will increase. Urine flow is scant or absent. Confusion and delirium may occur. (See Table 20-1.) An airway should be established if necessary

Administration of intravenous fluids is usually the first emergency treatment given to the severely burned patient. Many combinations of fluids may be used, depending on the physician's preference. For example, Ringer's solution plus albumin to combat protein loss and sodium bicarbonate to combat acidosis may be given. Fluids may be administered rapidly until urine flow is established, then regulated to maintain a urine output of 25 to 50 ml. per hour. The patient is catheterized, and it is the nurse's responsibility to measure the output, urinary pH, and specific gravity each hour.[8, 11] Almost every burned patient is extremely thirsty, but he must not be allowed to drink water, since this tends to dilute body electrolytes. The patient is NPO or is given intravenous fluids.

Initial treatment of the burn involves removing any debris or loose skin, cleansing with physiologic saline solution if necessary, and opening blisters. Strict asepsis is paramount to avoid wound contamination and subsequent infection. Morphine sulfate may be given to reduce pain and apprehension. Antibiotics and tetanus prophylaxis are usually given.

Environmental preparation. Large medical centers usually have a burn unit, but most hospitals admit the burned patient to a regular medical or surgical clinical unit. Ideally, the hospital should be notified of a pending admission of a burned patient; however, except in catastrophic fires, notification rarely occurs. If the patient's life is to be saved during the early critical hours, supplies and equipment must be available immediately. The nurse can provide valuable assistance in helping to secure the necessary equipment and supplies and in preparing the room to receive the patient. There will be some variation in equipment needed, depending on the treatment method used. The equipment listed should be available regardless of the method. If there is no burn unit, the patient should be placed in a private room in a clean area of the hospital. Patients are frequently placed on a Stryker frame or in a CircOlectric bed. Equipment needed may include the following:

Tracheotomy tray
Cutdown tray
Catheterization tray with retention catheter
Nasogastric tube
Suction equipment
Oxygen
Footboard
Bed cradles
Tetanus toxoid or tetanus antitoxin
Culture tubes
Ringer's lactate solution
Intravenous saline or glucose solution
Plasma
Intravenous and blood set
Intravenous stand
Tourniquet
Alcohol sponges
Sterile syringes, 30 and 50 ml., and needles
Sterile gloves
Sterile gauze dressings without cotton filling, various sizes

Each patient must be considered individually because the cause, depth, and extent of the burn, the patient's age, pre-existing disease, and the patient's emotional reaction to the injury will determine the method of treatment selected by the physician. Although different methods are employed, the basic objectives are always the same: (1) to save the patient's life, (2) to prevent infection, and (3) to restore normal function and appearance. The three most commonly used methods of treatment include (1) the exposure method using mafenide acetate (Sulfamylon acetate), (2) dressings continuously moistened with 0.5% silver nitrate solution, and (3) occlusive dressings. There are advantages and disadvantages to each technique, and often a combination of these may be used.

Exposure method. The exposure method of caring for burns leaves the burn exposed without dressings. Although opinions differ, in most situations the patient is placed on sterile sheets, and sterile sheets are draped over bed cradles or side rails. All persons entering the room must wash their hands thoroughly and wear a sterile gown, masks, and gloves.

Mafenide acetate (Sulfamylon acetate). A major factor in the death of burned patients is infection, and organisms most often involved include *Staphylococcus aureus*, hemolytic streptococci, and *Pseudomonas aeruginosa*. Mafenide has been found to be a safe, effective adjunct in preventing infection, and some believe that

it is more effective than silver nitrate.[3]

Mafenide acetate is a soft white cream that is soluble in water and can be easily washed off. It spreads easily, does not stain, and contains an antibacterial agent that controls wound infection and the growth of bacteria, thereby reducing mortality from infection.

One method for using mafenide acetate begins with a thorough washing of the burn with pHisoHex and physiologic saline solution. This may be done in a whirlpool or a Hubbard tank. Any blisters are opened, and loose skin is removed. If sedation is required, morphine or meperidine hydrochloride may be administered. The patient is then placed on a sterile sheet and 10% mafenide cream is spread 1/16 inch thick over the burned area using a sterile gloved hand. However, for small children or persons who may be sensitive about exposure a thin layer of gauze may be applied. The cream is reapplied to areas where it may have been rubbed off in about 12 hours, since the burned area must be kept covered with the cream. The patient is placed in the Hubbard tank or whirlpool daily and the cream washed off; debridement is carried out as necessary, after which the mafenide cream is reapplied. The procedure is repeated each day until new epithelial tissue appears in secondary burns or until the eschar separates and granulation tissue begins to appear in third-degree burns.

The patient must be observed for any increase in respiratory rate, since some patients may develop acidosis. If this should occur, the cream is washed off. If the complication is corrected within 72 hours, the treatment is resumed. If the acidosis continues longer than 72 hours, the treatment is discontinued. The patient may complain of a burning sensation when the cream is first applied; however, this gradually diminishes with each treatment. If a rash develops because of sensitivity to sulfonamides, an antihistaminic agent may be administered, but the treatment with mafenide cream is not discontinued.[9]

Silver nitrate method. The use of silver nitrate for treating burns is based on the fact that it is bacteriostatic and prevents infection. After thorough cleansing of the wounds the burns are wrapped with dressings saturated with a solution of distilled water containing 0.5% silver nitrate. The dressings must be thoroughly soaked and thick enough to hold large amounts of solution. The entire dressing is then covered with two layers of prebleached stockinette. The dressing must be rewet every 2 to 4 hours so that the solution is in direct contact with the skin at all times. The patient is covered with a dry sheet or blanket that must be changed often enough to keep a dry cover over the patient and thus prevent heat loss. The entire dressing is changed every 12 to 24 hours, and every second day the patient is placed in a bath of balanced salt solution (Locke's solution) for 20 minutes. The body is then rinsed with distilled water, and new silver nitrate dressings are applied.

When properly executed, treatment with silver nitrate appears to reduce the incidence of infection and permit early skin grafting. The primary disadvantage to its use is that silver nitrate stains everything that comes into contact with it. However, with care and the use of disposable equipment, most actual damage can be prevented.

Silver sulfadiazine is a relatively new ointment that can be smeared over the burned area. It does not appear to cause acidosis as does mafenide acetate.

Occlusive dressings. Occlusive dressings are used for burns of the extremities, for those burns treated on an outpatient basis, and occasionally for third-degree burns requiring grafting. A layer of petroleum gauze or gauze impregnated with antibiotic ointment is applied, followed by an absorptive bulky layer of fluffed gauze and pads. The dressings are applied evenly with compression and are held in place with an elastic bandage. This type of dressing protects the wound from bacteria in the environment, keeps the wound surface dry, and splints and supports the area. These dressings should be changed every 2 to 5 days. The use of this method enables the patient to move about more freely.

The nurse responsible for the dressings must position the extremity to prevent complications, prevent two skin surfaces from rubbing together (such as between toes and fingers), and check the circulation of the part frequently. Numbness, tingling, and pain indicate ischemia. Dead or con-taminated tissue should be removed carefully with each dressing change. Any signs of infection or an increased temperature and pulse rate should be reported to the physician. The physician may debride the area in the operating room, and skin grafts may be done.

Intake and output. One of the earliest aspects of treatment is the administration of intravenous fluids. Since large amounts of fluid, which may include blood, plasma, electrolytes, glucose, and physiologic saline solution, will be administered, a cutdown may be done. The amount of fluid administered and the rate of administration will be determined by the physician on the basis of extent of the injury and urinary output. The nurse must carefully regulate the rate of fluids according to the physician's directions. A urinary retention catheter will be inserted and connected to drainage. The urinary output is measured every hour for 24 hours and recorded. In the adult patient the output should be between 25 and 35 ml.[2] If the output falls below or rises greatly above this amount, it should be reported to the physician. Intravenous fluids may be continued for as long as a week.

Positioning the patient. Proper positioning of the patient is important to prevent contractures, decubitus ulcers, foot drop, and pulmonary complications. Turning the patient is facilitated when he is placed on a Stryker frame or in the CircOlectric bed, which offers many advantages in caring for the burned patient. Flotation therapy has been used successfully for severely burned patients. Flotation prevents pressure areas and allows blood flow to all areas of the body. This enhances nourishment of the cells, promotes healing, and helps to prevent decubitus ulcers. The sensation of floating is soothing and relaxing and lessens pain and tension, and the patient is able to move about more freely.[12] The physical therapist may assist with both passive and active range-of-motion exercises, and the patient should be encouraged to assist with his own exercises. The patient should not be placed in Fowler's position, and the knee gatch of the bed should not be elevated, since both will contribute to contractures. When the patient is in the supine position, hyperextension of the head will help to prevent contractures when the neck is burned. Splinting and exercise programs may be instituted to prevent deformities. A major objective of care is to encourage the patient to participate actively in his own care when his condition has stabilized.[19] Depending on the patient's condition, early ambulation is encouraged.

Prevention of infection. Some hospitals maintain plastic dressing rooms in which dressings are changed under aseptic conditions, or sometimes patients are taken to the operating room for dressing changes, and light anesthetics are administered. Medical centers and large hospitals are developing self-contained burn units. Regardless of the method of treatment used, all personnel caring for the patient should observe the practice of thorough hand-washing before providing any care. If the exposure method of treatment is used, a gown, mask, and sterile gloves must be worn, and the patient should wear a mask to protect himself from organisms present in his own respiratory tract. If visitors are allowed in the room, they should be required to follow the same procedure. Antibiotics are usually administered to the patient to aid in preventing infection. Treatment will depend partly on the conditions surrounding the injury. Persons with respiratory infections should not be allowed near the patient. When there are burns about the perineal area, care must be taken to prevent infection from fecal contamination. This may be especially important, but difficult, in children.

Relief of pain. When burns are severe, the patient will need medication for pain. When severe edema is present, medication to relieve pain should be given intravenously. Morphine may be diluted in 3 to 5 ml. of saline solution and injected slowly. If respirations are below 12 times a minute, the medication should be withheld because morphine depresses respirations. Meperidine hydrochloride (Demerol), barbiturates, dextropropoxyphene hydrochloride (Darvon) may be ordered.

Diet. Nothing is given by mouth for the first 24 to 48 hours. Many burned patients have nausea and vomiting, and a Levin tube is usually inserted to prevent abdominal distention and paralytic ileus. After 24 hours if there is no vomiting, oral fluids

may be started. If he can tolerate it, the patient may gradually progress to a high-caloric, high-protein diet in 7 to 10 days. Caloric requirements may exceed 5000 daily. The use of between-meal, high-protein drinks will aid in meeting caloric requirements. In the beginning, small, frequent feedings should be given, and protein may be added by the use of one of the commercial high-protein supplements.

Supportive nursing care. After admission of the patient, the bed should not be changed before the second or third day, and a sufficient number of persons should be available to assist. Medication for pain should be administered 30 to 45 minutes before beginning the procedure. Thereafter the bed is changed only as necessary. Vital signs are taken at frequent intervals, and when a blood pressure cuff can be applied, blood pressure is taken every 15 minutes until it is stable. The patient needs special mouth care, and lemon juice and glycerin may be used. If the lips are not burned, cold cream or a water-soluble jelly should be applied. A retention catheter is usually inserted, and care should be taken to prevent urinary tract infection by maintaining a sterile closed system of drainage.

If the feet have not been burned, ambulation is generally ordered as soon as possible for the patient. This helps to improve appetite and elimination and to raise the patient's spirits. Soaks or tub baths may be ordered to remove dressings and to prevent damage to the tissues or to remove eschar prior to skin grafting. The bathtub should be thoroughly scrubbed with soap and water and disinfected, and the temperature of the water should be 100° F.

Emotional care. The burned patient has many emotional problems, chief among which is probably fear of disfigurement. Since most burns are the result of carelessness, there are bound to be feelings of guilt. Most patients realize that long weeks of recovery lie ahead, and the worry over loss of income and expenses may cause endless anxiety. The patient's family have emotional problems and often guilt feelings. Both the patient and the family need opportunities to talk about their problems, and these opportunities may be provided by the nurse, the hospital social worker, or the religious counselor. Plans to assist a family financially may relieve worry. Diversional activities should be provided for the patient to help fill unused time and often may be helpful in preventing contractures. While patients are waiting for skin grafts to heal, they may be taken to solariums or moved near a nurses' station to relieve the monotony of always remaining in their room.

Skin grafting. Almost all severely burned patients will require skin grafting. However, burned patients are not the only persons for whom skin grafting may be done, and skin is not the only kind of body tissue that may be grafted. Any graft is living tissue taken from one part of the body or from another body and transferred to a new site to correct some defect. When a graft is taken from the same person to whom it is to be transplanted, it is called an *autograft*. When the graft comes from a different person, it is called a *homograft*. Occasionally skin grafts are taken from animals and are called *heterografts* or *xenografts*. Recently, porcine (pig) skin has been used successfully as a temporary biologic dressing prior to performing autografts. This treatment prevents fluid and protein loss, protects from infection, and prepares the site to receive the autograft.[17] In some institutions patients having full-thickness grafts for third-degree burns are taken immediately to the operating room, and the destroyed tissues are completely removed. Skin grafts are applied at once. The effects have been positive, particularly with burned children. They may be discharged healed within 3 weeks, barring any complications.[14]

Skin grafts are usually taken from the thigh, abdomen, back, or buttocks. There are several different techniques used in removing skin for grafts, and the particular method used depends largely on the purpose for the graft and the results desired. In skin grafting for burns the method most frequently used for moving the skin is the split-thickness graft. The skin may be removed by an electrically operated instrument called a *dermatome*. The graft taken this way is a half thickness of the skin and may vary in width up to about 2 inches.

When the burned patient is to have a skin graft, there are two factors that must be considered: the preparation of the donor site and the preparation of the burn site.

The nurse must understand the exact donor site to be prepared. The skin is washed and shaved in essentially the same way as in preparing the patient for any surgery. The burned area to be grafted must be free of all eschar and debris, since grafts will not grow unless the area is clean. The patient is usually placed in a tub of saline solution for periods as long as an hour. Depending on the amount of debridement necessary, several baths may be given, and the procedure may require several days. The nurse should wear a gown, mask, and sterile gloves while giving the bath. Debridement usually is done in the operating room.

The patient receives a general anesthetic, and on return from the operating room he will have two surgical sites to be cared for. There are various types of dressings used for the grafted area, including fine-mesh petroleum gauze held in place by cotton pads and bandage. Some physicians prefer that the area be left open to the air. If dressings are used, the nurse never removes them unless told to do so by the physician. In other cases dressings are applied so that a daily inspection may be done for evidence of infection. Since many methods are in use, the nurse will have to become familiar with the particular procedure desired by the physician. The care of the donor site will also vary. It may be covered with gauze and pressure bandages, or it may have a layer of fine-mesh gauze and be left open to the air. Analgesics may be needed for pain, and the ambulatory patient often finds that he has more discomfort from the donor site than from the grafted area. When the donor site is the thigh, walking may be difficult.

Not all grafted skin may grow, and repeat grafts may be required. The nurse should be careful to avoid discussing the success or failure of the graft with the patient. Specific questions should be referred to the physician.

Summary outline

1. Structure of skin
   A. Epidermis—outermost covering, which is constantly being shed
      1. Keratin—principal substance of epidermis
      2. Melanin—provides coloring of skin
   B. Dermis (true skin) contains numerous blood vessels and nerves

1. Sudoriferous glands (sweat glands) in dermis
   2. Sebaceous glands (oil glands)
   C. Subcutaneous tissue (superficial fascia)
   1. Supports dermis
   2. Maintains blood supply to dermis
   3. Contains large amount of fat and some sweat glands
   D. Appendages of skin
   1. Nails, hair, sebaceous glands, and sudoriferous glands
   E. Sebaceous glands—secrete sebum
   F. Sudoriferous glands—secrete oil and open on skin as pores
2. Function of skin
   A. Provides protective covering
   B. Acts as organ of excretion
   C. Regulates body temperature
   D. Provides information about environment
   E. Contributes to psychologic and mental health
3. Numerous causes of skin diseases and disorders
   A. Malfunctioning of other organs or systems
   B. Allergic conditions
   C. Side effects from drugs
   D. Chemicals, biologics, mechanical injury
   E. Heat and cold
   F. Nutritional indiscretions and deficiencies
   G. Invasion by pathogenic organisms
   H. Normal aging process
4. Characteristics of skin lesions
   A. Many types of skin lesions
5. Diagnostic tests and procedures
   Most disorders of skin can be diagnosed by careful history, general appearance, and distribution of lesions
   A. Bacteriologic study
   B. Biopsy for pathologic examination
   C. Examination of blood and urine
6. Specific aspects of nursing patient with diseases and disorders of skin
   A. Therapeutic baths
   1. Purposes
   a. Disinfection and deodorizing
   b. Relief of pruritus
   c. Soothing effects
   d. Softening and lubricating skin
   2. Substances used
   a. Soaps, oils, or medications
   b. Oatmeal, bran, starch, baking soda, or combination of these
   B. Wet dressings
   1. Purposes
   a. Cooling effect
   b. Relief of pruritus
   2. May be open or closed, hot or cold
   3. Solutions used
   a. Physiologic saline solution
   b. Boric acid solution
   c. Magnesium sulfate solution
   d. 0.5% aluminum acetate solution
   e. 1:4000 postassium permanganate solution
   C. Soaks may be used to loosen necrotic tissue and to promote suppuration
   D. Paste boots—commercial preparation of water, gelatin, glycerin, and zinc oxide
   E. Emotional support is necessary

7. Nursing patient with diseases and disorders of skin
   A. Bacterial diseases
   1. Furuncles, carbuncles, and felons
   a. Furuncles (boils) originate about hair follicle and are caused by staphylococcus
   b. Carbuncles occur when infection infiltrates into surrounding tissue, causing several boils; caused by staphylococcus
   c. Felon is infection of end of finger; streptococcus is frequent cause
   2. Impetigo contagiosa—superficial contagious skin disease caused by staphylococci and streptococci
   B. Fungus infections
   1. Tinea (ringworm)
   a. Tinea capitis—known as ringworm of scalp; primarily affects preadolescent children
   b. Tinea circinata—form of ringworm that occurs on nonhairy parts of body
   c. Tinea sycosis (barber's itch)—occurs in beard and may become serious condition involving cervical lymph nodes
   d. Tinea pedis (athlete's foot)—common disease of feet that may be transmitted to other persons
   (1) Prevention—keep feet dry, use medicated foot powder, wear clean socks
   C. Dermatitis of skin—inflammatory condition resulting from several causes
   1. Erythema intertrigo (chafing)—occurs when two skin surfaces rub together
   2. Miliaria (prickly heat)—caused by environmental and physiologic factors and occurs when persons are exposed to extremes of heat for long periods
   a. May occur in infants when they are kept too warm
   3. Dermatitis venenata (plant poisoning)—occurs from contact with certain plants
   a. Poison ivy, poison oak, poison sumac, poison elder
   4. Exfoliative dermatitis—may result from several causes, commonly from drugs containing heavy metals
   5. Dermatitis medicamentosa—term applied to skin disorders caused by drugs
   a. Nurses should observe patients carefully for evidence of skin lesions
   6. Psoriasis—incurable skin disease with unknown cause
   a. Characterized by remissions and exacerbations
   b. May be accompanied by form of arthritis
   c. No specific treatment
   7. Eczema—results from many causes and exhibits many different types of skin lesions
   8. Acne vulgaris—disease of adolescence believed to be caused by increased hormonal activity

      a. Condition is self-limiting and usually disappears by adult life

      b. Treatment nonspecific

      c. May interfere with personality development

D. Viral infections

  1. Herpes simplex (fever blister, cold sore)—caused by virus and self-limiting

  2. Herpes zoster (shingles)—often considered neurologic disorder, since lesions are located in spinal ganglia with involvement of skin supplied by nerve fibers

      a. Believed to be caused by virus

      b. Skin lesions usually occur in thoracic area

      c. Depression frequently accompanies disease

      d. If skin lesions are on face, patient should be observed for facial paralysis and disturbance of vision and hearing

E. Disorders of pigmentation

  1. Lentigo (freckles)—collections of skin pigment caused by quantitative changes in melanin

  2. Chloasma (liver spots)—not caused by liver disease

      a. May occur during pregnancy and at time of menopause

F. Disorders of glands

  1. Seborrhea (oily skin)—caused by excessive secretion of oil glands (sebum)

  2. Sebaceous cyst (wen)—often occurs on scalp and is caused by increase of sebum and obstruction of duct

  3. Hyperhidrosis (excessive sweating)

      a. Tuberculosis and hyperthyroidism

      b. Renal colic or other severe pain

      c. Shock

      d. Toxic conditions and fevers

      e. Antipyretic drugs

      f. Extremes of heat

      g. Severe physical exercise

  4. Anhidrosis (absence of sweating)

      a. Aging process

      b. Various skin diseases

      c. Administration of certain drugs

      d. Diabetes, hypothyroidism, and nephritis

G. Pruritus (itching)—symptom that accompanies many skin disorders, systemic diseases, and allergic conditions

  1. Complications may occur from scratching

H. Tumors of skin

  1. Benign tumors

      a. Keloid—tumor mass occuring at site of scar that consists of overgrowth of fibrous tissue

        (1) More common in blacks

      b. Angioma—benign skin tumor consisting of dilated blood vessels

        (1) Congenital (birthmark) or port-wine stain

        (2) Spider angioma occurs in persons with liver disease

      c. Nevus (mole)—nonvascular tumor that may be pigmented; there are many different types

        (1) Black moles may become malignant if irritated

      d. Verruca (wart)—benign tumor of skin; there are various kinds

        (1) One type seen in children is believed to be caused by virus

      e. Keratoses—many types of these lesions

        (1) Senile keratoses in elderly may be precancerous

  2. Malignant tumors—may develop from precancerous skin lesions exposed to irritation

      a. Carcinoma of skin responds to treatment by x-ray or radium therapy

I. Disorders of appendages

  1. Alopecia (loss of hair)—may be result of several causes

      a. Normal thinning with age

      b. Debilitating diseases

      c. Early syphilis

      d. Alopecia areata is sudden loss of hair with spontaneous recovery

  2. Hypertrichosis and hypotrichosis

      a. Hypertrichosis is excessive growth of hair that may be congenital or acquired and often results from endocrine disturbance

      b. Hypotrichosis is absence or deficiency of hair that may be skin disease or result of endocrine factors

  3. Nails—may indicate disease elsewhere in body, or disorders may be result of congenital defects

      a. Paronychia ("run-around")—infection at matrix of nail

      b. Fungus infections—respond poorly to ordinary methods of treatment

J. Infestations

  1. Pediculi (lice)

      a. *Pediculus capitis*—head louse

      b. *Pediculus corporis*—body louse

      c. *Pediculus pubis*—found in short, stiff hair as in genital area, eyebrows, and eyelashes

  2. Scabies (itch)—infectious skin disease caused by parasite that burrows under skin, causing itching

K. Burns—injuries to body tissue

  1. Caused by heat (dry or moist), electricity, chemicals, radiant energy

  2. Classification of depth of burn

      a. First degree

      b. Second degree

      c. Third degree

      d. Fourth degree

      e. Segmental charring

  3. Extent of burn is estimated by "rule of nine"

  4. First aid—apply cool water, wrap in clean sheet, and take to hospital

  5. Initial treatment

      a. Observe for and attempt to prevent shock

b. Give intravenous fluids
c. Remove debris or loose skin
d. Analgesics, antibiotics, and tetanus prophylaxis

6. Objectives of treatment
   a. To save patient's life
   b. To prevent infection
   c. To restore normal function and appearance
7. Environmental preparation
8. Methods of treatment
   a. Exposure method using mafenide acetate (Sulfamylon acetate)
   b. Silver nitrate method
   c. Occlusive dressings
9. Intake and output
10. Positioning the patient
11. Prevention of infection
12. Relief of pain
13. Diet
14. Supportive nursing care
15. Emotional support and diversional activities are important in recovery and rehabilitation
16. Skin grafting—graft is living tissue that is transplanted to another area of body
    a. Autograft—from same person to whom it is to be transplanted
    b. Homograft—donor is person other than recipient
    c. Heterograft or xenograft—donor is animal, usually a pig
    d. Split-thickness type graft frequently used for burns
    e. Variety of dressing methods for grafted area and donor area; nurse must understand physician's orders for care

Review questions

1. What are the purposes of therapeutic baths?
   a.
   b.
   c.
   d.
   e.
2. Why should external heat not be appiled to a hot wet dressing?
   a.
3. What is another name for a common boil?
   a.
4. What measures are recommended to prevent athlete's foot?
   a.
   b.
   c.
   d.
5. What are the two uppermost layers of the skin called?
   a.
   b.
6. What is the cause of herpes simplex?
   a.
7. What is the recommended treatment for *Pediculus humanus* var. *capitis?*
   a.
8. How are burns classified?

   a.
   b.
   c.
   d.
   e.
9. What are the three objectives in the care of the burned patient?
   a.
   b.
   c.
10. What is the difference between an autograft and a homograft?
    a.
11. How would you tell the difference between a second-degree burn and a third-degree burn?
    a.

Films

1. Early intensive therapy—burned hands—M-1632-X (15 min., sound, color, 16 mm.), Media Resources Branch, National Medical Audiovisual Center (Annex), Station K, Atlanta, Ga. 30324. Shows the treatment and early intensive therapy of first-, second-, and third-degree burned hands.
2. Metastasizing basal cell carcinoma (10 min., sound, color, 16 mm.), Squibb, 745 Fifth Ave., New York, N. Y. 10022. The story of a man who had a variety of lesions on the nose, cheeks, ears, arms, wrists, and trunk. The patient died, and the film stresses the need for early diagnosis and proper treatment for an ulceration on his leg, which could have saved his life.
3. Pustular psoriasis (15 min., sound, color, 16 mm.), Squibb, 745 Fifth Ave., New York, N. Y. 10022. Presents a patient and her history of psoriasis beginning at 4 years of age. At 51 years of age she had arthritis, and at 54 years her symptoms were generalized. Spontaneous remissions that lasted from weeks to months are described.
4. Special eye care (for burns) (11 min., sound, color, 16 mm.), Media Resources Branch, National Medical Audiovisual Center (Annex), Station K, Atlanta, Ga. 30324. Demonstrates the special eye care of patients suffering second- and third-degree burns of the face. Highlights nursing techniques and procedures before and after burn surgery to prevent eye infection and corneal ulceration.

References

1. Beeson, Paul B., and McDermott, Walsh, editors: Cecil-Loeb textbook of medicine, ed. 13, Philadelphia, 1971, W. B. Saunders Co.
2. Brunner, Lillian S., and Suddarth, Doris S.: Textbook of medical-surgical nursing, ed. 3, Philadelphia, 1975, J. B. Lippincott Co.
3. Claudia, Sister Mary: TLC and Sulfamylon for burned children, American Journal of Nursing 69:755-757, April, 1969.
4. Conn, Howard F., editor: Current therapy, 1976, Philadelphia, 1976, W. B. Saunders Co.
5. Emmons, Chester W., Binford, Chapman H.,

and Ulz, John P.: Medical mycology, Philadelphia, 1963, Lea & Febiger.

6. Fatal fires and explosions in the home, Statistical Bulletin **50**:9, Feb., 1969, Metropolitan Life Insurance Co.

7. Fitzpatrick, P. J.: Tumors of the skin, The Canadian Nurse **63**:45-47, Feb., 1967.

8. Hartford, Charles E.: The early treatment of burns, Nursing Clinics of North America **8**: 447-455, Sept., 1973.

9. Henley, Nellie L.: Sulfamylon for burns, American Journal of Nursing **69**:2122-2123, Oct., 1969.

10. Judd, Eloise: Herpes zoster: a nursing challenge, The Journal of Practical Nursing **19**: 27, Nov., 1969.

11. Luckmann, Joan, and Sorensen, Karen C.: Medical-surgical nursing, Philadelphia, 1974, W. B. Saunders Co.

12. Noonan, Joan, and Noonan, Lawrence: Two burned patients in flotation therapy, American Journal of Nursing **68**:316-319, Feb., 1968.

13. Shafer, Kathleen N., Sawyer, Janet R., McCluskey, Audrey M., Beck, Edna L., and

Phipps, Wilma J.: Medical-surgical nursing, ed. 6, St. Louis, 1975, The C. V. Mosby Co.

14. Sheehy, Elizabeth: Innovation in pediatric burn care, RN **37**:21-25, Aug., 1974.

15. Silverton, Alida: Psoriasis—the stubborn malady, The Canadian Nurse **65**:38-40, Nov., 1969.

16. Snively, W. D., Jr., and Beshear, Donna R.: Textbook of pathophysiology, Philadelphia, 1972, J. B. Lippincott Co.

17. Stinson, Velda: Porcine skin dressings for burns, American Journal of Nursing **74**:111-112, Jan., 1974.

18. Unger, Donald L.: Non-allergic drug reactions, American Journal of Nursing **63**:64-65, Jan., 1963.

19. Wagner, Mary: Positioning of burn patients, Nursing Care **7**:22-25, Aug., 1974.

20. Wexler, Louis: Gamma benzene hexachloride in treatment of pediculosis and scabies, American Journal of Nursing **69**:565-567, March, 1969.

21. Young, Clara G., and Barger, James D.: Introduction to medical science, ed. 2, St. Louis, 1973, The C. V. Mosby Co.

CHAPTER 21

Nursing the patient
with diseases and disorders
of the musculoskeletal
system

KEY WORDS

abduction *away from body*
adduction *toward body*
ankylosis *stiffening of a joint; develops fibrous*
arthrodesis *surgical fusion*
arthroplasty *plastic surgery to reshape the position of a diseased joint to increase mobility*
articulation *joint where 2 bones are joined*
contracture *muscle shrinkage*
countertraction *pulling in opposite direction*
external rotation *turn a limb away from body's midline*

internal rotation *turn a limb toward the body's midline*
lordosis *curvature of lumbar spine*
osseous *pertaining to bone*
osteotomy *cutting of bone to correct deformity*
prosthesis *artificial body part*
synovectomy *excision of the synovial membrane*
tophi *deposit of urates of a joint tissues in (gout)*

diaphysis - long shaft
epiphyses - ends of bone
medullary cavity - space in diaphysis
endosteum - lining of medullary cavity
periosteum - bone covering (except at joints)
articular cartilage - covering of ends of long bones

STRUCTURE AND FUNCTION OF THE MUSCULOSKELETAL SYSTEM
Structure

The musculoskeletal system is composed of the bones, joints, and muscles. The system also includes other tissues such as ligaments, which help to hold bones together at joints, and tendons, which attach the muscles to the bones. In some places, for example, between the vertebrae, another type of tissue called *cartilage* may join bones together.

Like any other tissue, bones are composed of living cells and an intercellular substance. Bone varies from other tissues in that the intercellular substance is calcified. It is this feature that gives bones their rigidity and strength. Children have bones that are more flexible and less brittle than adults, whose bones contain larger amounts of calcium. The aged person often has demineralization of bone, causing them to become brittle.

Each long bone consists of six major parts. The *diaphysis* is the long shaft of the bone, and the *epiphyses* are the ends of the bone. The *medullary (marrow) cavity* is the space that runs the length of the diaphysis. This is lined with the *endosteum* and consists of cells that form new bone as needed. The *periosteum* is the membrane that covers the bone except at the joints. The inner layer of the periosteum also contains bone-forming cells. Finally, each end of the long bone is covered with *articular cartilage* which cushions blows to the joint.

501

Bones are of various shapes. Long bones are found in the extremities; short bones may also be irregular and are found in the hands and feet. Flat bones protect vital structures such as the brain and organs located in the thorax. Irregular bones include the vertebrae and small irregular bones in other places in the body.

The nurse should have an understanding of joints to be able to put joints through a range of motion. Some joints are freely movable such as hinge joints in the elbows and knees, and the motions of these joints are called flexion and extension. The shoulder and hip joints are ball-and-socket joints and have a rotating motion. Other joints are slightly movable, for example, the joints between the vertebral bodies; the disks provide limited motion of the spine. Some joints are immovable and are found in many places such as the cranium. Only those joints that are freely movable can be put through a range of motion.

Although movement of the body depends largely on contraction of the muscles, it is actually a cooperative function of bones and muscles.

Function

The musculoskeletal system has other functions beside locomotion. The bony framework supports the body in an upright position and protects vital organs. Blood cells are formed in the marrow of bones, and bones deposit calcium, which may be used to supply a deficiency in the body fluids. Injury and disease may affect any part of the system and result in deformity or impairment of its functions. Some diseases involve both nerves and muscles and are called *neuromuscular diseases*.

POSITION, MOVEMENT, AND BODY MECHANICS

Considerable stress has been placed on proper positioning of the patient who is confined to a regimen of bed rest. This is a nursing function, and medical orders are unnecessary except in certain surgical procedures in which physicians' preferences vary. Many orthopedic patients are required to remain in plaster casts, traction, or other forms of immobilization over long periods of time. Nursing care must emphasize positioning to prevent contractures and the development of deformities. When possible, passive and active exercise and movement of joints through a range of motion (p. 170) must be faithfully done to prevent the development of fibrous tissue and to maintain muscle tone. Emphasis has been placed on the importance of turning patients to prevent pulmonary complications. Too often a comfortable patient objects to being disturbed, and more often the moving of an obese or comatose patient or a patient in a body cast or in traction presents a monumental task for the nurse. Research has confirmed the fact that turning the patient as little as 12 degrees is sufficient to prevent pulmonary complications, stimulate circulation, and prevent decubitus ulcers.

The tilt table is a device for helping the patient adjust to an upright position prior to ambulation. Patients confined to a bed rest regimen for long periods may develop hypotension when they are elevated to a sitting or standing position. When there is a gradual elevation using the tilt table, the problem may be overcome. The tilt table is helpful in preparing the patient for crutch walking and ambulation and in reducing osteoporosis that develops from immobilization. It may also help to reduce urinary tract infection by preventing the pooling of urine in the bladder that results when the patient remains in a supine position.

Nurses should consider their own body mechanics to conserve energy, prevent injuries to muscles, prevent fatigue, and work efficiently. After injuries to the musculoskeletal system many patients will need to be taught proper methods of standing, sitting, walking, stooping, and lifting. Nurses who use their bodies skillfully will be in a much better position to help teach patients body mechanics.

NURSING CARE OF THE PATIENT IN A CAST

It is important to take care of the cast so that the purpose for which it is intended may be fully realized. However, care of the cast is secondary to the care of the patient within its enclosure. The application of a plaster cast may be an elective procedure that has been carefully considered by the patient before its application. More often it is an emergency procedure, and the patient does not have the right of choice. The cast limits the patient's freedom of movement and interferes with his independence. It threatens his economic security by jeopardizing his job. The inability to attend school may be frustrating to an adolescent and of concern to parents, whereas a mother wonders how she will manage a home and who will care for the family. The emotional problems make the patient's adjustment to his situation extremely difficult. The nurse caring for the patient needs to have sympathy and understanding and should realize that seemingly unnecessary demands reflect the patient's emotional problems as well as his physical discomforts.

Nursing care should begin with preparation of the bed to receive the patient with a wet cast. Boards should be placed between the spring and mattress. If the cast is to be applied only to an extremity, hinged boards should be used so that the head of the bed may be elevated. The bottom of the bed is made as usual, and a cotton bath blanket is placed over the drawsheet covering the bed. Three pillows with plastic covers are placed crossways on the bed when a body cast is to be applied (Fig. 21-1). If a hip spica cast is being applied, one pillow is placed across the bed near the small of the back, and two pillows are placed lengthwise to support the leg (Fig. 21-2). When a long leg cast is applied to an extremity, the knee will be slightly flexed. The extremity should be supported and slightly elevated on pillows. Fig. 21-3 shows placement of the pillows. The patient must never be placed on a firm sur-

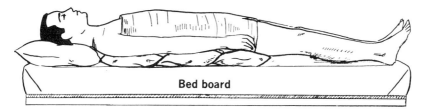

Fig. 21-1. Placement of pillows to receive a patient in a wet body cast.

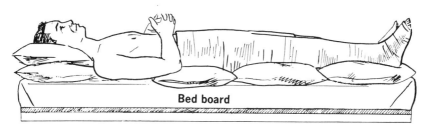

Fig. 21-2. Placement of pillows to receive a patient in a wet hip spica cast.

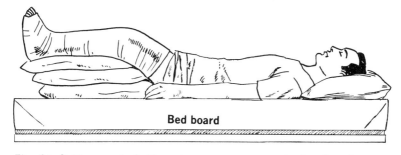

Fig. 21-3. Placement of pillows to support an extremity in a long-leg cast.

face while the cast is damp because it will become flattened and result in severe pressure over bony prominences.

When the patient is first placed on the bed, he must be lifted carefully onto it. Careless handling at this time may damage the cast and may affect the placement of the body that the physician has worked to achieve. The palmar surface of the hands must be used in lifting or in any moving of the patient as long as the cast is damp. Pressure from fingers may mold the cast and result in pressure on the skin. A small pillow should be placed under the patient's head and shoulders. The cast should not be covered, since it dries through evaporation of moisture into the air. Depending on size and thickness, the cast will dry in 24 to 48 hours. During the process of drying, heat is released and if the cast is large, the patient's temperature may rise slightly. Various methods to speed drying are sometimes employed, but heat should be used cautiously, since it dries the outside but may leave the inside damp, in which case evaporation is restricted. The added danger that a burn may occur is also present.

It is a fairly general policy that a patient in a body or hip spica cast should be turned to the prone position on the evening of the day the cast is applied to allow drying of the posterior cast. However, the patient should be turned only on the physician's written order to do so. The nurse must realize that the patient has dreaded this time and is afraid. He must be told exactly what is to be done. Three or four persons should be available for this turning. Later, when the cast is dry, the patient may help if a trapeze is placed above the bed so that one person can turn the patient.

The patient is moved to the side of the bed opposite the leg that is not in a cast; if surgery has been done, he will be turned toward the side that has not been operated on. The patient must not be pulled far enough to let the cast drop off the pillows. With care, dry cases may be placed on the pillows. The patient is instructed to place his arms at his sides, and the pillow is removed from under the head. A nurse places the palm of one hand on the patient's shoulder and the other palm on the patient's hip. A second nurse supports the extremity in the cast at the thigh and the ankle. Turning should always be done on the side that has not been operated on or the side that is not enclosed in a full cast. As the patient is gently turned to a prone position, a nurse on the opposite side of the

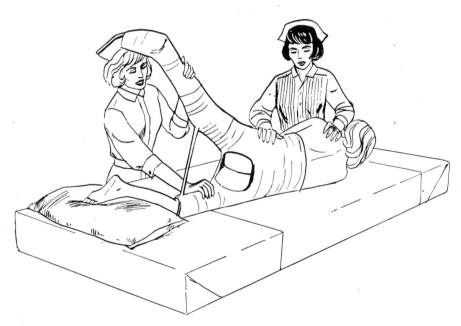

Fig. 21-4. Turning a patient in a hip spica cast.

bed assists by positioning the shoulder and the extremity (Fig. 21-4). The abduction bar should never be used at any time to turn the patient. Pillows should have been placed in position to receive the cast prior to turning. When the patient is in the prone position, care must be taken to see that the cast does not cut into the back, which may occur if too many pillows are under the head. When the patient is in the supine position, placing too many pillows under the head and chest may cause the cast to cut into the abdomen. Pillows should be placed under the feet to keep the toes off the bed.

The back and buttocks should be washed and gently massaged, and loose plaster should be removed from the bed. If the patient has been given a general anesthetic, his care is the same as that for any postoperative patient. In addition, the patient in a body or hip spica cast must be observed for abdominal distention. When casts are applied to extremities, circulation must be checked at intervals as long as the cast remains on the part. Pressure applied to a toe or finger will result in blanching (turning white), but immediately on releasing pressure, pinkness will return. If color should fail to return or be slow in returning, it must be reported immediately to the physician. The extremity should be observed for cyanosis, temperature, tingling, numbness, or edema, any of which may indicate pressure on blood vessels or nerves. The nurse should listen when the patient complains of pain at any place under the cast, since pressure may result in severe ulcer formation. Fingers and toes should be washed daily and carefully dried. Massaging the skin under the edges of the cast is often soothing and is appreciated by the patient.

When caring for the patient, the nurse should be alert to any foul odor about the cast. Perineal care is important, and it must be remembered that the patient in a body cast or hip spica cast often cannot give this care himself. When the nurse places the bedpan, the patient may help by lifting himself with the overhead trapeze, or he may be rolled onto the pan. A pillow should be placed under the back to support the cast at the level of the pan.

After the cast is dry the patient should be turned every 4 hours. He may be turned onto a stretcher and taken to a sun porch or near the nurses' station to provide relief from the monotony of his room. The patient's diet should be well balanced with adequate protein, minerals, and vitamins; however, excessive calories should be avoided to prevent weight gain. The head of the bed may be elevated on low blocks to make it easier for the patient to feed himself and to eat. Joints and extremities not enclosed in the cast should be given active exercise to maintain motion, strength, and muscle tone.

Care of the cast

The care of the cast should be directed toward maintaining cleanliness and preventing moisture, which may soften the plaster. Plaster from the raw edges of the cast will irritate the skin unless measures are taken to prevent it. No one has found a completely satisfactory method of keeping the outside of the cast clean. A slightly dampened cloth may be rubbed over a cake of abrasive soap and used to clean small areas. A stocking with the toes cut out may be pulled over a leg or arm. Stockinette tubing may be pulled over both the body cast and casts applied to the extremities. The cast may also be sprayed with a plastic substance for protection after it is thoroughly dry. However, in most cases the cast is left exposed. Adolescents enjoy having their friends autograph or draw caricatures on the cast, and the practice should not be discouraged.

The cast must be protected about the genital area from soiling by bowel and bladder elimination. This is particularly important in children, for whom protection must include the leg cast also. There are many ways to accomplish this. Oiled silk, waxed paper, and plastic may be cut into 4- to 5-inch strips, tucked inside the cast, and fastened on the outside with cellophane tape. In the home soft plastic materials are often available from dry cleaning bags or bags in which shirts are placed by the laundry. The bag may be washed in warm soapy water, dried, and cut to provide protection. Saran Wrap is soft and pliable, adheres to most surfaces, and may easily provide protection. Materials should be removed and replaced as necessary.

The edges of the cast are rough and may irritate the skin or cause pressure. Small particles of plaster may fall inside the cast and cause irritation or even abrasion. The edges may be finished by pulling the stockinette from the inside over the cast edge and fastening it with adhesive or a strip of plaster. The most common method is to cut round or oval petals from adhesive tape and bind all edges of the cast. Adhesive tape will not adhere to a wet cast; therefore the cast must be completely dry before the edges are finished. Any jagged edges should be smoothed before applying the binding.

The cast must not be allowed to become wet and must always be handled carefully to prevent cracking.

Removal of the cast

When the cast is removed, it may be bivalved, and the physician may wish the patient to lie in the shell for part or all of the time for a few days. After removal of the cast the body or extremity should be supported in the same position previously maintained by the cast. This may require the use of devices to keep the foot in position and to prevent the outward rotation of the leg. Extremities should be lifted carefully, supplying support to the joints. When the patient has been in a cast for a long period of time, varying amounts of decalcification have occurred, and the possibility of spontaneous fracture is always present. This should be kept in mind when turning or moving the patient.

The skin under the cast will be covered by an exudate consisting of secretions from the sebaceous and sudoriferous glands and dead skin. This may actually be a protective covering, and if another cast is to be applied, the physician may wish it to be left on the skin. No vigorous effort should be used in cleaning the skin. Gentle washing with a mild soap and warm water, followed by the application of lanolin or baby oil and gentle massage, is sufficient for cleaning the skin.

After removal of the cast from an extremity, the physician may wish some support given to the part, and an elastic bandage is applied as soon as the cast is removed. There will be some atrophy of muscles; the physician may order the patient to begin exercises to strengthen and restore muscle tone, and the patient may be referred to the physical therapy department. Often the patient will complain of joint discomfort after cast removal. Joint structures and muscles have become somewhat contracted from prolonged immobilization and disuse. The patient should be reassured that this is temporary and will improve as the joint is used. When the cast has been removed from a lower extremity, there should be no weight bearing until ordered by the physician.

Investigations have been made to determine whether other materials would be more suitable for casting than plaster of Paris. Materials such as plastics, metal, and fiberglass have been used in an attempt to develop a stronger cast. Fiberglass casts appear to have the most advantages and may eventually replace the plaster of Paris casts. These casts are stronger and lighter weight, may be immersed in water, and dry to a permanent set within 3 minutes when a black light is applied.[9]

NURSING THE PATIENT WITH AN ORTHOPEDIC DEVICE
Traction

Traction may be applied to any of the extremities, the cervical area, or the pelvic region. Cervical traction may be used when there is severe injury to the cervical vertebrae or the spinal cord. Pelvic traction may be indicated to relieve pain from injury of the lower back, frequently in the lumbar region. The purpose of traction may be to relieve muscle spasm, which often occurs because of disease or injury. For patients with certain kinds of fractures traction may be necessary to keep bones in place while healing of bones and soft tissues occurs. It may be used to reduce dislocations or to correct or relieve contractures.

Traction means "pulling"; therefore when traction is applied to a lower extremity because of a broken bone, it may be to pull the two ends of the bone into place. Traction may be applied as skin traction, in which some material with an adhesive surface is applied directly onto the clean dry skin, or as skeletal traction, in which various devices such as pins or wire are placed through a bone, or as Crutchfield tongs,

traction - purpose

Steinmann pin
Kirschner wire

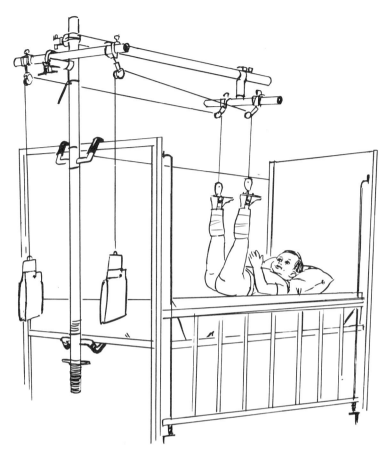

Fig. 21-5. Bryant's traction. Note that the hips are kept off the bed to provide counter-traction.

which are attached to the skull for cervical traction. Occasionally patients are placed in balanced suspension with a splint. This type of traction is often used to maintain an extremity in a specific position after surgery and may or may not involve skin or skeletal traction. In all types of traction there will be ropes, pulleys, weights, and provision for countertraction.

Some commonly used types of traction include Bryant's traction, which is used for young children with fracture of the femur (Fig. 21-5). In this type of traction the hips are flexed at about 90 degrees; the hips should be just off the bed, and traction is applied to both legs and usually maintained for 2 to 4 weeks. Often some type of restraint is required for young children. If Bryant's traction is used for children more than 2 years old, the legs should be carefully observed for decreased circula-

tion. Buck's extension (Fig. 21-6) is a type of traction in which adhesive material is attached to the skin. There is a footplate to which rope is attached, and the rope is placed over one pulley at the foot of the bed with weights attached at the end. This is a simple type of traction that can be easily adapted for home use. Russell traction consists of skin traction, often Buck's extension, in addition to a sling under the knee that is attached to ropes and pulleys to provide suspension. It may be used in fractures of the femur or hip, and countertraction is provided by elevating the foot of the bed (Fig. 21-7). When Russell traction is used, patients are able to move about more freely and nursing care can be given more easily, as with any suspension traction. There are other types of traction designed for specific purposes. It is not easy to understand traction, and it is not the

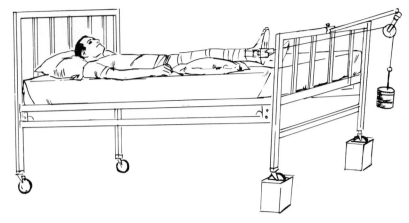

Fig. 21-6. Buck's extension.

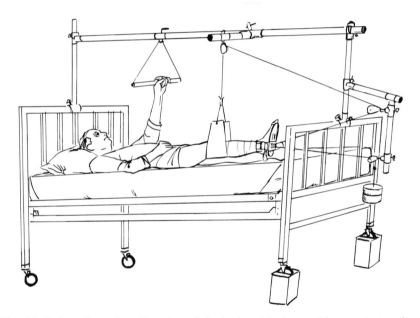

Fig. 21-7. Russell traction. Elevation of the bed on blocks provides countertraction.

responsibility of the nurse to construct traction. Many hospitals have personnel who are trained in the various types of traction and are responsible for setting up the type ordered by the physician. If such persons are not available, the physician assumes the responsibility for constructing the traction.

In many instances the patient will be required to lie flat in bed and may not be permitted to sit up or to turn to either side. The nurse caring for patients in traction must be familiar with the amount of movement that the physician allows the patient to have.

The quality of nursing care may in part be judged by the expertness of the nurse's observation. The skin around the edge of adhesive tape must be observed for irritation or abrasion. If the tape seems to be pulling or loosening, it must be reported. When pins or wire have been used, the area around the wound should be covered with sterile dressings and watched for evidence of infection. Extremities should be checked several times a day for color, numbness, cyanosis, pallor, pain, and edema. The skin about the ankles and the heel must be watched for pressure areas and

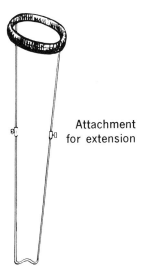

Attachment
for extension

Fig. 21-8. Thomas splint used with some kinds of traction. It may be used with a whole ring or half ring.

irritation. The patient's position and body alignment in bed are extremely important, as is avoiding internal or external rotation of extremities. When a Thomas splint (Fig. 21-8) is used, the area about the groin should be observed for pressure, and a sling as in Russell traction may wrinkle unless a felt pad is placed in the hammock. All weights must swing free and must never be removed without the physician's permission. Nothing may touch the ropes except the pulley over which they are placed. The nurse should be constantly alert for anything that may interfere with the purpose of the traction or that may retard the patient's progress and should report it immediately to the physician.

When giving morning care, several persons may be needed to lift the patient so that the back may be washed and massaged. Inspection of the sacral area for pressure points should not be overlooked. Massage of the area should be done several times a day and may be accomplished by running the hand under the back without lifting the patient. The bottom of the bed is changed from the unaffected side, and small pieces of blankets, small sheets, or split linen may be used to cover the patient when large ones interfere with placement of ropes or mechanical devices. An orthopedic bedpan and female urinal may

provide adequately for bowel and bladder elimination except in the case of an enema. When a larger pan is needed, a plastic-covered pillow should be placed lengthwise along the back when the patient is lifted onto the pan. In many cases an overhead trapeze is provided, and the patient can assist by lifting his hips. Good oral care and a diet high in calcium, protein, iron, and vitamins are important. Foods high in roughage may help to prevent constipation. The patient should be encouraged in coughing, deep breathing, and active exercise of the unaffected extremities; however, the affected extremity should not be exercised unless specifically ordered by the physician.

Frames

There are several types of frames that may be used for orthopedic, neuromuscular, or burned patients. The Balkan frame consists of a wooden or steel framework that attaches to the regular hospital bed. The frame has adjustable pulleys and a trapeze attached to an overhead bar. The Balkan frame is used for patients in traction and should be placed on the bed before traction is instituted.

The Bradford frame is a rectangular steel frame with two pieces of canvas stretched tightly and laced to the frame. A space is left between the pieces of canvas at the level of the buttocks to place the bedpan. The frame comes in several sizes and may be suspended to the bed with hooks, or it may be suspended in the bed on blocks or boxes. The canvas is usually covered with a sheet, or frame covers may be used which have tapes sewed to the sides so that they may be tied to the frame. If sheets are used, they must be tightened several times a day to avoid wrinkling under the patient. Since the frame is narrow and suspended, patients must be protected from falling. When children are placed on a Bradford frame, some type of restraint is required.

The Stryker frame and Foster frame are similar in that they provide for changing the patient's position from supine to prone without interfering with the body alignment. The frames are similar to the Bradford frame but fit onto a pivoting device at the head and foot of the frame, where they are held firmly by pins. There are two frames, a posterior and an anterior frame. The posterior frame has an opening in the canvas to allow use of the bedpan. Both frames have canvas covers over which a sponge rubber mattress cut the same size as the canvas may be placed and then covered with a sheet.

Nursing care of the patient on a Stryker or Foster frame is simplified in that the patient is easily turned, allowing for good skin care and frequent change of position. When giving morning care, the anterior part of the body is bathed. A pillow is placed lengthwise across the legs. The patient is covered with a sheet, and if a thin foam rubber mattress is used, it is placed over the sheet. The anterior frame is then placed on top of the patient. The frame is fastened at the top and bottom ends to the pivoting device, and straps are secured around both frames and the patient. It is recommended that two persons, one at the head and one at the foot, turn him. The pivot pins are removed, and the frame is slowly turned so that the patient is in the prone position. The pivot pins are replaced to hold the frame firmly in place, the straps are removed, and the posterior frame and bedding are removed. The posterior part of the body may then be washed and the back massaged and observed for any pressure areas.

The frame is equipped with armrests, footboard, and attachment for the head. When the patient is in the prone position, pillows should be placed on the armboards for the arms, and the toes should extend over the edge of the canvas. When the patient is in the supine position, the feet should be placed against the footboard at about a 90-degree angle; also, the bedpan may be placed under the patient below the frame and between the canvas space. The patient on a Stryker or Foster frame can do many things for himself, including his oral care, feeding himself, reading, or other diversional activities. Other nursing care is the same as that for any patient who is immobilized.

The CircOlectric bed is a vertical turning bed that may be operated electrically by one person. It also has an anterior frame, which is attached when the patient is to be turned to the prone position. As the patient is turned, his head rises and feet are lowered. The bed may be placed in a variety of positions, including the sitting and standing positions, and it may be used with traction (p. 100).

Splints

Splints are used to support or immobilize an area of the body in a specific position. They are made of a variety of materials such as plywood, light-weight aluminum, or plastic or casting materials. Plywood splints are generally used for first aid only. In treating a fractured finger or an injury in which immobilization of the finger is desired, a tongue blade is frequently used. Aluminum splints are made for right or left extremities and provide for support of the foot or thumb. They may be short for the lower leg or long enough to reach to the hip. The splint is usually held in place by elastic bandages and has the advantage of allowing wet dressings or care of ulcers or other superficial injuries. Occasionally casts are bivalved and made into removable shells. This allows access to the affected area, but immobilization is maintained.

There are other types of splints used for patients with specific orthopedic conditions. Some kinds of splints, such as the Thomas splint, are used in combination with traction (Fig. 21-8). When splints of any kind are used, the nurse must observe the skin for pressure areas and use care in handling the part.

Other orthopedic devices

Crutches and braces and their care were discussed in Chapter 10. Various types of heels are often used that may be incorporated into the cast and allow the patient to walk on the extremity. Sometimes an iron extending up into the cast is used, called a *walking iron*. Only certain kinds of fractures lend themselves to walking casts, and the orthopedic surgeon will decide if such a cast can be safely used. The patient must always be cautioned concerning the outward rotation of the foot when walking.

There are various types of collars or neck supports that are designed to immobilize the head and to take the weight of the head off the spine. They are generally used temporarily while healing occurs and may not be required at night.

Corsets and back braces are used to immobilize the spine and to prevent the patient from engaging in activities that would cause further harm to the spine. Braces may have steel supports in the back, and corsets usually lace in front but may lace in the back. The individual patient is measured for the support, which is made for him. A cotton T-shirt is worn under the brace, and the brace or corset should be put on with the patient in a recumbent position, before he arises in the morning.

Nursing care

The treatment of patients with orthopedic conditions is considered a surgical specialty, since many require minor or major operative procedures. Most patients will be cared for on an orthopedic service or on surgical wards. Certain basic aspects of nursing care apply to most orthopedic patients, and many of these procedures have been referred to in this and other chapters.

The nurse may be reminded that all patients with fractures should have bed boards, a firm mattress, and an overhead trapeze. Cast care is the same for all patients, regardless of the extent of the cast. Extreme care must be taken to protect devices such as traction equipment, splints, or tongs so that the corrective procedure may not be jeopardized. Skin care is a must for orthopedic patients, and since many patients are hospitalized for several weeks, the nurse should remember that good personal hygiene includes care of the nails and hair. The immobilized patient may have problems with elimination and adequate fluid intake; therefore a diet high in roughage or the use of mild laxatives or enemas may be necessary. Maintaining flexibility of unaffected joints, muscle tone, and function is important in preventing contractures and in fostering rehabilitation. Open surgery may be performed on bones, tendons, or muscles, and the immediate postoperative care is essentially the same as that for any surgical patient. All wounds must be protected from contamination.

NURSING THE PATIENT WITH DISEASES AND DISORDERS OF THE MUSCULOSKELETAL SYSTEM
Congenital deformities

Many congenital deformities affect bones, joints, and muscles. Some are readily recognized at birth, whereas others may not be observed for months or even years. Common congenital deformities may include clubbed feet or fingers, dislocated hips, webbing of fingers or toes, and spina bifida. Part or all of the extremities may be missing, multiple fingers or toes may be present, and multiple deformities may be present in the same child. When the pediatrician makes a thorough examination of the newborn infant soon after birth, defects are more likely to be discovered. The nurse assigned to work in obstetrics or in the nursery should watch for any unusual fold of tissue about the buttocks, failure to move extremities normally, or limitation of movement of a joint. The nurse should become suspicious if any of these signs is observed and should call it to the physician's attention.

The nurse should know that it is unnecessary for any child to go without treatment for orthopedic conditions. Assistance is available through the Department of Health, Education, and Welfare. The program of services to crippled children is administered through local health departments, and the parents may be advised to contact the public health nurse.

Clubfoot

Congenital clubfoot may affect only one foot or both feet and may be mild or severe. The condition involves an adduction and inward rotation of the foot. The foot resists being placed in a normal position when manipulated, and when released the foot will return to its former state. If the condition is mild, it may be overlooked. There seems to be a hereditary tendency toward clubfoot, and when it is present, the infant should be examined carefully, since other malformations are often present.[5] As in most congenital orthopedic disorders, early detection of clubfoot results in complete correction. The longer treatment is delayed, the longer the period of treatment and the less certain the outcome.

For patients who have mild cases, exercise may be all that is required. However, most patients are treated by application of plaster casts and by manipulation. Casts may be changed at frequent intervals in the beginning, and the intervals will be extended later. The parents should know that correction will take several months and the appointments for medical care should be faithfully kept. When the deformity has been corrected, the child will be fitted with special orthopedic shoes.

The care of the infant with casts on the feet requires frequent checking of circulation, as in all patients with casts. The casts should not be allowed to become wet or damp. Since the infant will be treated in the outpatient clinic or the physician's office, it is important for parents to be taught how to watch for pressure or circulatory disturbance, how to protect the top of the cast against moisture, and how to care for chafing of the skin. Young infants may outgrow the cast quickly, and chafing and irritation may result. Parents should be cautioned that close observation of the skin and the cast is necessary and to report to the physician any unusual condition that may occur.

When clubfoot fails to respond to treatment by manipulation and casts, surgery may be necessary.

Nurses who may be employed in public health departments may help parents to understand the importance of early treatment and continued medical supervision for several years after satisfactory correction has been achieved. There is always the possibility of the deformity recurring, and if neglected, treatment may require radical procedures.[5]

Torticollis (wryneck)

Torticollis, or congenital wryneck, may be observed during the first few weeks after birth. There is not general agreement as to its cause, although it is commonly believed to be the result of injury during birth. During birth the sternocleidomastoid muscle is torn, and hemorrhage resulting in a hematoma occurs. The result is a fibrotic mass of scar tissue in the muscle with loss of its elasticity and contraction of the muscle fibers. The ear on the affected side is pulled down toward the shoulder, with the chin pointed toward the opposite unaffected shoulder. If the defect is not recognized and treated early, deformity of the jaw and the face on the affected side will occur.

When the defect is discovered during the first few weeks of life, correction may be achieved by the use of heat, massage, and gentle stretching. Without treatment by the time the infant is about 8 months old, the

defect is considered permanent, and surgery is required.[5] After surgery a cast may or may not be applied, depending on the extent of the surgery and the technique of the particular surgeon. If a cast is applied, it may cover the chest, neck, and head, and after about 6 weeks it is replaced by an orthopedic collar that is worn for several weeks. Usually massage and stretching exercises are continued for several more weeks. When a cast is applied, it must be protected in the same way as all casts. Care should be taken not to let crumbs drop inside the cast and irritate the skin.

Dislocation of the hip

Congenital dislocation of the hip is a developmental error that usually is the result of poor development of the hip socket (acetabulum) into which the femur fits. Although the actual defect may be present at birth, often dislocation does not occur until the child begins to stand or walk. Early detection is important if good results are to be obtained from corrective measures.

Signs of the disorder vary according to age. It may be detected in the infant by abducting the hips or by placing the child's legs in a froglike position while lying on his back. Resistance or limited abduction is a meaningful sign. When this is done, a click is sometimes heard, and one knee may be lower than the other. As the child grows older, walking may be delayed, one leg may appear shorter, an extra gluteal fold may be observed, and a waddle or limp may be present.

When the condition is mild, treatment may consist of using extra diapers or a pillow to keep the legs in a position of abduction. The child may be given an anesthetic and the legs manipulated so as to place the head of the femur into the acetabulum, after which a cast is applied with the legs in the position of extreme abduction. After removal of the cast an adjustable abduction splint may be used. X-ray films are taken at frequent intervals to follow progress of the development of the joint. When walking is permitted, it should be undertaken as a gradual process.

The nursing care of the child depends largely on the corrective method used and the age of the child. Most children will be treated through the outpatient clinic or the physician's office, and the parents must understand the care. When a cast is applied, the care is the same as that for any patient in a cast. Perineal care for the child is especially important to prevent soiling and damage to the cast. When a cast is applied, the child is hospitalized for about 48 hours to permit drying. During this time the nurse has the opportunity to teach the parent how to care for the cast and the child and how to protect the cast from becoming wet. In some situations prior to open or closed reduction the physician may wish to have traction applied to bring the femoral head into a more satisfactory position for reduction and to avoid excessive manipulation.[5] (For more information consult a pediatric text.)

Arthritis

Arthritis belongs to a group of diseases commonly called *rheumatic disorders,* meaning inflammation of a joint. Exactly how many persons in the United States have some form of arthritis is probably unknown, although it is the number one crippling disease in the United States. Estimates vary widely, but it is believed that at least 50 million Americans are affected and at least 4 million of these are dependent and unable to work, attend school, or participate in social functions.[6] From these estimates it may readily be seen that not all persons with arthritis are completely incapacitated. Many go about their daily activities, including gainful employment, with only varying degrees of involvement and discomfort.

There are many types of arthritis, but the most common are rheumatoid arthritis, rheumatoid spondylitis, and osteoarthritis (degenerative joint disease). Forms of arthritis often accompany other diseases such as psoriasis (p. 483), rheumatic fever, infectious diseases such as gonorrhea, and gout, which is a metabolic disease. Basically, most types of arthritis have similarities, and the care of patients is essentially the same for all forms of the disease.

In providing care and services for the arthritic patient, goals should be established that include medical and nursing care during the acute stages and long-range plans to maintain the patient in the best

possible condition. Emphasis should be placed on prevention of infectious diseases that may be associated with arthritis, prevention and correction of deformity, teaching activities of daily living, and a psychosocial environment in which the patient and his family may accept and live comfortably with a chronic disability. To accomplish these goals many persons will be needed, including the physician, psychiatrist, psychologist, nurse, physical therapist, occupational therapist, religious counselor, social worker, vocational counselor, and the public health nurse. (See Chapter 10.)

Rheumatoid arthritis and rheumatoid spondylitis

Rheumatoid arthritis is the most serious form of the disease and leads to severe crippling. The disease may occur at any age, but it most frequently affects persons between 20 and 45 years of age. Rheumatoid arthritis in infants and children is a chronic systemic disease that affects many organs and tissues, including joints. Children between 2 and 4 years of age are most commonly affected.

Pathophysiology. Research has failed to find a specific cause of the disease, but a virus infection, autoimmune response, and abnormal metabolic states appear to be possible causative factors. The disease may develop rather insidiously, or it may have an acute onset. Remissions occur and symptoms subside, but subsequent attacks follow, and a chronic state slowly develops. The disease affects the joints, first causing an inflammation of the joint membrane. As the disease progresses, granulation tissue fills the joint and the normal joint cartilage is destroyed. The joint cavities fill with scar tissue and adhesions, causing stiffness and complete immobility.

The early symptoms of rheumatoid arthritis are loss of weight, loss of appetite, muscle aching, malaise, fever, and swollen painful joints. Complaints of joint stiffness, especially on arising in the morning, are common. During the early course of the disease considerable muscle spasm occurs, and any effort to move the affected joints is painful. Diagnosis is established by a variety of findings. The rheumatoid factor (RF) titer is elevated, indicating that an abnormal serum protein concentration is present. The erythrocyte sedimentation rate is elevated, and x-ray films show progressive damage.

Treatment and nursing care. The care of the patient is directed toward maintaining function, relieving pain, and preventing deformities. One of the most distressing factors in the treatment of rheumatoid arthritis is the patient's tendency to obtain unprofessional advice. As a result, the patient may wear copper bracelets, drink potions of vinegar and honey, wear beans or potatoes around his neck, or sit in uranium mines desperately hoping for relief of symptoms. Patients should seek medical attention early so that pain and joint deformity can be minimized.

During acute attacks rest is important, and the nurse should give special attention to good body alignment. Boards should be placed under the mattress to provide a firm bed. The extremities should be straight without pillows under the knees, and the Gatch bed should not be raised. A footboard should be placed at the foot of the bed and a bed cradle used to support bedclothing off painful joints. Sandbags or trochanter rolls should be used to prevent outward rotation of the extremities. The patient should be positioned so that the back is straight, and a small pillow is placed under the head. Hip and knee flexion is avoided.

Aspirin is generally considered to be the drug of choice to decrease both pain and inflammation. It may be given in fairly large doses and should be taken with food to avoid gastric upsets. The drug indomethacin (Indocin) is also anti-inflammatory and analgesic, although it appears to be no more effective than aspirin. Phenylbutazone (Butazolidin) has similar effects on the rheumatoid arthritic patient; however, effectiveness appears to be limited and serious side reactions can occur. Gold compounds are selected for some patients, usually those who are not responding to other forms of treatment. These medications are slow acting, and the patient must be carefully watched for side effects while receiving the drug. Adrenocorticosteroids

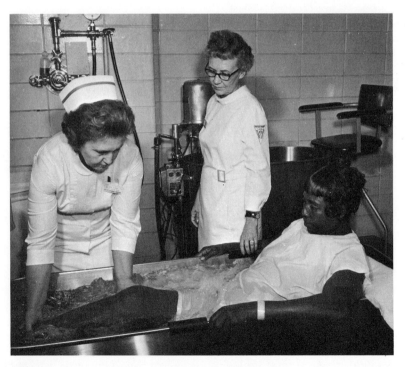

Fig. 21-9. Nurse assists physical therapist with whirlpool for arthritic patient. Note the support of the painful joint.

(cortisone, prednisone, hydrocortisone) are given after more conservative treatment has failed. These drugs may produce dramatic relief of symptoms, although they do not cure the disease. Rather severe side effects can result, however, and once the medication is discontinued, the patient may have a full return of original symptoms. Usually the patient is maintained on the lowest dose of corticosteroids that will produce an improvement in his condition. Hydrocortisone acetate injected into joints results in immediate relief of pain and a temporary halt of the destructive process, usually lasting for several weeks.

The use of heat is helpful in relieving pain and may include hot moist packs, hot tub baths, an electric blanket, heat cradles, paraffin baths, and whirlpool baths (Fig. 21-9). Some of the most severe joint deformities are caused by patients assuming a comfortably flexed position. Once the acute stage is passed, a program of physical therapy must be established for the individual patient. A planned program of rest and activity is important. Active exercise should be a part of the therapeutic plan so that normal functioning of the joints may be maintained. Exercises should be simple and may be taught by the physical therapist. There is no special diet for the arthritic patient, but he should have a well-balanced diet and should be encouraged to maintain good nutrition.

After recovery from acute attacks the patient may return to work and should be encouraged to remain active. Many patients with rheumatoid arthritis remain independent and self-sufficient for 20 or 30 years.

Rheumatoid spondylitis is an inflammation of the vertebrae and sacroiliac joints and may affect part or all of the spine, resulting in complete rigidity. The rheumatoid process may cause a bowing outward of the thoracic spine (kyphosis). Treatment of the condition is similar to that for rheumatoid arthritis except that the program of exercise is designed to prevent kyphosis. Exercises are planned to keep the spine straight and to maintain range of motion in the cervical spine. The patient should be positioned on a firm bed with bed boards and should not sleep on a pillow.

Osteoarthritis (degenerative joint disease)

Osteoarthritis is the result of the normal wear and tear placed on joints over the years. The process may be hastened by joint trauma or obesity. It is the most common form of arthritis and begins to make its appearance in persons past middle life. Most people have some degree of osteoarthritis by the time they reach 60 years of age. The disease damages the cartilage in the joints, and although pain and stiffness result, they usually do not cause crippling. Several factors contribute to development of the disease. Engaging in occupations in which prolonged strain is placed on joints, obesity, poor posture, and injury to a joint favor early development of osteoarthritis. The joints most often affected are the spine, knees, fingers, and hips.

Treatment for the disease should include reduction in weight if obesity is present and a regular program of exercise to maintain range-of-joint motion. Analgesics such as aspirin, 10 to 15 grains three or four times daily after meals, may be given to relieve pain. Also phenylbutazone (Butazolidin), 100 mg. two or three times daily, indomethacin (Indocin) or ibuprofen (Motrin), 400 mg. four times a day, may be ordered by the physician. In patients with severe joint pain, hydrocortisone acetate may be injected into the synovial cavity and will generally provide relief from pain for several weeks. The patient should have a program of rest, and joints should be protected from continuing wear and strain. The application of moist heat such as baths, soaks, packs, or paraffin baths may afford temporary relief.

Surgical treatment of arthritis. A variety of surgical procedures are available to prevent progressive deformities, relieve pain, improve function, and correct deformities resulting from rheumatoid or osteoarthritis. *Tendon transplants* can be done to replace damaged muscles. The excision of the synovial membrane of a joint, a *synovectomy*, is helpful in rheumatoid arthritis to maintain joint function. An *osteotomy*, a cutting of bone to correct bone or joint deformities, may be performed to improve function or relieve pain. Severe joint destruction may be treated with an *arthrodesis*, which is a surgical fusion of the joint in a functional position. An *arthroplasty* involves plastic surgery on a diseased joint such as the elbow, hip, knee, or shoulder to increase mobility. Sometimes an arthroplasty involves the removal of a portion of the joint and replacement with a prosthesis made of metal or synthetic material.[6]

A hip arthroplasty is a common procedure when arthritis involves the head of the femur and acetabulum. In this type of surgery a vitallium cup is cemented into the arthritic acetabulum to receive the head of the femur. The most recent development in hip reconstruction involves total replacement of both the acetabulum and the head of the femur with a plastic cup and corresponding vitallium femoral head. These prostheses are cemented into place with a plastic glue. The procedure may be done for damage resulting from trauma or congenital deformities as well as arthritis.

Principles of nursing care for patients having this type of surgery include maintaining the leg in a position of abduction, performing leg exercises as ordered, and preventing complications that accompany immobilization of the postoperative patient. Often suspension traction or Russell traction is used after surgery to provide support, maintain abduction, and provide comfort for the patient. The patient who has had a total hip replacement may be out of bed within a week and with the help of physical therapy will walk with crutches. Within 6 months the patient has a 95% chance of having minimal or no pain and relatively normal range of motion in the hip.[4, 5] Total knee replacements are now being done for arthritic conditions involving the knee, and procedures are being developed to replace other diseased joints of the body.

Gout (gouty arthritis)

Gout is a metabolic disease resulting from an accumulation of uric acid in the blood. The disease may be primary, caused by a hereditary metabolic error, or it may be secondary to some other disease process and to certain drugs. The disease usually appears in middle life. It does not occur before puberty in the male or before menopause in the female. It takes about 20 years for sufficient urates to accumulate in the body before causing symptoms.

Gouty arthritis can affect any joint in the body, but 20% of first attacks occur in a joint of the great toe. Although first attacks may occur in other joints, the great toe is involved in 80% of persons with the disease. Typically, the onset occurs at night with excruciating pain, swelling, and inflammation in the affected joint. The pain may be of short duration, returning at intervals, or it may be severe and continuous for 5 to 10 days. The patient may never have more than one attack throughout his entire life, or attacks may continue at intervals of months, gradually coming closer together.[1, 8]

Diagnosis is made on the basis of finding a high blood level of urates. Several drugs are used in the treatment of the disease. For acute attacks colchicine is administered orally or may be given intravenously. When administered orally, 0.5 mg. may be given hourly until twelve doses have been given. If gastrointestinal symptoms develop and if pain has been relieved, the drug may be discontinued. Other drugs that are equally effective in relieving pain are phenylbutazone and indomethacin.

A factor in the treatment of gout is the prevention of the formation of tophi and gouty arthritis. Tophi are deposits of uric acid that may form in various parts of the body, including the kidneys, where uric acid stones may occur that can destroy kidney tissue. Drugs may be given to prevent these disorders from occurring or to relieve them. Drugs in use include allopurinol (Zyloprim), probenecid (Benemid), and sulfinpyrazone (Anturane).[2] Each patient is treated on an individual basis, and the period during which these drugs are to be administered depends on the stage of the disease and the practices of the individual physician. The patient may need to continue receiving drugs over a period of several years. There is no special diet that has been found to be effective, although foods high in purine, such as liver, kidney, anchovies, sardines, and sweetbreads should be avoided. The diet should be well balanced, with a high water intake. During an acute attack the patient should be on a regimen of bed rest, and painful joints should be protected from bedcovers by a footboard or bed cradle.

Bursitis

The bursae are small sacs containing a small amount of fluid to lubricate areas in which movement may cause friction. They are located in the shoulder, elbow, knee, hip, and foot. The bursae may become inflamed, causing an acute bursitis, or inflammation extending over a long period of time may result in chronic bursitis and the formation of deposits of calcium salts. Bursitis is generally the result of injury, strain, or prolonged use of the bursae as in active exercise. It may also occur secondary to infection elsewhere in the body.

The subdeltoid region is the most frequent location of inflammation. Subdeltoid bursitis is characterized by severe pain that may radiate down the arm into the fingers. Treatment consists of supporting the arm in a sling and administering an analgesic for pain. X-ray therapy is frequently given, or hydrocortisone may be injected into the bursae. Several other methods of treatment may be used, including administering a local anesthetic, inserting needles, and washing out the calcium deposits. Range-of-motion exercises should be started as soon as possible. In chronic bursitis there is pain during use of the affected part; treatment includes analgesics to relieve pain and physical therapy. Surgical removal of hardened calcium deposits may be necessary.

Infectious diseases and disorders
Osteomyelitis

Osteo- is the prefix meaning bone; osteomyelitis is inflammation of the bone. The most common cause of the disease is the introduction of pathogenic bacteria into the bone in penetrating injuries such as gunshot wounds or in compound fractures with bones protruding. Acute osteomyelitis may result from infections elsewhere in the body, and the pathogenic bacteria are carried to the bone by the bloodstream. Since many infections are now treated with chemotherapeutic drugs, fewer cases of osteomyelitis result from bloodstream infection.

Chronic osteomyelitis may recur throughout life. In the past it was said "once an osteo, always an osteo" because the disease was certain to recur at intervals. Complete elimination of the disease depends on the thoroughness of the removal of dead bone and prolonged use of antibiotics.

There is no uniform method of treating patients with osteomyelitis. For some patients surgery may be done to remove necrotic bone, antibiotics are generally given, and immobilization may be helpful. Much depends on the age and condition of the patient.[5]

Good nursing care of the patient with osteomyelitis is most important. The wounds caused by the disease are painful, and the nurse should exercise gentleness in moving the affected part. Wounds are often irrigated with hydrogen peroxide or other antiseptic or antibiotic solution, and strict asepsis must be maintained. Contractures may easily occur unless care is taken to see that the patient is properly positioned. It is not unusual for a new focus of infection to develop, and the patient should be observed for any sudden elevation of temperature, which should be reported at once. The diet should be high in calories, in protein, and in vitamins. Since osteomyelitis patients are primarily children, some diversional activity to keep them occupied should be planned.

Tuberculosis of the bone

Tuberculosis caused by the tubercle bacillus may affect any bone or joint. The infection has usually been acquired from contact with infectious tuberculosis, but bone and joint tuberculosis is not infectious unless there are draining lesions or unless it is accompanied by infectious pulmonary tuberculosis. Tuberculosis of bones and joints occurs primarily in children between 2 and 12 years of age. Often it results from the child associating with older persons who have pulmonary tuberculosis. Tuberculosis of the spine (Pott's disease) is the most common form and accounts for more than 50% of bone and joint tuberculosis. Tuberculosis of the hip is next in frequency.

Pott's disease (tuberculosis of the spine). The symptoms of tuberculosis of the spine usually begin with muscle spasm, stiffness, and avoidance of any activity that would cause bending the back. The small child may be irritable and fretful and may cry out at intervals, particularly at night. The lower dorsal or the upper lumbar portion of the spine is most frequently involved. As the disease progresses with softening and destruction of bones, deformity occurs, giving a humped appearance known as gibbus, or kyphosis. Abscesses without inflammation may occur at various sites on the body, along the spine, hips, or in the groin.

An important factor in treatment is absolute immobilization of the spine. The child may be placed on a Bradford frame in hyperextension, or casts and braces may be used (p. 509). The administration of streptomycin, para-aminosalicylic acid (PAS), and isoniazid (INH) in addition to proper nutrition, sunshine, and fresh air is considered important in the plan of therapy. There is no shortcut to cure, and treatment must extend from months to years.

Tuberculosis of the hip. Tuberculosis of the hip may be observed in the very young child who limps and walks on the toes of the affected side. There may be stiffness of the joint and pain, which is often referred to the knee. In treating young children the hip is placed at rest, whereas the treatment of older children may include surgery followed by immobilization.[5]

The nursing care is the same as that for any patient in a cast, on a frame, or in traction. Good nutrition, immobilization, and rest are basic factors in the treatment of bone or joint tuberculosis. Patients are usually hospitalized initially and then discharged home. Parents must have specific instructions regarding care of the child, and demonstrations are particularly helpful. If the disease is diagnosed early, antituberculous drugs such as para-aminosalicylic acid, isoniazid, and streptomycin sulfate are effective in treating the disease. However, the disease is characterized by relapses and complicating factors.

Traumatic injuries

Traumatic injuries to the musculoskeletal system are responsible for a large number of hospital admissions among all age groups. Many less severe injuries, including contusions, sprains, and strains, are cared for in outpatient clinics or in the physician's office.

Contusions

Contusions are the most common and the simplest type of injury to the musculoskeletal system. Contusion is synonymous with bruise and is the result of an external injury to the soft tissues. The injury causes a rupture of small blood vessels, which bleed into tissues, resulting in the familiar discoloration often called a *black-and-blue spot*. When the contusion is severe, a large amount of blood may collect in the tissue, resulting in a hematoma.

The treatment generally includes elevation of the part and the application of cold, which may be in the form of cold compresses or an ice cap. After several hours if there is no further bleeding, heat may be applied to relieve muscle soreness.

Sprains

A sprain involves ligaments, tendons, and muscles and occurs as the result of twisting or wrenching a joint beyond its normal range of motion. When this occurs, ligaments are torn, and tendons may be pulled from the bone. Blood vessels are ruptured, causing bleeding (ecchymosis), and pressure on nerve endings results in pain. As the result of a disturbance of circulation and lymph drainage, muscle spasm occurs, with a tendency to edema.

Treatment should include x-ray examination to rule out the possibility of a fracture. Immediately after the injury the affected part should be elevated and an ice cap applied. The joint is then immobilized by a splint and Ace bandage or a cast if the sprain is severe. Occasionally, taping the foot will achieve enough immobilization for healing to occur. Usually the support is removed in 2 to 3 weeks. If the ankle joint is involved, minimal weight bearing is permitted at first and is gradually increased as the discomfort subsides. If the ankle has been casted, active exercises should be performed after cast removal prior to full weight bearing.

Dislocations

Dislocation may be congenital, as in the case of congenital dislocated hip discussed earlier in this chapter; it may be caused by a disease process in the joint; or it may be caused by trauma. A dislocation results in the temporary displacement of a bone from its normal position. It is accompanied by stretching and tearing of ligaments and tendons, and a fracture may sometimes occur at the same time. A dislocation results in severe pain, deformity, and loss of function.

The treatment of patients with dislocations is usually done with the patient under general anesthesia, and the displaced parts are manually manipulated into normal position. Sometimes the fluoroscope may be used to assist the surgeon. The affected part is then immobilized in splints, bandages, or a cast until the injured tissues have healed. When a fracture accompanies a dislocation, it may be difficult to secure as good a result as that achieved with dislocation alone.

The nursing care of the patient includes observation for signs of impaired circulation such as loss of sensation, pain, or tingling and numbness. The care of casts has been reviewed earlier in this chapter.

Fractures

A fracture is the same as a break and results from some violent external force. Pathologic fractures may result from disease such as metastatic cancer to the bone. Because of decalcification of bones and their brittleness in aged persons, a fracture may occur without any known cause. Frac-tures may occur directly at the place at which violence was applied, or the fracture may be some distance away from the point at which the force was applied. There are various kinds of fractures, and the method of treatment will vary with the location and kind. Whenever a fracture takes place, there is some injury to the soft tissues and some bleeding, since the bones have their own blood supply.

Fractures are most commonly classified as greenstick, comminuted, compound, spiral, or impacted (Fig. 21-10).

Greenstick fracture. A greenstick fracture, frequently seen in children, is an incomplete fracture, meaning that the break does not go completely through the bone.

Comminuted fracture. In a comminuted fracture the bone is splintered at the site of the break so that there are several fragments of the bone.

Compound fracture. The bone is completely broken when a compound fracture

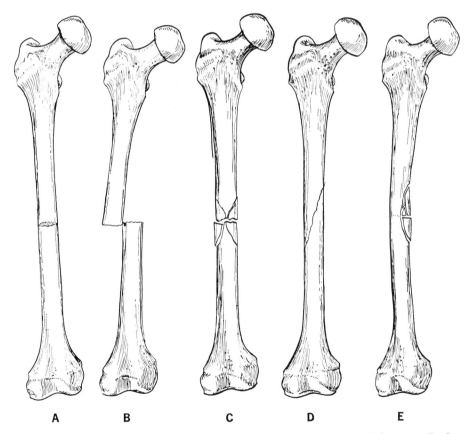

Fig. 21-10. Types of fractures. **A,** Impacted fracture. **B,** Compound fracture. **C,** Comminuted fracture. **D,** Spiral fracture. **E,** Greenstick fracture.

occurs, and the skin is also broken so that the fractured end of the bone may protrude through the skin. These fractures are especially serious, since contamination of the wound and the bone may occur.

Spiral fracture. A spiral fracture results when there is a twisting of the bone so that the fracture occurs in a longitudinal or oblique direction.

Impacted fracture. An impacted fracture, or compression fracture, occurs when the bone is broken, and the force drives one end of the bone into the opposite end. When this type of fracture occurs in long bones, there is always a shortening of the extremity. In some kinds of fractures the broken edges of the bones rub together, producing a grating that is called *crepitus.*

Fractures may occur in which the bone is completely broken, but the parts remain in their normal anatomic position. In some fractures the bone may be completely broken, with one part overriding the other.

Symptoms of fracture will vary with the type and location of the break. With some there may be deformity, pain, contusion at the site of injury, loss of motion, and muscle spasm; with others the symptoms may be lacking. Many times injury to other parts of the body occurs at the same time, and the patient may be admitted with severe shock and unconsciousness. The treatment of any general systemic condition takes precedence over treatment of the fracture.

An accurate diagnosis of the fracture is made by x-ray or fluoroscopic examination. The physician will also want to know exactly how the accident happened, since this has a bearing on the type of fracture and the method of treatment.

Fractures are treated by closed reduction or open reduction methods. In closed reduction the bones are manipulated into position and immobilized, whereas in open reduction the skin is opened and the bones exposed and usually fixed in position with some device. Various devices, including traction, splints, and casts, are used in the reduction and treatment of fractures. When open reduction is done, wire, screws, plates, nails, or bolts may be used. A combination of any of these devices may be used in the treatment of fractures.

The nursing care of patients with fractures is essentially the same as that given any surgical patient. The care of the patient in traction and in a cast has been reviewed earlier in this chapter. Nutrition and fluids, exercise of the unaffected joints, muscle-setting exercises, skin care, and elimination are important considerations in patient care. Internal fixation has simplified nursing care for many patients with fractures and shortened the period of hospitalization, but there will be many patients who must be hospitalized for several weeks. For these patients some form of occupational therapy should be available.

Fractures of the hip. Since people live much longer now, there is an increasing incidence of fractures of the hip among older persons. Because of the brittleness of bones, older people need only a slight fall to sustain a fracture of the hip or arm. Older persons are predisposed to complications when they must remain immobilized for long periods of time. Newer methods of treatment have made it possible for many patients to have greater mobility at an earlier period than was previously possible after hip fracture. Different kinds of fractures occur, and there is no one way in which all hip fractures may be treated. Basing the decision on x-ray examination, the surgeon determines the method to be used. The care of patients in casts and traction has been reviewed earlier in this chapter; a discussion of internal fixation by nailing is presented here.

Nailing means that a nail or rod made of stainless steel and vitallium is inserted through the marrow cavity of one bone fragment and driven across the site of the fracture into the marrow cavity of the other bone fragment, thus holding the fractured bones in correct anatomic position. Not all fractures can be nailed, but when this procedure is possible, it allows many patients to be out of the hospital in a few weeks, walking on crutches. The early ambulation results in fewer complications, permits some patients to return to work sooner, and makes nursing care easier. In some kinds of fractures a prosthetic device may be used. This is usually performed when the neck of the femur has been fractured and the blood supply necessary for healing has been disrupted. The head and neck of the femur are surgically removed and replaced with a ball and stem (Austin-

Moore prosthesis), which fits into the shaft of the femur. This enables the patient to bear weight directly on the leg in a short time. This technique offers the advantage of early ambulation and helps to prevent complications.[4]

Nursing care. After internal fixation with nails there is no danger in turning and moving the patient. The patient is given a general anesthetic for the procedure, after which vital signs are checked frequently until they are stable. The patient's position should be changed from side to side, and he may be made comfortable on the affected side. When the patient is turned on his unaffected side, the fractured extremity should be supported with pillows and remain in the same line as the rest of the body. When the patient is in the supine position, the knee may be slightly flexed, and the extremity should be supported from the hip to the ankle with sandbags or a trochanter roll to prevent outward rotation. A footboard should be used to support bedding and prevent foot drop. Pillows may be used to support the legs and keep the heels off the bed. Since physicians may vary in what activity they permit the patient, the nurse should understand exactly what the physician wishes done.

An orthopedic or pediatric bedpan may be more comfortable for the patient. The elderly patient should be observed for fecal impaction, and mild laxatives or small enemas may be ordered. Intake and output records should be maintained.

With the physician's permission the patient may be taught muscle-setting exercises such as quadriceps-setting exercises, exercises that tighten gluteal and abdominal muscles, plantar flexion, and dorsiflexion of the feet. All joints should be exercised, except the affected leg, and the patient may be encouraged to use the trapeze to move and exercise the arms. Exercise of the affected leg must be ordered by the surgeon.

In most instances the patient is out of bed in a chair on the day after surgery. Elderly patients may fatigue easily and should not be left sitting for long periods. Usually 1 hour two or three times a day is sufficient. Since the appetite may be poor, allowing the patient to be up at mealtimes may encourage him to eat better. Depend-

ing on the patient's age and progress, the use of crutches may be permitted in 3 to 6 months; weight bearing is allowed when healing is complete.

When a prosthesis is inserted into the joint, the limb is kept in a neutral position with slight abduction to prevent dislocation. If turning is permitted, the patient is placed on his unaffected side and abduction is maintained by placing pillows between his legs. Muscle exercises are encouraged. Partial weight bearing may be allowed in 10 to 14 days and full weight bearing in about 4 weeks.

Whiplash injuries

Whiplash injury to the musculoskeletal system is the result of an automobile accident in which a rear-end collision occurs. The injury may cause a compression fracture of the cervical vertebrae or result in tearing of muscles and ligaments. Although the injury may be severe enough to cause paralysis and loss of consciousness, most whiplash injuries do not produce immediate symptoms. Symptoms often do not appear until 4 or 5 days after the injury. At that time headache, spasm of neck muscles with loss of motion, and a drawing sensation in the back of the neck may be noticed. Pain may be referred from one side of the head to the base of the skull, and vision may be disturbed. If the injury has been severe enough to injure a nerve root, neurologic symptoms may occur.

Treatment should be secured immediately after the injury, since without treatment the conditon may become chronic. Methods of treatment vary; however, the patient may be admitted to the hospital for several days and placed on a regimen of bed rest. Cervical traction employing a head halter may be used, as well as the application of heat and massage. The patient may be fitted with a neck support to be worn when he is up. After approximately 4 weeks physical therapy and exercise are given to strengthen muscles. These patients are often misunderstood and need sympathy and understanding from all persons responsible for their care.

Rickets

Rickets is a disease that affects the bones, causing retarded growth and bone development. The disease occurs in infants and young children as the result of lack of vitamin D, which is associated with calcium-phosphorus balance in the body. The condition is more likely to develop in the presence of substandard hygienic conditions, inadequate nutrition, and lack of sunshine. Rickets sometimes results in severe orthopedic deformity.

Education and emphasis on infant care have done much to prevent the occurrence of rickets in the United States, but it remains prevalent in many parts of the world in which poor nutrition standards exist.

There are many symptoms characteristic of the rachitic child. Curvature of the long bones, which are soft because of the lack of mineral deposits, occurs; bowleg is an example of this bending. The head presents a square appearance and is often flattened in back or on the side if the infant lies too long in one position. The closure of the anterior fontanel and development of the dentition are delayed. Pigeon breast, knock-knee, and enlargement of the wrists and ankles may occur.

The treatment is administration of vitamin D, exposure to sunlight, and improvement in general nutrition.

Bone tumors

Tumors of the bone may be primary or secondary and may be benign or malignant. There are several types of benign tumors, and their cause is not always known. One type, *giant-cell tumor*, responds well to irradiation. Benign tumors do not metastasize to other parts of the body. There are usually few symptoms, with pain the most common complaint. Benign tumors are diagnosed by x-ray examination and biopsy. Some types are removed surgically.

There are several kinds of malignant bone tumors. One type of primary malignant tumor, *osteogenic sarcoma*, occurs in younger persons and metastasizes to the lungs, from which the malignant cells are carried throughout the body by the bloodstream. The long bones are usually affected, and amputation is often required.[3] Other types of malignant tumors affect the flat bones, often involving other types of tissues. Carcinoma of the prostate, lung, breast, thyroid, and kidney may metastasize to the bones, where destruction of the bone

and spontaneous fractures result. In most cases of bone tumor, both benign and malignant, pain and declining health are the primary symptoms. In some forms, anemia, elevation of temperature, swelling, and disturbance of the platelets occur. Treatment depends on the type of tumor, extent of involvement, its location, and the presence of malignant lesions in other parts of the body.

Amputation

The amputation of an extremity or a portion of it may be necessitated because of a malignant bone tumor, injury, diabetic gangrene, or any condition that threatens the life of the patient unless the procedure is performed. Occasionally amputation may be an emergency procedure performed when a severe accident has nearly severed the extremity. Generally it is an elective procedure, and the final decision rests with the patient. The exchange of a leg for a life, particularly when the life may not be too long, is not an easy decision to make. The patient needs all the emotional support and understanding possible. The patient should know preoperatively about prostheses, and often a visit from a person using a prosthesis may provide encouragement.

Preoperative care. The patient's general condition will be carefully evaluated, and routine laboratory examinations will be performed. If the patient is diabetic, an evaluation of his diabetic status will be determined. Other examinations such as an electrocardiogram and chest x-ray film may be ordered by the physician. Intravenous fluids may sometimes be given to combat dehydration, and blood transfusion may be ordered if anemia is present. The skin will be prepared according to the hospital procedure (Fig. 21-11). The surgery may be performed under regional hypothermia, in which case the extremity will be packed in ice for several hours preoperatively.

Postoperative care. Today the months of stump wrapping and conditioning prior to being fitted with a prosthesis have largely been eliminated. Patients are either fitted immediately after surgery with a rigid temporary prosthesis, or prosthesis fitting is delayed until the stump is healed and sutures removed. Every amputee should receive a temporary prosthesis as soon as pos-

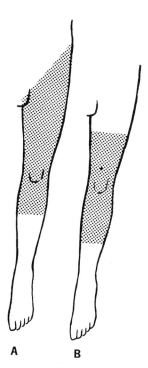

Fig. 21-11. Area of skin to be prepared for amputation. **A,** Midthigh amputation. **B,** Below-the-knee amputation.

sible after surgery. The patient benefits psychologically, and complications are prevented.

When the patient returns from surgery and prosthesis fitting is to be delayed, he should be watched for signs of shock, and vital signs should be checked at frequent intervals until they are well stabilized. The dressing should be observed for evidence of bright red blood, and a tourniquet should always be available for emergency use. In case of severe bleeding the nurse can apply the tourniquet tightly enough to stop the bleeding until the surgeon arrives. If oozing from the stump should occur, the nurse may reinforce the dressing but should never attempt to change it. Since many amputations are performed in persons between 60 and 70 years of age, the patient must be carefully observed for shock, pulmonary complications, or cardiovascular collapse. Suction equipment and oxygen should be at the bedside, and intravenous fluids and emergency drugs should always be available for immediate use if needed. Patients may be cared for in an intensive care unit where drugs and equipment are readily available. Often elderly patients have problems of urinary incontinence, and the dressing may have to be protected to prevent contamination of the wound.

Until the prosthesis can be fitted, the stump is wrapped in a cotton, elastic compression bandage. The stump may be elevated on a pillow for the first 24 hours, after which it should be removed to prevent flexion contractures. When the patient is in the supine position, the stump should rest flat on the bed. The patient should be encouraged to spend some time each day in the prone position with a pillow tucked under the lower trunk and the stump for support (Fig. 21-12). The stump should not be flexed over the good leg. When in the prone position, the patient may begin push-up exercises to strengthen arm and shoulder muscles. When in the supine position, the patient may begin exercises of the leg unless they would cause strain on the suture line.

The postoperative care of the patient patient with an amputation is directed toward preventing contractures of the hip or nearest joint, which would make wearing a prosthesis difficult, and preparing the stump for prosthesis. Before healing has occurred every effort must be made to prevent infection of the wound.

The patient may have little pain from the surgical procedure, but he may complain of pain in the amputated limb, or phantom limb pain, a phenomenon not completely understood. The patient may be allowed out of bed on the day after surgery, and if there are no complictaions, the wound may be healed, sutures removed, and a temporary prosthesis made of plastic or plaster of Paris provided in 2 to 3 weeks. At this time the patient is allowed partial weight bearing. Without complications the patient may bear full weight on his prosthesis within 6 weeks, and a permanent prosthesis may be supplied within 3 months.

With immediate postsurgical prosthetic fitting a sterile stump sock is pulled on over the stump when surgery is complete. Pressure areas are protected with felt pads. The stump is then wrapped with elastic plaster-of-Paris bandages to form a rigidly firm dressing, which prevents swelling and protects the stump from injury. As soon as the

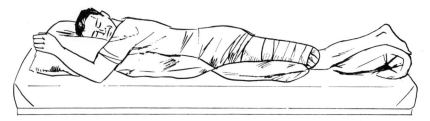

Fig. 21-12. Amputee in prone position. Note the position of the pillows.

dressing is dry, a prosthetic device with a foot is applied. The nurse must be alert for edema that may prevent weight bearing, and if the dressing is damaged or comes off, the physician must be notified immediately. Compression bandages should be applied until the physician arrives.[3] Brief ambulation with limited weight bearing is possible within 24 hours. Gradually ambulation is increased, although weight bearing is limited until healing is complete.[6] With this method rehabilitation is shortened, and the patient returns to an independent state much more rapidly. The method is not adaptable to all patients, however.

The patient may need to be taught balance and crutch walking before he leaves the hospital; he is often referred to the physical therapy department. It is important that he understand that the stump must be washed and dried thoroughly once a day when healing is complete. If any abrasion occurs, the patient should consult his physician immediately.

The child amputee. There has been considerable publicity given to congenital absence of limbs. This is not a new occurrence, since congenital malformations of this type are as common as other kinds of defects. Children of all ages may have amputations because of disease or injury. The meaning of the experience to the child depends on his age. For the adolescent it may be a profoundly traumatic experience. If the small child is treated by parents as an invalid, he may become completely dependent, rather than self-sufficient.

The child amputee faces some problems that must be recognized. When a prosthesis is fitted, regular medical supervision and changes must be made coincident with the growth process. The child with a prosthesis is likely to suffer from fatigue more readily than other children. Active children frequently suffer traumatizations of the stump, and edema may result from excessive pressure within the socket of the prosthesis. It is important that the socket fit properly because abrasions and irritations of the stump will occur if it does not. In some parts of the United States child amputee clinics are available to care for the child amputee.

Muscular dystrophy

The cause of muscular dystrophy is unknown, and at the present time there is no known cure. The disease is not reportable, thus the exact incidence is not known, but from studies that have been made it appears that the incidence may be lower than is generally believed. It is a disabling disease, and when it begins in childhood, most patients die before reaching adult life. There are several types of the disease, and the results of research indicate that it is inherited with the defective gene carried by the female and transmitted to the male. The childhood type may begin as young as 2 years of age, and nearly all will have their onset between 2 and 10 years of age and progress steadily without remission.

Muscular dystrophy affects voluntary muscles, which become weak, atrophy, and waste away. The gait is a waddling type with contraction of heel cords, and inward curve of the spine and a protuberant abdomen develop. Ultimately muscle function becomes so impaired that the individual is unable to maintain an upright posture. Often the person is able to be cared for in a wheelchair before bed rest becomes necessary. As in all rehabilitation, the child should be encouraged to do as many things as possible for himself as long as he is able. The nurse should know that the local chapter of the Muscular Dystrophy Association of America, Inc., may be able to provide assistance for the child with muscular dystrophy.

Cerebral palsy

Cerebral palsy is a name given to a neuromuscular disorder that may be caused by many different factors, including birth injuries. The disease results in motor disability and is characterized by spasticity and involuntary movements related to walking, talking, or any activity requiring muscular coordination. The disorder may be recognized soon after birth or during the first few months of life. Much can be done to help the child, but there is no treatment to correct the cerebral defect.

The person with cerebral palsy may have many disabilities in addition to motor function. Many have impairments of vision, hearing, and speech; convulsive disorders; and mental retardation. In addition, there are psychologic, emotional, and social problems. The care and treatment of the child with cerebral palsy requires the help of every person on the medical and nursing team. Teaching is basic to the program. The child may need speech therapy, and he may have to be taught how to walk, to eat, toilet training, how to relax, and all the activities of daily living. Work with parents is vitally important. In a study of 200 adults it was found that there was rejection of the child by parents in 20% of cases, whereas overprotection existed in 54% of cases. Unfavorable attitudes were found to exist in 81% of the persons studied. The child with cerebral palsy is barred from public schools and excluded from recreational and social activities, and 70% are never able to engage in competitive or sheltered work. The child and his parents live in a world of social isolation, and therapy must include the community, the neighborhood, the church, and the school.[7]

Summary outline

1. Structure and function of the musculoskeletal system
   A. Structure
      1. Composed of bones, joints, muscles, ligaments, tendons, and cartilage
      2. Bones—composed of living cells and a calcified intercellular substance
      3. Long bones comprise six parts—diaphysis, epiphyses, medullary (marrow) cavity, endosteum, periosteum, and articular cartilage
      4. Bones are various shapes—long, short, irregular, and flat
      5. Joints may be freely movable, slightly movable, or immovable
      6. Body movement depends on action of bones and muscles
   B. Function
      1. Locomotion
      2. Supports an upright position
      3. Protects vital organs
      4. Blood cells formed in bone marrow
      5. Deposits calcium for use in deficiency
2. Position, movement, and body mechanics
   A. Requirements for prevention of contractures and deformity and maintenance of muscle tone
      1. Proper positioning of patient
      2. Passive and active exercise
      3. Regular turning
         a. Turning patient 12 degrees is sufficient to prevent pulmonary complications, stimulate circulation, and prevent decubiti
      4. Tilt table—prepares patient for upright position
   B. Proper body mechanics—conserves energy, prevents muscle strain, prevents fatigue, and allows for more efficient work
3. Nursing care of the patient in a cast
   A. Enclosure in cast results in emotional problems for patient
   B. Preparation of bed—includes bed boards and firm mattress
      1. Use pillows to support wet cast
      2. Turn patient to prone position after 8 hours if in body or hip spica cast—physician's order required
      3. Give skin care
      4. Observe for abdominal distention, circulation, pain, and pressure
      5. Turn every 4 hours after cast is dry
4. Care of the cast
   A. Maintain cleanliness
   B. Keep dry
   C. Protect from soiling about genital area
   D. Bind raw edges
   E. Handle carefully to avoid cracking or breaking
5. Removal of the cast
   A. Cast may be bivalved; shell may be used for few days
   B. Support extremity carefully
   C. Skin may be washed with warm water and soap; apply oil and massage gently
   D. Elastic bandage may be applied
   E. Exercises may be given to strengthen muscles
6. Nursing the patient with an orthopedic device
   A. Traction—may be applied to extremities, cervical region, or pelvic region
      1. To relieve muscle spasm
      2. To keep bones in place while healing
      3. To reduce dislocations
      4. To correct or relieve contractures
   B. Skin traction—adhesive substance applied to clean dry skin
   C. Skeletal traction—uses pins, wires, Crutchfield tongs, etc.

D. Various kinds of traction
   1. Bryant's traction—used for children with fracture of femur
   2. Buck's extension—may be adapted for home use
   3. Russell traction—allows more freedom of movement
E. Frames
   1. Balkan frame
   2. Bradford frame
   3. Stryker frame
   4. Foster frame
F. Splints—used for immobilization and may be used with traction
G. Other orthopedic devices
   1. Various devices include crutches, braces, walking heel or iron, neck supports, corsets, and back braces
H. Nursing care
7. Nursing the patient with diseases and disorders of the musculoskeletal system
   A. Congenital deformities—may affect bones, joints, or muscles
      1. Clubfoot—may affect one or both feet and may be mild or severe
         a. Treated by exercise and application of plaster casts
      2. Torticollis (wryneck)—shortening of the sternocleidomastoid muscle fibers
         a. Treatment includes heat, massage, stretching, and sometimes surgery; condition may be treated with cast
      3. Dislocation of hip—may affect one or both hips
         a. Treatment is with pillows or splints to keep legs in abduction, application of cast, and use of abduction bar after cast removal
   B. Arthritis—rheumatic disorder resulting in inflammation of joints and adjacent tissue
      1. Rheumatoid arthritis and rheumatoid spondylitis are most serious forms and lead to crippling; no known cure
         a. Nursing care is directed toward maintaining function, relieving pain, and preventing deformities
         b. Treatment includes hot moist packs, hot tub baths, electric blanket, heat cradles, paraffin baths, active exercise, and aspirin for relief of pain
         c. Anti-inflammatory and analgesic drugs are used
      2. Rheumatoid spondylitis—inflammation of vertebrae and sacroiliac joints; may cause kyphosis, or humped back
      3. Osteoarthritis (degenerative joint disease)—result of normal wear and tear that occurs with aging process
         a. Treatment—reduction in weight if patient is obese, exercise, avoidance of cold and dampness, rest, and application of heat
      4. Surgical treatment of arthritis
         a. Tendon transplant
         b. Synovectomy
         c. Osteotomy
         d. Arthrodesis

   e. Arthroplasty
   f. Total joint replacement
      5. Gout—metabolic disease occurring usually in middle life
         a. Uric acid is retained in body
         b. Treatment includes administration of colchicine for relief of pain
         c. Tophi—deposits of uric acid in various parts of body
         d. Patient treated on individual basis
      6. Bursitis—inflammation of bursae
         a. Treatment is with x-ray therapy or hydrocortisone injected into bursae, analgesic drugs, rest, and support
         b. Calcium deposits may have to be surgically removed
   C. Infectious diseases and disorders
      1. Osteomyelitis—inflammation of bone; if chronic, may recur throughout life
         a. Treatment may be surgical or with antibiotics or immobilization; no uniform method of treatment
      2. Tuberculosis of bone—occurs primarily in children
         a. Pott's disease (tuberculosis of spine) usually affects lower dorsal or upper lumbar region
            (1) May result in softening of bone with destruction and deformity
            (2) Treatment is absolute immobilization of spine by casts, braces, the use of frames, and antituberculous drugs
            (3) Surgery may be done
         b. Tuberculosis of hip may affect very young child
            (1) Treatment is by immobilization and surgery
   D. Traumatic injuries
      1. Contusions—are like bruises
         a. If bleeding is severe, it may cause hematoma
      2. Sprains—involve twisting or wrenching of ligaments, tendons, or muscles
      3. Dislocations—may be congenital or result from disease or injury; temporary displacement of bone occurs
         a. Manual manipulation under general anesthesia is usually necessary, followed by immobilization with splints or cast
      4. Fractures—result of violent external force, of disease, or of decalcification in aged persons
         a. Classification of fractures
            (1) Greenstick—incomplete break
            (2) Comminuted—splintered bone
            (3) Compound—bone completely broken and protrudes through break in skin
            (4) Spiral—twisting of bone with longitudinal or oblique fracture
            (5) Impacted, or compression—one end of bone is driven into other end
         b. Fractures are treated by open or closed reduction

c. Patient may be in traction or cast
5. Fractures of hip—treatment usually consists of internal fixation, nailing, or prosthesis
   a. Permits earlier ambulation
   b. Fewer complications
   c. Return to work sooner
   d. Easier nursing care
   e. Nursing care
      (1) Position may be changed from side to side
      (2) Support to provide good body alignment
      (3) Intake and output records
      (4) Exercises
   f. Prosthetic device may be used
      (1) Patient progresses to weight bearing in 10 to 14 days
6. Whiplash injuries—result of automobile accident with rear-end collision
   a. May cause compression fracture of cervical vertebrae or tearing of muscles and ligaments
   b. Symptoms may be delayed several days
   c. Treatment includes heat, massage, and cervical traction; patient may be fitted with neck support
E. Rickets—disease occurring in infants and young children because of lack of vitamin D
F. Bone tumors—may be primary or secondary, benign or malignant
   1. Benign tumors do not metastasize to other parts of body
   2. Malignant tumors—several types may be primary and metastasize to other tissues
   3. Malignant tumors may be result of metastasis from other parts of body
   4. Treatment depends on type, location, extent of involvement, and lesions elsewhere in body
   5. Amputation of extremity may be necessary in some types
G. Amputation—performed when life of patient is threatened
   1. Preoperative care
      a. Psychologic preparation
      b. Laboratory examinations
      c. Treatment for dehydration, anemia if if necessary
      d. Chest x-ray film
      e. Electrocardiogram
      f. Regional hypothermia
   2. Postoperative care
      a. Methods of treatment
         (1) Delayed prosthesis fitting—patient should be fitted with temporary prosthesis as soon as possible
         (2) Immediate postsurgical prosthetic fitting—plaster of Paris is rigid dressing applied in operating room; temporary prosthesis attached
      b. Bed made like that for patient with fracture
      c. Observe patient for vital signs and hemorrhage
   d. Stump may be elevated for first 24 hours
   e. After first 24 hours stump should be placed flat in bed
   f. Patient should spend some time in prone position
   g. Phantom pain may be present
   h. Brief ambulation with limited weight bearing possible in 24 hours with immediate postsurgical prosthesis
   i. Patient should be instructed in home care of stump
   j. Patient should be referred to physical therapist for exercises, balancing, and crutch walking
   3. Amputation for child—may be necessary because of disease, trauma, or congenital absence of limbs
      a. Prosthesis must provide for growth
      b. Child may suffer from fatigue
      c. Traumatizations to stump may occur from excessive pressure
      d. Abrasions, edema, and irritation may occur if socket of prosthesis does not fit properly
H. Muscular dystrophy—of unknown cause but believed to be inherited
   1. Affects voluntary muscles, which become weak, atrophy, and waste away
I. Cerebral palsy—neuromuscular disorder that results in spasticity and involuntary movement in any activity requiring coordinated action of muscles

Review questions

1. After a cast is dry, how often should the patient be turned?
   a. *q 4 hrs.*
2. What six things should the nurse observe when an extremity has been placed in a cast?
   a. *skin color, numbness, edema, etc.*
   b. *infection around pins or wires*
   c. *rubbing of cast on skin*
   d. *pressure areas*
   e. *proper alignment in bed*
   f. *traction set up properly*
3. What are the reasons for the use of traction?
   a. *keep bones in place for healing*
   b. *reduce muscle spasm*
   c. *relieve pain*
   d. *reduce dislocations or correct contractures*
4. What type of traction is often used for young children with fracture of the femur?
   a. *Bryant's traction*
5. What are three common congenital orthopedic defects?
   a. *dislocated hip*
   b. *spina bifida*
   c. *clubbed fingers or feet*
6. What type of arthritis affects most elderly persons?
   a. *Osteoarthritis*
7. What is another name for a broken bone?
   a. *fracture*
8. How should the nurse position the stump when the patient has had amputation of a lower extremity?
   a. *elevated at first, then flat*

9. What analgesic is most commonly used for patients with arthritis?
   a. ASA
10. Why is it best to avoid the use of heat for drying a cast?
   a. *the outside would dry - preventing evaporation of H₂O from inside*
   b. *it must dry by evaporation*

Films

1. Bed care and positioning of the patient with arthritis (8 min., sound, color, 16 mm.), Media Resources Branch, National Medical Audiovisual Center (Annex), Station K, Atlanta, Ga. 30324. Demonstrates positioning and nursing care.
2. The homemaker with arthritis (28 min., sound, color, 16 mm.), Media Resources Branch, National Medical Audiovisual Center (Annex), Station K, Atlanta, Ga. 30324. Demonstrates techniques and equipment helpful to the homemaker as well as describing measures to protect joints and muscles from further deformity.
3. Home management of disability from arthritis (29 min., sound, black and white, 16 mm.), Squibb, 909 Third Ave., New York, N. Y. 10022. Home care service for chronically ill, medical and physical evaluation, and development of individual rehabilitation program reviewed. Patient treated in the home by visiting nurses and physical therapist. The role of the physician, nurse, patient, and family. Includes simple self-help devices.
4. One of sixteen million—M-1634-X (20 min., sound, color, 16 mm.), Media Resources Branch, National Medical Audiovisual Center (Annex), Station K, Atlanta, Ga. 30324. An animated story of a man with arthritis. Depicts common attitudes and a physician coming to grips with them. Warns against superstitions about arthritis cures, and explains what is known about arthritis.
5. Rheumatoid arthritis (29 min., sound, color, 16 mm.), Pfizer Laboratories, Film Library, 267 West 25th St., New York, N. Y. 10017. Several patients with severe arthritis are shown. The cause, treatment, prognosis, changes shown on x-ray film, and autopsy are presented.
6. Techniques for maintenance of range of motion—F-1471-X (Filmstrip, 19 min., color, 35 mm., 89 frames), Media Resources Branch, National Medical Audiovisual Center (Annex), Station K, Atlanta, Ga. 30324. Demonstrates various passive exercises applicable to any patient confined to bed because of a geriatric condition, burns, stroke, poliomyelitis, and cerebral palsy.

References

1. Barnes, Colin G.: Treatment of gout, Nursing Mirror **136:**21-24, April 6, 1973.
2. Beeson, Paul B., and McDermott, Walsh: Cecil-Loeb textbook of medicine, ed. 13, Philadelphia, 1971, W. B. Saunders Co.
3. Brunner, Lillian S., and Suddarth, Doris S.: Textbook of medical-surgical nursing, ed. 3, Philadelphia, 1975, J. B. Lippincott Co.
4. Davis, Ruth W.: Surgery for osteoarthritis of the hip, Bedside Nurse **5:**24-26, May, 1972.
5. Larson, Carroll B., and Gould, Marjorie: Orthopedic nursing, ed. 8, St. Louis, 1974, The C. V. Mosby Co.
6. Luckmann, Joan, and Sorensen, Karen C.: Medical-surgical nursing, Philadelphia, 1974, W. B. Saunders Co.
7. McCaritt, Martin E.: The cerebral palsied, Rehabilitation Record **7:**33-35, March-April, 1966.
8. Macgregor, P. A., and Woodbury, J. F. L.: Gout—the misunderstood malady, The Canadian Nurse **62:**26-29, Jan., 1966.
9. Urist, Marshall R.: Clinical orthopaedics and related research, Philadelphia, 1974, J. B. Lippincott Co.

CHAPTER 22

Nursing the patient with allergic conditions

KEY WORDS

allergen
allergist
antihistamine
atopic
autoimmune
desensitization
eosinophils
genetic
hypersensitivity

lacrimation
pollinosis
precipitin
rhinitis
sensitized
urticaria
wheal

The condition now known as allergy, or hypersensitivity, was first observed in 1832. However, it was not until 1890 that serious study was undertaken. Robert Koch was the first to observe and describe the allergic reaction after he administered the tuberculin test (p. 557). The term *allergy* was not used until 1906, when von Pirquet used it to describe changes associated with repeated contact with various antigenic substances. Since that time, allergy has been accepted to designate hypersensitivity in certain individuals. The terms *allergy* and *hypersensitivity* are used interchangeably.

Throughout the 1900s, study and research into allergic reactions has continued. During this period skin tests have been developed, passive immunity from mother to fetus was identified, and the production of extracts of antigenic substances for desensitization were produced. The treatment of allergic reactions with antihistaminic drugs and the use of corticosteroids was initiated. Allergic factors in asthma, hay fever, and urticaria were identified. The relationship of hypersensitivity to pathologic diseases and homograph rejection are areas under study.

Although many factors associated with immunity and hypersensitivity remain unsolved, research has accomplished a great deal in a short time. The diagnosis and treatment of allergic disorders is a medical specialty, and the physician treating these disorders is called an allergist.

CAUSES OF ALLERGY

It may be impossible to determine the cause of many allergic reactions; however, in general the cause is classified as hereditary, congenital, or contact.

529

The genetic transmission of the predisposition to allergy occurs in some families. If a parent has an allergic disorder, the offspring may develop an allergic condition at some period during their lifetime; however, it does not necessarily mean that the allergy will be the same type as the parent's allergy. When predisposition is present, contact with an allergen may be necessary for a reaction to occur. The homeostasis of the body plays an important role when the individual has an inherited predisposition to allergy. Any episode that disturbs the homeostatic balance, such as emotional and stress situations, severe infection, pregnancy, or endocrine dysfunction may cause some type of allergy to occur.

The congenital cause differs from the hereditary cause in that an allergen may be transmitted directly from the mother to the fetus in utero by the placental blood supply. When the infant has been sensitized in utero to a specific allergen, contact with the allergen after birth may cause an allergic reaction.

Contact allergy usually means that a person must have direct contact with an allergen for hypersensitivity to occur. Although the genetic factor may be important in contact allergy, an allergic disorder may occur in the absence of any predisposition. Contact allergens are classified as inhalants, ingestants, injectants, contactants, or bacterial. The most common inhalants are pollens from grasses, weeds, trees, grains, and dust. Allergy caused by inhaling these pollens is usually seasonal and occurs when flowering and pollination occur. The most common type of allergy caused by pollens

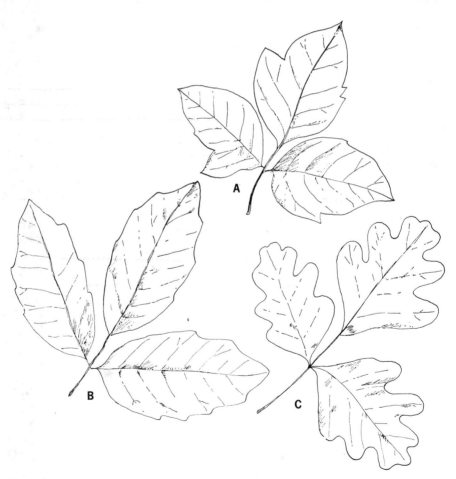

Fig. 22-1. Plants and shrubs that frequently cause severe skin reactions. **A,** Poison ivy. **B** and **C,** Types of poison oak.

No. 151

AN ACT

HB 129

Amending the act of May 22, 1951 (P.L.317, No.69), entitled, as amended, "An act relating to the practice of professional nursing; providing for the licensing of nurses and for the revocation and suspension of such licenses, subject to appeal, and for their reinstatement; providing for the renewal of such licenses; regulating nursing in general; prescribing penalties and repealing certain laws," changing definitions; changing the scope of activities permitted or prohibited by the act; authorizing the Board to establish educational standards and requirements and fees; regulating the issuance of licenses and further prescribing fines and penalties.

The General Assembly of the Commonwealth of Pennsylvania hereby enacts as follows:

Section 1.   Section 2, act of May 22, 1951 (P.L.317, No.69), known as "The Professional Nursing Law," is amended to read:

Section 2.   When used in this act, the following words and phrases shall have the following meanings unless the context provides otherwise:

(1)   **[A person engages in the "Practice of Professional Nursing," within the meaning of this act, who performs any professional services requiring the application of principles of the biological, physical or social sciences and nursing skills in the care of the sick, in the prevention of disease, or in the conservation of health.]** *The "Practice of Professional Nursing" means diagnosing and treating human responses to actual or potential health problems through such services as casefinding, health teaching, health counseling, and provision of care supportive to or restorative of life and well-being, and executing medical regimens as prescribed by a licensed physician or dentist. The foregoing shall not be deemed to include acts of medical diagnosis or prescription of medical therapeutic or corrective measures, except as may be authorized by rules and regulations jointly promulgated by the State Board of Medical Education and Licensure and the Board, which rules and regulations shall be implemented by the Board.*

(2)   "Board" means the State Board of Nurse Examiners.

(3)   "Approved" means approved by the State Board of Nurse Examiners.

(4)   "Diagnosing" means that identification of and discrimination between physical and psychosocial signs and symptoms essential to effective execution and management of the nursing regimen.

(5)   "Treating" means selection and performance of those therapeutic measures essential to the effective execution and management of the nursing regimen, and execution of the prescribed medical regimen.

(6)   "Human responses" means those signs, symptoms and processes which denote the individual's interaction with an actual or potential health problem.

2

Section 2.   The act is amended by adding a section to read:

Section 2.1.   The Board shall have the right and duty to establish rules and regulations for the practice of professional nursing and the administration of this act.   Copies of such rules and regulations shall be available for distribution to the public.

Section 3.   Section 3 of the act is amended to read:

Section 3.   **[Except as provided in section four, it shall be unlawful for (i) any person not licensed under this act, (ii) any person not holding a current license issued under this act, or (iii) any person whose license has been suspended or revoked, to practice professional nursing.]** *Any person who holds a license to practice professional nursing in this Commonwealth, or who is maintained on inactive status in accordance with section 11 of this act, shall have the right to use the title "registered nurse" and the abbreviation "R.N." No other person shall engage in the practice of professional nursing or use the title "registered nurse" or the abbreviation "R.N." to indicate that the person using the same is a registered nurse. No person shall sell or fraudulently obtain or fraudulently furnish any nursing diploma, license, record, or registration or aid or abet therein.*

Section 4.   Section 4 of the act, amended May 6, 1970 (P.L.353, No.118), is amended to read:

Section 4.   This act confers no authority to practice *dentistry, podiatry, optometry, chiropractic,* medicine or surgery, nor does it prohibit—

(1)   **[Services rendered by practical nurses, or home]** *Home* care of the sick by friends, domestic servants, nursemaids, **[companies,]** *companions,* or household aides of any type, so long as such persons do not represent or hold themselves out to be licensed nurses, licensed registered nurses, or registered nurses; or use in connection with their names, any designation tending to imply that they are licensed to practice under the provisions of this act *nor services rendered by any physicians, osteopaths, dentists or chiropractors, podiatrists, optometrists, or any person licensed pursuant to the act of March 2, 1956 (P.L.1211, No.376), known as the "Practical Nurse Law."*

[(2)   Gratuitous care of the sick by friends or members of the family.

(3)   Domestic administration of family remedies by any person.

(4)   Nursing services by anyone in case of an immediate emergency.

(5)   Nursing by a person temporarily in this State, in compliance with an engagement made outside of this State, which engagement requires that such person accompany and care for a patient while temporarily in this State: Provided, however, That said engagement shall not be of more than six (6) months' duration.

(6)] *(2)*   Care of the sick, with or without compensation or personal profit, when done *solely* in connection with the practice of the religious tenets of any church by adherents thereof.

[(7) Auxiliary services rendered by persons carrying out duties necessary for the support of nursing service, including those duties which involve minor nursing services for patients, performed in hospitals or elsewhere under the direction of licensed physicians or supervision of licensed registered nurses.

(8) Nursing services rendered by a student enrolled in an approved school of nursing, when these services are a part of the course of study.

(9) Nursing services rendered] *(3) The practice of professional nursing by a person temporarily in this Commonwealth licensed by another state, territory or possession of the United States or a foreign country, in compliance with an engagement made outside of this Commonwealth, which engagement requires that such person accompany and care for a patient while temporarily in this Commonwealth: Provided, however, That said engagement shall not be of more than six (6) months' duration.*

(4) The practice of professional nursing by a graduate of an approved [school] *program* of *professional* nursing in Pennsylvania or any other state, working under qualified supervision, during the period not to exceed one (1) year between completion of his or her [course of nursing education] *program* and notification of the results of a licensing examination taken by such person, and during such additional period as the Board may in each case especially permit.

[(10) Nursing services rendered] *(5) The practice of professional nursing* by a person who holds a current license or other evidence of the right to practice professional nursing, as that term is defined in this act, issued by any other state, territory or [province] *possession* of the United States or the Dominion of Canada, during the period that an application filed by such person for licensure in Pennsylvania is pending before the Board, [or] *but not* for a period of *more than* one (1) year. [whichever period first expires.

(11)] *(6)* The practice of professional nursing, within the definition of this act, by any person [lawfully qualified so to practice in another state, territory, province or country,] when such person is engaged in the practice of nursing as an employee of the United States. [, or, by a person . who is a foreign graduate nurse in the United States on nonimmigration status while enrolled in an approved, organized program of study as hereinafter provided.

The Board shall establish standards and approve organized programs of study offered to foreign graduate nurses in the United States on nonimmigration status who are studying in this Commonwealth. Initial approval shall be followed by at least annual survey and review of the program to assure maintenance of acceptable standards. Such programs shall be conducted only with approval of the Board. Each hospital maintaining an exchange visitor educational program for foreign graduate nurses shall pay a fee as established by the Board. Such fee shall be related to the actual costs incurred by the Board in rendering services in connection with such programs.]

Section 5.   Section 5 of the act is amended to read:

Section 5.   *(a)* The Board shall, once every year and at such other times and under such conditions as shall be provided by its regulations, examine all [applicants eligible for examination to determine whether they are qualified to be licensed, and shall authorize the issue to each person passing said examination to the satisfaction of the Board of a proper certificate setting forth that such person has been licensed to practice as a licensed registered nurse.] *eligible applicants for licensure; and shall, subject to the provisions of section 6 of this act, issue a license to each person passing said examination to the satisfaction of the Board.*

(b)   The Board may admit to examination any person who has satisfactorily completed an approved nursing education program for the preparation of registered professional nurses in Pennsylvania or such a program in any other state, territory or possession of the United States, considered by the Board to be equivalent to that required in this Commonwealth at the time such program was completed, and who meets the requirements of character and preliminary education.

(c)   The Board may admit to examination any person who has satisfactorily completed a nursing education program for the preparation of registered professional nurses in a country or territory not mentioned above who has been licensed, registered, or duly recognized there as a professional nurse provided such a program is considered by the Board to be equal to that required in this Commonwealth at the time such program was completed and who meets the requirements of character and preliminary education.

Section 6.   Section 6 of the act, amended May 29, 1968 (P.L.135, No.73), is amended to read:

Section 6.   No application for licensure as a registered nurse shall be considered unless accompanied by a fee of ten dollars ($10). Every applicant, to be eligible for examination for licensure as a registered nurse, shall furnish evidence satisfactory to the Board that he or she [is a citizen of the United States or has legally declared an intention to become such,] is of good moral character, has completed work equal to a standard high school course as evaluated by the [Department of Public Instruction] *Board* and has [graduated from a school of nursing which gives at least a two (2) years' course of instruction, or has received instruction in different schools of nursing and in other approved agencies with which such schools are affiliated for periods of time amounting to at least a two (2) years' course of instruction, and has then graduated. Such school or combination of schools of nursing must be on the approved list issued by the Board, as hereinafter provided. The course of instruction shall include, (1) principles of nursing based on biological, physical and social sciences; (2) responsible supervision of a patient involving skill in observation of symptoms and reactions and the accurate recording of the facts and carrying out of treatments and medication prescribed by a licensed physician; and (3) the application of such nursing procedures as involve understanding of cause and effect in order to safeguard life and health of a patient and others] *satisfactorily completed an approved program of professional nursing.*

Section 7. The act is amended by adding two sections to read:

Section 6.1. The Board shall establish standards for the operation and approval of nursing education programs for the preparation of registered professional nurses and for the carrying out of the rights given to the Board under this act. Programs for the preparation of registered professional nurses shall be established or conducted only with the approval of the Board.

The Board shall establish standards and approve organized programs of study offered to foreign graduate nurses in the United States on nonimmigration status who are studying in this Commonwealth. Initial approval shall be followed by at least annual survey and review of the program to assure maintenance of acceptable standards. Such programs shall be conducted only with approval of the Board. Each hospital maintaining an exchange visitor educational program for foreign graduate nurses shall pay a fee as established by the Board. Such fee shall be related to the actual costs incurred by the Board in rendering services in connection with such programs.

Section 6.2. The Board shall annually prepare and make available for public distribution a list of all programs approved and classified by it. Any student who shall be enrolled in any school which shall be removed from the approved list shall be given credit toward the satisfaction of the Board's requirements for examination for such of the requirements of the Board which any said student shall satisfactorily complete prior to the removal of said school from the approved list, and said student shall upon the satisfactory completion of the remainder of said requirements in any approved school be eligible for examination for licensure. The Board may withhold or remove any school from the approved list if the school fails to meet and maintain minimum standards, as established by regulation of the Board, of education, curriculum, administration, qualifications of the faculty, organization and function of the faculty, staff and facilities.

Section 8. Sections 7 and 8 of the act are amended to read:

Section 7. [(a)] The Board may [authorize the] issue [of] a license without examination to a graduate of a school of nursing [approved by the duly constituted agency in any other state, territory or province of the United States or the Dominion of Canada,] who has completed a course of study in nursing considered by the Board to be equivalent to that required in this State at the time such course was completed, and who [was] *is* registered or licensed *by examination* in [such] *any* other state, *or* territory [or province by examination] *of the United States or the Dominion of Canada,* and *who* has met all the foregoing requirements as to [age,] character, [citizenship] and preliminary education.

[(b)   The Board may admit to examination a graduate of a school of nursing in any other state, territory or province of the United States or the Dominion of Canada, which school was approved by the duly constituted agency thereof and is considered by the Board to satisfy current requirements of this State, and which graduate has met all the requirements as to age, character, citizenship and preliminary education, set forth in section six of this act.

(c)   The Board may admit to examination graduates of schools of nursing in other countries not mentioned above which are approved by the duly constituted agency thereof, provided such persons have been licensed or registered there and can meet current requirements in Pennsylvania.

(d)   The Board may license persons without examination, providing such persons are graduates or have graduated, prior to the effective date of this act, of or from approved schools of nursing or of organized courses of nursing study in hospitals or schools of nursing in Pennsylvania or any other state, territory or province of the United States or the Dominion of Canada, which school or course, at the time of graduation of such persons, required the satisfactory completion of a course considered by the Board to be equivalent to the minimum requirements then in effect in Pennsylvania for the preparation of registered nurses; and providing further, that application for such licensure shall be filed with the Board by such persons on or before the thirtieth day of September, one thousand nine hundred fifty-two.]

Section 8.   [Every person legally entitled to practice as a registered nurse and to use the letters "R.N." at the time this act becomes effective shall be considered as licensed to practice under this act, and may continue to practice as such and use the title registered nurse and the letters "R.N." until the expiration of his or her current certificate of record, and may obtain a license automatically thereafter by making application and paying the fee, as herein provided, for the renewal of licenses. Every holder of a valid license issued pursuant to the provisions of this act shall be] *The Board shall issue to each person who meets the licensure requirements of this act, a certificate setting forth that such person is licensed to engage in the practice of professional nursing and* entitled to use the title "registered nurse" [or "licensed registered nurse"] and the letters "R.N."

Section 9.   Sections 9 and 10 of the act are repealed.

Section 10.   Section 11 of the act, amended December 17, 1959 (P.L.1888, No.689), is amended to read:

Section 11.   [Each person, upon being licensed by the Board as a licensed registered nurse under the provisions of this act, shall, without additional fee therefor, be given a card to evidence such license, which shall be valid during the current renewal biennium.] *(a)* Licenses issued pursuant to this act shall expire on the thirty-first day of October of each biennium, or on such other biennial expiration date as [the Board may fix] *may be established by regulation of the Board.* Application for renewal of a license shall biennially be forwarded to each [active] registrant *holding a current license* prior to the expiration date of the current renewal biennium. The application form [shall] *may* be completed and returned to the Board, accompanied by the required fee of four dollars ($4); upon approval of each application, the applicant shall receive a renewal of license.

(b) Any registrant licensed under this act may request an application for inactive status. The application form may be completed and returned to the Board. Upon receipt of each application, the applicant shall be maintained on inactive status without fee and shall be entitled to apply at any time and to receive a current license by filing a renewal application as in subsection (a) hereof.

[The form and method of licensure and renewal shall be provided for by the Board in such manner as will enable it to carry into effect the purposes of this act. The Board shall maintain a record of all licenses issued under this act and of all renewals, as herein provided.]

Section 11.   Section 12 of the act is repealed.

Section 12.   Sections 13 and 14 of the act are amended to read:

Section 13.   Any person, or the responsible officers or employees of any corporation, copartnership, institution or association violating any of the provisions of this act, shall, upon summary conviction thereof, be sentenced to pay a fine of [not less than fifty dollars ($50) for the first offense; for the second and any subsequent offenses, not less than one hundred dollars ($100), nor more than two hundred dollars ($200)] *three hundred dollars ($300);* and in default of the payment of such fine and costs, to undergo imprisonment for a period [not to exceed thirty (30)] *of ninety (90)* days, *unless nonpayment of said fine is shown by affidavit made by the defendant to the court, to be the result of the defendant's indigency.*

Section 14.   The Board may suspend or revoke any license in any case where the Board shall find that—

(1)   The licensee is [guilty of gross immorality]   *on repeated occasions negligent or incompetent in the practice of professional nursing.*

(2)   The licensee is [unfit or incompetent by reason of negligence, habits, or other causes] *unable to practice professional nursing with reasonable skill and safety to patients by reason of mental or physical illness or condition or physiological or psychological dependence upon alcohol, hallucinogenic or narcotic drugs or other drugs which tend to impair judgment or coordination, so long as such dependence shall continue. In enforcing this clause (2), the Board shall, upon probable cause, have authority to compel a licensee to submit to a mental or*

physical examination as designated by it. After notice, hearing, adjudication and appeal as provided for in section 15, failure of a licensee to submit to such examination when directed shall constitute an admission of the allegations against him unless failure is due to circumstances beyond his control, consequent upon which a default and final order may be entered without the taking of testimony or presentation of evidence. A licensee affected under this paragraph shall at reasonable intervals be afforded an opportunity to demonstrate that he can resume a competent practice of professional nursing with reasonable skill and safety to patients.

(3) The licensee has wilfully or repeatedly violated any of the provisions of this act or of the regulations of the Board.

(4) The licensee has committed fraud or deceit in the practice of nursing, or in securing his or her admission to such practice.

(5) The licensee has been convicted, or has pleaded guilty, or entered a plea of nolo contendere, or has been found guilty by a judge or jury, of a **[crime or has been dishonorably discharged, or discharged under circumstances amounting to a dishonorable discharge, from the military forces of the United States or of any other country]** *felony in the courts of this Commonwealth or any other state, territory or country.*

[(6) The licensee is an habitual drunkard, or is addicted to the use of morphine, cocaine or other drugs having a similar effect, or if he or she has become mentally incompetent.

(7) The licensee is continuing to practice nursing when such licensee knows he or she has an infectious, communicable or contagious disease.

(8) The licensee has been guilty of unprofessional conduct, or such conduct as to require a suspension or revocation in the public interest.

(9)] *(6)* The licensee **[having obtained a license upon declaration of intention to become a citizen of the United States, has not become a citizen of the United States within seven (7) years after the date of such declaration of intention]** *has his license suspended or revoked in another state, territory or country.*

Section 13.   The act of June 8, 1923 (P.L.683, No.280), entitled "An act relating to the registration and reregistration of nurses and licensed attendants by the State Board of Examiners for Registration of Nurses, and the issuance of a license to practice nursing; making the violation of the provisions of this act a misdemeanor, and providing penalties therefor," is repealed in so far as it relates to the registration of registered nurses.

Section 14.   This act shall take effect immediately.

9

APPROVED—The 3rd day of July, A. D. 1974.

MILTON J. SHAPP

The foregoing is a true and correct copy of Act of the General Assembly
No. 151.

C. DeLoret Tucker

Secretary of the Commonwealth.

is hay fever. Ingestants are usually foods to which the individual may be hypersensitive. The most common offenders include the proteins of cow's milk, egg white, chocolate, strawberries, shellfish, and nuts. Among the injectants are drugs such as penicillin or other antibiotics. Horse serum that may be used in making antitoxins may cause severe reactions. The venom from a snake bite or stings from some insects may cause a reaction in a hypersensitive person. Some individuals may be sensitive to contactants such as laundry powders, cosmetic preparations and the sap from plants such as poison ivy or poison oak (Fig. 22-1). Factors related to infectants have been demonstrated in tuberculosis, typhoid fever, and anthrax. The role of bacteria in asthma has not been clearly substantiated.[2, 7]

ATOPIC ALLERGY

Atopic means to be displaced or out of place. Atopic allergy results from a wide variety of antigenic substances that are found normally in the environment. It has been assumed that each person has a threshold of tolerance for the many kinds of allergens to which he is exposed in day-to-day living. These allergens include the inhalants and digestants. However, the role of food as a cause of atopic allergy has received less study than inhalants, and the extent to which foods cause atopy is not always clear. The inherited predisposition is important in atopic allergy. When an individual reaches his level of tolerance for a specific allergen, he may develop some type of atopic allergy. Frequently the manifestations begin with homeostatic imbalance (p. 530). Atopic disease includes hay fever, urticaria, asthma, angioneurotic edema, and atopic dermatitis, and gastrointestinal disturbances or drug reactions may occur. The atopic individual may be hypersensitive to several different allergens; for example, a person may have asthma but also have a history of hay fever or dermatitis.[4, 10]

When hereditary factors are involved in hypersensitivity, it is considered to be natural and the disorders resulting from the sensitivity are called atopic disease. The atopic individual may experience allergy throughout his life; however, the antigenic substances to which he is hypersensitive and the manifestations of the atopic disease may not remain the same.[2]

TYPES OF ALLERGIC REACTIONS

Allergic reactions may be immediate or delayed. Antibodies circulating in the plasma react with the antigen to cause an immediate reaction. There are different kinds of antibodies. Precipitin antibodies are responsible for immediate reactions that occur causing serum sickness or anaphylactic shock. Other antibodies called reagins or skin-sensitizing antibodies have the capacity to become attached to tissue cells and to sensitize the cell. These antibodies are the ones usually involved in hay fever, asthma, and some atopic diseases. A third group of antibodies are within the cell and cause the delayed reaction seen in the tuberculin test.[4, 7]

Delayed reactions may be local or systemic and may be delayed from hours to days. The antibodies in the plasma are not significant in delayed reactions; the reaction is caused by the sensitized cells. There are several theories concerning the types of cells and their role in delayed reactions. Most authorities agree that more research is needed. The early work was done with the tuberculin test, which evoked a delayed reaction. Delayed allergic response occurs in other diseases, including bacterial, fungus, and viral infections. Delayed reactions have been observed after contact with plants such as poison ivy and with drugs. Homograft rejection is now believed to be delayed sensitivity.[4]

AUTOIMMUNE SENSITIVITY

Because of genetic differences, the human body rejects anything that is not of itself. This is the reason why human organ transplants are usually rejected by the recipient. It is also why skin for grafting is taken from a site on the recipient's own body and transferred to the site for grafting. Thus the individual is both the donor and the recipient. Recently considerable attention has been given to what is called autoimmune disease. Under usual conditions the body will suppress the production of antibodies that would injure its own body. For some reason not clearly understood the body loses self-identity and produces antigenic substances that stimulate antibody formation that will react against its own body. Diseases and disorders that result from this antigen-antibody reaction are called autoimmune diseases, and they may affect the eyes, skin, joints, thyroid gland, kidneys, brain, and vascular system. It may not be possible to cure autoimmune disease, but physicians are learning how to control these diseases. At the same time, intensive study and research is continuing to produce a better understanding of auto-immunity.[2, 9, 10]

PATHOPHYSIOLOGY

The pathologic response of the individual results from the antigen-antibody reaction, during which histamine and histamine-like substances are released. The histamine causes vasodilation of the peripheral blood vessels and constriction of the smooth muscles of the bronchioles. The dilation of the capillary vessels causes fluid to move from the plasma into the interstitial spaces. Edema and an increase in mucus from the mucus-secreting glands accompanied by itching and sneezing occur.

Symptomatically, allergic manifestations may vary from person to person and may vary in the same person from time to time.[6] Factors that influence symptoms include the type of allergen. Inhalants usually cause congestion of the nasal mucosa, sneezing, thin watery nasal discharge, red itching conjunctivae, and increased lacrimation. When the allergen is a digestant, gastrointestinal symptoms of nausea, vomiting, and diarrhea may occur. Various contactants cause urticaria and dermatitis. When histamine causes spasm and constriction of the bronchioles, bronchial asthma may occur. Some antigens cause serum sickness and anaphylactic shock) (p. 40). The individual may become sensitized to certain drugs such as penicillin, in which urticaria or anaphylactic shock and death may occur, whereas other reactions to drugs may cause fever and skin rash. Although penicillin has caused more fatalities, any drug, even aspirin, to which the individual is sensitive may cause a serious reaction.[7, 9]

DIAGNOSTIC TESTS AND PROCEDURES

The diagnosis of allergy includes (1) a complete family and personal history, (2) physical examination, (3) skin tests, (4) tests of mucous membrane sensitivity, and (5) elimination diets.

Previous reference was made in this chapter to genetic transmission and to congenital transmission of hypersensitivity. These factors are extremely important in helping to establish a diagnosis. The allergist will question the individual concerning any family members with an allergic disorder or any previous experiences that the individual may have had. If the patient is a female, the allergist will want to know about any allergy prior to, during, or after pregnancy, the type of allergic response, and its duration. The individual's history as it relates to tension-producing situations, history of infection, endocrine disturbance, and work-related activities may be significant. Geographic movement may be important because of change of climate or exposure to new kinds of allergens.

A complete physical examination is given, which involves a complete blood count, including the differential count (p. 232). Eosinophils are cells that normally occur in 1% to 3% of all persons. Primarily during an allergic reaction the number of eosinophils may be greatly increased. They may also be found in the nasal secretions during an allergic reaction.

Skin tests. There are several methods of doing skin tests, including the scratch test, intradermal test, and patch test. Testing is often started using the scratch test method. A small scratch is made through the skin with a blunt instrument, but not deep enough to cause bleeding. The allergin may be a powder, liquid, or paste. The allergen is applied to the scratch. When the test is done on the forearm, a control is placed on the other arm. After application of the allergen an area of redness and a wheal will appear in 15 to 30 minutes if the individual is sensitive to the antigen, whereas the control will not show any reaction.

The intracutaneous test may be used without prior use of the scratch test, or it may be used only for the antigens that failed to react to the scratch test. A minute amount (0.01 to 0.02 ml.) of the antigen is injected into but not through the skin with a tuberculin syringe and a No. 26 gauge needle. The test is read in about 10 minutes, and the sensitivity reaction is similar to that of the scratch test.

Patch tests may be used for suspected allergy to specific substances for which commercial allergens are not available. The allergen is applied to the skin, covered, and secured with adhesive tape. The patch is removed in 24 to 48 hours and the skin examined. If erythema or a wheal occurs, it indicates sensitivity to the allergen.

Mucous membrane sensitivity tests. Tests may also be made by placing the allergen into the conjunctival sac of the eye. Nothing is placed in the opposite eye, which serves as a control. If the test is positive, itching of the conjunctiva and increased lacrimation will occur. The eyes are then flushed with physiologic saline solution to remove the allergen, and 1 or 2 drops of a 1:1000 aqueous solution of epinephrine is placed in the conjunctival sac. The nasal cavity may also be used for testing, and the allergen is sprayed or sniffed into one nostril. The opposite nostril serves as a control. A positive reaction will cause sneezing, nasal congestion, and a thin watery discharge.

Elimination diets. When food is believed to be the cause of allergy, the patient may be given an elimination diet to determine the specific food causing the trouble. Either of two methods may be used. The patient may be asked to keep a record of all food eaten for a given period. Then one food such as milk, chocolate, or wheat products is eliminated from the diet. By gradually eliminating specific foods from the diet the food causing the allergy may be identified. The other method is to give the patient a diet consisting of foods that usually do not cause allergy. The diet is followed for a week, and if allergic symptoms continue, changes are made in the diet. If symptoms continue, it is generally considered that food is not the cause of the allergic reaction. However, if symptoms disappear, other foods are added to the diet until the patient develops allergic symptoms. That food is then considered to be the probable cause, and it is eliminated from the patient's diet.

DESENSITIZATION

Desensitization, or hyposensitization as it is sometimes called, is a form of immunization, the purpose of which is to neutra-lize the antibodies so that they will not react with the antigen. Small amounts of the extract of the antigen are administered at varying intervals for an extended period of time. The amount of the extract is gradually increased with each injection, until the largest dose that causes no reaction is given. This is considered to be the maintenance dose. Desensitization has been most effective in hay fever. Persons who are sensitive to seasonal allergy are advised to begin injections early before allergic symptoms appear.

DRUG THERAPY

Drugs commonly used in allergy are antihistamines: epinephrine, ephedrine, and corticosteroids. Histamine occurs normally in the body. As the result of the antigen-antibody reaction, histamine is released from the cells. Drug therapy is designed to counteract the effects of the histamine and prevent it from reaching its target site. Antihistamines are not effective for the symptoms caused by the histamine, or are they effective for all allergic disorders. They are most useful in allergic conditions affecting the nasal mucosa, such as hay fever, rhinitis, itching, and acute urticaria. The action of antihistamines is short, and they do not provide long-time relief. Although this chapter's chief concern is allergy, it may be pointed out that antihistamines are used for motion sickness, nausea and vomiting, vertigo, and sleeplessness.[1] The major side effect from these drugs is drowsiness. Persons who are taking any of this group of drugs are advised not to drive motorized vehicles. Other side effects include dizziness, dryness of mucous membranes, and weakness.[3] There are many antihistaminic preparations on the market. They may be administered orally, and some are available for parenteral injection or administration rectally. The most commonly used antihistamines include the following:

Chlorpheniramine (Chlor-Trimeton, Teldrin)
Diphenhydramine (Benadryl)
Promethazine (Phenergan, Fargan)
Tripelennamine (Pyribenzamine)
Chlorcyclizine (Di-Paralene, Perazil)
Dimenhydrinate (Dramamine); used in motion sickness
Trimethobenzamide (Tigan); used for relief of nausea and vomiting

Epinephrine (Adrenalin) has several uses. In allergy it is used for serious hypersensitivity such as anaphylactic shock. A 1:1000 aqueous solution is used for parenteral injection.

Ephedrine (racephedrine, I-sedrin) is a nasal decongestant, the action of which is similar to that of epinephrine but less potent. Its antiallergic effect causes shrinking of congested nasal mucous membranes; however, it also has several other uses in the body. The drug is available in tablet form for oral administration. Ephedrine is a constituent of most nasal sprays and drops and is widely used for relief of hay fever, colds, rhinitis, and sinusitis.[3]

Corticosteroids are not generally used in allergic disorders because of the serious side effects (p. 35). However, steroid preparations are marketed as ointments, creams, and lotions for topical application. They are used in allergic dermatosis and applied two or three times a day. Corticosteroids may be given to a patient with life-threatening asthma, but usually only after other forms of medication have failed. Corticosteroids are also administered in some immediate allergic reactions, including anaphylactic shock or allergic reaction to penicillin and other severe drug reactions.

PREVENTION AND ADAPTATION

To prevent allergic reactions it is necessary to identify the specific allergen and then to make whatever adaptation may be necessary. Sensitivity testing followed by desensitization may prevent reaction from some allergens. The most successful effort has been with hay fever. An individual may be hypersensitive to any number of substances within his environment. Identification of a specific antigenic substance may be impossible. When any antigenic substance can be identified and if there is no allergenic extract available for desensitization, the individual will need to avoid the substance involved. This may completely change a person's way of life. It may mean moving to another environment, a change in employment, or a change in the type of clothing worn. When animal dander is a factor, it may be necessary to dispose of household pets or to avoid contact with farm animals. Picnicking or hiking into the woods may have to be eliminated. Installing air-conditioning, damp mopping and dusting, and keeping windows closed may help to prevent some allergic attacks when caused by household dust or other allergens in the air. Rainy, damp, humid weather is often associated with asthma. The use of a humidifier to remove moisture from the air may be beneficial in preventing attacks of asthma. Individuals with allergy are advised to avoid exposure to infections. A common cold may be the trigger to precipitate an allergic reaction. Thus it may be seen from these examples that it may be necessary for the individual to make many adaptations to his environment and personal way of life. It should also be remembered that the adaptations made by the person with allergy may also affect members of the patient's family.

NURSING THE PATIENT WITH ALLERGIC CONDITIONS AND DISEASES

Many persons with allergic disorders are cared for in the physician's office or in an allergy clinic. Patients with severe reactions may require hospitalization. The nurse should understand the nature of the allergic reaction and appreciate the discomfort experienced by the patient. The nurse may be able to help the patient in identifying possible allergens and be able to make suggestions for avoiding the allergenic substances. The nurse may explain to the patient how infections, stress, and emotional problems contribute to allergic reactions. Sympathetic understanding and emotional support will help the patient.

Hay fever (pollinosis) and allergic and vasomotor rhinitis

Hay fever is the most common form of allergy and may affect children as well as adults. The condition may be seasonal, caused by a single pollen, such as ragweed or goldenrod, or it may be caused by several different pollens. However, many other inhalants cause hay fever. Allergic rhinitis may occur in persons with other types of allergy and may be seasonal, such as hay fever. The symptoms of vasomotor rhinitis are similar to those of allergic rhinitis; however, it is not seasonal and is not caused by allergens. Vasomotor rhinitis is a chronic disorder caused by irritants that affect the nasal mucosa. It may occur with prolonged use of nasal sprays or drops that contain phenylephrine (Neo-Synephrine) or ephedrine. Psychosomatic factors may also be involved. The disorder causes congestion of the nasal mucosa and an increase in nasal secretions that may show an increase in the number of eosinophils.[1]

Urticaria (hives and nettle rash)

Urticaria occurs in almost everyone who has any allergic reactions. Urticaria is an eruption of small papular wheals that are slightly red and associated with severe itching. They vary in size and pattern, with each wheal gradually disappearing and being replaced by others. The cause may be food, drugs, insect bites, serum reaction, or any other factor known to cause allergy. Urticaria may be treated by the subcutaneous injection of 1:1000 aqueous solution of epinephrine hydrochloride (Adrenalin hydrochloride) or by the oral administration of one of the antihistamines. Emollient baths consisting of starch or bran, which may be soothing and relieve itching, may be given several times a day for periods of 30 to 45 minutes. Ephedrine sulfate, 50 mg., may be ordered two or three times a day, and a sedative may be given for sleep and rest at night. In all cases the cause of urticaria should be determined if possible.

Eczema

Allergic eczema may be caused by the genetic predisposition to allergy. It may begin in infancy as infantile eczema and continue during the preschool years. Eczema may occur in the adult because of the inherited tendency for allergy. The adult who has eczema may also have had experiences with other types of delayed sensitivity reactions. The precipitating factors may be hypersensitivity to the proteins of cow's milk, egg white, certain fruits, or certain cereals.

The disease generally improves during the summer months and becomes worse in the winter. The lesions of eczema occur about the flexor surfaces of the knees, wrists, and elbows, and if the condition is severe, lesions may extend to the face and extremities. Eczema is characterized by redness and a dry, scaly, cracking type of lesion that may become raw and weeping. Moisture from the lesions becomes dry, and crusts may form. The eczematous lesions burn and itch, and the infant or young child will scratch most of the time unless restrained. It is important that an infant with eczema be protected from all forms of streptococcal and staphylococcal infections and not be vaccinated for smallpox while eczema is present.

Feeding the infant and young child who has eczema includes the use of various formula and elimination diets. Mild soap should be used in washing diapers, clothing, and sheets. Disposable diapers may be used. The infant may be bathed with special preparations such as a paste of powdered oatmeal; if the condition is mild, a superfatted soap may be used. Environmental stress conditions should be eliminated with as much tender loving care as is possible given to the infant. Eczema in the older child or the adult is treated much the same as in the infant.

Much of the treatment of both child and adult is concerned with providing relief from the itching and burning. Various types of lotions and ointments are used, and wet dressings may be ordered for some patients.

Drug allergy

An individual may be hypersensitive to a drug; however, most drug reactions may be attributed to the undesirable or unexpected side effects of the drug. Whenever a drug acts as an antigen and reacts with the antibodies in the body that have been produced as the result of a previous exposure to the drug, allergic symptoms such as urticaria, shock, or asthma may appear. Some drugs act in such a way that they release histamine from the body cells, and symptoms may occur that are similar to allergic reactions. True allergic reactions to drugs are usually progressive. A small dose may give rise to a mild reaction, but if administration of the drug continues, the reaction becomes increasingly severe, and shock and death may occur.[11] Reactions to drugs may affect every tissue, organ, or system of the body. Allergic reactions are most likely to occur when the drug is given in large doses or when it is administered over a long period of time. Drugs administered by the parenteral route are more likely to cause allergic manifestations than they are when given orally.

Bronchial asthma

When bronchial asthma is caused by an antigen-antibody reaction, it is referred to as extrinsic asthma or atopic disease. The genetic transmission of a predisposition is important in asthma caused by antigenic substances. (See Chapter 11 for more detailed information.)

Serum sickness and anaphylactic shock

Serum sickness and anaphylactic shock are examples of immediate reaction in which precipitin antibodies in the plasma and an antigenic protein cause an allergic reaction. Serum sickness is usually transient and without serious effects. However, anaphylactic shock causes a shocklike condition that may result in death. (See p. 40 for additional information.)

Allergic reactions from insects

The bites or stings of various insects may cause local or systemic reactions. The local reaction that occurs at the site of the bite or sting is not considered to be an allergic reaction. However, when systemic reactions occur, the symptoms are consistent with allergy. Stings caused by bees, wasps, hornets, and yellow jackets may produce systemic reactions that vary from mild urticaria and itching to respiratory embarrassment, shock, loss of consciousness, and death. The antigen-antibody reaction may be to all insects or only one specific insect. The same process of antibody formation occurs as with other antigens. The first sting may cause no trouble, but if the individual should be stung again, a reaction may occur. Reactions may be immediate or delayed, and the speed with which the reaction develops is in direct proportion to its severity. If a large number of stings occur at the same time, the reaction may be immediate and can be fatal because of the large amount of toxin injected. When the stinger is left in the skin, it should be scraped off and squeezing avoided. Persons who may be at risk from stings are advised to carry an emergency kit that contains the essential items for emergency care until medical care can be secured.

The immediate treatment includes the application of ice, rest, and elevation of the part to reduce edema. Antipruritic lotions such as calamine lotion or an antihistaminic drug may relieve the itching. Isoproterenol hydrochloride (Isuprel), 15 ml., or ephedrine may be administered. If a systemic reaction occurs, a 1:1000 solution of epinephrine is given subcutaneously. Adults may be given 0.3 to 0.5 ml., and children are given 0.2 to 0.3 ml. If bronchospasm occurs, aminophylline may be given intravenously, and oxygen may be required. When a systemic reaction occurs, the patient must be carefully observed because epinephrine is short acting, and symptoms may recur requiring additional treatment.[5]

Other types of insects such as flies, mosquitoes, fleas, chiggers, bedbugs, and grain itch mites may cause an allergic response in some hypersensitive persons. The severity of the reactions will vary with the individual. Urticarial wheals will usually develop soon after the bite, but reaction may be delayed for several hours. The immediate treatment is to administer epinephrine as previously discussed and to apply a lotion to relieve the itching and pain.

Summary outline

1. Allergy first established in 1832
   A. Robert Koch observed and described first allergic reaction
   B. The term *allergy* first used in 1906
   C. Accomplishments during 1900s
      1. Diagnostic skin tests
      2. Passive immunity from mother to fetus
      3. Production of extracts of antigenic substances
      4. Desensitization procedure
      5. Use of antihistamines
      6. Use of corticosteroids
      7. Allergic factors in hay fever, urticaria, and asthma identified
2. Cause of allergy
   A. Heredity—genetic transmission of predisposition to allergy occurs in some families
   B. Congenital—transmission of allergen from mother to fetus in utero
   C. Contact—must have direct contact with allergen
      1. Inhalants
      2. Ingestants
      3. Injectants
      4. Contactants
      5. Bacteria
3. Atopic allergy—atopic disease
   A. Inherited predisposition is important
   B. Atopic diseases
      1. Hay fever

2. Urticaria
3. Asthma
4. Angioneurotic edema
5. Atopic dermatitis
6. Gastrointestinal disturbance
7. Drug reactions
4. Types of allergic reactions
   A. Immediate—precipitin antibodies circulating in plasma
   B. Delayed—sensitized antibodies are attached to cells
      1. Reactions may be local or systemic
      2. Reactions may be delayed for hours or days
5. Autoimmune sensitivity
   The body produces antigenic substances that stimulate antibody formation that will react against its own body
   A. Autoimmune disease affects eye, skin, joints, thyroid gland, kidneys, brain, and vascular system
   B. Prognosis uncertain; control is possible
6. Pathophysiology
   A. Pathologic response to antigen-antibody reaction
      1. Release of histamine and histamine-like substances
      2. Vasodilation of peripheral blood vessels
      3. Histamine affects smooth muscles of bronchioles
      4. Fluid moves from plasma into interstitial spaces
      5. Edema of tissues
      6. Increase of mucus from mucus-secreting glands
   B. Physiologic manifestations
      1. Inhalants
         a. Congestion of nasal mucosa
         b. Sneezing
         c. Thin, watery, nasal discharge
         d. Red, itching conjunctivae
         e. Increased lacrimation
      2. Digestants
         a. Nausea and vomiting
         b. Diarrhea
      3. Contactants
         a. Urticaria
         b. Dermatitis
      4. Drugs
         a. Urticaria
         b. Fever
         c. Skin rash
7. Diagnostic tests and procedures
   A. Complete personal and family history
   B. Physical examination
   C. Skin tests
      1. Scratch tests
      2. Intracutaneous test
      3. Patch test
   D. Mucous membrane sensitivity tests
   E. Elimination diets
8. Desensitization
   A form of immunization
   A. Extracts of antigenic substances are injected over extended period of time
   B. Most successful in hay fever
9. Drug therapy

Purpose is to counteract effects of histamine
   A. Antihistamines
   B. Epinephrine
   C. Ephedrine
   D. Corticosteroids
10. Prevention and adaptation
    A. Identification of allergen necessary
    B. Desensitization
    C. Avoidance of antigenic substances involved
    D. Persons may need to change their way of life
11. Nursing the patient with allergic conditions and diseases
    Nurse should appreciate discomfort experienced by patient
    A. Hay fever (pollinosis) and allergic and vasomotor rhinitis
       1. Hay fever most common
       2. Usually seasonal
       3. Caused by one or several pollens
    B. Allergic rhinitis
       1. May be seasonal
       2. Person may have other types of allergy
    C. Vasomotor rhinitis
       1. Not caused by allergens
       2. Caused by irritants that affect nasal mucosa
    D. Urticaria (hives and nettle rash)—eruption of small papular wheals that are red and itchy
       1. Treatment is with epinephrine, emollient baths, ephedrine, and antihistaminic drugs
    E. Eczema—may begin in infancy and continue into preschool years
       1. Adult with eczema may have other types of delayed hypersensitivity
       2. Causes may be hypersensitivity to proteins of cow's milk, egg white, certain fruits, and certain cereals
       3. Disease is characterized by dry, scaly, cracking lesions that may become red and weeping with crust formation
    F. Drug allergy—reactions usually are undesirable side effects
       1. True drug allergy usually progressive
    G. Bronchial asthma—extrinsic or atopic disease
    H. Serum sickness and anaphylactic shock
       1. Precipitin antibodies in plasma and antigenic protein cause severe allergic reaction
    I. Allergic reactions from insects—local reaction is not allergic
       1. Allergic reactions are systemic
       2. Bites of bees, wasps, hornets, and yellow jackets may produce systemic reactions resulting in urticaria, itching, respiratory difficulty, shock, and death
          a. Persons at risk should carry emergency kit
          b. Immediate treatment—application of ice, rest, antipruritic lotion, isoproterenol hydrochloride (Isuprel), or ephedrine
          c. Systemic reaction—1:1000 solution of epinephrine given subcutaneously, aminophylline, and oxygen

538   Total patient care

3. Flies, mosquitoes, fleas, ticks, chiggers, bedbugs, or grain itch mites may cause allergic reaction
   a. Treatment is with epinephrine and skin antipruritics

Review questions

1. In general, what are the three classifications of allergic disorders?
   a. *contact*
   b. *congenital*
   c. *heredity*
2. What factor is important in atopic allergy?
   a. *inherited predisposition*
3. What are the two types of allergic reaction?
   a. *immediate*
   b. *delayed*
4. What two allergic disorders may occur in an immediate reaction?
   a. *serum sickness*
   b. *anaphylactic shock*
5. What groups of drugs are widely used in the treatment of allergic disorders?
   a. *antihistamines*
6. What substance is released from the cells when there is an antigen-antibody reaction?
   a. *histamine*
7. List four procedures used to diagnose allergic disorders.
   a. *skin test*
   b. *elimination diet*
   c. *physical exam*
   d. *test mucous membrane sensitivity*
8. List several symptoms characterized of seasonal pollinosis.
   a. *sneezing*
   b. *lacrimation*
   c.
   d.
9. List three pathologic conditions that result from an antigen-antibody reaction.
   a. *urticaria*
   b. *shock*
   c. *asthma*

Films

1. Rejection of renal transplant—T-1746 (18 min., sound, black and white, 16 mm.), Media Resources Branch, National Medical Audiovisual Center (Annex), Station K, Atlanta, Ga. 30324. Discusses acute or hyperacute, intermediate, and chronic rejection of renal homografts.
2. The specificity of antigen-antibody reactions—T-1509 (33 min., sound, black and white, 16 mm.), Media Resources Branch, National Medical Audiovisual Center (Annex), Station K, Atlanta, Ga. 30324. Presents the basic principles of immunology and immunologic specificity.

References

1. Beeson, Paul B., and McDermott, Walsh: Cecil-Loeb textbook of medicine, ed. 13, Philadelphia, 1973, W. B. Saunders Co.
2. Beland, Irene L.: Clinical nursing pathophysiological and psychosocial approaches, ed. 2, New York, 1970, The Macmillan Co.
3. Bergersen, Betty S.: Pharmacology in nursing, ed. 13, St. Louis, 1976, The C. V. Mosby Co.
4. Burdon, Kenneth L., and Williams, Robert P.: Microbiology, ed. 6, New York, 1968, The Macmillan Co.
5. Conn, Howard F., editor: Current therapy 76, Philadelphia, 1976, W. B. Saunders Co.
6. Kintzel, Kay C., editor: Advanced concepts in clinical nursing, Philadelphia, 1971, J. B. Lippincott Co.
7. Luckman, Joan, and Sorensen, Karen C.: Medical-surgical nursing, Philadelphia, 1974, W. B. Saunders Co.
8. Samter, Max, editor: Immunological diseases, Boston, 1965, Little, Brown & Co.
9. Smith, Alice L.: Microbiology and pathology, ed. 11, St. Louis, 1976, The C. V. Mosby Co.
10. Snively, W. D., Jr., and Beshear, Donna R.: Textbook of pathophysiology, Philadelphia, 1972, J. B. Lippincott Co.
11. Unger, Donald L.: Nonallergic drug reactions, American Journal of Nursing 63:64-65, Jan., 1963.

CHAPTER 23

Nursing the patient with infectious disease

KEY WORDS

coalesce
concurrent disinfection
desquamation
epidemiology
host
incubation period
infectious disease
isolation
Koplik's spots
opisthotonos

orchitis
Peyer's patches
quarantine
rose spots
strawberry tongue
syndrome
terminal disinfection
vector

[handwritten annotations:] sun together / continuous / inflammation of testes / typhoid fever in sm. intestine / isolation / typhoid spot / pink abdomen / scarlet fever / a group of symptoms / release of pt. / an insector animal carrying diseases infecting humans / time between exposure to + appearance of symptoms / able between exposure to transmitted / white spots in throat in measles / rigid arched spine / a scaling of the skin / study of epidemics

CAUSES OF INFECTIOUS DISEASE

In this brief study of infectious disease the nurse should review Chapters 1 through 4 to understand factors related to the destruction of pathogenic organisms and prevention of disease through immunization, immunity, and medical asepsis.

In studying infectious diseases the nurse should become familiar with certain factors concerning them.

1. Some diseases are transmitted from person to person such as measles or pertussis.

2. Some diseases are transmitted from animals to humans, such as rabies.

3. Some diseases are transmitted to humans through an intermediate vector, such as malaria, or they may be transmitted from a reservoir of infection through some vehicle such as water.

There are also different ways through which an infectious disease may be transmitted:

1. Direct contact. A disease may be transmitted from person to person by close association while one person is in an infectious state.

2. Indirect contact. The individual may contract a disease by coming in contact with contaminated objects such as contaminated dressings or bedding soiled with vomitus. Infection may be the result of hand-to-mouth transfer of the infectious material. Infection may be transferred by the nurse's hands when they are not washed after being contaminated.

3. Vectors transmit disease by inoculation. For example, the infected mosquito bites a well person, introducing the malaria parasite through a puncture wound.

[handwritten:] i.e. - incephalitis

539

4. There are numerous vehicles through which disease organisms may be transmitted, including water, milk, food, contaminated intravenous fluids, blood and blood products, and prepackaged supplies (p. 62).

5. Some microorganisms are suspended in the air as droplets or droplet nuclei, resulting from coughing, sneezing, talking, etc. It is also believed that some may remain in dust over a fairly long period of time.

There are various classifications of infectious disease according to causative agent, and as science reveals more about diseases and their causes, changes in classification may occur. For practical purposes the causative agents will be classified here as (1) bacteria, (2) viruses, (3) rickettsiae, and (4) protozoa.

Infectious disease is caused by various kinds of pathogenic bacteria such as the streptococcus, staphylococcus, bacillus, and spirilla. Some infectious diseases are caused by viruses about which little has been known until recently. Also, infectious disease may be caused by rickettsiae, which are neither bacteria nor viruses but are believed to hold an intermediate position between bacteria and viruses. The transmission of disease caused by rickettsiae is through a vector such as an insect. In addition, other diseases are caused by single-celled animal parasites called *protozoa*. Some are caused by other animal parasites called *metazoa*, which will not be included in this chapter (Chapter 1).

PREVENTION OF INFECTIOUS DISEASE

The control of infectious disease has been one of the accomplishments of the twentieth century. It has been brought about through the cooperation of many agencies such as the United States Public Health Service, state and local health departments, and voluntary organizations. Scientists have played a major role in the development of serums and vaccines for both prophylactic and therapeutic treatment of disease. Improved sanitation in the disposal of excreta, improved water and milk supplies, better methods of handling food, and public enlightenment and education have been significant factors in the control of infectious disease. In all these activities nurses have played an active and important role. As the result of these combined efforts and eternal vigilance, many diseases have been almost eliminated and others controlled. However, infectious disease prevention and control is a continuing program. There always remains a large reservoir of susceptible persons, and no community can ever be made completely safe.

As nurses assume increasing responsibility for patient care, there should be an understanding of the ways in which infectious diseases are contracted, spread, and ways in which the causative organism can be destroyed. When the nurse is responsible for supervision of persons with lesser understanding of infectious diseases, the nurse must be able to interpret to them why precautions are necessary and how measures to prevent their spread are maintained. The nurse also has a responsibility to the family and the community by promoting an active program of immunization in the community.

DIAGNOSTIC TESTS AND PROCEDURES

The diagnosis of infectious disease can generally be made by the history and clinical manifestations or characteristics of the symptoms. A history of exposure and knowledge of the duration of the incubation period often provide significant information.

Laboratory examinations may include leukocyte count, agglutination or complement-fixation tests, dark-field examination of suspected syphilitic lesions, sedimentation rate, smears, and cultures. Stool examinations are done in diagnosing many diseases, and in some diseases inoculation of animals may be necessary to confirm a diagnosis. Special kinds of skin tests are done for tuberculosis and histoplasmosis and infrequently may be done to determine immunity to certain specific infectious diseases such as diphtheria and rubella.

NURSING RESPONSIBILITIES

Medical asepsis. Principle: Contain within a given area and destroy all pathogenic organisms to prevent their spread.

The nursing care of the patient with infectious disease involves the basic principles of medical asepsis, as well as the physiologic and psychologic care of the patient. The principles of medical asepsis are the same whether the patient is in a special infectious disease hospital, in a clinical unit of a general hospital, or in the home. There are no uniform procedures, and many details of medical asepsis will vary with the hospital and the specific disease. Many adaptations will have to be made when caring for a patient in the home, but the basic principles are the same. The duration of isolation will vary with the disease, the hospital, and the state laws and regulations.

Many changes have taken place in the care of patients with infectious diseases. The trend is away from special infectious disease hospitals and toward admitting patients to general hospitals. Some general hospitals may have a clinical unit for infectious diseases, but most hospitals will place the patient in a ward, cubicle, or private room on a medical service. Nurses assigned to care for patients with infectious disease should know how the disease is spread, how to protect themselves, and how to protect other patients. Nurses must understand which areas are clean and which are contaminated. In general, the area surrounding the patient and the inside of sinks and hoppers are considered contaminated. All other areas are clean. Nurses must know how to handle all contaminated equipment and materials to avoid contaminating a clean area and to prevent spreading the infection.

Nurses must be familiar with the policy of the hospital concerning the use of gowns, caps, and masks. There is no sound argument that a gown protects against the transfer of microorganisms, and it may provide a false sense of security. However, if the policy of the hospital requires the use of a gown, nurses should be familiar with the procedure of caring for it. Opinions differ concerning the use of long-sleeved or short-sleeved gowns, but it is agreed that any gown worn must provide for a wide lap in the back (Fig. 23-1). The use of caps and masks will depend on the particular institution and the disease. A properly constructed and properly worn mask

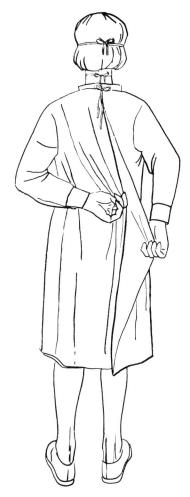

Fig. 23-1. The gown worn by the nurse caring for patients in isolation must lap at least 12 inches in the back.

may provide partial protection to the wearer but should never be considered absolute protection. Nurses should consult a textbook on basic nursing for gowning procedure.

Careful washing of the hands is one of the most important aspects of infectious disease control, whether in the hospital or in the home (Fig. 23-2). The hands must be washed after every contact with the patient or with any contaminated object (Chapters 3 and 4).

In communities that have public sewerage systems it is generally permissible to place bowel and bladder discharges into the system. When such facilities are not available, all waste from bowels or bladder,

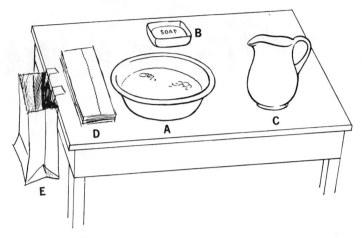

Fig. 23-2. Method of washing hands in the home. **A,** Ordinary washbasin. **B,** Bar of soap in soap dish. **C,** Pitcher of water. **D,** Paper towels. **E,** Paper bag for used towels. Water is poured from the pitcher over the hands, which are thoroughly lathered with soap. Rinsing is accomplished by pouring water over the hands. The hands should not be immersed in the washbasin of water.

vomitus, or liquids from food must be placed in a covered container and disinfected. Various disinfecting agents are used such as full-strength Wescodyne, a 5% chlorinated lime solution, or a 5% solution of creosol.

Discharges from the nose and throat and any disposable supplies such as tissues and paper cups, plates, straws, or dishes should be placed in a paper bag and burned.

In the hospital, linens are placed in a bag and autoclaved. When hospital laundries use boiling water and a detergent, contaminated linen may be washed with other hospital laundry except in the case of spores, for which autoclaving prior to washing is necessary. Nondisposable equipment—such as sphygmomanometers, thermometers, plastic, or other delicate equipment should be wiped with a germicidal agent. In the home, linens should be placed in a large covered wash boiler and boiled. Dishes should be boiled and paper supplies burned.

Any environmental area used for patients with infectious disease must be screened and protected from flies or other vermin that may carry the disease.

The daily handling and disposal of contaminated material or equipment is called *concurrent disinfection*. After the patient's recovery, death, or release from isolation the room must be thoroughly cleaned. The mattress and pillows should be exposed to the sunlight or sterilized, and all bedding, including blankets, should be washed. The room should be thoroughly aired for at least 8 hours. This procedure is called *terminal disinfection*. The terminal cleaning of a room or contaminated area requires only the usual cleaning given by good housekeeping practices. Emphasis is placed on regular and thorough concurrent disinfection.

Quarantine is a procedure imposed by the health department in controlling certain infectious diseases. It requires all persons to remain on the premises and prohibits anyone from entering the home. The quarantine may be lifted only by the health department. The present-day control of infectious disease places greater emphasis on good isolation procedures and less on rigid measures such as quarantine.

Isolation. Isolation is a procedure of segregating a person sick with an infectious disease from well persons to prevent spread of the disease. It also means that all infectious material and equipment must be confined to a specific area and cared for according to the basic principles of medical asepsis.

Beginning in 1965, the Center for Disease Control has been engaged in a program of surveillance and control of hospital infections. The data appear to indicate that different infections, that is, infectious diseases and nosocomial infections, need different kinds of isolation procedures. The necessity for isolation may vary from strict isolation, as in staphylococcal pneumonia, to infections that require no isolation but only special care in handling of dressings.[5]

It is the responsibility of the physician to order isolation, and it should be in writing. It is also the duty of the physician to determine when isolation may be terminated. The duration of isolation is usually the period that the disease is infectious. For some diseases isolation is terminated only after laboratory examination has shown that the pathologic organism is no longer present. Some diseases require limited isolation when the patient is receiving a chemotherapeutic drug. In some diseases the patient's symptoms may subside and he appears well, but he may carry the infectious organism in his body for weeks or even months, as in typhoid fever.

The physician should prepare the patient for isolation, but often the patient and his family fail to understand the necessity for isolation. The nurse should know what the physician has told the patient and should be able to interpret and reemphasize it. It is best not to simply tell the patient that isolation is the hospital policy. Most patients will be more cooperative if they understand the real reasons why precautions are being taken.

Physiologic care. The physical care of the patient includes the same supportive care given to any sick patient. The use of chemotherapeutic drugs has greatly altered the course of some infectious diseases, whereas in others they are ineffective. During the acute stage of the disease bed rest is usually indicated, and measures to provide comfort for the patient should be employed. When there is a high temperature, measures to reduce it such as alcohol sponges, antipyretic drugs, and tepid sponge baths may be ordered by the physician. The use of throat irrigations or ice collars may provide relief from painful throat conditions. Intravenous infusions may be given to supply fluids during the acute stage, and blood transfusions may be necessary. Urinary output must be watched, since kidney complications may occur in patients with some diseases. Diet may be liquid or consist of foods tolerated by the patient, but the diet is generally kept fairly light.

Emergency conditions may arise in which a tracheotomy is necessary to save the patient's life. Regular checking of vital signs with particular attention to the pulse, which may indicate heart complications, is important especially for patients with diphtheria.

Since many of the infectious diseases affect children under 10 years of age, the problem of keeping a child in bed and amused is always present. The nurse in the hospital or the parent in the home must be prepared to spend considerable time with the child. Reading, games, scrapbooks, color books, a magazine, scissors, and a jar of paste may provide interesting amusement for the child.

Psychologic care. Within this century patients with infectious disease were cared for in the "pest house" located at the outskirts of the city, often surrounded by a high fence to keep the patients in. There was no need to worry about visitors, for no one ever went near. In fact, not long ago a quarantine sign on a house meant that people passed on the opposite side of the street. Although the care of patients with infectious disease has made tremendous progress, the isolation unit is too often surrounded by a high fence, and the isolation sign is equivalent to a quarantine sign.

Many patients know little about infectious disease and do not understand the precautions taken, which may seem unnecessary to them. It may mean an extra gown or an extra handwashing if the isolated patient is to receive psychologic support and care. Nurses caring for the patient can plan patient care to make more frequent trips to the room. When nurses understand how the disease is spread and the period of communicability, many adjustments can be made in caring for the patient. In many situations nurses may enter the unit without contaminating themselves, such as in handing the patient a glass of juice, serving a tray, and offering a few cheerful words. An understanding of the purpose of isolation and a few minutes spent with the patient several times a day may be more valuable than technical competence in carrying out a rigid procedure.

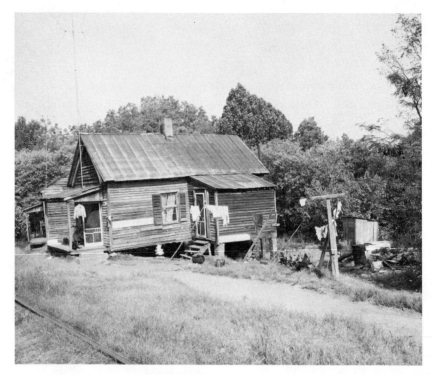

Fig. 23-3. Social problems contribute to the spread of infectious diseases.

Fear, anxiety, and apprehension are emotional components of many infectious diseases. When hospitalization is prolonged or convalescence long, economic factors create worry and tension. Some diseases may affect the self-image of the person, or he may believe that his social status is being threatened. Emotional behavior often occurs during community epidemics such as meningitis or encephalitis; the slightest indisposition of apparently well persons may cause apprehension and fear. Nurses caring for patients with infectious disease may find them irritable, depressed, and critical. The nurse should understand and realize that this behavior reflects the patient's feelings of frustration and anxiety.

Sociologic factors. Sociologic factors may have a profound effect on the incidence of certain infectious diseases. In low economic areas where there is inadequate housing, sanitary facilities, and refuse collection, a potential reservoir of infection may exist (Fig. 23-3). Infectious skin diseases, tuberculosis, and venereal disease are frequently components of the social milieu. Poor nutritional standards decrease resistance to disease and provide the opportunity for pathogens to invade the human organism. The social picture is often one of apathy and lack of motivation, coupled with lack of transportation and availability of medical and clinical services. This contributes to the failure to secure immunization of young children and provides for the potential epidemic of infectious disease. The high mobility of the population means that a person exposed to an infectious disease or who is a possible source of disease may be miles from the point of contact in a few hours.

Contraindications for immunization. Most children and adults have no adverse reactions to vaccines or serums administered as protection against infectious diseases. There are a few persons in whom they must be administered with caution or in whom they are contraindicated.

1. Hypersensitivity to egg protein
2. Altered immune states
   a. Lymphoma
   b. Leukemia
   c. Generalized malignancy
   d. Dysgammaglobulinemia

3. Immunosuppressive drugs
   a. Steroids
   b. Antimetabolites
   c. Alkylating drugs
   d. Radiation
4. Skin disorders
   a. Eczema
   b. Chronic dermatitis
5. Pregnancy in some instances
6. Febrile illness—delay administration of vaccine until recovery

NURSING THE PATIENT WITH INFECTIOUS DISEASE
Bacterial diseases
Scarlet fever

Scarlet fever is an acute infectious disease caused by a strain of the hemolytic streptococcus bacterium. It occurs most frequently during the winter months in children under 10 years of age. The disease is spread through secretions from the nose and throat and from suppurative complications. The incubation period is from 2 to 5 days and rarely as long as a week.

The onset of the disease is abrupt, with chills, vomiting, headache, and elevated temperature ranging from 102° F. to as much as 106° F., rapid pulse, and an extremely sore throat. In approximately 24 hours an erythematous rash may be observed behind the ears and on the sides of the neck. The rash gradually spreads over the entire body except the face. The tongue has a furred appearance that gradually disappears, and it takes on the characteristic red appearance known as *strawberry tongue*. The cervical lymph nodes become enlarged, and there is leukocytosis.

In approximately 7 days the rash begins to fade, and desquamation of the body begins. A fine scaling occurs on the body, with large flakes of skin desquamating from the palms and soles of the feet. Desquamation may continue for 2 weeks or longer.

Treatment and nursing care. The speed with which the acute symptoms are relieved depends on early treatment. When penicillin is administered, the early relief of symptoms and disappearance of the streptococcus bacterium may be expected within 48 hours. Palliative care for relief of symptoms may include warm throat irrigations or the application of an ice collar to the throat. Tepid sponge baths or alcohol sponges may

be given to reduce the elevated temperature. Little soap should be used, and after desquamation begins warm oil rubs may be given.

The patient should be observed carefully for complications, which may appear throughout the course of the disease. Otitis media, abscess of the cervical lymph nodes, and kidney and heart complications are the most frequent. A rheumatic complication similar to rheumatic fever with heart involvement often occurs.

The disease is most infectious during the early stages, and it is not transmitted from the desquamating skin. The Dick test is used to determine immunity; however, active immunization against the disease is not generally recommended because of the severe reaction from the immunizing agent. Some physicians recommend a prophylactic dose of penicillin for those who have been in close contact with the patient. Scarlet fever is not quarantined, and isolation is generally unnecessary after 7 days.

Diphtheria

Diphtheria is an acute infectious disease caused by the diphtheria bacillus. The disease rarely affects children under 1 year of age but usually occurs in children under 10 years of age. However, susceptible adults may contract the disease. The disease is transmitted through the nose and throat secretions of an infected person or by a diphtheria carrier. The incubation period is 1 to 5 days after exposure.

The disease involves the mucous membranes of the nose, throat, larynx, or trachea, and in patients with severe cases secondary involvement of the nervous system and the heart may occur. Four forms of the disease are recognized: tonsillar diphtheria, nasal diphtheria, nasopharyngeal diphtheria, and laryngeal diphtheria.

The onset of the disease is insidious, with a slight sore throat and low-grade fever. Temperature gradually increases to 102° or 103° F., and a characteristic grayish white or yellow membrane that firmly adheres to the tonsils and pharynx develops. Any effort to remove the membrane leaves a red, raw surface beneath. Enlargement of the cervical lymph nodes may occur. In nasal diphtheria there is a thin watery discharge from both nostrils. In the nasopharyngeal form the membrane spreads into the nasopharynx and may extend into the nasal mucosa, sometimes appearing at the external nares. Children with nasopharyngeal diphtheria are often seriously ill, and the danger of complications is greater than it is with other forms.

Laryngeal diphtheria, sometimes called *membranous croup,* is the most dangerous form of the disease. The membrane extends downward, resulting in hoarseness and dyspnea, and may seriously affect the airway. Because of the edema, there may be a cough, the respirations may become noisy and labored, the pulse is rapid, and cyanosis develops. An emergency tracheotomy must be done or death will occur.

Treatment and nursing care. The treatment for diphtheria is administration of a sufficient amount of antitoxin. The patient should be tested for sensitivity to horse serum prior to administration of the antitoxin.

The nursing care of the patient is extremely important, and every effort must be made to keep him quiet and to avoid exertion on his part. A strict isolation procedure must be carried out. The patient is on a regimen of complete bed rest and is not permitted to participate in any part of his care, not even to feed himself, for 2 weeks. Warm saline solution throat irrigations may be given, and an ice collar may be applied to the throat for relief of discomfort. During mouth hygiene, care must be taken to prevent gagging. The temperature is taken every 4 hours, and during the acute stage the blood pressure and pulse and respiration rates are taken at intervals of 15 to 30 minutes. There usually is some increased elevation of temperature after the administration of the antitoxin. If the edema in the throat is severe, a liquid diet or a diet of suitable consistency should be offered. Tube feeding may sometimes be necessary, or parenteral fluids may be given if there is vomiting. When an emergency tracheotomy is necessary, suction equipment and oxygen must be available at the bedside. The patient is not released from isolation until the results of two or more throat and nose cultures taken at intervals of 48 hours are negative for the causative organism.

Complications. Myocarditis is a serious complication of diphtheria that may occur between 1 and 2 weeks after the onset of the disease. The nurse caring for the patient should be alert for any change in the pulse rate, epigastric pain, or vomiting and report such signs immediately. The nervous system may be affected, causing paralysis of the palate and muscles of the eyes and extremities. The paralysis may affect the entire body so that respirator care will be needed.

A 2-year-old child with diphtheria had been ill for more than a week and appeared to be recovering. The child asked the mother for milk, and as the mother placed her arm under the child's head and lifted it for her to drink the milk, the child suddenly died from a heart complication. A 20-year-old cousin of the child who also contracted diphtheria suffered a nervous system complication with paralysis of the eye muscles.

Prophylaxis. The conquest of diphtheria in the United States has been dramatic because of immunization procedures; however, the disease still exists. During the first 28 weeks of 1975, 204 cases were reported by the Center for Disease Control, whereas for a similar period of 1974, 148 cases were reported.[17] The immunization procedure recommended by the Public Health Service Advisory Committee on Immunization Practices is as follows. Three injections of diphtheria and tetanus toxoid and pertussis vaccine (DTP) should be given at intervals of 4 to 6 weeks. The first injection should be given at 2 or 3 months of age. A reinforcing dose should be given a year after the last injection. When the child enters school, he should be given a booster injection of DTP. School-age children and adults should be given only tetanus and diphtheria toxoid (Td), and an injection is recommended at 10-year intervals.[11] Injections for children under 3 years of age should be given in the gluteal muscle, and may be given in the deltoid muscle for children over 3 years of age. The nurse can contribute to an active program of diphtheria immunization by inquiring of parents whether a child has been protected. The nurse should be familiar with the facilities in the community and be able to refer parents to a physician or clinic.

Whooping cough (pertussis)

Pertussis is an acute infectious disease caused by the *Bordetella pertussis* that occurs in very young children, although it may occur in older children and adults. Mortality rates in infants are often high, and death may be the result of complications such as bronchopneumonia, intestinal infections with diarrhea and dehydration, and convulsions. The incubation period is 7 to 21 days, the average being 10 days.

Pertussis affects the upper respiratory tract and the bronchi, and the germs are carried by minute droplets or droplet nuclei expelled by the patient during paroxysms of coughing. The disease with symptoms similar to those of an ordinary cold, with a slight cough occurring only at night. The disease is highly infectious during this early stage. The coughing gradually increases in frequency, duration, and intensity, and large amounts of mucus are expectorated. The coughing generally occurs in paroxysms accompanied by gagging and vomiting. Coughing attacks often follow a meal, and the food eaten is lost. Approximately 2 weeks from the onset the characteristic "whoop" develops, which is diagnostic. The whoop is heard on inspiration of air and results in a crowing sound. At this stage the paroxysms of coughing are so severe that cyanosis may occur, the face becomes extremely red, the veins of the neck stand out, and the child may strangle. Finally there is a gradual decrease in the paroxysms of coughing, which become less frequent, milder, and shorter in duration. The disease usually lasts for about 6 weeks, during which time the child should be isolated from other children.

Treatment and nursing care. There is no specific treatment for pertussis. Chemotherapeutic drugs are of value only in preventing complications. Several doses of hyperimmune pertussis gamma globulin may be given and may be helpful for some patients. Cough mixtures that depress the cough are not recommended. Depending on the severity of the disease, bed rest may be indicated. The room should be well ventilated but not cold; increased humidity thins secretions and makes expectorations easier. When weather is warm and sunny, the child may be outside but must not be allowed to become chilled. The child's nutrition must be watched carefully, since during the vomiting stage so much food may be lost that the child becomes malnourished. Small feedings of nourishing food should be given, and food may be retained if it is given after a paroxysm of coughing. All children with pertussis should be under medical supervision throughout the course of the disease. Most children with pertussis are cared for at home; however, infants or children with severe cases should be hospitalized. Pertussis antibodies do not cross the placenta in sufficient amounts to provide passive immunity for young infants, and the disease is often serious in infants under 1 year of age.

Prophylaxis. Active immunization is of no value once exposure has taken place. Active immunization is combined with diphtheria and tetanus toxoid, and the schedule is the same as that described for diphtheria (p. 546). Full protection does not develop until 1 month after the last immunizing dose. The immunization of premature infants should depend on their physical progress. Although the full recommended dose is necessary for protection, fractional doses may be given with more trips made to the physician. It may be necessary to keep the infant quiet the day after the treatment, to reduce the amount of food, and to avoid overheating. In spite of the availability of pertussis immunization, there were 3,402 cases of the disease reported in the United States in 1974. However, this does not represent the total number of cases that occurred because reporting is incomplete.[13]

Typhoid fever and paratyphoid fever

Typhoid fever is caused by the typhoid bacillus (*Salmonella typhosa*). The disease has often been referred to as the *disease of filth*, since its source is the feces and urine from infected persons, and it is spread by food or drink contaminated by the organism. Although the disease is prevalent throughout the world, it has become rare in the United States. During 1974 there were 437 cases of typhoid fever in the United States, most of which were caused by the ingestion of contaminated food.[13] About 2% to 5% of all persons with cases of typhoid fever will become carriers.[9]

The incubation period may be no more than 7 days, or it might be as long as 21 days; however, it usually is between 10 and 14 days. The onset is gradual, with headache, weakness, malaise, cough, and chilly sensations, and there may be nosebleed. There is loss of appetite, and constipation or diarrhea may occur. By the end of a week the temperature has risen to 103° to 105° F. by a gradual day-by-day increase. Abdominal distention with tenderness and enlargement of the spleen are present. Small rose-colored spots begin to appear in a croplike sequence on the abdomen (rose spots). In contrast to the high temperature, the pulse rate is slow, often under 90 beats per minute. Areas of lymphoid tissue on the mucous membrane of the small intestine become elevated and inflamed, causing what is called *Peyer's patches*. The lesions may become ulcerated and perforate. The temperature remains high until about the third week, when it begins to fall by lysis. The patient is usually dehydrated and may be incontinent, and delirium may occur.

Treatment and nursing care. The treatment of typhoid fever has been greatly facilitated by the use of chloramphenicol (Chloromycetin). After its administration the patient is clinically well in 4 or 5 days. However, the typhoid bacillus may remain in the intestinal tract and be excreted in the feces and urine for 50 days or longer, and unless the administration of the drug is continued over a long period of time, relapses may occur. In May, 1973, the Center for Disease Control reported fifty-two cases of typhoid fever originating from a source outside of the United States. The strain of *Salmonella typhosa* isolated was found to be resistant to chloramphenicol and several other antibiotics including ampicillin. A new drug presently under investigation is co-trimoxazole, which may be effective in typhoid fever that is resistant to chloramphenicol and ampicillin.[12] Intravenous fluids are administered to overcome the dehydration.

If the nurse cares for a patient with typhoid fever, it is well to remember the four Fs—fingers, feces, food, and flies. There may be differences of opinion concerning isolation procedure when the patient is receiving antimicrobial therapy; however, the four Fs may never be overlooked. Whether the patient is cared for in the hospital or home, the room must be well screened against flies. Whoever cares for the patient should not handle food or participate in its preparation. The hands must be thoroughly washed after giving any care to the patient, and special care must be given to areas under and around the nails. When the patient is receiving antimicrobial drugs, feces may be placed in a public sewerage system. When such systems are not available, bowel and bladder discharges must be disinfected.

The nursing care of the patient is the same as that given to any febrile patient. Tepid sponges, an ice cap to the head, and alcohol sponges may be used to help in the reduction of fever. The environment should be quiet and provisions made for uninterrupted rest. Diet will vary with the physician's orders, but it may be high in calories, with roughage and gas-forming foods avoided. Laxatives are generally not used, but small low enemas may be ordered. During the acute stage of the disease rectal temperature is taken every 2 or 3 hours. Special mouth care, frequent turning, and skin care are important aspects of nursing care. If delirium occurs, the patient must be watched carefully and protected from injury.

The patient should be observed for signs of complications, which include perforation of the intestine and hemorrhage. If perforation occurs, there will be abdominal pain, and the slightest complaint of pain should be reported.

Prophylaxis. Vaccination for typhoid fever has been in use for many years, but only recently has research been conducted outside the laboratory to determine its effectiveness. Routine immunization in the United States is not recommended except under the following conditions:

1. Foreign travel where typhoid fever is known to occur
2. Exposure to a known typhoid carrier as in the home
3. If an outbreak should occur in the community or in an institution

Immunization for children under 10 years of age consists of two injections of 0.25 ml. given subcutaneously, separated by 4 weeks. Adults are given two injections of 0.5 ml. separated by 4 weeks. If the person is at continued risk, a single booster dose is advised every 3 years. Every case of typhoid fever should be thoroughly investigated to determine the source and all household contacts examined and immunized.[11]

Paratyphoid fever is caused by a bacillus that belongs to the same strain as the typhoid bacillus *(Salmonella paratyphi)*. The characteristics and method of spread are like those of typhoid fever. The symptoms appear abruptly and reach their height more quickly than in typhoid fever, and the course of the disease is shorter. The treatment and nursing care of patients with paratyphoid fever is the same as that for patients with typhoid fever.

Bacillary dysentery

Bacillary dysentery is an acute inflammatory diarrheal disease of the colon caused by the bacillus bacterium. The specific type of bacillus belongs to the *Shigella* genus. The inflammatory condition, which may also involve portions of the ileum, results in severe ulceration and, if sufficiently severe, may destroy the mucous membrane of the colon, although perforation may not occur. The disease is spread by the same routes as is typhoid fever, that is, through contaminated water, food, or feces. It usually occurs in crowded areas in which sanitary conditions are poor (Fig. 23-4).

The incubation period is usually between 1 and 7 days, with an abrupt onset. A highly acute infection may terminate fatally within a few days. Although recovery may be expected within 2 or 3 weeks, the disease may become chronic, resulting eventually in ulcerative colitis. The primary symptom is severe diarrhea with abdominal cramping. The diarrhea results in loss of fluids and electrolytes, and the patient becomes severely dehydrated. The stools contain blood, pus, and mucus. The temperature may range from low-grade elevation to 102° to 104° F. in the afternoon. Urination may be painful, and the patient has a constant desire to defecate.

Treatment and nursing care. A problem in the treatment of bacillary dysentery has been the resistance of the organisms to various antimicrobial drugs. At present chloramphenicol and tetracycline are considered to be the most effective. Intravenous fluids and electrolytes are given to combat dehydration, and paregoric and morphine may be ordered to relieve abdominal discomfort and the constant desire to defecate.[3] The patient should be isolated and the same precautions taken as for typhoid fever. A gown should be worn when giving nursing care. A low-residue diet is

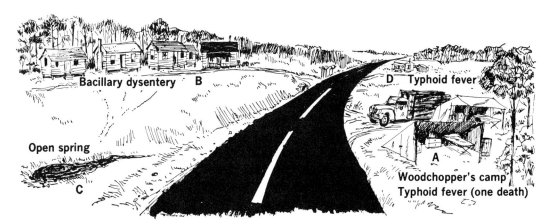

Fig. 23-4. A, Woodchoppers' camp, where approximately fifteen persons, including children, lived in open tents. A 2-year-old child died from typhoid fever. **B,** About twenty families lived on a slight elevation, none of whom had any sanitary facilities for excreta disposal. All excreta were deposited on the ground. Thirty-five stool specimens collected were positive for bacillary dysentery. **C,** Open spring at the foot of the elevation from which all families dipped water with a pail. **D,** An 18-month-old child had typhoid fever but survived after a debilitating illness. (From the author's personal experience.)

offered, and the use of milk and cream should be avoided. The disease is considered to be self-limiting, and mortality is low when treatment is secured.

Tetanus (lockjaw)

Tetanus is a highly fatal disease caused by the tetanus bacillus, which gains entrance to the body through a puncture wound. The causative organism will grow only when air is excluded; thus puncture wounds provide an optimum environment for its growth. The organism may develop a spore-bearing form, producing a powerful toxin that has an affinity for nervous tissue. The tetanus bacillus normally lives in the intestinal tract of certain animals, particularly the horse and cow. In areas in which there are large numbers of animals, the soil is likely to be highly contaminated. In certain sections of the country the disease occurs with relative frequency, and the mortality rate is high, usually from 50% to 60%, with death resulting within the first 4 days.

The incubation period varies and may be as short as 5 days or as long as several weeks. It is generally believed that the length of the incubation period has a direct bearing on the outcome of the disease. The shorter the incubation period the more likely is the disease to be fatal. The early symptoms include headache, restlessness, apprehension, irritability, sometimes profuse sweating, and pain or tenderness about the area of the wound. As the toxin gradually spreads to motor and sensory nerves, spasms of the jaw occur so that the mouth cannot be opened. The neck becomes rigid, spasms of the abdominal muscles occur, and the spine becomes rigid, producing an arching of the body (opisthotonos) (Fig. 23-5). There are also spasms of the larynx, and gradually muscular spasm involves the entire body; the slightest external stimuli may cause violent convulsions. Dyspnea and cyanosis occur, and the patient may become incontinent without losing consciousness.

Treatment and nursing care. Large doses of tetanus antitoxin are given by both the intravenous and intramuscular routes. A skin sensitivity test should precede its administration. The tetanus antitoxin will not have any effect on the tetanus toxins already in the nerves but will neutralize toxins that have not become fixed in the nerves. The second aspect of treatment is to administer analgesics and muscle relaxants to relieve the muscle spasm. Many different drugs are used, and close medical supervision is necessary. An antibiotic may be given to prevent secondary infection.

The patient is isolated in a darkened,

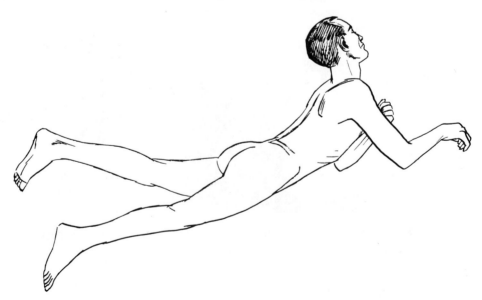

Fig. 23-5. Opisthotonos. Arching of the back, which may occur in patients with meningitis and tetanus.

well-ventilated room, and absolute quiet must be maintained. This cannot be overemphasized, since the slightest noise may cause the patient to have severe muscle spasms or convulsions. The patient must be carefully protected from injury. The diet should be adequate, but no solid food should be given. It may be necessary to administer feedings by nasogastric tube. The fluid intake should approximate 3000 ml. in 24 hours and may be given by intravenous infusion. A retention catheter in the urinary bladder is connected to gravity drainage. The patient may have a tracheotomy; suctioning is used to maintain an open airway, and oxygen may be administered. If the patient survives the first week, recovery may occur, but convalescence will be gradual, extending over several weeks.

Prophylaxis. Tetanus is preventable through active immunization with tetanus toxoid. The inoculations are given to infants with diphtheria toxoid and pertussis vaccine (DPT). Adults may be immunized with tetanus toxoid. If a wound occurs, a booster dose of toxoid is given if more than 1 year has elapsed since the last injection of the initial series of injections. If the individual has no history of prior immunization or has incomplete immunization, a series of primary injections of toxoid is given. Whether tetanus antitoxin should be administered in the case of a wound occurring in an unimmunized person is a medical decision. If in the judgment of the physician passive immunity is necessary, it is recommended that 250 units of tetanus immune globulin (human) be given. If antitoxin made from animal serum is used, the person must be carefully tested for sensitivity because serious or fatal reactions can result. The usual dose of antitoxin is 3000 to 5000 units.[11]

Gas gangrene

Gas gangrene is a serious infection caused by a gas bacillus, which is a spore-forming type of organism that produces a gas and a toxin. The specific organism lives in the intestinal tract and may find its way into a wound through soiled clothing. The gas bacillus, like the tetanus bacillus, has the power to live in the absence of air. Thus it may infect penetrating wounds such as gunshot wounds and is always a dreaded complication of compound fractures.

The onset is usually sudden and may occur within a few hours after injury. Severe pain and edema develop, and although there may be little fever, the pulse rate may be rapid, weak, and thready. The respiratory rate is increased, and the blood pressure may fall. The nurse caring for the patient may notice a peculiar odor from the wound, which may be the first indication of the infection. [*gas gangrene*] The slightest unusual odor should be reported immediately to the physician. As the infection extends into the surrounding muscles, skin color change and gas bubbles may be seen at the site of the wound or may be expressed from the muscles. Unless it is treated promptly, the disease is fatal.

Treatment and nursing care. The most important aspect of treatment is the excision of all infected tissue. Gas gangrene antitoxin is given, and antibiotic therapy is started. Supportive treatment may include blood transfusion and intravenous fluids. When an extremity is involved, amputation may be necessary to save a patient's life. The patient must be isolated, and rigid medical asepsis must be carried out. The nurse must remember that spore-forming bacteria are not destroyed by ordinary disinfecting methods and that contaminated equipment and linens must be autoclaved. Gas gangrene is dangerous and may spread to other patients unless precautions are taken.

Viral diseases
Measles (rubeola)

Measles (rubeola) is a highly infectious and often severe disease occurring in young children. Although measles is preventable through active immunization, during the first 44 weeks of 1975, 21,808 cases were reported in the United States by the Center for Disease Control. Measles is often complicated by bronchopneumonia, otitis media, and encephalitis. Encephalitis accompanies rubeola in about one of each 1000 children affected and causes brain damage and mental retardation.[13]

The onset of measles is usually sudden after an incubation period of 7 to 14 days. The disease occurs primarily in children under 10 years of age, with epidemics starting in the late winter or early spring. In the beginning the disease is often taken for a severe cold. Coryza, lacrimation of the eyes, which are red and sensitive to light, sneezing, and a bronchial cough appear. The child may have fever, with temperature ranging from 103° to 105° F., and often appears severely ill. During this period examination of the throat may reveal small white spots with a reddened base, which are called *Koplik's spots*. In approximately 4 days a macular type of rash begins to appear about the face and gradually extends over the entire body. The rash gradually coalesces to form a slightly elevated eruption that reaches its height in approximately 48 hours, after which it begins to fade. After disappearance of the rash a fine desquamation of the skin occurs.

With the development of the rash the acute symptoms begin to subside, and if complications do not develop, recovery may be expected in 10 to 14 days.

Nursing care. The child with measles should be isolated from other children, and care should be taken in the disposal of nose and throat secretions. The patient is usually more comfortable in a darkened room because of the sensitivity to light. Sponge baths may be given to reduce fever, and fluids should be encouraged. Bed rest is indicated, and exposure to drafts or respiratory infections should be avoided. The nurse should be alert to complaints of earache or enlargement of the cervical lymph nodes, and if they should occur, the physician should be notified. During the febrile period the diet should be liquid or soft. Cough medicines have little effect on the cough, and antibiotic therapy does not alter the course of the disease.

Prophylaxis. For children who have not had measles, active immunization should be given at 12 months of age. If the child has been exposed to measles, no protection will be derived from immunization unless it is given on the day of exposure.

Two types of vaccine are available: live attenuated measles virus vaccine (the original Edmonston B) and the further attenuated strain (Attenuvax).[11] The administration of human immunoglobulin is not necessary with Attenuvax. If the original Edmonston B type is used, human

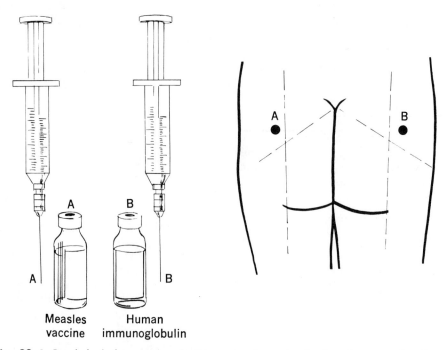

Measles vaccine   Human immunoglobulin

Fig. 23-6. Prophylaxis for measles. **A,** Edmonston B vaccine is given in one syringe in one site. **B,** Human immunoglobulin is given in another syringe in a different site.

immunoglobulin should be administered simultaneously to reduce the febrile reaction that may result if the vaccine alone is given (Fig. 23-6). Results are equally satisfactory with the Schwarz strain without the use of human immunoglobulin. When the vaccine is given between 9 and 12 months of age, some failures will occur. The vaccine should not be given during febrile illnesses or to a child with active tuberculosis. If a child has received human immunoglobulin, measles vaccine should not be given until 3 months have elapsed. Adults may be immunized with live attenuated measles virus vaccine but should not receive the vaccine during pregnancy.[11]

Combination live virus vaccines have recently been licensed, which are measles-mumps-rubella, measles-rubella, and rubella-mumps vaccines. These vaccines are considered to be effective; however, combining one manufacturer's vaccine with another manufacturer's vaccine has not received sufficient testing for recommendation of their simultaneous administration at this time.[11]

German measles (rubella)

German measles is sometimes called *3-day measles* because of the short duration of the disease. The symptoms may be similar to those of rubeola but are usually much milder, and Koplik's spots are absent. Some cases may be so mild that the rash is the first and only significant indication of the disease. The lymph nodes behind the ears are almost always enlarged.

The incubation period of the disease is from 10 to 21 days. Bed rest is indicated, depending on the severity of the disease. Isolation and careful handling and disposal of respiratory secretions are important during the course of the disease.

In pregnancy. The occurrence of rubella during pregnancy has been found to present a major hazard to early fetal development. Prior to 1941 rubella was looked on as a mild innocuous disease of short duration with few, if any, complications. It has now been definitely established that rubella during the first trimester of pregnancy may cause abortion and malformation in surviving infants. It has been estimated that during the last epidemic of rubella in 1964-1965, 30,000 children were

born with defects. The rubella virus infects the placenta and spreads to the fetal circulation. The time of gestation and the length of time that the virus survives and continues to grow in fetal tissue will determine the effects on the fetus. The greatest incidence of defects takes place between the second and the sixth week of gestation. After 8 weeks defects involving the heart, cataracts, and glaucoma decrease, but those of the brain and the ear may continue to occur into the second trimester of pregnancy. Fetal defects do not develop during late pregnancy.

Rubella epidemics occur in cycles of 7 to 10 years. During 1974, 11,917 cases of rubella were reported. During the same period 44 infants were reported to have congenital rubella syndrome.[13] During the first 44 weeks of 1975, 15,301 cases of the disease were reported, and for the same period 20 cases of congenital rubella syndrome were reported.[18] Since 75% of rubella cases occur in school-age children, they represent the reservoir of infection for exposure of pregnant women and women of childbearing age.

Prophylaxis. In 1969 the United States government licensed rubella virus vaccine live for general distribution. One injection of the vaccine is recommended for all children between the ages of 1 year and puberty. Children in kindergarten and early grades are frequently the source of community epidemics and should be high on the priority list to be immunized.[17]

The vaccine should not be given to pregnant women, adolescent girls, or women who may become pregnant within 2 months of receiving the vaccine. Each adolescent girl or adult woman should be considered individually. Many persons cannot confirm having rubella. Screening for susceptibility should be expanded, and if found to be susceptible, immunization may be considered during the immediate postpartum period.

The immunization of male adolescents and adults is useful only in preventing and controlling epidemics.[11] The rubella vaccine contains neomycin; thus persons sensitive to that drug should not receive the vaccine.

Since rubella vaccine is in general use, several factors are important: (1) surveillance of epidemics, (2) accurate diagnosis and reporting of cases, and (3) reporting of all birth defects related to rubella.

Rubella syndrome. A syndrome is a group of symptoms that occur together and that are characteristic of a disease. Although rubella immunization has eliminated a large reservoir of rubella infection, a small number of cases of the disease continue to occur among pregnant women. Infants born to these mothers may have congenital rubella and exhibit some symptoms of the disease. Although the condition may be observed or suspected in the newborn infant, frequently the infant is readmitted to the hospital at some later time when the parent has observed signs of defective development. When admitted to the hospital, the infant should be isolated. The rubella virus may be excreted from the nasopharynx and in the urine for weeks or even months. It has been suggested that all personnel assigned to the nursery and obstetric services should be tested to determine their immunity and that only immune persons should be assigned to these clinical areas.[20]

Chicken pox (varicella)

Chicken pox is an acute, infectious childhood disease caused by a virus. The incubation period is 14 to 21 days, and in many cases the only symptom is the skin rash. The rash goes through a series of stages, beginning with a macule, then progressing to a papule, vesicle, and crust. If secondary infection occurs, scar formation may result; however, in the absence of infection, the crust dries and drops off. The rash is superficial and appears first on the chest, abdomen, and back, gradually extending to other parts of the body. The lesions appear in crops, and small reddened spots may often be observed in the throat before the rash appears on the skin. There may be an elevation of temperature, the extent of which may be closely related to the extent of the skin rash. Headache, loss of appetite, and malaise are commonly associated with the disease. There is often pruritus, causing scratching that may lead to secondary infection and scarring.

The diagnosis of chicken pox is made on the basis of the clinical signs. The disease is self-limiting, and there is no specific treatment. There is no vaccine to produce

[handwritten margin note: no vaccine no isolation no complications]

immunity. Isolation is generally considered unnecessary, but concurrent disinfection of nose and throat discharges should be carried out. There usually are no complications with chicken pox unless secondary infection results from scratching.

Smallpox (variola)

As of June 10, a total of 15,031 cases of smallpox were reported to the World Health Organization for 1975, a decrease of 89% compared to the same period of 1974. Bangladesh accounts for 80% of the world incidence, with an increase of 3% compared to the same period of 1974.[16] (See Fig. 23-7.)

The last confirmed case of smallpox in the United States occurred in 1949. According to the Center for Disease Control,[13] "A declining probability of smallpox importation, and occasionally untoward side effects of vaccination justify discontinuing routine vaccination of school children in the United States." At the present time only persons traveling to areas where smallpox is endemic are required to be vaccinated before leaving the United States. Hospital personnel are considered to be high-risk groups, and a regular program of revaccination every 3 years is recommended for all hospital and medical personnel and public health and allied professions.[13]

Mumps (parotitis)

Mumps is an infectious disease caused by a specific virus that primarily affects children; however, susceptible adults may contract the disease. Mumps is characterized by inflammation and swelling of the parotid glands on one or both sides, and the salivary glands may be affected. The incubation period is 14 to 21 days but may extend beyond 21 days. The disease is transmitted through droplet infection from the upper respiratory tract.

Symptoms depend on the severity of the attack, which may include slight to moderate elevation of temperature, with general malaise and pain on moving the jaw or opening the mouth. A characteristic condition associated with mumps is an acute sensitivity to acid substances.

Occasionally other glands in the body may become involved, the most common being the testes in the male past puberty.

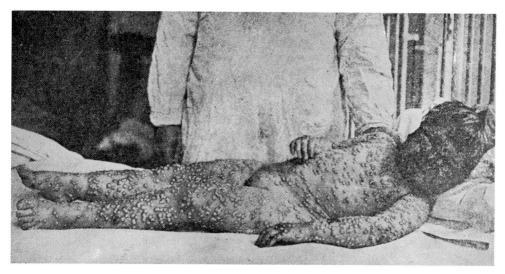

Fig. 23-7. Smallpox in a young child. Note how the pustules run together. (From Monthly Bulletin of Detroit Department of Health, April-May, 1925.)

The question of mumps occurring during early pregnancy as a possible cause of fetal malformations has come under investigation.

Treatment and nursing care. The patient should be isolated until all symptoms of the infection have subsided. Bed rest is indicated and is especially important in the case of adults. The use of a commercial suspensory for the adult male patient is desirable as a routine procedure, and if orchitis develops, an ice bag may be applied. Heat may be applied to swollen, tender salivary glands. The diet should be liquid or soft, and any food or drink with tart or acid taste should be avoided. If it remains uncomplicated, the disease may run a course of approximately 7 to 10 days.

Prophylaxis. Immunization with a single dose of mumps virus vaccine live is recommended for all children over 1 year of age. Although there is no contraindication for administering the vaccine after exposure to mumps, there is no indication that it will offer any protection. It is considered best not to administer the vaccine to women during pregnancy. Mumps vaccine combined with measles vaccine is now available (p. 553).

Rabies

Rabies is an acute infectious disease caused by a virus that attacks the nervous system. It is transmitted to humans through the bite of an animal that has the disease. Rabies can exist in all types of warm-blooded animals, but the dog is the most common source of the infection in the human. Rabies among wildlife in the United States is considered endemic, especially in skunks, foxes, and raccoons. The public is cautioned against catching or handling animals caught wild and that they do not make safe pets. The virus is contained in the saliva of the animal, which is injected into the human through the broken skin caused by the bite. The virus travels along the nerve pathways, eventually reaching the brain. Bites occurring about the face, head, neck, and especially about the mouth are the most serious because of the increased nerve supply in these areas. The incubation period in humans may be as short as 5 days or as long as 2 years.

The disease is characterized by three phases. In phase one there is mental depression, headache, irritability, and increased sensitivity about the area of the bite, and there may be a sensation of tingling or numbness in the extremities. Phase two is marked by excitement, restlessness, irritability, dyspnea, muscle spasms, and convulsions. The patient may be unable to swallow, and laryngeal spasm occurs; the patient is unable to stand the sight or sound of water. The symptoms gradually increase in severity, and drooling and spitting occur. The temperature becomes elevated, the pulse rate irregular, and the eyes staring; the patient is apprehensive, and death may occur. Phase three is the paralytic phase, and when the convulsions cease, paralysis occurs. The temperature may be elevated to as much as 108° F. rectally, and although the patient remains conscious, he is unable to talk. Death takes place within 18 hours.

Treatment and nursing care. Prior to 1970 no one who contracted rabies was known to recover. Late in 1970 a 6-year-old boy in Ohio was bitten by a rabid bat. Extensive laboratory tests failed to prove human rabies. However, clinical and epidemiologic features of the case indicated that the child had human rabies. The boy recovered and was dismissed from the hospital late in January, 1971.[17] However, in September, 1973, a man who was bitten on the ear by a bat died, and antemortem examination confirmed a diagnosis of rabies.[15] In January, 1975, a man was bitten by a cat and died from rabies.[17a]

Treatment is usually only supportive. The patient is given drugs to relieve anxiety and excitement and to control convulsions. Intravenous fluids may be administered to prevent dehydration. The patient may be isolated as a means of providing a quiet environment, but the disease is not transmitted from person to person. However, a gown and gloves are worn, since it has been possible to isolate the virus from the saliva. The patient should be protected from injury, and during stages of extreme excitability restraints may be necessary. The patient must have continuous nursing care. He should not be bathed, and no water should be brought near the patient or faucets turned on within his hearing. Absolute quiet should be maintained. In the beginning the patient may be given a soft diet, but as swallowing becomes more difficult, he will be unable to eat.

Prophylaxis. More than 30,000 persons in the United States receive postexposure antirabies treatment each year. Treatment may be both passive and active. Two types of rabies vaccine are available: duck embryo vaccine (DEV) and nervous tissue vaccine (NTV), also known as Semple type. High-risk persons such as veterinarians, wildlife rangers, and dog wardens are advised to secure preexposure immunization. Postexposure prophylaxis treatment may be administered with or without hyperimmune serum. The serum is of equine origin, and 20% of persons receiving it may have serum sickness. Hyperab, a new human rabies immune globulin (HRIG), has been available since September, 1974, and may be given to persons hypersensitive to serum of equine origin. When serum is not given, fourteen daily injections of the vaccine are administered. When serum is given, twenty-one injections of the vaccine are given. The immediate first-aid care of all wounds or scratches is thorough washing with large amounts of soap and water.[11]

Infectious mononucleosis

The cause of infectious mononucleosis is unknown; however, it is believed to be caused by a virus. The disease seems to have a low degree of communicability, but it frequently occurs among physicians, nurses, and other hospital personnel. It often occurs among groups of young people living together, as in college dormitories. The disease has been referred to as the "kissing disease" because transmission appears to be by the oral route and the exchange of saliva. The name *mononucleosis* was derived from the atypical lymphocytes among the white blood cells[6] (p. 244).

The disease is characterized by sore throat, fever, enlarged lymph nodes, headache, and vomiting, and in persons with severe cases the spleen may be enlarged or jaundice may occur. The incubation period is believed to be 4 to 14 days but may be as long as 6 weeks.

Treatment and nursing care. There is no specific treatment for the disease, which is self-limiting. During the acute phase the patient should be confined to bed. Mild analgesics such as aspirin may be given to relieve the discomfort from the sore throat and enlarged glands. Warm saline solution throat irrigations may also provide relief. Corticosteroid therapy has been effective in severe cases. Antibiotics have no effect on the course or the outcome of the disease.[6] Although serious complications are possible, their occurrence is considered rare.

Patients with infectious mononucleosis do not have to be isolated, and there is no prophylactic therapy for contacts.

Pulmonary tuberculosis

Tuberculosis is an infectious disease that was known to exist long before Christ. However, it was not until 1882, when Robert Koch discovered the tubercle bacillus as the causative organism, that modern treatment became possible. Tuberculosis has been one of the most devastating diseases of all time, and unlike other infectious diseases, it may attack any organ and tissue in the body and can result in years of chronic invalidism or death. Tremendous advances have been made in the treatment and control of the disease, and it appears that its elimination as a health problem is within reach. Nurses who work in tuberculosis hospitals will need special training in the care of the patient and specific procedures. In this book no attempt is made to cover all the various aspects of the disease; the following discussion will deal only with tuberculosis of the lungs.

Incidence. The number of new cases of tuberculosis (all forms) has shown a gradual decrease. During 1974 a provisional report showed 30,000 new cases of active tuberculosis. The rate for new active cases dropped to 14.3 per 100,000 population, which was 46% lower than for 1964.[18]

Mode of transmission. The tubercle bacillus is contained in the sputum of persons with tuberculosis, and the disease is contracted through inhaling the organism. When a person with tuberculosis coughs, sneezes, or expectorates, the germs are carried into the air as droplets and droplet nuclei. The disease may also be contracted by kissing a person with tuberculosis.

The tubercle bacillus is not killed by ordinary disinfectants but may be destroyed by boiling, autoclaving, and exposure to ultraviolet light. If a person with the tubercle bacillus in his sputum expectorates in a place not exposed to the sun, the organism may live for months.

Symptoms. There are no early symptoms in tuberculosis, and when symptoms do appear, they may be the result of toxic manifestations produced by the infection or by the lesions in the lung. In either case it may mean that the disease has progressed to a stage at which cure may be difficult. Toxic symptoms may include slight elevation of temperature, which is not considered particularly significant, since a person may have fever from a variety of causes. Fatigue, malaise, and gradual weight loss are among the more common symptoms. Profuse sweating occurs at night, commonly called *night sweats*. There may be some increase in the pulse rate, and the patient frequently complains of various digestive discomforts. Febrile

As in most respiratory diseases, when anything interferes with normal breathing, there will be some indication of respiratory distress. In tuberculosis of the lungs there generally is some coughing, which may be slight or severe and may or may not be productive. Dyspnea may be present, and tuberculosis may cause other conditions such as pleurisy or fluid in the pleural cavity, resulting in pain and further interference with respiration. The spitting of blood or frank hemorrhage (hemoptysis) may occur when cavitation extends into a blood vessel. There is a wide variety of symptoms in tuberculosis, and there is no specific pattern in which they occur.

Diagnostic procedures. The most valuable tool in the diagnosis of pulmonary tuberculosis is the chest x-ray film. Various types of chest x-ray films may be taken, Acid fast smear Bronchoscopy and films are also taken from various positions. The fluoroscope may be used both for diagnosis and to follow the course of the disease. Frequent sputum examinations are often required to isolate the tubercle bacillus, and failure to find it does not always rule out the diagnosis of tuberculosis but may indicate the need to look for some other disease. Under some conditions it may not be possible to secure sputum for examination; a gastric lavage is then done, and the gastric contents are examined. A bronchoscopic examination is often done to secure secretions from the bronchial tree or directly from portions of the lung. When tuberculosis is suspected, there must be a complete history and physical examination, including routine laboratory examination. A history of exposure is of special significance.

Treatment. It is recommended that all patients with tuberculosis be admitted to a hospital for extensive tests and examination.

The stage of the patient's disease is evaluated, and an individual schedule of treatment is planned. Most patients will not have to be in the hospital for longer than 3 to 6 months.

Tuberculosis is treated with chemotherapeutic drugs; the drugs used are classified as primary drugs and secondary drugs. The primary drugs include streptomycin, para-aminosalicylic acid (PAS), isonicotinic acid hydrazide (isoniazid), ethambutol, and rifampin. These are the most commonly used drugs; however, not all patients respond to the same drugs, and sensitivity tests should be done prior to beginning treatment so that the most effective drug may be used. Often a combination of drugs is given. Any treatment considers the stage of the disease, its activity, and the patient's resistance to the drug. There are several secondary drugs, including pyrazinamide, kanamycin, cycloserine, and ethionamide. Some of these drugs may be used in combination with primary drugs, or they may be given when there is resistance to the primary drugs. They are also used for some kinds of atypical tuberculosis.

Certain toxic symptoms may occur, and the patient must be observed because it may be necessary to change or discontinue the drug. Numbness, tingling, and weakness of the extremities are toxic signs that may be observed when isoniazid is being given. Streptomycin may cause deafness, dizziness, unsteadiness of gait, ringing in the ears, or severe headache. The most common symptoms of toxic reaction to PAS are gastrointestinal complaints such as diarrhea. Toxic symptoms are more likely to occur in older persons or in those who have been taking the drug for several years. Since patients with tuberculosis often receive chemotherapeutic drugs over a prolonged time, regular laboratory examinations are important. These examinations may include urinalysis, blood urea nitrogen test, liver function tests, and serum glutamic oxaloacetic transaminase test. In addition, visual acuity and hearing tests should be done at intervals.[1, 2] In February, 1974, the Center for Disease Control advised that persons with tuberculosis who completed adequate chemotherapy should be considered cured and that periodic reexamination is unnecessary. All complaints and symptoms should be reported to the physician. Not all patients will respond to chemotherapy; they may need prolonged hospitalization, and some may require surgery such as lobectomy or pneumonectomy (Chapter 11).

Case finding. Everyone should have an annual examination for tuberculosis. All adult persons should have a chest x-ray film as a part of the examination, and children should have a chest x-ray film if they have a positive tuberculin test. If the tuberculin test is negative, it should be repeated every 3 months for medical and nursing personnel to check for conversion. There is an increasing incidence of tuberculosis among older persons, and annual chest x-ray films for these persons are assuming greater importance.

The tuberculin test is a diagnostic aid that indicates the presence of infection but does not necessarily indicate the presence of disease. The tuberculin test is presently used as a screening method to detect persons with the disease and to rule out persons who do not have tuberculosis. Considerable emphasis is being placed on the testing of children under 6 years of age. If the child has a positive test, it may indicate that there is a case of tuberculosis in the home or in some other close contact.

Commonly used methods of tuberculin testing include the intradermal (Mantoux) test, in which 0.1 ml. of old tuberculin (OT) or purified protein derivative (PPD) in the proper concentration is injected on the surface of the forearm. The jet injector is a method of using a jet gun that injects PPD intradermally under high pressure. Multiple puncture tests are done using the Sterneedle and the tine test method. The Mantoux and jet injector tests should be read between 48 and 72 hours after the administration of the test. If the site of induration is 0 to 4 mm., the test is considered negative; if the induration is 5 to 9 mm., it is doubtful; and if it is 10 mm. or more, it is positive. The tine test is considered to be positive if the induration of the laregst puncture area measures 5 mm. or more. If the reaction is negative, there will be no area of induration. If a reaction occurs with the Sterneedle, it should be followed with an intradermal test. In the absence of any reaction the test is negative.[4]

Prophylaxis. A vaccine known as BCG

may be administered to certain persons such as student nurses who have a negative tuberculin test. The vaccine must be administered by persons who are familiar with the technique. If used, it is given only to persons who have a negative tuberculin test. It is generally believed that administration of BCG vaccine is not necessary in the United States; however, under certain conditions it may be given.

The use of chemotherapeutic drugs for known contacts exposed to tuberculosis who do not have the disease is now recommended.

Tuberculosis in the general hospital. Fewer patients are being admitted to specialized tuberculosis hospitals, and more patients are being admitted to general hospitals. For some reason nurses in general hospitals seem to be frightened of tuberculosis, and hospital policies tend to emphasize factors of little or no real significance while ignoring the most important factors. The patient needs a comfortable physical and emotional environment but is frequently made uncomfortable by outdated procedures. The nurse needs to understand the following factors concerning tuberculosis:

1. Tuberculosis is not a highly infectious disease.

2. The nurse needs to have a clear understanding of how the disease is spread.

3. Isolation is unnecessary, and the use of gowns and caps is unnecessary.

4. Good ventilation is important in the patient's environment.

5. A planned program of teaching for the patient and his family is necessary.

6. Chemotherapy limits the release of tubercle bacilli into the air within a few days after therapy has been initiated.

When the patient coughs or sneezes, moist droplets are carried into the air. Some droplets will fall into the immediate environment, whereas others will remain suspended in the air as droplet nuclei. Good ventilation will carry droplet nuclei on air currents where they may be killed by sunlight or ultraviolet light. When the patient is taught to cover his nose and mouth when coughing or sneezing, the dissemination of moist droplets into the environment is reduced or eliminated. When the patient understands the importance of this procedure, cooperation may usually be expected.

Tissues used to cover coughs or to collect sputum may be placed in public sewerage systems or into a paper bag and burned.

Basic to the care of all patients in the general hospital is an admission x-ray examination. Early detection of the disease means that therapy may be initiated, even before the patient is releasing the organism into the environment. The employee health service should conduct tuberculin tests on all employees and take x-ray films of any person with a positive tuberculin test. When the test is negative, a retest should be done at regular intervals. If conversion occurs, chest x-ray films are taken, and the individual may be given prophylactic therapy.[7]

Research is underway at the Trudeau Institute at Saranac Lake, New York, concerning the body's ability to resist infection. Some of the findings appear to indicate that there is an immune response to reinfection and that therapy has no effect on the duration of the immunity. It is believed that this research may be the key to the total eradication of tuberculosis.[21]

Rickettsial diseases

Several diseases are caused by the rickettsia, a minute organism whose specific classification remains to be determined. Diseases caused by rickettsiae are transmitted by the bite of an insect, and the rickettsiae are probably kept alive by some animal. Only one of the well-known rickettsial diseases will be reviewed here.

Rocky Mountain spotted fever tick bite

The nurse might believe from the name that this disease exists only in the far western part of the United States, specifically in the Rocky Mountain area. Actually, this is not the case; it has been reported in every state and wherever there are ticks that bite human beings.

It has been reported that the incidence of Rocky Mountain spotted fever is greater along the eastern seaboard and in the southeastern states than in the Rocky Mountain area. During 1974 a total of 754 cases of the disease occurred. The figure includes cases of typhus fever, which is also a tick-borne disease.[11]

Rocky Mountain spotted fever is an acute infectious disease transmitted by the bite of an infected tick. There are three types of ticks that may be responsible for the disease: the American dog tick, the Rocky Mountain wood tick, and the Lone Star tick. The disease is seasonal, being more common from April to August, and in some areas presents an occupational hazard. When occupations take persons into areas heavily infested with ticks, the risk is greater. The disease is frequently contracted by persons vacationing or picnicking in areas in which ticks exist. If the disease is untreated, the fatality rate is high. The incubation period is 3 to 10 days.

Symptoms. The disease may be mild, with the person remaining ambulatory, or it may be severe, with death occurring within a few days after its onset. Early symptoms may be loss of appetite, malaise, irritability, and vague aches and pains. The disease may have an abrupt onset, beginning with a chill, severe headache, an elevation of temperature to 104° F. or more, and severe aching. There may be an unproductive cough, nosebleed, and abdominal pain with nausea and vomiting. The face is flushed, there is profuse sweating, the mouth is dry, and the tongue is coated. In persons with severe cases there may be rigidity of the neck, mental confusion, delirium, incontinence, constipation, and severe prostration; convulsions and coma may occur. On about the third or fourth day a rash appears, beginning on the wrists and ankles but gradually spreading over the body, and it may include the scalp and the mucous membranes of the mouth and throat. The rash is petechial in type and tends to fade on pressure; it is rose colored in the beginning but darkens as the disease continues. The acute illness may last for 2 or 3 weeks, with the temperature remaining high for as long as 10 days. The pulse rate is usually slow in relation to the amount of fever present, but in persons with severe cases it may become weak and rapid.

Treatment and nursing care. The treatment of Rocky Mountain spotted fever is with chloramphenicol (Chloromycetin), which should be administered early in the disease, preferably with the beginning of the skin rash. Chlortetracycline and oxytetracycline are also used. The use of antibiotic therapy may bring about remarkable improvement in the symptoms and will reduce the febrile period. Other treatment

consists of administering intravenous fluids if sufficient fluid is not taken orally. Blood transfusions may sometimes be indicated.

The nursing care is the same as that for any patient with febrile disease. The patient is on a regimen of bed rest, and measures to control temperature such as giving sponge baths and administering antipyretic drugs are instituted. Enemas may be used to provide for bowel elimination, and special mouth care and eye irrigations may be necessary. The diet should be high in protein with extra between-meal feedings that are also high in protein.

Prophylaxis. Rickettsia rickettsii vaccine is available and may be administered in three injections at 7- to 10-day intervals. It should be given prior to the beginning of the tick season and requires an annual booster dose. Persons whose work requires them to go into tick-infested areas in which there is considerable risk are advised to avail themselves of the protection.[8] Persons who go camping or picnicking in areas in which they may be exposed to ticks should use tick repellents, avoid sleeping on the ground, and inspect clothing and skin carefully. Areas such as the hairline and under the arms should be given special attention. In removing ticks it is important to avoid crushing them or leaving the head embedded in the skin. The greatest danger of infection occurs after the tick has fed for 6 to 8 hours.

Protozoal disease
Malaria

Malaria is a worldwide problem; the disease is transmitted from person to person by a mosquito known as the *Anopheles quadrimaculatus* (Fig. 23-8). Control of the disease in the United States has been brought about by many factors, chief of which have been destruction of breeding places and adequate treatment of persons with malaria. In 1963 only ninety-nine cases of malaria were reported in the United States. The incidence rose to 3102 cases in 1969, primarily because of servicemen returning from malarial areas. The incidence dropped to 742 cases in 1972,[13] and for 1974, 293 cases were reported to the Center for Disease Control.[13] For the first 44 weeks of 1975, 352 cases have been reported. Between 1963 and 1972, forty-two

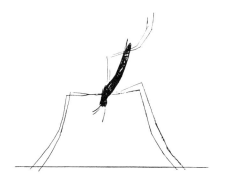

Fig. 23-8. *Anopheles quadrimaculatus* mosquito, the vector for malaria.

fatal cases of malaria were reported in the United States, thirty-seven of which were caused by a form known as *Plasmodium falciparum.* This form of the disease requires immediate diagnosis and treatment, or it may terminate quickly in death. Most cases have occurred in persons returning from travel to areas where the disease still exists.[14]

Malaria protozoa undergo a complicated reproduction cycle within the human body, and the clinical symptoms are closely related to this cycle. After exposure to the disease the first symptoms occur 12 to 14 days later.

Symptoms. In tertian malaria, the most common form in the United States, symptoms begin with headache and a gradually increasing fever. The typical malaria pattern soon develops; there is a severe chill, followed by a high fever, with temperature ranging from 103° to 105° F., and a rapid fall in temperature followed by profuse sweating. This sequence may repeat itself every 48 hours, and between the episodes the patient may be reasonably well. However, over a period of time without adequate treatment there is a gradually developing anemia with enlargement of the spleen.

Treatment. Quinine sulfate has long been considered a specific drug in the treatment of malaria. During World War II, when quinine could not be obtained, a synthetic drug, quinacrine hydrochloride (Atabrine), was used as a substitute. In recent years several new drugs have been developed for the treatment of malaria, including chloroquine (Aralen), which is administered both orally and intramuscularly, and chloroguanide (Guanatol, Paludrine, Proguanil), which are available for oral administration.

Venereal diseases

Five diseases are classified as venereal diseases: syphilis, gonorrhea, chancroid, lymphogranuloma venereum, and granuloma inguinale. All five diseases are spread through sexual contact; however, syphilis and gonorrhea are by far the most prevalent, and only these two venereal diseases will be reviewed here.

Infectious syphilis and gonorrhea are reported to have reached epidemic proportions in the United States. During 1974, 83,771 new cases of infectious syphilis and 898,943 cases of gonorrhea were reported from the venereal disease branch of the Center for Disease Control. The largest number of cases of syphilis and gonorrhea occurred in the 20- to 24-year-old age group. For 1975, 21,111 cases of infectious syphilis and 822,626 cases of gonorrhea have been reported as of Nov. 1.

Syphilis

Syphilis is the most serious of the venereal diseases, since it attacks the vital organs of the body. It damages the heart and blood vessels, affects the central nervous system, and may cause blindness and deafness. An untreated pregnant woman may transmit the disease to the fetus through the placenta.

Syphilis is contracted almost exclusively through sexual contact and is caused by a spirochete, *Treponema pallidum.* The disease is described in three stages, which are called the primary, secondary, and latent stages.

Primary syphilis. The incubation period for syphilis is 10 to 90 days, with an average of 21 days. The first sign of the disease is a single lesion (chancre), which appears on the male prepuce or the female vulva. In the female the lesion may occur on the cervix. The lesion occurs at the point of inoculation and is painless, and the serologic blood test is usually negative at this time. During the primary stage the disease is highly infectious. The primary lesion disappears in 3 or 4 weeks with or without treatment, and no topical application will hasten its healing. Positive identification of the specific spirochete may be made at this time by a dark-field examination (special attachment on the microscope). When adequate treatment is given early during the primary stage, the serologic test may remain negative. After approximately a week without treatment the serologic test becomes reactive, and the disease enters the secondary stage.

Secondary syphilis. As a result of the invading organisms, several symptoms develop, including a rash. The rash may be a slight erythema or may be extensive, with macular, papular, or pustular lesions. Lesions called *mucous patches* appear about the mouth and lips, and the throat may be sore. A papular type of lesion (condyloma latum) appears about the genitals. All moist lesions are infectious, and positive dark-field examination may often be secured from these secondary lesions. Other symptoms include alopecia, pain in the bones, gastric disturbances, inflammation of the eyes, loss of appetite, and malaise. Without treatment the symptoms of secondary syphilis may disappear slowly and recur at intervals for as long as 2 years, and the disease is considered highly infectious during this stage.

Latent syphilis. The latent stage is generally considered to cover a period of 4 years or more from the time of onset of the disease. During this period there is no clinical evidence of the disease after disappearance of secondary lesions except the reactive serologic test. However, it is during this time that the organism is attacking the vital structures and causing an inflammatory condition. The body's defenses may be sufficient to overcome the destructiveness of the organism; however, there is no way to determine which individuals may ultimately suffer severe disability. The serologic test remains reactive, and the disease is potentially infectious through sexual contact. After 15 or 20 years the late manifestations of the disease may begin to appear. The central nervous system and the cardiovascular system may be affected, and these disorders have been reviewed in other chapters of this book.

Congenital syphilis. Mothers with untreated syphilis often have a history of repeated abortions. If the pregnancy is completed, the fetus may be stillborn, or if the infant survives, it may have syphilis. An infant with congenital syphilis may have a rash on the face, palms of the hands, soles of the feet, and buttocks, with the latter often taken for diaper rash. There may be mucous patches in the mouth and a nasal stuffiness and rhinitis (snuffles), and the bones and abdominal organs are often involved. The syphilitic lesions of the infant are infectious, just as are those of the adult. The child who survives may develop complications at any time before 16 years of age. These complications include changes in the bones, deformed permanent teeth, interstitial keratitis, and eighth nerve deafness. The central nervous system may be involved, and mental retardation may occur in a small number of children.

Treatment. The present treatment of syphilis is administration of penicillin. At the present time there is no evidence that the syphilitic organism is becoming resistant to penicillin; however, caution must be exercised because more individuals are becoming sensitive to penicillin. The same care should be exercised as when administering penicillin to a patient for any condition. Treatment may extend over a period of several days or may be given in one divided dose. Patients who are sensitive to penicillin may be treated with tetracycline or erythromycin.

Gonorrhea

Gonorrhea is caused by the *Neisseria gonorrhoeae* (gonococcus bacterium), and its prevalence is much greater than that of any of the other venereal diseases. The disease is transmitted through sexual contact. Research has indicated that the female is a significant reservoir of infection. Symptoms in the male are more readily detected than in the female. As a result, many women go untreated and spread the infection.[8]

Symptoms. The characteristic symptoms begin with burning, urgent, and painful urination. There may be redness and edema of the urinary meatus. After the initial symptoms a purulent urethral discharge occurs in the male, and a discharge may be expressed from the vaginal glands, ducts, and the urethra in the female. In the absence of treatment or with inadequate treatment the disease may become chronic and lead to complications. Epididymitis and prostatitis may occur in the male, and salpingitis may occur in the female. An acute inflammatory condition in the fallopian tube may result in atresia and sterility.

Treatment. The treatment for gonorrhea consists of administering penicillin. However, there is evidence that certain strains of the gonococcus are becoming less sensitive to penicillin. For persons who are sensitive to penicillin or when the organism is resistant to penicillin, other antibiotics may be administered. A new drug minocycline (Minocin), a semisynthetic derivative of tetracycline, has been used as an alternative agent to treat gonorrhea. A new semisynthetic penicillin carbenicillin (Geopen, Pyopen), has been found effective in treating males with gonococcal urethritis.[19]

Sociologic factors and trends

The venereal diseases have frequently been termed "social diseases" because of the factors in society that have contributed to their existence, including poverty, poor housing, low income, ignorance, and in more recent times, the high mobility of people, increased consumption of alcohol, ease of treatment, and a breakdown of moral standards. All these factors have resulted in an increase in the incidence of infectious syphilis and gonorrhea. Primary and secondary syphilis have continued to increase. Most new cases of syphilis occur in persons under 25 years of age. The rates per 100,000 population are significantly higher across the South Atlantic United States.

For the fiscal year of 1972, $16 million in federal funds was made available for activities against syphilis and gonorrhea. A massive campaign was initiated to locate, diagnose, treat, and investigate the diseases and to educate physicians, teen-agers, schoolchildren, and others considered to be at risk.[22]

Summary outline

1. Causes of infectious disease
   A. Transmission of infectious disease
   B. Classification of causative agents
      1. Bacteria
      2. Viruses
      3. Rickettsiae
      4. Protozoa
      5. Metazoa—not reviewed in this chapter
2. Prevention of infectious disease
   A. Development of vaccines and serums for prophylactic and therapeutic use
   B. Improved sanitation in disposal of excreta, improved milk and water supplies, and improved methods of handling food
   C. Public enlightenment and education
   D. Continuing program needed because large reservoir of susceptible persons always exists
   E. What nurses should know
      1. How infectious diseases are contracted and spread
      2. How causative organisms can be destroyed
      3. How active immunization programs can be promoted
      4. How to protect themselves and others when caring for patient with infectious disease
3. Diagnostic tests and procedures
   A. History and clinical manifestations, characteristic symptoms, history of exposure, and knowledge of duration of incubation period
   B. Laboratory examinations of blood, secretions, sputum, stools, and lesions
   C. Inoculation of animals
   D. Skin tests
4. Nursing responsibilities
   A. Medical asepsis: Principle—contain within a given area and destroy all pathogenic organisms to prevent their spread
      1. Knowledge of how disease is spread
      2. Trend away from special hospitals for infectious diseases—patients being admitted to general hospitals
      3. Frequent and thorough handwashing
      4. Care in collecting, handling, and disposing of discharges
      5. Care of equipment and linens in hospital and home
      6. Protection of environment from flies
      7. Concurrent disinfection—daily care, handling and disposing of contaminated material
      8. Terminal disinfection—thorough cleaning of environment after patient's release from isolation
      9. Quarantine—restriction of entering or leaving of all persons by health department regulation
   B. Isolation—segregation of sick person from well persons to prevent spread of disease
      1. Physician writes order for isolation
      2. Physician determines duration of isolation
      3. Physician should prepare patient for isolation
      4. Patient more cooperative when he knows purpose of isolation
   C. Physiologic care—like that given any sick patient
   D. Psychologic care
      1. Isolated patient should not be left alone for long periods; frequent visits to patient by nurse provide emotional support
   E. Sociologic factors
      1. Potential reservoir of infection may exist in some areas

2. Failure to secure immunization of young children
    a. Apathy, lack of motivation, lack of transportation, or lack of medical and clinical services
3. High mobility of population
F. Contraindications for immunization
5. Nursing the patient with infectious disease
    A. Bacterial diseases
        1. Scarlet fever
            a. Caused by hemolytic streptococcus bacterium and spread through nose and throat secretions and suppurating complications
            b. Treatment should be given early with penicillin
            c. Incubation period is 2 to 5 days
            d. Isolation is required for approximately 7 days
            e. Patient should be observed carefully for complications
        2. Diphtheria
            a. Caused by diphtheria bacillus and transmitted through nose and throat secretions
            b. Four forms are recognized
                (1) Tonsillar diphtheria
                (2) Nasal diphtheria
                (3) Nasopharyngeal diphtheria
                (4) Laryngeal diphtheria
            c. Antitoxin should be administered as soon as possible
            d. Patient should be observed for complications of heart and nervous system
            e. Strict isolation is necessary until two or more negative throat and nose cultures 48 hours apart have been secured
            f. Prophylaxis with diphtheria toxoid (DPT) should be started at 2 or 3 months of age
        3. Whooping cough (pertussis)
            a. Caused by *Bordetella pertussis* and transmitted through nose and throat secretions
            b. No specific treatment for disease
            c. Isolation is required for approximately 6 weeks
            d. Prophylaxis should be started at 2 or 3 months of age (DTP)
        4. Typhoid fever
            a. Caused by typhoid bacilli (*Salmonella typhosa*) from feces and urine of infected person or carrier and spread through contaminated food or drink
            b. Treatment is with chloramphenicol (Chloromycetin) co-trimoxazole
            c. Patient is observed for complications
            d. Isolation depends on hospital policy
            e. Prophylaxis given during certain situations
                (1) Foreign travel where disease is known to occur
                (2) Exposure as in home
                (3) If outbreak occurs in community or institution

f. Paratyphoid fever is caused by bacillus of same group as typhoid bacillus (*Salmonella paratyphi*)
    (1) Disease is similar to typhoid fever but less severe
    (2) Treatment is same
5. Bacillary dysentery
    a. Acute inflammatory disease of colon caused by bacillus organism
        (1) Incubation period is from 1 to 7 days
    b. Treatment is administration of chemotherapeutic drugs; paregoric or morphine for abdominal discomfort
    c. Isolation—technique is same as in typhoid fever
6. Tetanus (lockjaw)
    a. Highly fatal disease caused by tetanus bacillus
        (1) Disease attacks nervous system
        (2) Incubation period is from 5 days to several weeks
    b. Treatment consists of giving large doses of tetanus antitoxin
    c. Patient is isolated to provide quiet and rest
    d. Prophylaxis should be given through administration of tetanus toxoid (DTP), beginning when child is 2 or 3 months of age, and booster dose should be given in case of injury if more than 1 year since last injection
7. Gas gangrene
    a. Serious infection caused by gas bacillus bacteria
        (1) Infection may develop within few hours after injury
    b. Rigid medical asepsis must be carried out
    c. Infection is treated with special antitoxin and antibiotics
    d. Amputation of extremity may be necessary
    e. Spore-forming gas bacillus is not destroyed by ordinary disinfection methods
B. Viral diseases
    1. Measles (rubeola)
        a. Primarily disease of children under 10 years of age
            (1) Incubation period is 7 to 14 days
            (2) Disease is transmitted through nose and throat secretions
        b. Isolation is required
        c. Otitis media, encephalitis, and bronchopneumonia are frequent complications
        d. Prophylaxis—at 12 months of age
            (1) Edmonston B strain given with human immunoglobulin
            (2) Use separate syringes and needles and give in different sites
            (3) Edmonston further attenuated strain (Attenuvax)
            (4) Schwarz strain given without human immunoglobulin
            (5) Combination vaccines may be used

2. German measles (rubella)
   a. Similar to measles but milder and of shorter duration
      (1) Incubation period is from 10 to 21 days
      (2) Disease is transmitted by direct contact
   b. Isolation required
   c. German measles (rubella) in pregnancy
      (1) Cause of fetal malformation or abortion during first trimester of pregnancy
   d. Prophylaxis
      (1) Single injection of live rubella virus vaccine may be given from 1 year of age to puberty, or combination vaccine may be given
      (2) Not to be given to adolescent girls, pregnant women, and women who may become pregnant within 2 months of injection
   e. Important factors to be considered
      (1) Surveillance of epidemics
      (2) Accurate diagnosis and reporting of all cases
      (3) Reporting all birth defects related to rubella
   f. Rubella syndrome
      (1) Congenital rubella may exhibit same symptoms as primary rubella
      (2) Isolation of infant
      (3) Testing of personnel in nursery and obstetrical service to determine immunity
         (a) Only immune persons should be assigned to these areas
3. Chicken pox (varicella)
   a. Caused by virus
      (1) Occurs in children and is rare in adults
      (2) Incubation period is 14 to 21 days
      (3) Disease is transmitted by direct contact
   b. There is no prophylaxis
4. Smallpox (variola)
   a. Still exists in some countries and is dangerous disease
   b. Vaccination of schoolchildren should be discontinued
   c. Hospital personnel considered high-risk group and should be vaccinated
5. Mumps (parotitis)
   a. Caused by virus
      (1) Occurs in children and susceptible adults
      (2) Incubation period is 14 to 21 days
      (3) Disease is spread through discharges from upper respiratory tract
   b. Isolation is required until all symptoms have disappeared
   c. Prophylaxis
      (1) Single injection of mumps virus

vaccine live for all children over 1 year of age, or combination vaccine may be given
      (2) Not recommended for pregnant women
6. Rabies
   a. Caused by virus that attacks nervous system
      (1) Disease is transmitted by bite of animal having disease
      (2) Incubation period is from 5 days to 2 years
      (3) Death is almost inevitable
   b. Isolate patient to provide quiet environment
   c. Vaccines available for preexposure and postexposure protection
      (1) Duck embryo vaccine (DEV)
      (2) Nervous tissue vaccine (NTV), Semple type
   d. Hyperimmune serum may be given with vaccine or human rabies immune globulin (HRIG)
   e. High-risk groups should receive preexposure immunization
7. Infectious mononucleosis
   a. Of unknown cause and has low degree of communicability; believed to be caused by a virus
      (1) Incubation period is from 4 to 14 days but may be 6 weeks
   b. No specific treatment
C. Pulmonary tuberculosis
   1. Caused by tubercle bacillus
   2. Disease is transmitted in sputum of persons with disease and through droplet infection and droplet nuclei
   3. Tubercle bacillus is not killed by ordinary disinfectants
   4. Diagnosis of disease is made through x-ray examination, sputum examination, bronchoscopy, gastric washings, history, and physical examination
   5. Treatment—chemotherapeutic drugs
      a. Classification of drugs
         (1) Primary drugs
         (2) Secondary drugs
      b. Laboratory examinations
   6. Case finding through annual x-ray films of chest and tuberculin testing is important in eliminating disease
      a. Mantoux test—intracutaneous test
      b. Sterneedle test
      c. Tuberculin tine test
      d. Jet injector
   7. Prophylaxis may be given with BCG vaccine to persons with negative tuberculin test
   8. What nurse should know about tuberculosis
      a. Tuberculosis is not highly infectious
      b. How the disease is spread
      c. Isolation unnecessary; gowns and caps unnecessary
      d. Importance of good ventilation
      e. Planned program of teaching patient and family
      f. Chemotherapy limits release of

tubercle bacilli within few days after therapy is initiated

9. Admission x-ray examinations of all patients

10. Tuberculin tests and x-ray examinations of all hospital personnel

D. Rickettsial diseases—caused by minute organisms with characteristics of both bacteria and viruses

1. Rocky Mountain spotted fever
   a. Transmitted by bite of infected tick
   b. Treatment is administration of chloramphenicol (Chloromycetin), chlortetracycline, and oxytetracycline
   c. Prophylaxis with *R. rickettsii* vaccine may be given to persons whose work requires them to be in infested areas

E. Protozoal disease

1. Malaria
   a. Caused by malaria protozoan
      (1) Disease is transmitted by bite of *Anopheles quadrimaculatus* mosquito
      (2) Incubation period is 12 to 14 days
   b. Treatment may be with quinine sulfate or with one of several new drugs

F. Venereal diseases—include syphilis, gonorrhea, lymphogranuloma venereum, chancroid, and granuloma inguinale

1. Syphilis
   a. Caused by *Treponema pallidum*
      (1) Disease is transmitted through sexual contact
      (2) Primary syphilis
      (3) Secondary syphilis
      (4) Latent syphilis
      (5) Congenital syphilis
      (6) Incubation period is from 10 to 90 days with average of 21 days
   b. Treatment is administration of penicillin

2. Gonorrhea
   a. Caused by *Neisseria gonorrhoeae* (gonococcus bacterium)
      (1) Disease is transmitted through sexual contact
      (2) Incubation period is from 3 to 5 days
   b. Treatment is administration of penicillin, minocycline, carbenicillin

3. Sociologic factors and trends
   a. There is alarming increase in incidence of infectious syphilis
   b. There is increased incidence of venereal disease in persons under 25 years of age
   c. Social factors related to venereal disease
      (1) Poverty
      (2) Poor housing
      (3) Low income
      (4) Ignorance
      (5) High mobility
      (6) Increase in use of alcohol
      (7) Breakdown in moral standards

Review questions

1. What four types of infectious agents cause infectious diseases?
   a. *bacterial*
   b. *viral*
   c. *Rickesttial*
   d. ~~venereal~~ *Protozoa*
2. What is the daily care of contaminated material called?
   a. *concurrent disinfection*
3. What diseases is the infant immunized for when he receives DTP?
   a. *diphtheria*
   b. *tetanus*
   c. *whooping cough - pertussis*
4. Why should gas gangrene be considered a dangerous disease?
   a. *often fatal*
5. At what age should a child be immunized for measles?
   a. *12 mo.*
6. Why should all young children be immunized against rubella?
   a. *to prevent infection - epidemic disease*
7. How are drugs used in the treatment of tuberculosis classified?
   a. *primary*
   b. *secondary*
8. If you were given an intradermal tuberculin test and the area of induration was 0 to 4 mm., what would this indicate?
   a. *negative reading*
9. What principle is involved in medical asepsis?
   a. *Isolation*
10. What is the difference between droplets and droplet nuclei?
    a. *droplets - from a cough or sneeze*
    b. *d.N - material suspended in the air.*

Films

1. A case against rubella (10 min., sound, color, 16 mm.), Smith, Kline & French Laboratories, 1500 Spring Garden St., Philadelphia, Pa. 19101. Reviews danger of rubella. Shows children with defects from rubella being treated and educated. The history of rubella is reviewed.

2. Life history of the Rocky Mountain wood-tick—M1716-X (18 min., sound, color, 16 mm.), Media Resources Branch, National Audiovisual Center (Annex), Station K, Atlanta, Ga. 30324. Reviews life-span of vector of Rocky Mountain spotted fever in the West.

3. Tuberculin tine test—Mis-973 (5 min., sound, color, 16 mm.), Media Resources Branch, National Audiovisual Center (Annex), Station K, Atlanta, Ga. 30324. Shows how to administer the tine test and how it may be included as part of a regular health checkup. Explains the technique of interpreting the test.

4. Tuberculin testing, part 2, administration techniques—M-1017 (6 min., sound, color, 16 mm.), Media Resources Branch, National Audiovisual Center (Annex), Station K, Atlanta, Ga. 30324. Shows the equipment and technique of the Mantoux tuberculin test.

References

1. Alexander, Stewart, Braxton, Olivia, Curry, Eleanor, and Besmond, Marie: Caring for the tuberculous patient, Part 1, The Journal of Practical Nursing 21:22-26, Jan., 1971.
2. Alexander, Stewart, Braxton, Olivia, Curry, Eleanor, and Besmond, Marie: Caring for the tuberculous patient, Part 2, The Journal of Practical Nursing 21:22-26, Feb., 1971.
3. Beeson, Paul B., and McDermott, Walsh, editors: Cecil-Loeb textbook of medicine, ed. 13, Philadelphia, 1973, W. B. Saunders Co.
4. Diagnostic standards and classification of tuberculosis, New York, 1969, American Lung Association.
5. Garner, Julia S., and Kaiser, Allen B.: How often is isolation needed? American Journal of Nursing 72:733-737, April, 1972.
6. Giesbrecht, Edith: Infectious mononucleosis —the kissing disease, The Canadian Nurse 68: 37-40, Feb., 1972.
7. Gosselin, Marie: Tuberculosis: why cling to isolation practices? The Journal of Practical Nursing 22:22-25, March, 1972.
8. Lenz, Philomene E.: Women, the unwitting carriers of gonorrhea, American Journal of Nursing 71:716-719, April, 1971.
9. McInnes, Mary Elizabeth: Essentials of communicable disease, ed. 2, St. Louis, 1975, The C. V. Mosby Co.
10. Morbidity and mortality weekly report, week ending Feb. 20, Atlanta, 1971, Center for Disease Control.
11. Morbidity and mortality weekly report; collected recommendations of the Public Health Service Advisory Committee on Immunization Practices, Atlanta, 1972, Center for Disease Control.
12. Morbidity and mortality weekly report, week ending May 26, Atlanta, 1973, Center for Disease Control.
13. Morbidity and mortality weekly report, annual supplement summary 1974, reported incidence of notifiable diseases in the United States, 1974, Atlanta, 1974, Center for Disease Control.
14. Morbidity and mortality weekly report, week ending Sept. 1, Atlanta, 1973, Center for Disease Control.
15. Morbidity and mortality weekly report, week ending Sept. 29, Atlanta, 1973, Center for Disease Control.
16. Morbidity and mortality weekly report, week ending June 28, Atlanta, 1975, Center for Disease Control.
17. Morbidity and mortality weekly report, week ending July 12, Atlanta, 1975, Center for Disease Control.
17a. Morbidity and mortality weekly report, week ending Feb. 15, Atlanta, 1975, Center for Disease Control.
18. Morbidity and mortality weekly report, week ending Nov. 1, Atlanta, 1975, Center for Disease Control.
19. Nelson, Morton: Carbenicillin in the treatment of gonorrhea in males, Health Services Reports 87:762-764, Oct., 1972.
20. Reid, Winifred M.: Congenital rubella—one approach to prevention, The Canadian Nurse 67:38-40, Jan., 1971.
21. Resistance of body to reinfection with tuberculosis, Health Services Reports 88:681, Aug.-Sept., 1973.
22. Wilson, Vernon E.: New era in VD control, Health Services Reports 87:392-393, May, 1972.

CHAPTER 24

The nurse in first aid, emergency, and disaster

KEY WORDS

abuse
addiction
cannulation
drug dependency
emergency
flashback
ghetto - *slum*
hallucinogenic
hashish - *drug*
illicit *illegal*

lysergic acid diethyla-
    mide (LSD)
marihuana (Cannabis
    sativa)
mescaline
methadone
opiates
psilocybin
withdrawal

ACCIDENT PREVENTION

The prevention of accidents is the responsibility of every citizen, whether in the home, on the farm, at the lake, on the highway, or in the hospital. Most accidents result from human error, carelessness, or indifference. Children are often the innocent victims of poisoning, which claims several hundred lives each year. Nearly all such poisonings occur in the home, with the accidental ingestion of drugs, particularly aspirin, a major cause of death. Household cleaning aids, insecticides, and cosmetic preparations are only a few of the possible dangerous products found in the home. There is no known antidote for many of the new poisonous products being developed. It must be remembered that children are curious and will climb to reach their objective. The practice of putting bleach preparations such as Clorox into soft drink bottles is an invitation to young children. It is estimated that 75% of poisoning caused by drugs and household aids is the result of leaving such substances in sight and reach of children and that three of every four poisonings are due to parental carelessness and negligence.

The "old swimming hole" still exists in some places, but it mostly has been replaced by private and public swimming pools. In recent years the emphasis on water sports has led to increased boating and swimming activities and therefore an increase in accidental drownings.

All types of motorized or pedaled equipment are potential hazards. Whole families may be wiped out in a few seconds on the highway. Farm tractors, bicycles, motorized bikes, and lawn mowers are a few examples of machines that take thousands of lives each year.

Falls in the home due to scatter rugs and rickety stepladders are common. Grease fires, smoking in bed, electricity, or lighted burners may result in painful and fatal burns.

Every person must assume a fair share of responsibility in helping to prevent and reduce accidents. Some precautions that should be taken include the following:

1. Find out if there is a poison control center in your community. Write the telephone number on a slip of paper and attach it to the medicine cabinet or the telephone, along with the telephone number of your physician.
2. Read the label on all household aids. The Federal Hazardous Substance Act of 1960 requires that products used about the home carry information to protect and warn users. Poisonous substances must also carry a warning to keep the product out of reach of children.
3. Keep all medicines in a locked cabinet. Dispose of all unused medicines by flushing them down the toilet. Do not place them in the trash can. Keep all medicines separate from other products. Always turn on the light when taking or giving a medication. Never take a drug from the cabinet in the dark.
4. Do not place dangerous laundry or cleaning agents in bottles or cups. Keep them in their original containers.
5. Avoid taking any medication in the presence of children. If interrupted while in the process of taking a drug, take the bottle with you or place it out of the reach of children. Do not leave drugs such as aspirin on bedtables or lying about the room.
6. When administering a medication to a child, do not offer bribes, refer to it as candy, or play games. Administer any medication as a serious procedure.[1]
7. Do not drive any motorized vehicle while under the influence of alcohol or tranquilizing drugs that may cause drowsiness or if extremely fatigued or under severe emotional stress. Keep the vehicle at a safe speed, watch highway signs, and obey them.
8. Do not permit children to ride bicycles two on a bike, avoid allowing children to ride after dark, and be sure the bicycle fits the child.
9. Attach a reflectorized tag to children's coat zippers and see that they are worn at night as recommended by the American Academy of Pediatrics.
10. Avoid smoking in bed or using matches to hunt in closets or other dark places. Never touch appliances with wet hands, and replace all damaged or worn electric cords.
11. Be certain that all burners are turned off when not in use and that room heaters are turned off at night and are in proper working condition. Remember that fumes may be fatal. Keep a carbon dioxide fire extinguisher near the stove to smother fires. Plan the easiest escape route from your home in case a fire should occur.[8]

STATISTICS

During 1974 there were 106,000 accidental deaths in the United States. This was approximately 11,000 less than in 1973. Most of the decrease came from a decrease in motor vehicle accidents. Catastrophic accidents in which five persons or more lost their lives accounted for 1,150 deaths, slightly higher than in 1973.[2]

FIRST AID IN THE HOME

Medicine cabinet. The medicine cabinet may be a wall type and should be placed in an accessible location where there is good lighting. Most new homes constructed today do not make provision for medicine cabinets. Any type of cabinet should be locked, and this is especially important if bathroom or kitchen cabinets are used. It is important to remember that a child may climb onto a kitchen counter to reach a cabinet. The following is a suggested list of supplies that may be kept in the home medicine cabinet:

1 box table salt or 10-grain sodium chloride tablets
1 box baking soda or 5-grain sodium bicarbonate tablets
4 2-inch roller gauze bandage
4 1-inch roller gauze bandage
1 box assorted Band-Aids

4 2 × 2 sterile gauze pads
4 4 × 4 sterile gauze pads
1 roll 2-inch adhesive tape
2 triangular bandages
1 box absorbent cotton balls
1 box cotton swabs
Soap for cleansing such as pHisoHex
2 to 4 ounces antiseptic—tincture of thimerosal (Merthiolate) or 1:1000 benzalkonium chloride (Zephiran chloride) solution
2 ounces aromatic spirits of ammonia
6 large safety pins
1 medicine glass
1 medicine dropper
1 pair of tweezers
1 set measuring spoons
12 wooden tongue blades—one padded for mouth gag
Paper cups
Flashlight with extra batteries

Small injuries occur in every home. Most involve minor cuts, abrasions, scratches, bruises, scuff burns, and burns. Children are the usual victims of these injuries, which occur during play. Treatment includes tender loving care by the parent to support the child's emotional reaction to the injury and treatment of the injury to prevent infection.

Abrasions, scuff burns, scratches. The objective is to prevent infection. Cleanse the wound with soap and water or pHisoHex, apply tincture of thimerosal (Merthiolate), and cover with a sterile Band-Aid.

Minor cuts. The objective is to control bleeding and prevent infection. If the cut is on an extremity, elevate it. Cleanse the area and apply a sterile Band-Aid snugly. If bleeding continues, apply pressure.

Minor burns. The objective is to relieve pain and prevent tissue damage. Cool the wound by placing in cold water or apply cold compresses until pain is relieved. Do not cover.

Bruises. The objective is to prevent edema. Apply cold or iced compresses to constrict blood vessels, and elevate the part.

Foreign body in eye. The objective is to prevent injury to the cornea and conjunctiva. Hold the lids apart and flush with cool water. If the foreign body is under the lower lid, pull the lid down and remove the foreign body with a cotton swab. If the foreign body is under the upper lid, evert it, and remove the object with a cotton swab. If the object is not easily removed, secure medical care.

Puncture wounds. The objective is to prevent infection. All puncture wounds are potentially dangerous. Cleanse with soap and water, apply a sterile Band-Aid, and secure medical care.

Animal bites. The objective is to prevent infection. All animal bites are potentially infective. Wash with soap and water, apply a sterile dressing, and secure medical care. Report the incident to the local health department.

Insect stings. The objective is to relieve pain. If the stinger is left in the skin, remove it with tweezers. Pain may be reduced by applying a 10% solution of household ammonia. Watch for signs of hypersensitivity and secure immediate medical care.

Fainting. If the fainting is transitory, the objective is to return the person to consciousness; if it is habitual, secure medical care. Keep the person lying down, moisten a cotton ball with aromatic spirits of ammonia, and hold near nostrils. One teaspoonful of aromatic spirits of ammonia in 1 ounce of cool water may be given to the patient to drink if he is conscious. Do not attempt to give the mixture to an unconscious patient.

Convulsions. The objective is to prevent injury. Keep the person lying down, place a padded tongue blade between his teeth prior to onset of the seizure, and secure medical care.

Poisons. Different poisons require different antidotes. In every case immediate medical care should be secured. If the ingested material is known, call the poison control center for instructions. Always take the containers or bottle to the physician or hospital with the patient.

Heat stroke. Move the patient to a cool place, apply iced compresses, and sponge the body with alcohol. Medical treatment is necessary. Call a physician or ambulance and transport the patient to the hospital.

Heat exhaustion. Move the patient to a cool place. If the pulse is weak, give the patient strong black coffee. If weakness develops, call the physician or take the patient to the hospital.

Snake bite. Apply a tourniquet about 2 inches above the bite just tight enough to prevent venous return partially. Make cross cuts through the fang marks and apply suction. Keep the patient quiet. The tourniquet should be loosened every 15 to 20 minutes for 1 to 2 minutes. Take the patient to a physician or hospital immediately. Continue first-aid treatment while en route.

To avoid delay it is suggested that the telephone number of the poison control center and the physician be placed on the door of the medicine cabinet and if possible on the telephone.

EMERGENCY DEPARTMENT

During the past decade emergency care has been undergoing many changes. Some states have enacted legislation establishing standards for equipping ambulances and training ambulance personnel to provide emergency care at the scene of an accident or serious illness. Emergency departments are caring for an increasing number of persons, estimated to be increasing between 5% and 10% each year. Special training and practice programs for all hospital personnel are being initiated to prepare them to operate efficiently during any major emergency.

Nurses are assigned to the emergency department with increasing frequency. In many instances the outpatient clinic is now part of the emergency department. It has been reported that one third of persons seen in the emergency department during 1969 were outpatients.[15, 18] Many of these patients have minor or major medical and/or surgical conditions requiring emergency care. Some will be admitted to the hospital for observation or further care, whereas others will be treated and returned to their homes.

In large medical centers it may be expected that a physician will be in residence. Some hospitals will have a physician on call, and in some rural hospitals there may not be a physician readily available. The nurse may be responsible for saving a life, but to do so it is necessary to recognize the extent of the emergency and the indications for initiating life-saving measures. The nurse must be able to differentiate between minor and major emergencies or illnesses and to understand that what appears to be a minor complaint may actually foretell a serious complication because of an underlying disease or condition.[19] The nurse should carefully secure the patient's history and review the complaint. Special attention

should be given to infants, young children, and elderly persons. Vital signs are often a guide in determining illness. The often-heard expression that "he looks sick" may be a clue to illness. When a patient looks sick, invariably he is sick.[9]

The care that the nurse may give in the emergency department should be carefully defined in written hospital policies. Consideration must be given to the availability of a physician, and when there is no resident physician, one who is on call should be reached.

Although the nurse in the emergency department will care for a variety of patients with minor conditions, there will be many with serious injuries or illnesses. The basic principles are the same for each individual: (1) to reduce suffering, (2) to save life, (3) to prevent worsening of the condition until medical care can be secured, and (4) to provide emotional support for the patient and his family.[4]

Airway. Many patients will be in respiratory difficulty, and the first consideration is to restore breathing. This may be accomplished in some cases by removing foreign material from the mouth with a piece of gauze wrapped about the finger, grasping the tongue and pulling it forward, and pushing the lower jaw upward and forward. If this fails, artificial respiration should be started. Dentures should be removed and mouth-to-mouth resuscitation started (Fig. 24-1). In the hospital, oxygen may be administered when the airway is clear of foreign material or objects. (See Chapter 11.)

Efforts should be made to determine whether the heart is beating. If no pulse can be felt and a heartbeat cannot be heard by placing the ear directly over the apex of the heart, closed-chest cardiac massage may be done by the physician or a person trained in the technique (Fig. 13-2).

Cardiac arrest is an acute emergency and requires immediate treatment. A physician is not always available. In many places training programs have been established to train nurses and ambulance attendants in the technique of closed-chest cardiac massage (Fig. 13-2). The patient with cardiac arrest should not be turned to the side for drainage of secretions. Since the restoration of cardiac function must be accom-

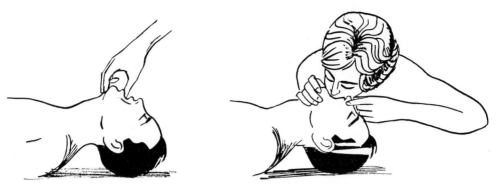

Fig. 24-1. Mouth-to-mouth resuscitation.

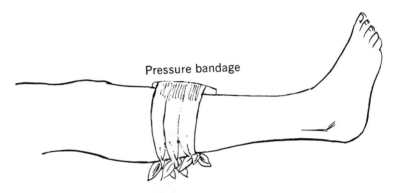

Pressure bandage

Fig. 24-2. A sterile dressing and pressure bandage will control most bleeding.

plished quickly to prevent cerebral damage, the nurse should endeavor to master the technique of closed-chest cardiac massage. Until trained, the nurse should not undertake the procedure (p. 259).

Bleeding. The nurse may realize that the control of bleeding is sometimes given precedence over respiration. It must also be realized that the patient cannot live without oxygen, but blood can be replaced. Each situation must be evaluated quickly in relation to the amount of bleeding and the immediate necessity to relieve respiratory distress. Most bleeding can be relieved by direct pressure at the site of the bleeding. The nurse in the hospital or physician's office may cover the wound with a sterile dressing and apply a pressure bandage (Fig. 24-2). A properly applied pressure dressing makes the use of a tourniquet rarely necessary. The use of a tourniquet, although saving a life, may result in the loss of a limb, whereas careful and proper

handling of bleeding may save both the life and the limb.

The patient in the hospital may suffer severe bleeding from the stomach, lungs, or uterus. A hemorrhage may occur after amputation of an extremity or any surgical procedure. In each case an emergency is created, and the life of the patient may depend on the nurse knowing what to do at the exact moment. These situations have been covered in the appropriate chapters.

Shock. Shock may be caused by hemorrhage, fractures, and severe wounds. The signs of shock and nursing responsibilities have been discussed in Chapter 9. When an emergency occurs outside the hospital and signs of shock are present, the accident victim should be kept lying down and warm, and injuries such as bleeding should be controlled, and attention should be given to wounds and fractures. In severe injury an ambulance should always be called. The accident victim should never

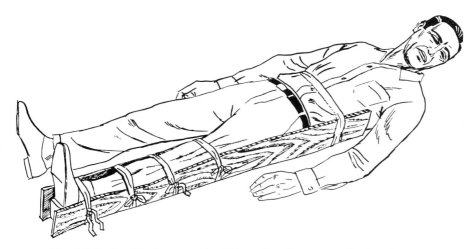

Fig. 24-3. Possible fractures should be splinted to prevent further damage.

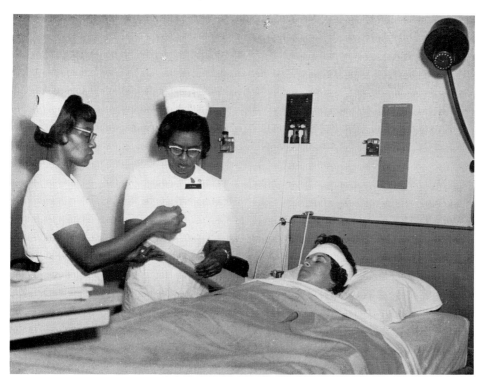

Fig. 24-4. Nurses applying a splint to a patient's injured arm. (Courtesy Medical Center, Columbus, Ga.)

be placed in an automobile to be taken to the hospital. Most ambulance personnel are trained in emergency care and proper handling, and the ambulance carries equipment to support life until the person reaches the hospital. In some areas work is being done with the use of helicopters to transport victims, particularly highway accident victims, to the hospital.

Fractures and wounds. The nurse has learned in first-aid courses how to apply splints to possible fractures to prevent further damage and to help relieve pain (Figs. 24-3 and 24-4). When a fracture has occurred, there may be other injuries such as lacerations or possible internal injuries, and the patient may be in shock. The patient should always be kept lying down and warm until an ambulance arrives. Persons with possible fractures of the spine or the head must be handled extremely carefully (Chapter 18). When there is possible injury to the cervical spine, the head must be held with slight traction applied when moving the patient in an effort to prevent damage to the spinal cord. The patient should not be turned to the side for drainage of secretions. Wounds may be minor such as scratches and abrasions, or they may be massive, including the chest or abdomen. If the wound is on an extremity, elevating the affected part helps to control bleeding. All wounds should be covered with a sterile dressing; if sterile dressings

are not available, the wound should be covered with any clean material (Fig. 24-5).

Identification. Persons who are victims of accidental injuries may not always be conscious. Accident victims may have diabetes or epilepsy, or they may be taking steroids or anticoagulant drugs. If these facts are not known, the person's life may be seriously jeopardized. Therefore the nurse should always look for some identification such as a Medic Alert emblem, card, or other device that may provide information. The Medic Alert Foundation* maintains a central file that gives detailed information about everyone enrolled in the program. If the person is wearing a Medic Alert emblem and is unconscious, a collect call may be made any time of the day or night to the foundation and identifying information obtained.[7] The nurse should look for contact lenses; if there is evidence that they are still in the eye, a strip of adhesive tape should be attached to the forehead with the words "contact lens" printed on it (Fig. 19-3).

Air pollution. Air pollution may create emergency situations for patients with chronic pulmonary disease such as emphysema or chronic cardiovascular disease when the atmospheric index of pollutants

*Turlock, Calif. 95380.

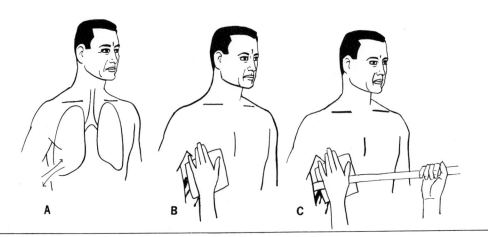

Fig. 24-5. Sucking types of chest wounds should be closed to prevent collapse of the lung. **A,** Air enters the chest cavity. **B,** Apply sterile dressing over the wound. **C,** Pull edges of wound together and fasten with wide strips of adhesive tape.

is high. The patient may be admitted to the emergency department because of acute symptoms. The nursing care is essentially the same as that outlined for these conditions in other chapters of this book. However, in emergency respiratory care a tracheotomy may be required. A respirator may be necessary to assist the patient with pulmonary ventilation. Patients with chronic respiratory or cardiac disorders may suffer an exacerbation of the disorder when the air pollution index is high. These patients should be advised as follows:

1. Remain indoors with windows closed and, if possible, use some form of air-conditioning or air-filtering device.
2. Avoid smoking or any activity that would raise dust such as dusting, vacuuming, using a fireplace, or remaining in a room where others are smoking.
3. Avoid overexertion, exposure to cold, or exposure to any substance known to cause allergic reactions.
4. Take medication early before symptoms have become established, or call a physician for instructions.

HOSPITAL ACCIDENTS

Most accidents occurring in the hospital are caused by falls, fires, or errors in the administration of drugs. Although the hospital is generally a safe place, under certain conditions it may present hazards. It should be remembered that hospital accidents may result in lengthy litigations, and the nurse may be involved. Falls are frequent causes of accidents. When floors are highly waxed and polished, they become dangerous for ambulatory patients, visitors, and personnel. Anything spilled on floors should be cleaned up immediately to prevent slipping. Side rails should be placed on the bed for all elderly patients to prevent them from falling out of bed. High-low beds for elderly persons should be kept low except when giving nursing care.

Fires may be caused by smoking in bed. The sedated patient may fall asleep with a lighted cigarette in his hand. When administering a sedative to the patient, the nurse should encourage him not to smoke unless someone is staying with him. It is always well to recheck the patient after the sedative has been given.

When an error occurs in administering a drug, it may be serious or even fatal. Nurses who administer medications should remember the basic principles that they have been taught concerning reading directions and measuring drugs. If an error does occur, it should be admitted and reported immediately. The nurse should also be alert for medications that the patient may bring to the hospital from home and keep at his bedside. An explanation should be made to the patient and such drugs sent home with a member of the family unless the physician approves their use in the hospital.

Explosive gases are used throughout the hospital, and care should be exercised in their use; the nurse should realize their potential danger.

Because of technology, a whole new area of hospital accidents now exists. They involve the use of equipment such as electrocardiac monitoring devices, defibrillators, electric beds, pacemakers, and other electrically operated equipment. It has been reported that 1200 persons are electrocuted in hospitals annually. If nurses understood the hazards associated with electrical equipment, much of this loss could be prevented. The nurse should be alert to any malfunction in the cardiac monitoring system, such as poor electrocardiographic tracings or failure of the alarm system to operate properly. Electrically operated beds should not be used in units where other electronic equipment is in use. When disconnecting equipment, the nurse should grasp the plug at the outlet to remove and avoid pulling on the cord. All plugs and outlets should be of the three-way type. The nurse should watch for any damaged cord or overheating, which may be detected if the cord or plug feels hot to the touch or if there is an odor of burning. The slightest malfunction should be reported at once.[20]

The team. When an emergency patient arrives in the hospital, his care may require the services of many persons. The team may consist of physicians, nurses, laboratory technicians, x-ray technicians, an anesthesiologist, social workers, and often many other workers in the health field. Other persons who are not specifically a part of the health service may also be included. The nurse who has learned to give good care to medical and surgical patients may be a valuable member of the team. The responsibilities of the nurse will vary with each situation, the number of emergencies, the available professional personnel, and the policies of each institution. In many small rural hospitals the physician and nurse may comprise the team.

Most of the activities of the nurse will include procedures learned in basic nursing and medical-surgical nursing. The nurse may carry out various procedures under the direction of the physician, including catheterization, injection of tetanus toxoid, skin testing, lavage, and administration of antibiotics, analgesic drugs for pain, oxygen, and antidotes for poisoning. The nurse may assist the physician in securing supplies and equipment, applying a plaster cast, setting up sterile tables, or assisting the physician with minor surgical procedures such as caring for lacerations. The nurse must remember not to administer any injection or medication except under the specific order of the physician. In emergency situations it may not always be possible to write orders before they are carried out, and care must be exercised in carrying out verbal orders. The nurse assisting with emergency nursing must recognize the importance of maintaining records, since legal aspects are often involved, especially in motor vehicle accidents. The nurse should also be familiar with the policies of the hospital concerning the care of the dead. The nurse should be aware that many persons such as law enforcement officials, newsmen, the family, and curiosity seekers may be asking for information. The nurse should be courteous but refer all questions to the physician.

DISASTER NURSING

Kinds of disaster. In this atomic age most people think of disaster as bombing by nuclear weapons. Few realize that disaster and destruction occur almost daily throughout the land as the result of fires, tornados, hurricanes, water accidents, floods, transportation mishaps, and explosions.

Kinds of injuries. Most casualties from disaster will be surgical in nature, and the nursing care will be largely the same as that given to any surgical patient. There will be all kinds of contusions, lacerations, fractures, often multiple, crushing injuries, burns, and severe hemorrhage from wounds. Many patients will be suffering from shock, and persons uninjured physically will be suffering from psychologic shock. In addition, a large group of curious onlookers who feel they must know what is going on are always present.

Disaster nursing differs from emergency nursing only in the number of persons who must be cared for. Every effort should be made to protect the individual from further injury and infection, but in the care of mass casualties the precise techniques that the nurse has learned may require considerable modification.

In many communities the Office of Civil Defense has organized community agencies to provide various services. Agencies often involved include the fire and police departments, the Red Cross, Salvation Army, Department of Family and Children Services, Public Health Department, hospitals, clinics, and other agencies. In many disasters the local hospital and medical facilities are adequate for the emergency. However, emergency first-aid centers may be established in schools or churches to care for those with minor injuries and to refer those suffering from more serious injuries to the hospital. If the disaster has caused many deaths, a temporary morgue may have to be set up.

The nurse in the community. The nurse may assist in various community activities when a disaster occurs. Centers are often established to immunize large numbers of persons when water supplies have been contaminated. Temporary shelters to house, feed, and care for large numbers of persons may be set up in various types of buildings. The shelter may have infants, young children, and elderly persons. The nurse needs to understand the anxiety and concern of families who may have lost all of their material possessions or their grief over the fate of a missing family member. When large numbers of persons are crowded together in shelters, there may be health problems. The nurse should be careful to check for respiratory infections, diarrhea, or elevation of temperature. Such persons should be referred for medical care, and in some instances it may be necessary to provide for temporary isolation. The nurse should be familiar with persons receiving regular medication for conditions such as cardiac or respiratory disease and make certain that their medication is available. It is necessary to remain calm and reassuring and to cooperate with social workers and community agencies that are working to restore normal family living.

DRUG DEPENDENCY

The nurse will encounter patients who have drug problems of varying degrees. These persons will be seen in the emergency department, in clinical units of the hospital, in mental health centers, in drug treatment centers, and in psychiatric units. A differentiation is sometimes made between the person who becomes dependent on a drug that is taken frequently or regularly and the individual who uses drugs continuously and has serious withdrawal symptoms when the drug is discontinued. The terms *dependency* and *addiction* are frequently used interchangeably. It has been suggested that *drug dependency* is a more accurate term to use.[11] Drugs have an important place in modern medicine, and without them thousands of persons would die every year. Most physicians prescribe drugs for legitimate purposes, but every year thousands of doses of drugs that are manufactured find their way into illicit channels. It has been reported that 50% of all amphetamines manufactured find their way into illicit channels.

Sociologic factors. Drug dependency is not new in this society. It has existed for hundreds and even thousands of years on this and other continents. History has recorded the smoking dens of some oriental societies where groups met and smoked opiate drugs. The sniffing parties of the early 1800s led to the eventual discovery of ether as an anesthetizing agent. In society today people have become dependent on alcohol, cigarettes, tranquilizers, and sleeping pills, and even the obese person who is a compulsive eater may be so dependent on food that he is unable to control the desire for food. It has been estimated that adults consume 20 tons of aspirin every day and that every person in this society receives sixty doses of a prescription drug annually.[10] In addition, it has been stated that 2.5 billion dollars are spent on over-the-counter drugs annually.[16]

The abuse of drugs is not confined to any particular segment of society. It may be found among all social, economic, and ethnic groups and among a wide range of age groups. One study found the median age to be 30 years with a range from 19 to 61 years of age[12]; other studies have found a large proportion of persons under 13 years of age. The incidence of drug dependency varies widely with geographic area and the number and kind of drugs used. Problems of drug dependency are frequently greater in large urban centers than in rural areas. Society has looked on drug dependency as a stigma and has associated it with the ghetto and certain segments of society. Attitudes are changing, and people are beginning to focus attention on causal factors, education, prevention, and treatment.

Most states have laws prohibiting the sale, possession, and use of certain drugs. If a person violates the statutes and is apprehended, he may be sentenced to a prison term. An individual may be so dependent on drugs that he is led to commit serious crimes to secure money to purchase drugs.

Drug dependency usually affects the family. A mother may neglect her children and home responsibilities when under the influence of drugs. A father may be unable to secure employment if he is known to be using drugs. Young persons may run away from home, causing parental worry and concern. Some young people leave home and set up their own "pad," where they have freedom and independence of action. Drug dependency, as with alcohol dependency, may cause disintegration of the family and lead to separation and divorce.

Causes. Persons working with drug dependency problems agree that there is no single cause but that multiple factors are usually involved. Some of the factors that have been cited include (1) excessive or lax parental discipline, (2) permissiveness of modern society, (3) rebellion against established social standards, (4) social pressures to conform, (5) lack of self-esteem and self-confidence, and (6) curiosity leading to experimentation.[10] There are many other factors in society that may lead a person to drugs as an escape from reality or because of the inability to solve his problems.

Classification of drugs. Following is a major classification of most frequently abused drugs:

1. Opiates—derived from opium
   a. Heroin
   b. Codeine
   c. Morphine *downers*
2. Barbiturates—both short acting and long acting *uppers*
3. Amphetamines
4. Hallucinogenic drugs
   a. Lysergic acid diethylamide (LSD)
   b. Mescaline
   c. Psilocybin
5. Marihuana and hashish are classified as hallucinogens
6. Tranquilizers

A variety of other agents are used when major drugs are unavailable; solvents such as gasoline, glue, ether, chloroform, nail polish, lighter fluid, and benzene may be sniffed. Morning glory seeds and nutmeg are also used.[11] Recently a tranquilizing agent piperidine (PCP) used to put animals to sleep has been used as a substitute for cocaine and mescaline.[6]

Physiologic effects. The aforementioned drugs affect the central nervous system in varying ways. The opiates and barbiturates depress the central nervous system, whereas amphetamines stimulate the central nervous system. Tranquilizers are classified as minor and major drugs and act on both the central nervous system and the autonomic nervous system. Depressant drugs cause a feeling of contentment, relaxation, relief from anxiety, and calmness. The individual's response is so depressed that he feels no necessity to satisfy other biologic needs such as food. Therefore the person using heroin is usually malnourished and in general poor physical condition. Depressant drugs affect the cardiovascular system and the respiratory system. Pulse and respiration rates decrease, and motor activity decreases. If untreated, the person may lose consciousness with collapse of these systems.

A new nonbarbiturate called methaqualone (Quaalude, Sopor, Parest-400) is a tranquilizer and causes depressed vital signs. Is has rapid and long-lasting effects, and recent reports indicate that it is being used with heroin. When the availability of heroin is limited, methaqualone is combined with heroin, and the combined use increases the effectiveness of the heroin and delays the withdrawal syndrome.[5]

Amphetamines stimulate the central nervous system, and their action is primarily on the cerebral cortex. They cause the individual to be alert, fatigue will be relieved, there may be aggressiveness, and the person may be hyperactive, exhausting his normal reserve of energy. The exhilarated feeling and euphoria cause the individual to lose sleep and rest and to feel little need for food.

The hallucinogenic agents are mind-altering or mood-changing drugs. As with other drugs that are abused, they act on the central nervous system. They may cause a complete personality change. The individual experiences altered changes in colors and in auditory and gustatory senses. His behavior is irrational, and all hallucinogens may cause hallucinations and exhilaration or depression, and they may lead to psychic manifestations and suicidal or homicidal tendencies.

Marihuana (*Cannabis sativa*) and hashish are classed as hallucinogenic agents and act on the central nervous system. They depress the higher centers of the brain, and there is some evidence that they may have a mind-altering effect. Although considerable controversy surrounds the use of this drug, limited controlled research indicates that its use causes exhilaration and relaxation. It is believed that dependence is psychic and not physical but leads to antisocial behavior and may lead to the use of other drugs.[3, 17]

Withdrawal syndrome. Most of these drugs cause mild to serious symptoms when they are discontinued. Most symptoms begin with restlessness, increase in nasal and lacrimal secretion, weakness, vomiting, and diarrhea; there may be twitching, tremor, headache, and dizziness. Symptoms may progress to hypotension and cardiovascular collapse or respiratory arrest. The withdrawal symptoms from marihuana are usually less severe and of shorter duration than those from other drugs. Symptoms from barbiturate withdrawal may be serious, leading to confusion, convulsions, coma, and death.

Although use of the hallucinogen LSD is

not believed to result in withdrawal symptoms when it is discontinued, the important factor is its latent effect. After weeks or months the individual may have a recurrence of certain aspects of his original experience with the drug (flashback). If the person has completely discontinued the use of the drug, the frequency and intensity of the flashback may decrease with time.

Treatment. There is no specific treatment for drug dependency. The goal of any therapy program is psychosocial and vocational rehabilitation. Through mental health counseling and guidance and the desire of the individual to "kick the habit," it may be possible to assist him in forming new patterns of living.

A second approach is through drug therapy. Under controlled conditions a drug may be administered in decreasing doses, keeping the dosage just above the threshold of the withdrawal syndrome, until the drug is eventually completely discontinued. Persons using heroin may be treated with methadone (Dolophine), which is a synthetic narcotic analgesic agent. When it is administered to replace heroin, it blocks the desire for heroin. If the person takes heroin while receiving methadone, he will not experience the pleasurable effects of the heroin. Methadone will not cure heroin dependency, but it may enable the individual to function better in society and to benefit from psychosocial therapy.

Methadone is an addictive drug, and to prevent it from reaching illicit channels the federal government has recently established new regulations concerning its distribution and use.[14] Much more research is needed concerning the use of methadone. The present indications are that some individuals may be rehabilitated and withdrawn from the drug, whereas others may require it indefinitely.

Nursing care. The nurse's first contact with the drug-dependent patient may occur in the emergency department. The patient may have taken an overdose of heroin or barbiturates and may be dead on admission. He may appear to be asleep, in a stupor, or in a coma, depending on the extent of the overdose. Barbiturates are often used in a suicidal attempt and are most often involved in drug overdose. It is often necessary to act quickly to save

the patient's life. The nurse should monitor all vital signs promptly and give special attention to rate, depth, rhythm, and the presence of apnea and hypotension. The nurse should be ready to assist the physician in establishing adequate ventilation. Oxygen, an endotracheal catheter, and some type of mechanical ventilator should be available. A cutdown tray should be ready to provide for cannulation of a vein to provide a route for fluids and intravenous drugs. Blood specimens may be required for laboratory examination, central venous pressure, and electrocardiographic monitoring for cardiac rhythm and to assess and evaluate therapy and the state of the cardiovascular system. The patient is usually transferred to the intensive care unit, where the nurse may provide continuous monitoring of the patient's condition.

Patients may be seen in the emergency department in a state of acute anxiety, and suicidal or homicidal tendencies may be present that are caused by a hallucinogenic drug. The first responsibility of the nurse is to keep the patient from injuring himself or others. The patient is suspicious and may overreact to environmental stimuli. The nurse should be calm and reassuring, and if possible, the patient should be placed in a quiet area away from the noise and confusion of the department. Depending on the patient's condition and need for treatment, he may be transferred to the psychiatric unit.

The nurse may assist in the methadone treatment centers. In this capacity the nurse has the opportunity to assess the patient's reaction and tolerance to the drug. The nurse should be alert to signs of other illness such as hepatitis B and should be familiar with the withdrawal syndrome. The face-to-face contact with the person on a daily basis provides the opportunity for encouragement and friendliness. Nurses working with patients having drug dependency problems must examine their own feelings concerning the problem. The patient looks to nurses for sympathy and understanding, and a negative attitude on their part will cause rejection on the patient's part. Most persons with drug dependency problems know more about drugs than nurses, and this knowledge and understanding should be respected.[13] Nurses should never moralize, realizing that they cannot change the patient's behavior.

PSYCHOLOGIC CARE

Any emergency or disaster is a crisis situation for the persons involved. When the unexpected happens, most persons are shaken, frightened, and unsure of themselves. Each one will have his own way of reacting to the fear and anxiety created by the emergency. Some persons may demonstrate emotional types of behavior, whereas others may appear dazed and wander about helplessly. Parents may exhibit remorse and feelings of guilt when a child has been seriously injured. The nurse must be prepared to deal with all these behavior symptoms and to realize that the emotional care of the injured is just as important as the physical care. The nurse can do much to calm emotional behavior by applying knowledge with skill and self-confidence and maintaining a calm, collected attitude and efficient behavior. To provide reassurance to the patient and his family the nurse must recognize and believe in the true worth of the person and be able to convey to him that people really care what happens to him.

In major disasters it may be necessary to segregate emotionally disturbed persons to prevent their spreading panic among others. Often it is helpful to assign persons to tasks that make them feel useful and that will help channel their anxiety into more constructive behavior.

Summary outline

1. Accident prevention—responsibility of every citizen
   A. Causes of accidents
      1. Poisoning—drugs, household cleaning aids, insecticides, and cosmetic preparations
      2. Drowning
      3. Motorized and pedaled equipment
      4. Falls
      5. Fires
   B. Precautions to prevent accidents
      1. Check for poison control center in community
      2. Read labels on all household cleaning aids
      3. Keep medicine in locked cabinet
      4. Keep laundry and cleaning preparations in original container
      5. Avoid taking medicines in presence of children

      6. Administer medications to children as a serious matter
      7. Do not drive motorized vehicle if taking tranquilizers or alcohol, if fatigued, or if under emotional stress
      8. Do not permit children to ride double on bicycle
      9. Put reflectorized tag on zipper of children's coats
      10. Avoid smoking in bed
      11. Turn off burners and room heaters
      12. Keep carbon dioxide fire extinguisher near stove
      13. Plan escape route from home if fire should occur
2. Statistics
   A. Fatal accidents in 1974—106,000
      1. Catastrophic accidents resulting in death increased to 1,150 in 1974
3. First aid in the home
   A. Medicine cabinet
   B. First aid for minor injuries
      1. Abrasions, scuff burns, and scratches
      2. Minor cuts
      3. Minor burns
      4. Bruises
      5. Foreign body in eye
      6. Puncture wounds
      7. Animal bites
      8. Fainting
      9. Convulsions
      10. Poisons
      11. Heat stroke
      12. Heat exhaustion
      13. Snake bite
4. Emergency department
   A. Changes in emergency care
      1. Legislation
         a. Establishment of standards for equipping ambulances
         b. Training ambulance personnel
      2. Increase in number of persons cared for in emergency department
      3. Training and practice programs for all hospital personnel
      4. Outpatient care part of emergency department
      5. There may be resident physician, physician on call, or no physician available
      6. Nurse must assess each patient
         a. Secure history
         b. Review complaint
         c. Give special attention to infants, young children, and elderly
         d. Check vital signs
         e. Consider physical appearance of patient
      7. Defined written hospital policies
   B. Objectives
      1. Reduce suffering
      2. Save life
      3. Prevent worsening of condition
      4. Provide emotional care
   C. Priority of care
      1. Provide patent airway
      2. Control bleeding
      3. Care for or prevent shock
      4. Care for wounds and fractures

D. Identification
E. Air pollution
5. Hospital accidents
   A. Falls
   B. Fires
   C. Errors in drug administration
   D. Explosive gases
   E. Electrically operated equipment
      1. Electrocardiac monitoring devices
      2. Defibrillators
      3. Electric beds
      4. Pacemakers
      5. Nurse should be alert to slightest malfunction and report it immediately
   F. The team
6. Disaster nursing
   A. Kinds of disaster
   B. Kinds of injuries
   C. Civil Defense
   D. The nurse in the community
      1. Immunization centers
      2. Temporary shelters
         a. Understand anxiety and concern
         b. Observe for health problems
         c. Be familiar with persons needing regular medication
         d. Cooperate with social workers and community agencies
7. Drug dependency
   A. Drug addiction or drug dependency
   B. Sociologic factors
   C. Causes
   D. Classification of drugs
   E. Physiologic effects
   F. Withdrawal syndrome
   G. Treatment
   H. Nursing care
8. Psychologic care
   Emergency or disaster creates crisis situation
   A. Each person reacts differently to situation
   B. Nurse should apply knowledge with skill and self-confidence and maintain calm collected attitude and efficient behavior

Review questions

1. What drug is a major cause of poisoning in young children?
   a. *ASA*
2. List the four objectives of emergency care.
   a. *save lives*
   b. *reduce suffering*
   c. *prevent further injury*
   d. *provide emotional support*
3. List in the order of priority the principles of emergency care.
   a. *provide airway* A
   b. *control bleeding* B
   c. *prevent shock* C - (circulation)
   d. *care of wounds & fractures.*
4. How can most external bleeding be controlled?
   a. *direct pressure*
5. If you came on a highway accident and found a person with signs of shock, what could you do while waiting for an ambulance?
   a. *keep pt. warm & covered & lying down*
   b. *control bleeding*

6. If a disaster should occur, what are two areas of community service in which the nurse may assist?
   a. *immunization centers*
   b. *temporary shelter mngm*
7. List all of the groups of drugs that are most commonly abused.
   a. *opiates*
   b. *barbiturates*
   c. *amphetamines*
   d. *halucinogens*
   e. *marihuana*
   f. *tranquilizers*
8. What physiologic effect would you expect heroin to have?
   a. *CNS depressant*
9. What drug is being used to treat heroin dependency?
   a. *methadone*
10. What is the possible danger from this drug?
    a. *more addiction*

Films

1. Bridge to no place (22 min., sound, color, 16 mm.), secure through local Blue Shield Insurance Co. Presents an overview of drug addiction, who addicts are, methods of treatment, research, problem of imprisonment, and need to reform laws.
2. Narcotic deaths, part 1—T-1898-A (38 min., sound, black and white, 16 mm.), Media Resources Branch, National Audiovisual Center (Annex), Station K, Atlanta, Ga. 30324. Reviews narcotic deaths, drugs used, symptomatic changes, external and internal. Demonstrates devices involved in using narcotics. Pictures of victims of overdose and effects on veins and subcutaneous tissues.
3. No margin for error (30 min., sound, black and white, 16 mm.), Film Library, William S. Merrell Co., 1269 Gest St., Cincinnati, Ohio 45203. Presents case histories that deal with major causes of in-hospital liability actions such as mixup in patient identification, error in medication dosage, and loss of sponge during surgery.
4. The best care (30 min., sound, color, 16 mm.), Film Library, William S. Merrell Co., 1269 Gest St., Cincinnati, Ohio 45203. Film is designed to alert hospital personnel to steps necessary in accident prevention.
5. Marijuana—L.F.L. (34 min., sound, color, 16 mm.), Eli Lilly & Co., Audio-visual Film Library, Indianapolis, Ind. 46206. Examination of facts and claims about the use of marijuana.

References

1. Arena, J.: A physician advises on poison prevention, The Journal of Practical Nursing 17:34-35, May, 1967.
2. Accident death toll drops sharply in 1974, Statistical Bulletin 56:6-8, Jan., 1975, Metropolitan Life Insurance Co.
3. Bergersen, Betty S.: Pharmacology in nursing, ed. 13, St. Louis, 1976, The C. V. Mosby Co.
4. Brunner, Lillian S., and Suddarth, Doris S.:

Textbook of medical-surgical nursing, ed. 3, Philadelphia, 1975, J. B. Lippincott Co.

5. Distasio, Carol, and Nawrot, Marcia: Methaqualone, American Journal of Nursing **73:** 1922-1925, Nov., 1973.
6. Drug pushers sell LSD guised as artwork, Health Services Reports **87:**508-509, June-July, 1972.
7. Fish, Shirley A.: Medic Alert: it will speak when you can't, The Journal of Practical Nursing **20:**29-30, March, 1970.
8. Handle yourself with care, Washington, D.C., 1969, Government Printing Office.
9. Jackson, Edgar B.: In the screening clinic, American Journal of Nursing **72:**1398-1400, Aug., 1972.
10. Kaufman, Karl L.: Drug abuse—Who? Why? How? Bedside Nurse **4:**18-23, Dec., 1971.
11. Kaufman, Karl L., and Salerni, O. L.: Today's drugs of abuse, Bedside Nurse **4:**13-19, Sept., 1971.
12. Lucas, Warren C., Grupp, Stanley E., and Schmitt, Raymond L.: Single and multiple drug opiate users: addicts or nonaddicts? HSMHA Health Reports **87:**185-192, Feb., 1972.
13. Nelson, Karin: The nurse in a methadone maintenance program, American Journal of Nursing **73:**870-874, May, 1973.
14. New regulations for use of methadone in drug-addiction treatment, FDA Consumer **7:** 28, Feb., 1973.
15. O'Boyle, Catherine: A new era in emergency service, American Journal of Nursing **72:** 1392-1397, Aug., 1972.
16. Ray, Oakley S.: Drugs, society, and human behavior, St. Louis, 1972, The C. V. Mosby Co.
17. Rich, Joseph D.: Medical aspects of drug abuse, Bedside Nurse **5:**29-32, July, 1972.
18. Taubenhaus, Leon J.: Planning today's emergency department, American Journal of Nursing **72:**2050-2053, Nov., 1972.
19. Wagner, Mary M.: Assessment of patients with multiple injuries, American Journal of Nursing **72:**1822-1872, Oct., 1972.
20. Walker, Patricia H.: Detecting electrical hazards in the hospital, Nursing Care **6:**11-14, March, 1973.

Glossary

AARP American Association of Retired Persons.

abduction Movement of the extremity away from the midline of the body.

abortion Expulsion of the contents of the pregnant uterus before 20 weeks of gestation.

abscess A localized infection with an accumulation of pus.

abuse To use wrongly or excessively.

acceptance Approval or the willingness to accept.

acromegaly A chronic disease caused by an oversecretion of the growth hormone of the pituitary gland. In the adult it may be caused by a tumor.

acuity Clearness as in seeing sharply or clearly.

adaptation Modification to meet a new or changed situation.

addiction Term used interchangeably with dependency to describe the condition of a person who uses drugs continuously.

adduction Movement of the extremity toward the midline of the body.

adhesion Joining of two parts by an abnormal fibrous band.

ADL Activities of daily living.

aerobic Describes a pathogen that requires free oxygen to live.

aerosol A suspension of a drug that can be atomized into a fine spray for inhalation.

alienation A separation from others or estrangement from friends.

alkalosis A condition in which the alkalinity of the body is increased.

alkylating agent A drug such as nitrogen mustard and related compounds used in the treatment of cancer.

allergen Any substance to which some individuals react abnormally.

allergist A physician trained in the diagnosis and treatment of allergic diseases and disorders.

alopecia Loss of hair.

ambulation Not confined to bed; walking.

amenorrhea Absence of menses; normal before puberty and during pregnancy.

amputee A person who has lost one or more of his extremities.

anabolism A constructive process by which food is converted into living cells.

anaerobic Describes a pathogen that will not live in the presence of oxygen.

analgesic A drug that will relieve pain.

anaphylaxis An immediate reaction from sensitivity to a foreign protein.

anemia A blood disorder caused by a reduction of erythrocytes and hemoglobin.

anesthesia Administration of a substance that causes loss of bodily sensations.

anesthesiologist A physician trained in administering anesthesia.

aneurysm Dilation of blood vessel into a sac-like bulge.

anger An emotion that indicates agitation and and displeasure.

angina pectoris Paroxysms of pain caused by decreased blood supply to the myocardium.

anhidrosis Lack of sweating.

ankylosis Stiffening of a joint caused by infection or irritation, and the development of fibrous tissue in the joint.

anorexia Loss of appetite.

antibody An immune substance produced within the body in response to a specific antigen.

anticoagulant A drug that lengthens the prothrombin time and helps to prevent thrombosis and embolism.

antiemetic A drug that helps to control nausea and vomiting.

antigen A substance that causes the body to manufacture antibodies against it.

antihistamine A drug used in the treatment of allergic disorders and motion sickness.

antimetabolite An agent that is used primarily in treating leukemia in children.

antipruritic An agent that reduces fever and relieves itching.

antiseptic Any agent that retards the growth of bacteria.

antispasmodic A drug used to relieve spasms of smooth muscles.

antitoxin A serum that is used to combat the toxin produced by a microorganism.

anuria Failure of the kidneys to secrete urine.

aphasia Loss of the ability to speak.

apnea A temporary absence of breathing.

apoplexy Cerebrovascular accident.

appendicitis Acute inflammation of the appendix.

arrhythmia Any deviation from the normal rhythm of the heart beat.

arteriosclerosis Hardening of the arteries caused by the formation of fibrous (plaques) and loss of elasticity.

arthrodesis Surgical fusion of a joint in a functional position.

arthroplasty Plastic surgery on a diseased joint to increase mobility.

articulation Point at which two bones are joined together as in a joint.

Ascaris A genus of large roundworm similar to the earthworm.

ascites Accumulation of fluid in the peritoneal cavity.

asepsis A condition of freedom from pathogenic organisms.

asphyxia Suffocation caused by a decrease of oxygen and an increase of carbon dioxide.

asthma A chronic bronchial disease caused by spasm of the bronchial tubes accompanied by edema.

astigmatism A defect in the curvature of the cornea or the lens of the eye.

ataxia A lack of coordination of motor movements.

atelectasis Collapse of the lung; may be total or partial.

atherosclerosis a degenerative process of the blood vessels characterized by fatlike deposits along the walls of the vessels.

atopy Hypersensitivity to an antigen that is related to hereditary susceptibility.

atresia Narrowing or closure of a normal opening.

atrophic Wasting away of an organ or part of the body.

atrophy To waste away or decrease in size.

atropine An alkaloid of belladonna; may be administered with a narcotic as preoperative medication.

attenuate To weaken.

audiologist A person trained in the detection of hearing problems and the administration of hearing tests; advises persons in the use of hearing aids.

aura A visual sensation experienced by the epileptic person prior to having a seizure.

auricular fibrillation An arrhythmia of the atria characterized by rapid irregular rate of contraction.

autoclave An apparatus using steam and pressure to sterilize.

autogenous Made from within the body. A vaccine made from organisms taken from a person is an autogenous vaccine.

autograft Tissue taken from the same donor as the recipient.

autoimmunity A condition in which antibodies are produced by one's own body, causing immunization against the body's own proteins.

bacteremia Presence of bacteria in the bloodstream.

bacterial endocarditis Infection affecting the valves and the lining of the heart.

bactericidal Describes an agent that kills bacteria.

bacteriophage A virus that attacks bacteria.

bacteriostatic Describes an agent that prevents multiplication of bacteria.

bargaining A mutual agreement.

barium A silver white chemical agent used as a contrast medium in x-ray examination of the gastrointestinal tract.

basal metabolism A breathing test to determine the amount of oxygen used by the body in a fasting state at rest.

bath itch Disorder caused by dryness of the skin and causing severe itching.

bends Abdominal cramps caused by a rapid change from increased atmospheric pressure to normal pressure.

benign Describes a nonmalignant growth or tumor.

bereavement Deprivation, such as in loss by death.

bilateral On both sides.

biliary Relating to the gallbladder, liver, and their ducts.

biliary colic Acute pain caused by obstruction of the cystic duct, usually because of a stone.

biopsychosocial The interrelationship of physical, emotional, and social factors.

bleb An irregular elevation of the epidermis filled with serous fluid.

blood dyscrasias Diseases of the blood and the blood-forming organs.

body image Way in which a person views his body; may mean his acceptance in care of a deformity.

boil Cutaneous superficial infection of short duration.

braces Mechanical device used for support, usually of an extremity.

bradycardia A cardiac arrhythmia marked by an unusually slow heart beat.

bronchiectasis A chronic disease of the lungs in which there is a dilation of the bronchi; may affect both lungs or only a portion of one lung.

bronchitis An inflammatory condition of the bronchial tubes.

bronchography X-ray examination of the bronchi using a radiopaque substance.

bronchoscopy Examination of the bronchi and a portion of the lungs with a lighted instrument.

bursitis Acute or chronic inflammation of a bursa caused by injury, disease, or unknown factor.

calibrated Marked or graduated to provide for accurate measurement.

cannulation Procedure of placing a cannula into the body as into a vein.

capsule Mucilaginous envelope surrounding some forms of bacteria.

carbuncle A boil with infiltration into adjacent tissues finally opening in several places on the skin.

carcinogenic Anything capable of producing cancer.

carcinoma A malignant growth with a tendency to infiltrate or metastasize to other tissues.

cardiogenic shock Interference with pumping action of the heart causing insufficient vascular circulation.

cardiogram A tracing of the electrical activity of the heart.

cardiospasm A spasm of the cardiac valve between the esophagus and the stomach; generally a functional disorder.

carrier A person who harbors germs of a disease and transmits the disease to others while having no symptoms of the disease himself.

casualty A person injured in an accident that is usually fatal.

catabolism Destructive process by which complex substances are broken down into simpler ones; opposite of anabolism.

cataract An opacity of the lens or the capsule of the eye.

catastrophe A great or sudden disaster. Prolonged costly illness may be referred to as a catastrophic illness.

central venous pressure A measurement to determine the ability of the right side of the heart to receive and pump blood.

cerebral palsy A chronic neuromuscular disorder affecting motor coordination.

cerumen Secretion of the sebaceous glands of the external auditory canal.

chancre Lesion of primary syphilis occurring at the point of inoculation.

chemotherapy Treatment of disease with chemical drugs.

Cheyne-Stokes respiration Respiration in which the rhythm and depth vary with periods of apnea.

cholangiography X-ray examination of the biliary tree after injection of a radiopaque dye.

cholecystectomy Surgical removal of the gallbladder.

cholecystitis Inflammation of the gallbladder.

cholecystography X-ray examination of the gallbladder by use of a radiopaque dye to determine the shape and position of the organ.

cholelithiasis A condition in which calculi are present in the gallbladder or one of its ducts.

cholesterol A substance present in all body tissues and fluids. It may be increased and is thought to be a factor in the development of atherosclerosis.

chronic disease A disease involving structure or function or both and may be expected to continue over an extended period of time.

cilia Hairlike projections in nasal cavities, trachea, and bronchi.

CircOlectric A type of electrically operated bed that permits easy turning and moving of the patient.

circumvent To go around or to prevent.

cirrhosis Disease characterized by death of liver cells and their replacement by scar tissue.

climacteric Synonymous with menopause.

clonic Describes alternate contraction and relaxation of muscles.

coalesce To run together as in measles.

coccidioidomycosis A disease of the lungs caused by inhaling spores of fungi from the soil.

colectomy Surgical removal of part or all of the colon.

collagenase (ABC) ointment; found to be effective in the treatment of decubitus ulcers.

colostomy A surgical procedure for the purpose of providing an artificial passageway for fecal material from the colon to the outside.

coma A deep sleep from which the person cannot be aroused.

comedomes Blackheads.

communicable disease See *infectious disease.*

concurrent disinfection Daily handling and disposal of contaminated material or equipment.

concussion A violent shaking of the brain against the skull.

congenital Existing at birth.

conical Shaped like a cone.

conization A surgical procedure in which a cone-shaped piece of tissue is removed from the cervix.

conjunctivitis Inflammation of the conjunctiva of the eye.

contamination Soiling with any infectious material.

continuity Uninterrupted connection, succession, or union.

continuum Something that is continuous, the parts of which cannot be separated.

contracture A shortening or tension of a muscle that affects the extension.

contusion Bruise; black and blue spot caused by rupture of small blood vessels.

convulsion Involuntary contraction of voluntary muscles.

Coramine Trade name of a drug that acts on the central nervous system and results in stimulation of respiration.

corpuscles Synonymous with white blood cells.

coryza An acute upper respiratory infection; a common cold.

countertraction An opposing force or pulling in the opposite direction.

craniotomy A surgical opening of the cranium for exploration or removal of a tumor or blood clot.

cretinism A condition resulting from complete absence of the thyroid gland or its secretion at birth.

crisis A crucial point; an emergency in which the outcome may be in doubt.

crossinfection Transmission of an infection from one patient to another patient who is already ill with another disease.

crust A dry exudate, commonly called a scab.

cryoprecipitate A fraction of fresh blood plasma; used to control bleeding in hemophilia.

cryptorchism A condition of an undescended testicle.

culdoscopy A diagnostic procedure; an incision through the posterior cul-de-sac and inserting of a culdoscope to visualize the pelvic organs.

curettage A surgical procedure in which a cavity is scraped with an instrument called a curet.

cutdown Incision through the skin for the purpose of placing a needle or catheter into a vein.

cyanosis A bluish color of the skin caused by inadequate oxygenation of the blood.

cyst Saclike, nonmalignant tumor; may contain fluid or cheeselike material.

cystectomy Removal of the urinary bladder.

cystitis Inflammation of the urinary bladder.

cystocele Protrusion of the bladder into the vagina.

cystography X-ray examination of the urinary

bladder after injection of a radiopaque substance.

cystoscope Lighted instrument for examination of the inside of the urinary bladder.

cystostomy A surgical opening of the urinary bladder through an abdominal incision and drainage by a catheter through the abdominal wound.

cytologic Refers to the examination of the cells.

debridement Removal of infected or necrotic tissue from a wound.

decompression Reduction of pressure.

decubitus ulcers Necrotic ulcers caused by pressure over bones where there is little fat and subcutaneous tissue.

defibrillation Application of a current countershock to the chest wall to stop ventricular fibrillation.

degeneration Gradual deterioration of the normal cells and body functions.

dehiscence Separation of a surgical incision.

dehydration Loss of fluids from the tissues.

delirium A mental state in which there is a disturbance of cerebral function and disorientation occurs.

delirium tremens A form of alcoholic psychosis.

demineralization A decrease of mineral or inorganic salts that occurs in some diseases.

denial Refusal to accept a situation.

depilatory cream A preparation to remove hair from the body.

depression Feeling of inadequacy or sadness.

deprivation The loss or taking away, as of a loved one taken away by death.

dermatologist A physician trained in the diagnosis and treatment of skin diseases and disorders.

dermis True skin just below the epidermis.

dermatomycosis Superficial mycotic infections of the skin, hair, and nails.

desensitization Injection of extracts of antigenic substances causing immunization against specific antigens.

desquamation A scaling or flaking of the skin after certain infectious diseases or in psoriasis.

diabetic A person with diabetes caused by a deficiency of insulin being secreted by the islands of Langerhans.

dialysis Process of separating or removing certain substances from the blood when the kidneys fail to perform their normal function.

diaphoresis Excessive sweating.

diaphragmatic hernia Protrusion of an abnormal organ, usually the stomach, through the diaphragm into the thoracic cavity.

digitalization Administration of digitalis in doses sufficient to achieve the maximum physiologic effect without toxic symptoms.

dignity Feeling of worth.

diplopia A condition of the eye in which a person sees double.

disaster Any catastrophic occurrence that causes serious damage or injury to many persons.

disease Any condition in which either the physiologic or psychologic functions of the body deviate from what is considered to be normal.

disengagement Release or detachment of oneself from other persons or responsibilities.

disinfectant A chemical that when applied to inanimate objects will destroy microorganisms.

dislocation Separation of a bone in a joint from its normal position.

diuresis Increase in urinary output.

diuretic A drug used to increase urinary output.

donor A person who gives or furnishes blood, skin, or body organs for use by another person.

dorsiflexion A bending backward from a neutral position.

droplet nuclei Minute particles of infectious material that remain suspended in the air and are carried by air currents.

droplets Infectious material contained in the spray from coughing, sneezing, or talking.

drug dependency Continuous use of a drug and withdrawal symptoms if the drug is discontinued.

dwarfism Abnormal smallness of body caused by undersecretion of the growth hormone from the the anterior pituitary gland.

dyscrasias Diseases of the blood.

dysmenorrhea Painful menstruation.

dysphagia Difficulty in swallowing.

dyspnea Shortness of breath or difficult, labored breathing.

ecchymosis Large amount of bleeding into the tissues.

eclampsia A condition occurring in pregnancy characterized by convulsions, hypertension, and edema.

electrocardiogram Graphic recording of the electric potential resulting from the electric activity of the heart.

electroencephalograph Graphic recording of brain waves within the deep structures of the skull.

electrolytes Salts of various minerals that are in solution in the body.

embolectomy Surgical removal of a blood clot from a vein.

embolism Foreign substance in the bloodstream; may be fragment from a blood clot or an air bubble.

embryonic Pertaining to the embryo.

emergency A sudden, unexpected occurrence.

empyema Presence of pus in the pleural cavity.

endemic Describes the presence of a few cases of a disease in a community continuously.

endogenous From within.

endometriosis A disease caused by groups of cells growing in the pelvic cavity. The cells are similar to those of the uterine mucous membrane.

endotoxin A toxin that is released when the cell disintegrates.

enteritis Inflammation of the intestines.

enterotoxin A toxin contained in contaminated food that causes nausea, vomiting, and diarrhea; food infection.

enucleation Surgical removal of the eyeball.

enuresis Involuntary voiding of urine; bedwetting.

eosinophils Granular leukocytes. Number is increased during an allergic reaction.

epidemic Occurrence of a large number of cases of a disease in a specific area at a given time.

epidemiology Study of factors related to epidemics of disease, their control, and methods of spread.

epididymitis Inflammation of the epididymis.

epinephrine A hormone secreted by the adrenal medulla; prepared commercially as Adrenalin.

epispadias A congenital malformation in which the male urethra opens on the underside of the penis.

epistaxis Nosebleed.

erythema A redness of the skin.

erythroblastosis A congenital blood disease of the newborn in which there is a reaction of the Rh-negative antibodies of the mother with the Rh-positive antibodies of the infant.

erythrocytes Red blood cells.

erythropoiesis Production of erythrocytes.

eschar Slough of tissue resulting from a burn.

Escherichia coli A species of organism found in the intestinal tract of humans and animals.

esophagoscopy Examination of the esophagus by the use of the endoscope.

estrogen A hormone secreted by the ovaries.

ethylene oxide A gas used in sterilization of surgical supplies and equipment.

etiologic Describes the cause of diseases or disorders.

eustachian tube Tube connecting the middle ear with the pharynx.

euthanasia The intentional death of a person suffering from an incurable disease; mercy death.

evisceration Opening of a surgical incision permitting the viscera to protrude to the outside.

exacerbation Increase in the symptoms of the disease.

excoriation An abrasion or denuded area of the skin.

exfoliative cytology Microscopic study of cells that have been shed from the body.

exogenous From outside the body.

exotoxin A toxin or poison secreted by an organism.

expertise Skill and knowledge of a person by reason of special training.

external rotation Turning away of a limb from the midline of the body.

extracellular Applied to body fluid outside the cells.

extracorporeal Outside the body; used to describe a method of bypassing a patient's heart and lungs by using the heart-lung machine; used in open heart surgery.

extrasystole A form of cardiac arrhythmia in which heartbeats occur sooner than expected.

extrinsic Coming from the outside.

exudate Pus containing dead cells, phagocytes, bacteria, and tissue fluids.

filter A device for separating one substance from another.

fimbriated Demonstrating fingerlike projections at the end of the fallopian tubes.

fissure A crack or slit in the skin.

flaccid Limp; cannot be controlled.

flagella Hairlike projections extending from some bacterial cells making them capable of movement.

flashback A recurrence of a previous experience with a hallucinogenic agent.

flatulence Accumulation of gas in the intestinal tract.

flotation therapy Semiweightlessness produced by various types of equipment; used in prevention and treatment of decubitus ulcers.

fomite Any object or material that may hold or transmit pathogenic organisms.

frostbite Freezing caused by exposure to extreme cold.

fungi Microbes from the plant kingdom, of which there are many different kinds. Some are harmless and some cause disease.

fusion Joining together, as in joining two or more vertebrae to make solid and prevent motion.

gait A way of walking.

gamma globulin A protein substance obtained from human plasma; now called immunoglobulin.

gangrene Necrosis of tissue caused by cutting off the blood supply.

gas gangrene A serious infection caused by the gas bacillus; occurs in wounds such as compound fractures.

gastrectomy Partial or complete surgical removal of the stomach.

gastritis Inflammation of the stomach generally caused by ingestion of contaminated food.

gastroscopy A direct visualization of the stomach with a gastroscope.

genetic Pertaining to origin or inherited.

geriatrics A medical specialty dealing with problems of aging and the aged.

germicide An agent that destroys bacteria.

gerontology Study of the aged and aging.

ghetto An area in which ethnic or racial groups live.

gigantism Excessive growth of long bones caused by an oversecretion of the growth hormone from the anterior pituitary gland.

glaucoma An eye disease caused by increased intraocular pressure; may cause blindness if not treated.

glomerulonephritis A type of nephritis in which the glomerulus of the kidney is involved.

glycosuria Presence of sugar in the urine.

goiter Any abnormal enlargement of the thyroid gland.

gonads Sex glands; testes in the male and ovaries in the female.

gram negative Term used in identifying bacteria after staining with a dye. Color can be removed with a solvent.

gram positive Term used in identifying bacteria after staining with a dye. Color cannot be removed after staining.

granulocytes Leukocytes identified by shape of the nuclei and coloring of their cytoplasm. About 50% 70% of leukocytes are granulocytes.

grief Emotional suffering caused by loss.

gumma A tumorlike lesion that is similar in appearance to an abscess.

gynecology A medical specialty concerned with diseases and disorders of the female reproductive system.

habitat Natural environment where a plant or animal, including humans, resides.

hallucination A mental aberration based on seeing or hearing things that do not exist in reality.

hallucinogenic Describes an agent that causes changes in personality or causes hallucinations.

hashish A resinous mixture contained in the flowering tops of *Cannabis sativa* plant.

helminth A worm.

hematemesis Vomiting of blood.

hematocrit A measure of the volume of red blood cells and the plasma.

hematogenic shock A shock state caused by loss of blood or plasma internal or external.

hematuria Blood in the urine.

hemiplegia Paralysis affecting one side of the body.

hemodialysis Artificial method of removing urea and nitrogenous wastes from the blood when the kidneys fail to function normally.

hemoglobin electrophoresis A test used to identify various abnormal hemoglobins in the blood; may indicate genetic disorders such as sickle cell anemia.

hemophilia A group of hereditary bleeding disorders.

hemoptysis Hemorrhage that may be from the lungs, trachea, or larynx.

hemorrhoids Varicosities of the anal canal; may be internal or external.

hepatic coma Comatose condition caused by liver failure; believed to result from accumulation of nitrogenous substances in the blood, especially ammonia.

hepatitis Inflammation of the cells of the liver; two types—hepatitis A and hepatitis B.

herniorrhaphy Surgical repair of a hernia.

herpes simplex Cold sore or fever blister.

herpes zoster Shingles; caused by a virus that affects the nerve roots of the posterior ganglia; same virus that causes chicken pox.

heterograft Tissue taken from an animal or a species other than a human donor.

hiatus hernia Protrusion of a structure through the diaphragm about the esophageal opening.

high risk Applied to groups of persons considered to be more susceptible to infections or diseases than other individuals.

histoplasmosis A benign disease of the lungs caused by a fungus.

Hodgkin's disease A malignant disease affecting the lymph nodes; once considered highly fatal but is now being cured.

Homemaker service A service to provide assistance in the home for elderly or sick persons; federal program under the Older Americans Act.

homeostasis Relative stability of the normal environment of the human body.

homicide Killing of one individual by another.

homograft A graft taken from a person other than the recipient.

hormone A chemical substance secreted by an endocrine gland; some prepared commercially.

host An organism, which may be a human, from which another obtains its nourishment.

hydrocele A collection of fluid in the testicle.

hydrolysis Splitting of a compound into parts by adding water. In digestion, enzymes reduce large molecules into small particles so that they may be absorbed.

hydronephrosis Distention of the kidney pelvis with urine caused by an obstruction along the urinary route.

hyperalimentation A method of providing complete nutritional requirements by the intravenous route.

hyperbaric oxygen Oxygen at a pressure greater than atmospheric pressure.

hyperglycemia Increase above normal of the amount of glucose in the blood.

hyperopia Farsightedness.

hyperplasia Increased number of cells causing a part to be enlarged.

hypersensitivity An abnormal sensitivity to certain substances.

hypertension A consistent elevation of blood pressure above normal.

hypertrophic Enlargement of an organ that may or may not be due to disease.

hypnotic A drug that produces rest and sleep.

hypochromia Below normal color, as in a low index of the color of hemoglobin.

hypospadias Congenital malformation of the male urethra.

hypostatic pneumonia Pneumonia caused by a person's remaining in the same position for long periods of time.

hypothermia An adjunct to anesthesia produced by lowering the body temperature below normal. It may be local or general.

hypoxia A deficiency of oxygen in the tissues.

hysterectomy Surgical removal of the uterus; may be abdominal or vaginal; may be total or partial.

icterus index A test to measure the amount of yellowness in the blood serum.

ileal conduit Method of urinary diversion. Ureters are implanted into a section of the ileum and brought out through the abdomen as an ileostomy.

ileostomy A surgical procedure in which an artificial passage from the ileum to the outside of the abdomen is constructed.

illicit Unlawful.

immunity Resistance to a specific disease.

immunization Process of becoming immune to certain diseases; usually refers to injections to develop active acquired immunity.

immunoglobulins (Ig) Serum proteins that include several groups of globulins; formerly called gamma globulins.

immunologist A person trained in the science of immunity.

impetigo contagiosa Contagious skin disease.

incontinence Inability to retain urine in the bladder.

incubation period Time between exposure to a disease and the appearance of the first symptoms.

infectious disease A disease that may be transmitted from person to person either by direct or indirect contact.

infiltration Passing of fluid through, as when intravenous fluid passes into the tissues; usually caused by needle being displaced from the vein.

internal rotation Turning of limb toward the midline of the body.

intravenous therapy Administration of fluids and/ or drugs into the general circulation through a venipuncture.

intrinsic Coming from within.

intussusception Telescoping of the intestine; may involve any part of the small or large intestine.

iodophor An antiseptic or disinfectant agent that combines iodine with another agent, usually a detergent.

irreversible Permanent and cannot be changed.

ischemia A temporary interruption of the blood supply to any area causing anemia of the part affected.

isolation Separation of a sick person from a well person, usually when an infectious condition is present.

isometric exercise Exercise done by the patient in which he contracts and relaxes a muscle.

isotonic saline Saline solution that is compatible with the normal tissue by having the same osmotic pressure.

isotope A chemical element that has been made radioactive.

jaundice A condition in which a yellow color affects the skin and the sclera of the eyes caused by an accumulation of bile pigments in the blood.

keloid A benign overgrowth of fibrous tissue.

keratitis Inflammation of the cornea of the eye with formation of ulcers.

keratoplasty Synonymous with corneal transplant.

ketosis Presence of acetone or ketone bodies in the urine and occurs in diabetic acidosis.

Klebsiella aerogenes A species of bacteria that lives in the intestinal tract and may cause serious infections.

Koplik's spots White spots on a reddened base found in the throat in measles.

kyphosis Curvature of the spine backward causing what is called humpback.

labyrinthitis Inflammation of the labyrinth of the inner ear.

lacrimal fluid Tears secreted by the lacrimal glands.

lacrimation Increased secretion from the lacrimal glands.

laminectomy Surgical procedure for ruptured intervertebral disk or for fusion.

laparoscopy Examination of the interior of the abdomen with the laparoscope.

laparotomy Any surgical procedure for which the abdomen is opened.

laryngectomy Surgical procedure for the removal of the larynx.

lethargic Abnormally drowsy.

leukemia Serious and usually fatal disease of the blood.

leukocyte White blood cell.

leukocytosis Great increase in leukocytes occurring in many kinds of infections.

leukopenia A reduction in the number of leukocytes.

leukoplakia White spots formed on the mucous membrane of the mouth that may become malignant.

leukorrhea White or yellow vaginal discharge.

life-island A plastic bubble enclosing a bed that is used to provide a germ-free environment.

ligature Suture used in surgery to tie or ligate a blood vessel.

lithiasis Formation of stones or calculi.

litigation Lawsuit.

live attenuated vaccine A vaccine containing live organisms which have been weakened so that they will not cause disease.

living will A written agreement between a patient and the physician to withhold heroic measures if his condition is irreversible.

lobectomy Surgical removal of a lobe of a lung.

lordosis An abnormal inward curvature of the lumbar spine.

lumen Passageway within a tube such as the lumen of blood vessels.

lymph nodes Small structures of lymphatic tissue containing lymphocytes, the function of which is filtration and phagocytosis.

lymphangitis Inflammation of one or more lymph vessels.

lymphoma A malignant type of tumor.

lysergic acid (diethylamide) (LSD) A hallucinogenic agent causing changes in mood and personality.

lysis A gradual decrease of symptoms of a disease, also a laboratory procedure to indicate decomposing of an agent by another agent.

macrophage Large phagocyte cell that wanders about.

macule A discolored spot on the skin that may be of various colors and shapes. It is neither raised or depressed.

malaria A disease caused by a protozoan and transmitted by the *Anopheles* mosquito.

malformation Abnormal development of a part of the body.

malignant Describes a disease that is a threat to life, usually applied to cancer.

mammary gland Synonymous with the female breast.

mammography X-ray examination of the breast.

marihuana (*Cannabis sativa*) Same plant as hashish but contains less resin and is less psychoactive.

mastectomy Surgical removal of the breast; may be simple or radical.

mastitis Inflammation of the breast.

mastoiditis Inflammation of the cells of the mastoid process.

Meals-on-wheels Program designed to prepare food and take hot meals to elderly or physically handicapped persons.

mediastinum Space between the lungs that contains the heart.

Medicaid Federal- and state-supported program to provide hospital and medical care for certain eligible persons.

Medicare Federal program to provide hospital and medical care for persons 65 years of age or older.

menarche First menstruation occurring at the time of puberty.

meninges Membrane enclosing the brain and spinal cord.

meningitis Infection and inflammation of the meninges.

menopause Climacteric or the cessation of menses representing the end of the reproductive period.

menorrhagia Excessive menstrual flow either in quantity or duration.

mental retardation A condition in which there is an absence of normal mental growth and development.

mescaline Derivation of peyote cactus and classified as a hallucinogenic agent.

metabolism Sum of all processes that go on within the body, including the breaking-down and wearing-out processes and the regeneration and building-up processes.

metastasis Spreading of cancer cells by the bloodstream or lymph from one part to another part of the body.

Metazoa Multicellular animals.

methadone Synthetic narcotic analgesic agent used to replace heroin; considered addictive.

metrorrhagia Bleeding between regular menstrual periods.

microphage A phagocyte that ingests and carries away bacteria by the blood and lymph systems.

microscopic Describes microorganisms that may be observed only with the aid of the microscope.

micturition Urination.

miotic A drug that causes contraction of the pupil of the eye.

molecule Smallest particle of an element or compound.

monitor A device used to provide continuous checks on the physiologic condition of the patient.

mononucleosis An infectious disease characterized by swelling of the lymph nodes, especially the cervical nodes.

motivation Providing an incentive to cause a person to move or to act in a particular way.

mycotic Pertaining to a disease caused by a fungus.

mydriatic A drug that will dilate the pupil of the eye.

myelography X-ray examination of the spinal column after injection of a radiopaque substance.

myocardial infarction Disorder caused by obstruction or thrombus of a coronary artery or its branches depriving the myocardium of its blood supply and causing death of the tissue affected.

myopia Nearsightedness.

myxedema Hypothyroidism in adults causing changes in the physical appearance and mental apathy.

narcotic A drug that may be an opium derivative or synthetic narcotic-like agent used to relieve pain and produce sleep. All narcotic drugs are habit forming and under government control.

nebulization A method of spraying a drug into the respiratory passages; may be used with or without oxygen to carry the drug to the lungs.

necrosis Death of tissue.

necrotic tissue Death of tissue or dead small groups of cells.

Nematoda Roundworms.

neobladder Urinary diversion by transplanting the ureters into a constructed segment of the sigmoid colon.

neoplasm Abnormal tumor growth; may be benign or malignant.

nephrectomy Surgical removal of a kidney.

nephritis Inflammation of the kidney; may be acute or chronic.

nephron Nephron and its component parts comprise the structural and functional unit of the kidney.

nephrosclerosis Sclerosis of the blood vessels of the kidney, usually associated with hypertension.

nephrosis (**nephrotic syndrome**) Degeneration of renal tissue with inflammation; may occur with glomerulonephritis.

nephrostomy Surgical wound on the flank and placement of a catheter into the kidney pelvis for the purpose of drainage.

nodule Small solid node that can be detected by touch.

noninfective vaccine A vaccine in which organisms have been killed by heat or chemicals.

nosocomial Refers to a hospital-acquired infection.

nystagmus A continuous movement of the eyeball; may be associated with labyrinthitis.

occlusion Blockage of a passageway.

oliguria Decreased urinary output.

oophorectomy Surgical removal of an ovary.

opacity Omitting light or opaque to light rays.

ophthalmia neonatorum Infection of the eyes of the newborn with the gonococcus organism.

ophthalmologist A physician trained in the diagnosis and treatment of eye diseases and the correction of vision defects with lenses.

opiate Drug derived from opium.

opisthotonos Arching of the body caused by rigidity of the spine.

opportunist Microorganism capable of adapting to a tissue or host other than the normal one.

orchitis Inflammatory condition of the testes caused by infection, injury, or malignancy.

orthopedic Describes disorders of the musculoskeletal system.

oscilloscope An instrument that records a visual wave on a screen.

osmotic pressure Pressure of a fluid that determines its ability to pass through a semipermeable membrane.

osseous Pertaining to bone.

osteoarthritis A degenerative type of arthritis affecting the joints; characteristic of the aging process.

osteomyelitis Infection and inflammation of a bone.

osteoporosis Chronic condition of vertebrae caused by demineralization or absorption of minerals from the bone; may result from prolonged immobilization and is common in women past menopause.

osteotomy Cutting of bone to correct joint or bone deformities.

otitis media Abscess of the middle ear.

otologist A physician trained in the diagnosis and treatment of diseases and disorders of the ear.

otosclerosis A disease of the middle ear in which changes in the stapes occur that prevent transmission of sound to the inner ear.

ovulation Discharge of a mature ovum from the ovarian follicle.

pacemaker A mechanical device used to provide electrical stimulation in heart block; may be temporary or permanent.

palliative Giving temporary relief but not cure.

pancreatitis Inflammation of the pancreas.

pandemic A disease that is widespread in a geographic area or throughout the world.

panhysterectomy Surgical removal of the uterus and the cervix.

Papanicolaou smear test A cytologic test for the detection of cancer cells.

papule A small solid elevation on the skin varying in size from a pinhead to a pea.

paraplegia Paralysis of the lower part of the body below a point of injury to the spinal cord.

paroxysm Spasmodic attacks that recur at periodic intervals.

paroxysmal atrial tachycardia Very rapid heartbeat beginning suddenly and ending abruptly.

Pasteur treatment A series of injections given to a person who may have been exposed to rabies.

patency A state of being open or sufficiently large to permit passage.

pathogen An organism capable of causing disease.

pathologic Describes the presence of a disease condition.

pathophysiology Changes in the physiologic function when a pathologic disease is present.

penicillinase An enzymelike substance produced by some bacteria that affects the antimicrobial properties of penicillin.

peptic ulcer An ulcer occurring in the wall of the stomach or the duodenum.

perfusion Procedure of introducing a chemical drug to an isolated part of the body by way of the bloodstream.

peripheral Near the outside of the surface of the body.

peristalsis Involuntary wavelike contraction of muscles of the gastrointestinal tract.

permeable Able to penetrate or to go through.

pertussis Whooping cough.

pessary A device used to support the uterus in a normal position.

petechiae Small pinpoint hemorrhagic spots on the skin.

Peyer's patches Areas of lymphoid tissue on the mucous membrane of the small intestine that become elevated and inflamed in typhoid fever; may become ulcerated and rupture, causing hemorrhage.

phagocyte Cell that engulfs and ingests bacteria or other material.

phagocytosis Presence of phagocytes that ingest and digest bacteria at the scene of an infection.

phenylketonuria Hereditary disease in which there is a faulty utilization of the amino acid phenylalanine.

phimosis A narrowing of the prepuce opening so that the foreskin of the penis cannot be retracted.

phlebotomy Incision of a vein for the purpose of removing blood.

phobia Abnormal fear.

pinna Auricle of the ear, or the cartilaginous external ear.

pinworm Small parasitic worm that matures in the large intestine and crawls to outside of rectum to deposit its eggs.

plaques Fatty deposits found in the intima of blood vessels; often the coronary arteries are affected.

plasmapheresis Process of separating the plasma and the red blood cells.

Platyhelminthes Flatworms.

pleurisy Inflammation of the pleura.

pneumonectomy Surgical removal of a lung.

pollinosis An allergic condition; same as hay fever.

polyp A small tumorlike growth projecting from a mucous membrane.

polyuria Increased urinary output.

postoperative Refers to period after a surgical procedure.

precipitin Antibody that causes precipitation of the antigen. Precipitin antibodies in the plasma react with the antigen to cause anaphylactic shock.

preoperative Refers to the period just prior to a surgical procedure.

priority In the order of importance.

proctoscopy Examination of the rectum, anus, and sigmoid colon with a proctoscope.

prognosis Expected outcome of a disease.

prostatic hypertrophy Enlargement of the prostate gland.

prostatitis Inflammation of the prostate gland.

prosthesis Any artificial device used to replace a missing part of the body.

prosthetist A person skilled in making and fitting prostheses.

prostration Great exhaustion.

Proteus morganii A species of bacteria that may cause infectious diarrhea in infants.

Proteus vulgaris A species of bacteria found in feces, water, and soil; a frequent cause of urinary tract infection.

Protozoa A phylum of unicellular organisms.

pruritus Itching of the skin.

Pseudomonas aeruginosa Microorganism found on the skin or in the intestinal tract of humans; may be the cause of hospital-acquired infections. It is resistant to most antibiotics.

psilocybia Active agent of the *Psilocybe mexicana* mushroom; classified as a hallucinogenic agent.

psoriasis A chronic skin disease characterized by scaly patches and desquamation.

psychosomatic Refers to disorders for which no pathologic condition can be found.

ptosis A dropping from the normal position, such as ptosis of the eyelid in facial paralysis.

puberty Period at which the ability to reproduce begins.

pulmonary edema A condition in which left ventricular heart failure occurs, causing a slowing of the systemic circulation and back up of returning blood; a serious condition.

pulmonary embolism A condition that is usually caused by a blood clot that breaks away from its place of origin and travels by the bloodstream to the lungs, where it lodges in a small vessel.

pulmonary emphysema A chronic obstructive disease of the lungs in which there is an overdistention of the alveoli.

pulse deficit Difference between the radial pulse rate and apical pulse rate.

pulsing therapy Method of administering a drug at intervals to achieve selected toxicity.

Purkinje fibers Continuation of the bundle of His that extends into the muscle walls of the ventricles.

purpura Bleeding into the skin.

purulent Describes a discharge containing pus.

pustule An elevated skin lesion containing pus.

pyelitis Inflammatory condition of the kidney pelvis.

pyelography X-ray examination of the kidney pelvis and may include the ureters after injection of a radiopaque medium.

pyelonephritis An inflammatory condition that involves the kidney pelvis and extends into kidney tissue.

pyloric spasm Severe and painful spasm of the pyloric valve.

pyogenic Pus producing.

pyuria Pus in the urine.

quadriplegia Paralysis of all four extremities.

quarantine Isolation for a given period of time that prohibits person-to-person contact.

Queckenstedt test A test used in the diagnosis of obstruction of the spinal cord.

radioactive substance Any substance capable of giving off rays resulting from disintegration such as radium.

radiopaque A substance that cannot be penetrated by any form of radiation; used in x-ray examination of internal structures.

reflex An involuntary act.

refraction Bending of light rays entering the eye; also used in correction of abnormal bending of light rays by the ophthalmologist.

regression Going backward.

regurgitation Usually applied to the return of food or fluids from the stomach.

rehabilitation Process of assisting an individual after a disabling event has occurred.

reminiscing Recalling past events or experiences.

remission Relief from symptoms or temporary improvement; opposite from exacerbation.

residual Refers to the part remaining, such as urine remaining in the bladder after catheterization.

reticuloendothelial system Main bodily defense to protect humans from harmful agents; responsible for phagocytosis and elimination of cellular debris in inflammatory conditions.

retirement Period in a person's life when he leaves his job and enters another phase of life.

rhinitis Inflammation of the nasal mucosa.

rickettsiae Small bodies that occupy an intermediate position between bacteria and viruses.

ringworm A disorder caused by a fungus.

roentgen Unit for measuring radiation, such as in x rays.

rose spots Small rose-colored spots on the abdomen occurring in typhoid fever.

sarcoma A type of malignant tumor.

scale A small thin flake of dry epidermis.

scar A mark left on the skin after repair of tissue.

Schick test A subcutaneous skin test to determine immunity to diphtheria.

scintillator A device used to measure the amount of radioactive material in a part of the body.

scolex Segment of the tapeworm that forms the head with hooks or suckers.

sebaceous glands Oil glands that secrete sebum.

seborrhea An increased secretion of sebum from the sebaceous glands.

sebum Secretion from the sebaceous glands.

sedimentation rate Rate at which red blood cells settle when blood is placed in a test tube.

seizure A sudden loss of consciousness, such as in epilepsy.

senescence Process of becoming old, or old age.

senility Old age with physical or mental changes; term is rarely used today.

sensitized Describes tissues that have been made susceptible to antigenic substances.

septicemia A bloodstream infection resulting from invasion of the blood by bacteria or their toxins.

serum sickness Immediate response to the introduction of a foreign protein into the body, such as horse serum.

shearlings Sheepskins used on the bed to help prevent decubitus ulcers.

sickle cell disease Congenital disease marked by sickle-shaped red blood cells; occurs most commonly in blacks.

sigmoidoscopy Examination of the sigmoid colon with a sigmoidoscope.

sinoatrial node Cells located in the right atrial wall that contract to set the rate the heart will beat; initiates electrical conduction system of the heart; called the pacemaker.

sinus bradycardia A slowing of the heart action to 60 beats per minute or less.

sinus tachycardia Rapid beating of the heart in excess of 100 beats per minute.

sordes A foul accumulation of secretions and crusts about the teeth and gums caused by lack of oral care.

spasm A severe muscular contraction.

spastic Describes involuntary muscular contractions resulting in rigidity.

sphincter Muscles that are circular in shape and that constrict an anatomic opening, such as the anal sphincter.

spirometer Mechanical device to measure vital capacity.

splenectomy Surgical removal of the spleen.

splenomegaly Enlargement of the spleen.

spores Bacilli that are capable of changing into resistive forms that can exist at high temperatures and in the presence of ordinary disinfectants.

stapedectomy Surgical procedure to correct otosclerosis, a disorder that prevents sound from reaching the inner ear.

Staphylococcus aureus Species of bacteria often responsible for hospital-acquired infections.

stasis Slowing or stopping the normal flow.

stenosis Narrowing or constriction of a passageway, such as in the valves of the heart, mitral stenosis.

sterilization Process of destroying all pathogenic microorganisms.

stigma A mark of disgrace.

stimulus Any action or agent that causes changes or action in an organ or part.

stoma An opening onto the skin created by an artificial passageway; may also apply to the normal opening of a pore.

stomatitis Inflammation of the mucous membranes of the mouth.

strabismus Crossed eyes.

strawberry tongue Strawberry-like appearance of the tongue in scarlet fever.

stump Distal portion of an extremity after amputation.

stuporous Describes deep sleep with diminished sense of feeling and responsiveness.

subculture An ethnic, regional, economic, or social group with characteristic patterns of behavior that distinguish it from the larger culture or society.

suicide Self-destruction.

sunstroke Disorder caused by overexposure to the sun.

surgical scrub Washing of hands and forearms prior to a surgical procedure using a prescribed method.

surveillance Supervising or watching a person or a condition.

syndrome A group of symptoms.

synovectomy Excision of the synovial membrane of a joint.

tachycardia A cardiac arrhythmia that results in a very rapid beating of the heart.

tenacious Describes secretions that are sticky and stringy and tend to hold together.

terminal disinfection Cleaning of equipment and airing of room after the release of a person who has had an infectious disease.

tetany A paroxysmal type of spasm involving the extremities.

thanatology Study of death and dying.

thermography Technique of determining surface temperature of the body through photography.

therapist A person skilled in various therapeutic techniques.

thoracotomy A surgical opening into the thoracic cavity.

thrombophlebitis Inflammation of a vein caused by a thrombus.

thrombosis Presence of a blood clot.

thrush An infection of the mouth and throat caused by a fungus; usually occurs in infants.

tonic Refers to tension or contraction.

tonsillectomy Surgical removal of the tonsils.

tophi A deposit of urates in tissues about the joints in gout.

toxemia Presence of toxins or poisons in the blood.

toxicity State of being poisonous.

tracheostomy Permanent opening into trachea after tracheotomy.

tracheotomy A surgical incision into the trachea to provide a patent airway.

transected Cut across or severed.

transplantation Surgical transfer of an organ from a donor to a recipient.

Trendelenburg position Elevation of the lower extremities above the level of the heart.

trephine Removal of small circular disks of bone from the skull.

trichinosis Infection with trichina, a worm found in pork.

trichomoniasis Infection with the *Trichomonas* parasite.

ulcer An open lesion on the skin with loss of deep tissue.

uremia Accumulation of urinary constituents in the blood causing a general toxic condition.

urticaria Hives; an allergic reaction characterized by the appearance of wheals on the skin.

vaccine A pathogen whose virulence has been reduced and which is used as prophylaxis against a disease.

vaginitis Inflammation of the vagina.

varicocele A varicosity or dilation of veins in the spermatic cord.

varicosities Dilated veins.

vector An insect, rodent, or arthropod that carries disease and transmits it to humans.

vegetative bacteria Bacteria that do not form spores.

ventricular fibrillation Disorganization of the heartbeat that may cause cardiac arrest without prompt treatment.

ventricular tachycardia Rapid contraction of the ventricle with reduced cardiac output.

ventriculogram A diagnostic procedure in which air is injected into the cerebral ventricles and x-ray films are taken.

vertigo A sensation characterized by the movement of objects or of self-movement; an extreme form of dizziness.

vesicle A blisterlike elevation on the skin containing serous fluid.

vesiculation Formation of vesicles.

virology Study of viruses.

virulence Strength of an organism to produce disease.

viruses Infective agents that cause several diseases.

viscosity Thickness of a fluid that causes it to resist flow.

vital capacity Amount of air that can be retained in the lungs after a full inspiration.

vulvovaginitis Inflammation of the vagina, the vulva, and usually the vulvovaginal glands.

Wangensteen suction A suction-siphonage method to remove secretions from the stomach.

wen A cyst that often occurs on the back of the scalp.

wheal An elevated type of rash on the skin, such as in urticaria.

withdrawal syndrome A syndrome of serious symptoms when the use of a drug is discontinued.

Index

Alum-precipitated toxoid, 38
Alveoli, 186
Ambulation
  of geriatric patient, 136-137
  after heart surgery, 286
  postoperative, 155
Amenorrhea, 368
  secondary, 368
Ammonium compounds for disinfection, 49
Amputation, 522-524
  in children, 524
  pillow placement after, 524
  postoperative care in, 522-524
  preoperative care in, 522
  prone position after, 524
  skin preparation for, 523
Anal sphincter spasm, 323
Analgesic blocks, 147
Anaphylactic shock, 536
Anaphylaxis, 40-41
Anastomosis of stomach to small intestine, 319
Anemia, 238-243
  hemorrhagic, 238-240
    emergency care, 239
    follow-up care, 239
    nursing care, 239-240
    pathophysiology, 238-239
  iron-deficiency, 240-241
    iron preparations and dosages in, 241
    nursing care, 240-241
    pathophysiology, 240
    treatment, 240
  pernicious, 241-242
    nursing care, 241-242
    pathophysiology, 241
    treatment, 241
  primary; *see* pernicious *above*
  sickle cell, 242-243
    pathophysiology, 243
    treatment, 243
Anesthesia, 146-148
  inhalation, 146
  intravenous drugs, 147
  rectal, 147
  spinal, 147
  types of, 146-149
Aneurysm, 276-277
  fusiform, 277
  saccular, 277
Anger and death, 115
Angina pectoris, 273-274
  pain of, 273
  treatment and care, 273-274
Anginal syndrome; *see* Angina pectoris
Angiocardiography, 265
Angiography, 265
  cerebral, 421
  cholangiography, 299
Angioma, 77
  of skin, 487
Anhidrosis, 486-487
Animal bites, first aid for, at home, 570
Animalcules, 4
Anomalies; *see* Congenital malformations
Anopheles quadrimaculatus mosquito, 561
Antibiotics, 33
  partial list of, 34-35

Antibody(ies), 37
  heterophil, test, 236
Antigen, 37
Antiseptics, 47-50
  definition, 47
Antitoxins, 39-40
Anvil of ear, 455
Aortic stenosis, 271-272
Aphasia, 435-436
  expressive, 435
  receptive, 435
Apnea, 187
Apoplexy, 433-437
Appendectomy, 302
Appendicitis, 309-310
  pathophysiology, 309-310
  treatment and care, 310
Aquamatic K pad, 442
Aqueous humor, 454
Arm
  emergency splint for, 573
  exercises after mastectomy, 381
Arrhythmia, cardiac, 256-257
Arteries
  coronary; *see* Coronary artery
  intra-arterial perfusion, 378
Arteriosclerosis, 268
  aging and, 135
  treatment and care of, 268
Arthritis, 513-517
  gouty, 516
  osteoarthritis, 515
  rheumatoid, 513-515
    pathophysiology, 513-514
    treatment and care, 514-515
  surgery of, 515-516
  whirlpool for, 514
Arthrodesis in arthritis, 515
Arthroplasty in arthritis, 515-516
Articular cartilage, 501
Artificial airways, 149-150
Ascaris, 10
Asepsis, 46-47
  medical, 46-47, 540-542
  in staphylococcal infection, 66-67
  surgical, 47
Asphyxia, 187
Asthma, 205, 208-210
  bronchial, as drug allergy, 536
  extrinsic, 208
  intrinsic, 208
  pathophysiology, 208-209
  treatment and care, 209-210
Astigmatism, 459
Ataxia, locomotor, 429
Atelectasis, 211-212
  treatment and care, 212
Atherosclerosis, 268
  aging and, 135
  treatment and care, 268
Atopic allergy, 531
Atrial fibrillation, 257
Atrial tachycardia, paroxysmal, 258
Audiometer, 456
Auditory canal, 455
Auscultation of heart, 262
Autoclaves, 52